Neural Basis of Motivational and Cognitive Control

Neural Basis of Motivational and Cognitive Control

edited by Rogier B. Mars, Jérôme Sallet, Matthew F. S. Rushworth, and Nick Yeung

The MIT Press
Cambridge, Massachusetts
London, England

For information about special quantity discounts, please email special_sales@mitpress.mit.edu

This book was set in Times Roman by Toppan Best-set Premedia Limited. Printed and bound in the United States of America.

Library of Congress Cataloging-in-Publication Data

Neural basis of motivational and cognitive control / edited by Rogier B. Mars . . . [et al.].
   p.   ; cm.
Includes bibliographical references and index.
ISBN 978-0-262-01643-8 (hardcover : alk. paper)
1. Motivation (Psychology)—Physiological aspects. 2. Cognition—Physiological aspects. 3. Frontal lobes. I. Mars, Rogier B.
[DNLM: 1. Motivation—physiology. 2. Cognition—physiology. 3. Frontal Lobe—physiology. QP 409]
QP409.N48 2012
612.8′233—dc22

                                        2011010089

10 9 8 7 6 5 4 3 2 1

Contents

Preface

This volume deals with a simple question: How does the brain choose efficiently and adaptively among available options to ensure coherent, goal-directed behavior? Hidden behind this question are many problems that necessitate a multidisciplinary approach. Indeed, to understand how humans and other animals solve this problem, we need answers from researchers versed in anatomy, traditional psychology, learning theory, neuroimaging, and mathematical modeling. The goal of this book is to provide the reader with an overview of key approaches that researchers are currently pursuing in this quest.

How This Volume Came About

This volume was inspired by a meeting of the same name held at St. John's College, Oxford, June 2 through 4, 2010. The meeting was the fourth in a series that started around the turn of the century with a meeting in Jena, Germany, organized by Michael Coles and Wolfgang Miltner. That first meeting was motivated by an upsurge of research interest in the error-related negativity (ERN), a component of the human event-related brain potential that is elicited in the anterior cingulate cortex following errors in simple choice reaction-time tasks. The discovery of the ERN by Michael Falkenstein and colleagues in the early 1990s provided a clearly observable neural correlate of a key aspect of cognitive control: the ability to monitor ongoing thought and action to identify situations in which effortful, intelligent control is required.

The Jena meeting was followed in 2003 by a meeting in Dortmund, Germany, organized by Markus Ullsperger and Michael Falkenstein. By the time of this meeting, two prominent theories of the ERN had been proposed—the reinforcement learning theory of Holroyd and Coles, and the conflict monitoring hypothesis of Botvinick, Carter, and Cohen—giving rise to the meeting's title: "Errors, conflicts, and the brain." Both theories were grounded in formal computational models that could account for a number of behavioral and physiological phenomena observed in the psychological literature and that proposed possible underlying neural architectures. Meanwhile, the ERN was being investigated in an increasing number of research fields, extending from traditional cognitive neuroscience to developmental psychology and psychopathology. This meeting resulted in a book edited by the organizers and published by the Max Planck Institute for Human Cognitive and Brain Sciences.

A third meeting, "Errors, conflicts, and rewards," was organized in 2006 in Amsterdam, the Netherlands, by Richard Ridderinkhof, Sander Nieuwenhuis, and Rogier Mars. Reflecting the growing scope of research on cognitive control and performance monitoring, this meeting also included researchers working on nonhuman primate and rodent models of control. The title of the meeting also featured the word "reward," signifying the increasingly evident convergence between research on performance monitoring and cognitive control, on the one hand, and studies of reward-guided learning and decision making on the other. Ridderinkhof, Nieuwenhuis, and Todd Braver edited a special issue of the journal *Cognitive, Affective, and Behavioral Neuroscience* (2007, 7:4) with contributions from speakers at this meeting.

The fourth meeting, held in Oxford in 2010, followed these trends of increasing the scope of the research presented while maintaining an emphasis on conceptual and methodological convergence in studies of the motivational and cognitive control of behavior. In addition to psychologists and cognitive neuroscientists, the speaker list included a zoologist, a behavioral economist, an anatomist, and a number of researchers with a background in engineering and machine learning. From a meeting focused on developments around a small number of event-related potentials, the meeting has expanded into a medley of approaches, each addressing the same underlying question: How does the brain choose efficiently and adaptively among available options to ensure coherent, goal-directed behavior? We have invited contributions to this volume from researchers working in a wide range of fields, reflecting the spectrum of approaches present at the meeting.

Organization of the Book

This book is aimed at a graduate audience in all fields of research that deal with motivational and cognitive control. We hope that, besides providing an overview of cutting-edge research in the area, the volume will serve as a handbook that can be used by psychologists, biologists, economists, and neuroscientists alike. The contributors have been asked to situate their own findings and theories in the context of authoritative overviews of the relevant fields. For ease of further study, each chapter includes boxes with suggestions for further reading and questions that are outstanding in the field. In addition, interim summaries between the parts aim to integrate their contents into the wider literature.

The book begins with a consideration of the anatomical basis of control. The three chapters in part I each deal separately with one core component of the control system: the mechanisms of high-level control within the prefrontal cortex; the mechanisms of motivated action selection and learning in the basal ganglia; and the mechanisms of modulatory control by monoamine neurotransmitter systems. In the first chapter, Sallet and colleagues focus on anatomical aspects of the interaction between lateral and medial prefrontal cortex, a prominent feature of many models of cognitive control. The chapter by Haber focuses on the connectivity of basal ganglia circuits, which are increasingly recognized as providing a crucial point of convergence between cognitive and motivational influences on behavior. Haber describes the various pathways of communication within reward circuits of the brain and between reward and association circuits, and the interactions among these networks. In the third chapter, Ullsperger describes the role of modulatory neurotransmitters in control, focusing primarily on dopamine, serotonin, and norepinephrine.

Part II addresses the contributions of the cerebral cortex to control. Building on the anatomical perspective taken in the first section, these chapters focus on the functional architecture of cortical control. The chapters by Boorman and Noonan and by Kennerley and Tobler provide complementary perspectives on the contributions of subregions within prefrontal cortex to action selection and choice based on reinforcement value. Laubach focuses on the frontal cortex in rats, providing a basis for the expanded cortex in human and nonhuman primates discussed in the following chapters. Mars and colleagues look at how the prefrontal cortex exerts control via modulation of activity in posterior brain areas. Pearson and colleagues extend the field of focus from the frontal lobes to the posterior cingulate cortex, a region of the brain often seen in imaging experiments of control but thus far largely neglected in the literature.

Part III considers the many ways in which subcortical brain regions underpin the control functions of the cortex. Two of the contributions focus on the role of the basal ganglia: Liljeholm and O'Doherty review evidence on the role of the basal ganglia in instrumental behavior, while Greenhouse and colleagues discuss the contribution of these structures to a hallmark feature of cognitive control: response inhibition. In the other chapters in the section, the focus is on the role of monoamine neurotransmitter systems: Walton and colleagues provide an in-depth look at the most widely studied neurotransmitter in the field of motivational control, dopamine. In the final chapter, Nieuwenhuis reviews work on the locus coeruleous norepinephrine system, which influences cortical functioning through its widespread network of cortical connections.

Whereas most chapters in this volume focus on group-averaged data, assuming that the neural systems in question operate in a similar manner across individuals, the contributions in part IV focus on three types of individual differences in control. First, Van den Bos and Crone look at changes in neural control of social decisions during the development from adolescence into adulthood, showing how neural functioning and behavior undergo substantial changes during this period. Ridderinkhof and colleagues then review evidence regarding individual differences in control in the adult population. Their chapter specifically focuses on how incorporating individual differences into one's research can shed new light on the interface between motivational and cognitive control. Finally, De Bruijn and Ullsperger discuss performance monitoring in patient populations, showing how various neurological and psychiatric conditions are associated with specific and identifiable disturbances in cognitive control.

Research on cognitive and motivational control has historically benefitted greatly from the use of explicit computational models of neural functioning. Part V takes a closer look at recent developments in computational approaches that have been particularly influential in this regard. Ribas-Fernandes and colleagues provide an overview of formal models of learning, proposing a hierarchical reinforcement model of behavior. This focus on reinforcement learning is followed in chapters by Cockburn and Frank and by Holroyd and Yeung. Both chapters consider the relationship between the basal ganglia and prefrontal cortex in motivational and cognitive control, while presenting somewhat contrasting accounts of the respective roles of the basal ganglia and anterior cingulate cortex. The chapter by Khamassi and colleagues provides a complementary perspective on "meta-control" and the mechanisms by which the control system is itself optimized. Once again, the focus is on lateral and medial prefrontal regions. Finally, Shenoy and Yu adopt a Bayesian approach that considers paradigmatic response inhibition tasks within a rational decision-making framework.

The concluding part VI comprises three chapters that highlight recent overarching trends in the literature. Chierchia and Coricelli discuss the influence of concepts and methodologies from economic decision theory on theorizing and experiments in the study of control. Hunt and Behrens discuss how the approaches apparent in this volume are now starting to be used to solve problems in more complex and applied domains, focusing in particular on the neuroscience of social decision making. Finally, Bestmann and Mars look at how computational models such as those proposed in part V can be formally linked to the experimental data obtained in neuroimaging and electrophysiology experiments.

Acknowledgments

As Jared Diamond and James Robinson state in their recent edited volume (*Natural Experiments of History*, Harvard University Press, 2008), completing an edited book costs each editor on average two friends, because of the various levels of stress involved in the process. We are grateful that this has not proven true in our case. We thank all of our contributors, as well as the speakers and attendees of the Oxford meeting, for making both the meeting and this book a success. We are tremendously grateful to the International Brain Research Organization, the UK Neuroinformatics Node, the Guarantors of Brain, and the McDonnell Network of Cognitive Neuroscience at the University of Oxford for their generous financial support, and to the staff at St John's College, Oxford, for their warm hospitality at the June meeting. We thank MaryAnn Noonan, Laurence Hunt, and Vanessa Johnen for their able assistance in organizing that meeting. We are delighted to be able to publish this book with MIT Press, and would like to thank specifically Susan Buckley and Robert Prior, who have provided unwavering support to a group of first-time editors. Finally, we would like to thank our colleagues, friends, and families for their support during periods of stress and strain as we worked on this volume deep into the night.

I ANATOMICAL BASIS OF CONTROL

The chapters in this section provide an overview of neuroanatomical and neuro-modulatory systems at the core of control processes. In the first two chapters, the focus is principally on two prefrontal regions—the anterior cingulate cortex (ACC) and the dorsolateral prefrontal cortex (dlPFC)—and a basal ganglia region, the ventral striatum. The last chapter of this section takes a complementary approach to the classic neuroanatomical one by addressing the role of the different neuro-transmitter systems in monitoring performance.

One cannot understand the neural basis of control process without carefully considering the architecture of the brain. As Richard Passingham stated: "Anatomy is not tedious: it is fundamental."[8] One of the core criteria for subdividing the cortex is its cytoarchitectonic properties, an endeavor that started with the pioneering work of Brodmann and Von Economo. With the appearance of modern computational and databasing techniques, it is now possible to compare individual differences and create large databases and probabilistic maps of not only cytoarchitecture, but also chemoarchitecture and connectivity.[5] Indeed, connectivity has received much attention recently, with demonstrations that each cortical area has a unique con-nectivity fingerprint that constrains the information to which it has access.[9] Neglect-ing these fine anatomical properties of networks may prevent the identification of functional subdivisions within each area, and then preclude any clear understanding of integrated systems.

Chapters in this section emphasize the complexity of the connectivity patterns: for instance, the clustering organization of prefrontal connectivity, the poor under-standing of the interarea connectivity at a microscopic level, and the complex convergent-divergent connections within basal ganglia pathways. Those results show that a lot remains to be done to achieve a level of understanding of control networks comparable to that of the visual system.[2,6,11] Although recent progress in imaging tools has allowed researchers to address the issue of the connectivity in the human brain,[4] most methods are constrained by the resolution of a voxel. Thus, work on animal models remains essential,[7] especially in order to understand brain mechanisms at infra-voxel resolution—that is, at cortical layers, cell, and synaptic levels. Furthermore, understanding the microarchitecture of a network also implies one has to determine the neurochemical nature of the connections. For instance, dopamine (DA) is a key molecule in many models of motivational and cognitive control. In the reinforcement learning theory of performance monitoring,[3] it is suggested that DA acts on ACC pyramidal cells via D1 receptor. In the prefrontal cortex, D1 and D5 receptors can be found on medium spiny neurons, with D5 receptors also found on aspiny neurons typical of cholinergic interneurons.[1] Those receptors are principally found in layers I through III. Because DA effects within the prefrontal cortex are complex and vary depending on the family of DA receptors,[10] it is important to determine how DA is acting in the considered network.

In this section, but also in the wider literature, the focus is primarily on the prefrontal cortex and the basal ganglia. However, other areas are thought to play important roles in cognitive or motivational control. The pre-supplementary motor area (pre-SMA), inferior frontal junction (IFJ), intraparietal cortex, and insula have all been suggested to play an important role in control mechanisms. However, apart from pre-SMA, none of the aforementioned structures correspond to a specific cytoarchitectural territory. The IFJ refers to the region at the junction of the inferior frontal sulcus and the inferior branch of the precentral sulcus. In humans, caudal to this precentral sulcus lies the rostral premotor cortex, in front of it and ventral to the inferior frontal sulcus is area 44, and dorsal to this last sulcus is area 8. In monkeys, these sulci do not exist, making identification of between-species homologs difficult, although an equivalent area exists around the inferior branch of the arcuate sulcus. Furthermore, the term *intraparietal cortex* refers to a number of cytoarchitectonic areas lying within the intraparietal sulcus. In monkeys, those areas include the ventral, lateral, medial, and anterior intraparietal areas (VIP, LIP, MIP, and AIP). Although multiple areas are also found within the human intraparietal sulcus, the precise homologs in humans and monkeys remain a topic of debate. Finally, the term *insula* does not refer to only one cortical territory. On the basis of their degree of lamination, three areas can be distinguished: agranular, dysgranular, and granular insula. It is suggested that the insula, in interaction with the ACC, plays a role in motivational control. As with the anterior cingulate and dorsolateral prefrontal cortex and basal ganglia, which are the topic of this section, the terms *insula, intraparietal cortex,* and *IFJ* should be used very carefully, as the ambiguity in the application of anatomical labels complicates our understanding of the neuroanatomical basis of control.

References

1. Bergson C, Mrzljak L, Smiley JF, Pappy M, Levenson R, Goldman-Rakic PS. 1995. Regional, cellular, and subcellular variations in the distribution of D1 and D5 dopamine receptors in primate brain. *J Neurosci* 15: 7821–7836.

2. Douglas RJ, Martin KA. 2004. Neuronal circuits of the neocortex. *Annu Rev Neurosci* 27: 419–451.

3. Holroyd CB, Coles MG. 2002. The neural basis of human error processing: reinforcement learning, dopamine, and the error-related negativity. *Psychol Rev* 109: 679–709.

4. Johansen-Berg H, Rushworth MF. 2009. Using diffusion imaging to study human connectional anatomy. *Annu Rev Neurosci* 32: 75–94.

5. Mazziotta J, Toga A, Evans A, Fox P, Lancaster J, Zilles K, Woods R, et al. 2001. A probabilistic atlas and reference system for the human brain: International Consortium for Brain Mapping (ICBM). *Philos Trans R Soc Lond B Biol Sci* 356: 1293–1322.

6. Nassi JJ, Callaway EM. 2009. Parallel processing strategies of the primate visual system. *Nat Rev Neurosci* 10: 360–372.

7. Passingham R. 2009. How good is the macaque monkey model of the human brain? *Curr Opin Neurobiol* 19: 6–11.

8. Passingham RE. 2007. Commentary on Devlin and Poldrack. *Neuroimage* 37: 1055–1056.

9. Passingham RE, Stephan KE, Kotter R. 2002. The anatomical basis of functional localization in the cortex. *Nat Rev Neurosci* 3: 606–616.

10. Seamans JK, Yang CR. 2004. The principal features and mechanisms of dopamine modulation in the prefrontal cortex. *Prog Neurobiol* 74: 1–58.

11. Vezoli J, Falchier A, Jouve B, Knoblauch K, Young M, Kennedy H. 2004. Quantitative analysis of connectivity in the visual cortex: extracting function from structure. *Neuroscientist* 10: 476–482.

1 Neuroanatomical Basis of Motivational and Cognitive Control: A Focus on the Medial and Lateral Prefrontal Cortex

Jérôme Sallet, Rogier B. Mars, René Quilodran, Emmanuel Procyk, Michael Petrides, and Matthew F. S. Rushworth

Understanding the neural mechanisms of control regulation requires delineating specific functional roles for individual neural structures, and consequently their functional relationships. Higher-order control over behavior has traditionally been seen as the function of the prefrontal cortex (PFC). Models of various aspects of control, including top-down processing, decision making, and performance monitoring focus primarily on two subdivisions of the PFC, namely, the dorsolateral prefrontal cortex (DLPFC) and the medial frontal cortex, particularly the anterior cingulate cortex (ACC). Within these frameworks, DLPFC is allocated a role in the maintenance of representations of goals and means to achieve them in order to bias processes that depend on posterior brain areas,[58] while medial frontal areas, again especially ACC, participate in performance monitoring, action evaluation and detection of events that indicate the need for behavioral adaptation and action revaluation.[75,76] Furthermore different hierarchical levels of cognitive control are thought to be supported by different prefrontal subdivisions.[4,46,47,68]

One prominent example of framework of control is the conflict model proposed by Cohen et al.[15] This model posits that the ACC tracks evidence for a need to increase cognitive control and sends this information to the DLPFC, which then exerts control over the processes occurring in posterior brain areas. The ACC-DLPFC interactions can be direct[11] or indirect.[15] A related model proposed by Brown and Braver also posits that the activity of the ACC regulates the activity of structures involved in implementing cognitive control.[14] A rather different model, based on the principles of reinforcement learning has been proposed by Holroyd and Coles and ascribes to the ACC a role in action selection[37,38] in response to a dopaminergic teaching signal.[38] For simplicity's sake these models either supposed the existence of a homogenous ACC and DLPFC, or else they are focused on sometimes undetermined subdivisions of these two regions. Furthermore, most models have emphasized a unidirectional flow of information between the structures; in some cases, however, the direction emphasized is from the ACC to the DLPFC,[11,14,15] while in other cases it is from the DLPFC to the ACC.[38]

A feature of these computational models is that they often do not consider all aspects of the underlying neuroanatomy of these cortical regions. However, a more detailed analysis of the connections between these brain areas may be of extreme importance to the functionality of models. Indeed, as Passingham et al. suggest, each cytoarchitectonic area has a unique connectivity pattern that is likely to be related to its function.[65] Thus, paying careful attention to the details of the anatomical properties of networks may facilitate the identification of functional subdivisions within each area, which may in turn generate a clearer understanding of integrated system function. In this chapter, we review neuroanatomical data concerning two key nodes in cognitive and motivational control models, the ACC and the DLPFC. Our aim is to review neuroanatomical data related to these two regions in the hope that it may help improve our understanding of control networks and how structures within these networks are interacting. Furthermore, we discuss the degree of correspondence in the anatomy of these areas in the human brain and the monkey brain, a model on which much of our knowledge is based.

Cytoarchitecture of ACC and DLPFC

Though both terms are commonly used, neither ACC nor DLPFC corresponds to a unique cortical area. They refer to a collection of areas (or subareas) with distinct cytoarchitectonic properties and connectivity profiles.

The abbreviation ACC commonly refers to cytoarchitectonic areas 24 and 32 (figure 1.1a). Based on cytoarchitectural properties and quantification of neurotransmitter receptors it has been proposed that the ACC in monkeys extends to the middle of the dorsal bank of the cingulate sulcus,[53,54,61,88] or lies just ventrally to the bottom of the cingulate sulcus.[12,20,87] Vogt et al. consider that most of the cortex on the dorsal bank of the cingulate sulcus belongs to the adjacent medial frontal cortex.[87] Area 32 is located rostrally to area 24. Petrides and Pandya proposed that the latter area extended caudally to form, on the dorsal bank of the cingulate sulcus, a transition area between the ACC and the medial prefrontal cortex.[68] Some disagreement also exists over the nature of the cingulate cortex. While Petrides and Pandya distinguished an agranular (area 24) and granular ACC (area 32), others considered area 32 to be dysgranular, and argued that area 24,[8] or at least the area 24c subdivision,[20] was dysgranular. Similar discrepancies also exist concerning the number of subdivisions of the ACC. Various studies find from four to nine subdivisions[54,87] in ACC area 24. Vogt et al. divide area 24 into an anterior division (the ACC) and a posterior division, which they call the midcingulate cortex (MCC).[87] The ACC then corresponds to areas 24a, b, and c; the MCC corresponds to subdivisions 24a', b', c', and d.

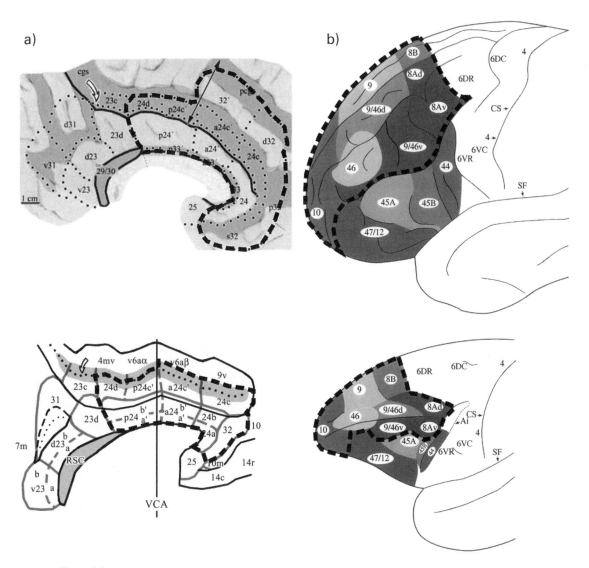

Figure 1.1
Cartography of medial and lateral prefrontal cortex. (a) Cytoarchitecture maps of human (top) and monkey (bottom) medial prefrontal cortex (adapted from Vogt et al.[83,87] by permission of Oxford University Press). (b) Cytoarchitecture maps of human (top) and monkey (bottom) lateral prefrontal cortex (adapted from Petrides and Pandya[69]). The dashed lines on the left and right figures correspond to the boundaries of the ACC and DLPFC, respectively. VCA, vertical line through the anterior commissure.

Although most of these debates have concerned the nature of ACC in the macaque, similar debates concern the human ACC. The presence of an additional sulcus known as the paracingulate sulcus, dorsal to the cingulate sulcus, further complicates the problem.[84] This sulcus is present in only 30 to 60% of cases[29] and, when present, shows highly variable morphology across individuals.[84] The morphology of the paracingulate sulcus affects the extent of areas 24 and 32 and is suggested to be related to performance in demanding cognitive tasks.[30] One hypothesis explaining the interindividual differences in sulcal anatomy is that they reflects differences in the connectivity between dorsal ACC and DLPFC.[30] As in monkeys, several subdivisions of the area 24 can be distinguished, and a similar organization has been proposed[63,86] (figure 1.1a).

The DLPFC is also a heterogenous region (figure 1.1b). In monkeys, it is located within the principal sulcus and extends dorsally. Based on cytoarchitectonic properties, one can distinguish multiple areas: areas 8A and 8B, area 9, area 46. Some authors proposed even further subdivisions, including transition areas around the lip of the principal sulcus and subdivisions based on the position in the principal sulcus. Those areas are labeled area 9/46 dorsal and ventral,[68,69] and a distinction is often made between area 46 ventral and dorsal.[3,7] Finally, area 8 is subdivided into area 8A, located at the level of the genu of the arcuate sulcus, and area 8B dorsal to it.

As is immediately apparent, the human lateral prefrontal cortex is more folded than that of the monkey (figure 1.1b). Instead of one sulcus (the principal sulcus), there are three: the superior frontal sulcus, the complex intermediate frontal sulcus, and the inferior frontal sulcus.[70] The inferior frontal sulcus is suggested to be the ventral boundary of the DLPFC. Despite this discrepancy between humans and monkeys, Petrides and Pandya proposed similar organization of the DLPFC.[69]

Connectivity of ACC and DLPFC

Mediolateral Prefrontal Cortex Connectivity in Monkeys

Before discussing DLPFC-ACC connectivity, it is important to underline the fact that it is difficult to perfectly describe the relationships between cingulate cytoarchitectonic areas and connectivity patterns. Indeed, in the literature most of the tracers injected in the cingulate cortex targeted either the cingulate gyrus (area 24a, b) or the rostral/caudal cingulate motor areas (rCMA, cCMA). rCMA and cCMA are cingulate subregions defined by their projections to the primary motor area (M1), the spinal cord, and their excitability.[51,59,73] In the interest of clarity, we consider the portion of area 24 that includes all the cingulate motor areas as the posterior ACC (pACC). Area 24 rostral to pACC is referred to as the rostral ACC (rACC). Connectivity of area 32 is considered separately.

A number of models of control emphasize interactions between ACC and DLPFC.[11,14] Surprisingly, the emphasis on the ACC-DLPFC functional relationships in fact relies on relatively weak anatomical connections (figure 1.2). For instance, pACC receives roughly 20 to 40 times more projections from the preSMA and cCMA than from area 46,[36] and area 46 projects more to medial prefrontal areas (areas 8B, 9) than to rCMA.[80] Note that the rACC also receives projections from the DLPFC,[7,72] and the ACC projects back to the DLPFC. Despite a lack of fully quantitative data, the anterior part of area 24 (and area 32) seems to project more to the principal sulcus than its caudal part.[50]

This last result suggests that the connectivity patterns between the ACC and the DLPFC differ between cytoarchitectonic areas. Labeled cells often form clusters and are not evenly distributed across the entire area. Note that the clustering organization of connections may reflect a modular organization of the prefrontal cortex.[49] For instance, area 8B but not area 8A projects to the rACC.[64,71] However, area 8A is interconnected with pACC and receives afferents from rACC.[1,39,89] The efferents from area 8A to pACC are limited to two separate clusters—one just anterior to rCMA and one adjacent to the ventral cCMA—that are then defined as cingulate eye field rostral and caudal, respectively.[89] Note that no projection in the cingulate sulcus was found after an injection of isotope specifically in the ventral subdivision of area 8A.[71] Areas 8A and 8B also present different connectivity patterns with other areas of the DLPFC. They are connected to each other as well as to areas 10, 9, and 9/46d; however, only the rostral part of area 8A is connected with area 46d, whereas area 8B is connected with area 46v.[64,71]

ACC receives projections from areas 10, 9, 46, and 9/46d.[6,7,42,59,60,71,72,85] But even within one cytoarchitectonic territory, the projections are not even. For instance, the connectivity of the ACC with the medial part of areas 9 and 8B is stronger than that with their lateral parts. Indeed, while area 8B and medial area 9 project to both the sulcal and gyral part of the rostral ACC, the lateral part of area 9 only projects to the rostral cingulate sulcus.[6,60,71] The dorsal part of area 46 receives projection from area 32, rACC and pACC, but only the ventral part of area 46 receives afferent inputs, from pACC.[1,7] The projections from area 10 to the ACC principally target the cingulate gyrus and are reported to be organized in columnar manner.[72] Area 10 projections to the cingulate sulcus area are restricted to its more rostral part.[72] Note that only the rACC and area 32 project back to area 10; no projection from pACC to the frontopolar cortex has been reported.[1,6,85] Finally, rACC (at the depth of the cingulate sulcus) and pACC (only the more ventral subdivision) project to 9/46v[66]; only pACC receives inputs from area 9/46v.[77]

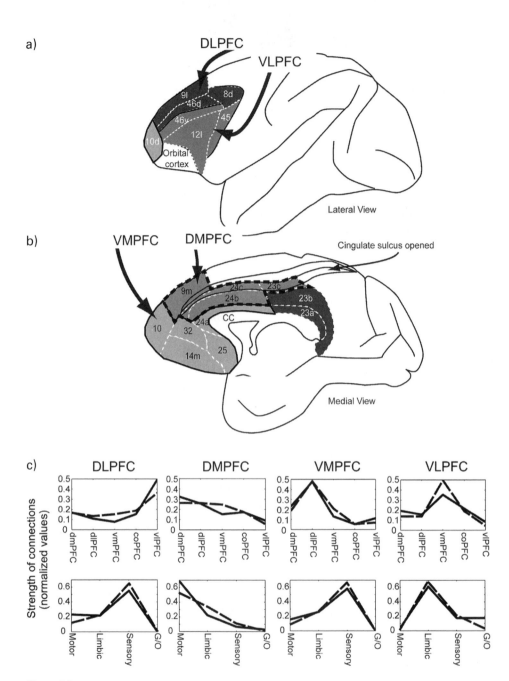

Figure 1.2
Connectivity of medial and lateral prefrontal cortex. (a,b) Lateral (a) and medial (b) view of macaque prefrontal areas. Clustering of prefrontal areas based on their connectivity patterns (adapted from Averbeck and Seo[3]). (c) Profile of inputs characterizing the five clusters illustrated in (b). The y-axis corresponds to the proportion of the connections. The top row represents the prefrontal interconnections; the bottow row corresponds to connections with extraprefrontal systems (adapted from Averbeck and Seo[3]). Note that DMPFC-DLPFC interconnections represent only between 20 and 30% of their prefrontal connections; connections that are themselves a subset of the total connections of these clusters.

This overview of the mediolateral prefrontal connectivity shows the expected interconnectivity between the different areas but also highlights the complexity of the connection patterns. Consistent with this, a meta-analysis of prefrontal cortex connectivity based on the COCOMAC database (<http://cocomac.org>) reveals that the ACC and DLPFC do not simply correspond to two different entities[3] (figure 1.2). Instead, a cluster analysis suggested that one can consider the medial part of area 9, the cingulate sulcus (24c), and part of the cingulate gyrus (area 24b) as a dorsomedial prefrontal cortex whereas areas 24a and 32 form part of a ventromedial prefrontal cortex. On the lateral surface areas 8A, 46d, and the lateral part of area 9 form the dorsolateral cluster.

Microarchitecture of Mediolateral Prefrontal Cortex Connectivity

Not merely the presence of connections, but also their laminar distribution pattern is important. Indeed, it may reflect some key functional properties of the network.[9,16,25,82] A simplified approach is to consider terminations that principally target layer IV as driving or feedforward projections. Terminations that principally target supragranular (layers I to III) or infragranular (layers V and VI) layers are considered as modulating or feedback projections, respectively. A similar logic could be applied depending on the localization of the cell bodies of efferent projections. If the majority of the cell bodies are found in the supragranular layers or in the infragranular layers, the projections are feedforward or feedback, respectively. This hierarchical organization originally proposed for the visual system has been proposed for the prefrontal cortex as well.[19]

As is the case for the presence of the projections, their laminar patterns are also heterogenous. The afferents to rACC (areas 24a, b) from area 9 are distributed throughout the different cortical layers.[1] But rACC afferents from the principal sulcus are denser in supragranular layers than in the infragranular layers.[1,85] The same pattern is observed in pACC.[50,85] However, rACC efferences to both areas 46 and 9 are distributed over all cortical layers with a lower density in area IV.[1] Note that cingulate (area 32) projections to DLPFC originate mainly in the deep layers, layer V and VI.[5]

A quantitative analysis of connectivity analogous to that applied in interpreting the neuroanatomy of the visual system[9,82] might potentially be applied to the study of the prefrontal cortex. Nevertheless, the data available concerning ACC-DLPFC connectivity suggest that ACC may modulate DLPFC activity (feedback projections), while the DLPFC may drive ACC activity (feedforward projections). One can go a step further and try to understand how these two structures are interacting at a synaptic level.

At a more microscopic level, the literature is principally concerned with the intrinsic connectivity, that is, the intra-areal connectivity, of the DLPFC or the ACC each in isolation.[21,22,32,33,61,74] In recent experiments, Medalla and Barbas addressed the issue of the mediolateral prefrontal connectivity at a synaptic level.[56,57] In a first experiment they injected tracers in areas 32 and 46 and examined the labeled axon terminals in layers I through III of area 9.[56] Both areas predominantly formed single synapses on the spines of spiny dendrites of excitatory cells. However, area 32 had more synapses with inhibitory neurons in area 9 than area 46 had, and the nature of inhibitory neurons receiving afferents from those two pathways was also different. Although the majority of synaptic boutons were small, those from area 32 were bigger than those from area 46, suggesting the synapses had a higher efficacy. The interneurons receiving projections from area 32 are thought to be involved in the enhancement of the signal-to-noise ratio (calbindin-positive cells, or CB cells), or in the enhancement of signals (calretinin-positive cells, or CR cells) in highly demanding cognitive situations. In their subsequent experiment Medalla and Barbas also investigated area 32 connectivity with area 10.[57] Area 32 is also connected with area 10; however, some features of the pathway were distinct from the one that links area 32 and area 46. For instance, area 32 projections largely target the area 10 excitatory cells. This suggests that, instead of enhancing inhibition, area 32 enhances excitatory activities in area 10. These results highlight the importance not only of inferring the existence of connections, but also of understanding the nature of these connections.

Mediolateral Prefrontal Cortex Connectivity in Humans

Our knowledge of connectivity patterns comes principally from studies on animal models. The recent development of the diffusion tensor imaging (DTI) method enables investigation of connectivity in the human brain.[43] There is a strong similarity between the results obtained with classic labeling (injection of tracers) and those obtained with DTI.[17,78] Apart from methods assessing structural connections, functional connectivity and effective connectivity, as assessed using functional magnetic resonance imaging (fMRI), provide another route to information about the connectivity of the human brain. Functional connectivity is thought to reflect temporal correlations between areas; effective connectivity refers to the influence of one neural system over another.[79] Although these can be modulated by polysynaptic connections, patterns of effective and functional connectivity have often been related to direct anatomical connections.[28]

A recent DTI study in humans confirmed the heterogeneity of the cingulate cortex (figure 1.3a). The study reported that the ACC could be divided into different regions on the basis of their probability of interconnection with the rest of the brain.[10] One cluster corresponded to the supracallosal part of the cingulate gyrus (cluster 7), and one is likely to include area 32 (cluster 2). Three other clusters correspond to different regions of the cingulate sulcus and paracingulate sulcus.

The caudal clusters have been suggested to be the cingulate motor areas (clusters 4 and 5).

Studies of cingulate functional connectivity at rest revealed that ACC activity is correlated with DLPFC activity, but again emphasized that parts of the ACC are differently correlated with the DLPFC.[34,52] The most striking result of a recent study by Margulies et al.[52] is the difference between ventral and dorsal cingulate regions (figure 1.3b). Unfortunately, it is difficult to infer from the results presented in their study with which different DLPFC regions ACC activity correlates. Nevertheless the caudal ACC (x = 5, y = 14, z = 42, MNI space) did not correlate with the frontopolar cortex whereas the more anterior ACC did. Two patterns of functional connectivity with the DLPFC could be observed for anterior regions at coordinates [5 25 36], [5 34 28], and regions at coordinates [5 42 21], [5 47 11]. The two most anterior regions are unlikely to contain the cingulate motor areas and showed less correlation with the middle frontal gyrus. Note that the cCMA also showed less correlation with the DLPFC than rCMA. Furthermore, the DLPFC region showing correlation with cCMA activity was more posterior [-30 37 32] than the one [-28 44 32] for which correlation was observed with rCMA activity.[34]

Not only at rest, but also during the performance of a variety of tasks are the ACC and DLPFC coactivated. Paus and Koski's meta-analysis of positron emission tomography (PET) studies revealed that supracallosal cingulate cortex activations, more precisely area 24c and 32, were very often associated with activation in the middle frontal cortex.[47] In addition, they distinguished within this supracallosal activity a caudal cingulate region (y < 10) in which activations co-occurred more frequently with activations in the precentral gyrus and the medial frontal gyrus than was the case for the more rostral cingulate region (y > 10) did.

For modeling purposes, one is probably more interested in effective connectivity than in structural connectivity. Not only coactivation but also interactions have been reported between rCMA and the middle frontal gyrus, peaking at (44, 30, 24), while subjects were performing a flanker task.[24] According to Kouneiher et al.,[48] interaction between these two regions is related to motivational control, rather than cognitive control. Caudal paracingulate activity predicting behavioral adaptation did not interact with the middle frontal gyrus activity associated with behavioral adjustements.[40,44,45]

In summary, resting state functional connectivity confirmed the existence of networks linking the ACC to the DLPFC in the human brain. It also confirmed the fact that different regions of the ACC are communicating with different regions of the DLPFC (see figure 1.3b). Task-related activity in fMRI and PET functional studies suggested that a network centered on rCMA and middle frontal gyrus (areas 46 and 9/46) is of particular interest.

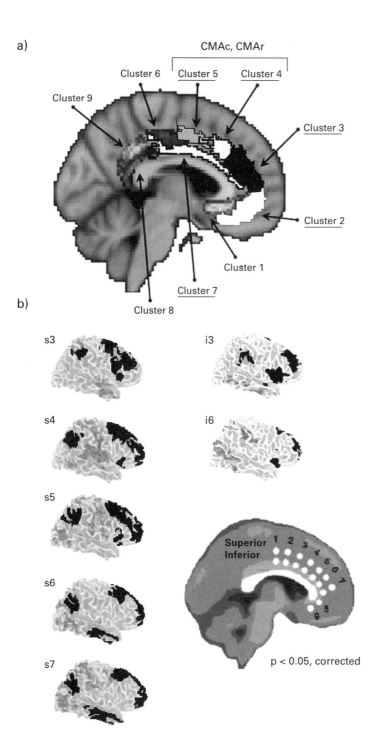

a)

CMAc, CMAr

Cluster 6   Cluster 5   Cluster 4

Cluster 9

Cluster 3

Cluster 2

Cluster 1

Cluster 7

Cluster 8

b)

s3   i3

s4   i6

s5

Superior
Inferior   1 2 3 4 5 6 7 8 9

s6

s7   p < 0.05, corrected

Beyond the ACC or the DLPFC

This chapter principally focused on the ACC and the DLPFC; however, we are aware that motivational and cognitive control processes do not simply rely on these two regions. For instance, noradrenergic (NA) and dopaminergic (DA) systems both play a critical role in cognitive control[2,15,38] (see chapter 3, this volume).

The locus coeruleus and its two modes of response (tonic and phasic) are proposed to induce alternation between explorative and exploitative behaviors. This structure projects to the entire neocortex and receives projections back from the rACC and adjacent medial prefrontal areas, but not the lateral prefrontal areas.[2] The interactions between ACC, DLPFC, and the DA system are quite complex. The DA has direct (mesocortical pathway) and indirect influences on the ACC and DLPFC via the striatum (nigrostriatal pathway) or the thalamus (nigrothalamocortical pathway).[35,41,90,91]

The conflict-monitoring model developed by Cohen et al. focuses on the effect of DA on the DLPFC, while the model developed by Holroyd and Coles is centered on DA inputs to the ACC.[15,38] Nevertheless, both of them implied the involvement of the direct mesocortical pathway. Though both ACC and DLPFC receive direct DA afferents, there is a regional difference in the origin of the inputs.[91] Similarly, ACC and DLPFC send sparse projections to the midbrain DA nuclei with a similar spatial organization.[31] The DLPFC receives more afferents from more lateral DA midbrain nuclei, the distribution of ACC afferents originates more in the medial midbrain nuclei. The topographic segregation of DLPFC and ACC projections is more obvious in the caudal part of the midbrain nuclei while they tend to overlap more anteriorly.

This anatomical compartmentalization could reflect a functional compartmentalization. Indeed, in a recent study, Brischoux et al. found some functional differences between dorsal and ventral VTA in rats[13] and along a dorsoventral axis in monkeys DA midbrain nuclei.[55] Some DA cells discharge preferentially for positive outcome related events,[13,27,55,80] but some DA cells discharge also, or preferentially for negative events.[13,55] Earlier studies also reported functional heterogeneity in VTA/SN

Figure 1.3
Connectivity-based parcellation and functional connectivity at rest of the human cingulate cortex. (a) Connectivity-based parcellation of human ACC (adapted from Beckmann et al.[10]). The ACC(/MCC) corresponds to clusters 2, 3, 4, 5 and part of cluster 7. (b) Functional connectivity at rest of cingulate regions (adapted from Margulies et al.[52]). Positive correlations ($p < 0.05$, corrected) of different cingulate regions, or seeds (represented on the medial view) are shown in black on cortical surface maps for superior (s3, s4, s5, s6, s7) and inferior seeds (i3, i6). Inferior seeds are located 5 mm from the corpus callosum, starting at $y = -10$ mm, and spaced 10 mm apart along the curve parallel to the corpus callosum. Superior seeds are located 15 mm from the corpus callosum along the radial axis from each of the first seven inferior seeds.

cells. Not only were cells that discharged to visual or outcome-related events found, but also cells that discharged to arm or mouth movement.[23,62] Finally, although often described as relatively independent systems, non-DA and DA VTA cells have been shown to project to the LC,[18] and LC cells also project to the VTA.[26] Furthermore, stimulation of VTA cells induces discharge of LC cells.[18]

Altogether the topographic segregation of mesocortical projections and the heterogeneity of DA cell activities may have to be taken into account in refining models of cognitive control. More specifically, the existence of VTA cells encoding either appetitive or aversive cues may need to be implemented in models such as those proposed by Holroyd and Coles.[38]

Conclusion

Our intention was to propose some comments on computational models of control based on a review of neuroanatomical data. Reviewing this literature reveals not only the huge amount of work that has been done but also the huge amount of work that remains to be done. The identities of the principal subdivisions of the macaque brain, the most frequently used model for understanding the architecture of the human brain, are still being discussed, and quantitative analysis of prefrontal cortex connectivity remains largely to be done. Nevertheless, we suggest, on the basis of anatomical connectivity studies in monkeys and functional and effective connectivity studies in humans that models of cognitive control might more precisely incorporate descriptions of regions than just "ACC" and "DLPFC."

Outstanding Questions

• What is the detailed topography of mediolateral prefrontal connections, at both meso- and microscopic levels?

• What, if any, is the correspondence between the primate and the rat medial prefrontal cortex and dorsolateral prefrontal cortex?

Further Reading

Vogt BA, ed. 2009. Cingulate Neurobiology and Disease. Oxford: Oxford University Press. A comprehensive volume for more detailed reviews of cingulate structures and functions.

Schmahmann JD, Pandya DN. 2006. Fiber Pathways of the Brain. Oxford: Oxford University Press. This book gives a nice overview of the major fiber pathways in the primate brain.

Johansen-Berg H, Behrens TEJ, eds. 2009. Diffusion MRI: From Quantitative Measurement to In-Vivo Neuroanatomy. Amsterdam: Academic Press. The first comprehensive overview of diffusion MRI techniques and their applications.

References

1. Arikuni T, Sako H, Murata A. 1994. Ipsilateral connections of the anterior cingulate cortex with the frontal and medial temporal cortices in the macaque monkey. *Neurosci Res* 21: 19–39.

2. Aston-Jones G, Cohen JD. 2005. Adaptive gain and the role of the locus coeruleus-norepinephrine system in optimal performance. *J Comp Neurol* 493: 99–110.

3. Averbeck BB, Seo M. 2008. The statistical neuroanatomy of frontal networks in the macaque. *PLOS Comput Biol* 4: e1000050.

4. Badre D, D'Esposito M. 2009. Is the rostro-caudal axis of the frontal lobe hierarchical? *Nat Rev Neurosci* 10: 659–669.

5. Barbas H. 1986. Pattern in the laminar origin of corticocortical connections. *J Comp Neurol* 252: 415–422.

6. Barbas H, Ghashghaei H, Dombrowski SM, Rempel-Clower NL. 1999. Medial prefrontal cortices are unified by common connections with superior temporal cortices and distinguished by input from memory-related areas in the rhesus monkey. *J Comp Neurol* 410: 343–367.

7. Barbas H, Pandya DN. 1989. Architecture and intrinsic connections of the prefrontal cortex in the rhesus monkey. *J Comp Neurol* 286: 353–375.

8. Barbas H, Zikopoulos B. 2007. The prefrontal cortex and flexible behavior. *Neuroscientist* 13: 532–545.

9. Barone P, Batardiere A, Knoblauch K, Kennedy H. 2000. Laminar distribution of neurons in extrastriate areas projecting to visual areas V1 and V4 correlates with the hierarchical rank and indicates the operation of a distance rule. *J Neurosci* 20: 3263–3281.

10. Beckmann M, Johansen-Berg H, Rushworth MF. 2009. Connectivity-based parcellation of human cingulate cortex and its relation to functional specialization. *J Neurosci* 29: 1175–1190.

11. Botvinick MM, Braver TS, Barch DM, Carter CS, Cohen JD. 2001. Conflict monitoring and cognitive control. *Psychol Rev* 108: 624–652.

12. Bozkurt A, Zilles K, Schleicher A, Kamper L, Arigita ES, Uylings HB, Kotter R. 2005. Distributions of transmitter receptors in the macaque cingulate cortex. *Neuroimage* 25: 219–229.

13. Brischoux F, Chakraborty S, Brierley DI, Ungless MA. 2009. Phasic excitation of dopamine neurons in ventral VTA by noxious stimuli. *Proc Natl Acad Sci USA* 106: 4894–4899.

14. Brown JW, Braver TS. 2005. Learned predictions of error likelihood in the anterior cingulate cortex. *Science* 307: 1118–1121.

15. Cohen JD, Aston-Jones G, Gilzenrat MS. (2004) A systems-level perspective on attention and cognitive control. In: Cognitive Neuroscience of Attention (Posner MI, ed), pp 71–90. New York: Guilford.

16. Crick F, Koch C. 1998. Constraints on cortical and thalamic projections: the no-strong-loops hypothesis. *Nature* 391: 245–250.

17. Croxson PL, Johansen-Berg H, Behrens TE, Robson MD, Pinsk MA, Gross CG, Richter W, Richter MC, Kastner S, Rushworth MF. 2005. Quantitative investigation of connections of the prefrontal cortex in the human and macaque using probabilistic diffusion tractography. *J Neurosci* 25: 8854–8866.

18. Deutch AY, Goldstein M, Roth RH. 1986. Activation of the locus coeruleus induced by selective stimulation of the ventral tegmental area. *Brain Res* 363: 307–314.

19. Dombrowski SM, Hilgetag CC, Barbas H. 2001. Quantitative architecture distinguishes prefrontal cortical systems in the rhesus monkey. *Cereb Cortex* 11: 975–988.

20. Dum RP, Strick PL. 1991. The origin of corticospinal projections from the premotor areas in the frontal lobe. *J Neurosci* 11: 667–689.

21. Elston GN, Benavides-Piccione R, Defelipe J. 2005. A study of pyramidal cell structure in the cingulate cortex of the macaque monkey with comparative notes on inferotemporal and primary visual cortex. *Cereb Cortex* 15: 64–73.

22. Elston GN, Benavides-Piccione R, Elston A, Zietsch B, Defelipe J, Manger P, Casagrande V, Kaas JH. 2006. Specializations of the granular prefrontal cortex of primates: implications for cognitive processing. *Anat Rec A Discov Mol Cell Evol Biol* 288: 26–35.

23. Fabre M, Rolls ET, Ashton JP, Williams G. 1983. Activity of neurons in the ventral tegmental region of the behaving monkey. *Behav Brain Res* 9: 213–235.

24. Fan J, Hof PR, Guise KG, Fossella JA, Posner MI. 2008. The functional integration of the anterior cingulate cortex during conflict processing. *Cereb Cortex* 18: 796–805.

25. Felleman DJ, Van Essen DC. 1991. Distributed hierarchical processing in the primate cerebral cortex. *Cereb Cortex* 1: 1–47.

26. Fields HL, Hjelmstad GO, Margolis EB, Nicola SM. 2007. Ventral tegmental area neurons in learned appetitive behavior and positive reinforcement. *Annu Rev Neurosci* 30: 289–316.

27. Fiorillo CD, Tobler PN, Schultz W. 2003. Discrete coding of reward probability and uncertainty by dopamine neurons. *Science* 299: 1898–1902.

28. Fonteijn HM, Norris DG, Verstraten FA. 2008. Exploring the anatomical basis of effective connectivity models with DTI-based fiber tractography. *Int J Biomed Imaging* 2008: 423192.

29. Fornito A, Whittle S, Wood SJ, Velakoulis D, Pantelis C, Yucel M. 2006. The influence of sulcal variability on morphometry of the human anterior cingulate and paracingulate cortex. *Neuroimage* 33: 843–854.

30. Fornito A, Yucel M, Wood S, Stuart GW, Buchanan JA, Proffitt T, Anderson V, Velakoulis D, Pantelis C. 2004. Individual differences in anterior cingulate/paracingulate morphology are related to executive functions in healthy males. *Cereb Cortex* 14: 424–431.

31. Frankle WG, Laruelle M, Haber SN. 2006. Prefrontal cortical projections to the midbrain in primates: evidence for a sparse connection. *Neuropsychopharmacology* 31: 1627–1636.

32. Gabbott PL, Bacon SJ. 1996. Local circuit neurons in the medial prefrontal cortex (areas 24a,b,c, 25 and 32) in the monkey: I. Cell morphology and morphometrics. *J Comp Neurol* 364: 567–608.

33. Gabbott PL, Bacon SJ. 1996. Local circuit neurons in the medial prefrontal cortex (areas 24a,b,c, 25 and 32) in the monkey: II. Quantitative areal and laminar distributions. *J Comp Neurol* 364: 609–636.

34. Habas C. 2010. Functional connectivity of the human rostral and caudal cingulate motor areas in the brain resting state at 3T. *Neuroradiology* 52: 47–59.

35. Haber SN, Fudge JL, McFarland NR. 2000. Striatonigrostriatal pathways in primates form an ascending spiral from the shell to the dorsolateral striatum. *J Neurosci* 20: 2369–2382.

36. Hatanaka N, Tokuno H, Hamada I, Inase M, Ito Y, Imanishi M, Hasegawa N, Akazawa T, Nambu A, Takada M. 2003. Thalamocortical and intracortical connections of monkey cingulate motor areas. *J Comp Neurol* 462: 121–138.

37. Holroyd C, Nieuwenhuis S, Mars RB, Coles MGH. 2004. Anterior cingulate cortex, selection for action, and error processing. In: Cognitive Neuroscience of Attention (Posner MI, ed), pp 219–231. New York: Guilford Press.

38. Holroyd CB, Coles MG. 2002. The neural basis of human error processing: reinforcement learning, dopamine, and the error-related negativity. *Psychol Rev* 109: 679–709.

39. Huerta MF, Krubitzer LA, Kaas JH. 1987. Frontal eye field as defined by intracortical microstimulation in squirrel monkeys, owl monkeys, and macaque monkeys. II. Cortical connections. *J Comp Neurol* 265: 332–361.

40. Hyafil A, Summerfield C, Koechlin E. 2009. Two mechanisms for task switching in the prefrontal cortex. *J Neurosci* 29: 5135–5142.

41. Ilinsky IA, Jouandet ML, Goldman-Rakic PS. 1985. Organization of the nigrothalamocortical system in the rhesus monkey. *J Comp Neurol* 236: 315–330.

42. Jacobson S, Trojanowski JQ. 1977. Prefrontal granular cortex of the rhesus monkey. I. Intrahemispheric cortical afferents. *Brain Res* 132: 209–233.

43. Johansen-Berg H, Rushworth MF. 2009. Using diffusion imaging to study human connectional anatomy. *Annu Rev Neurosci* 32: 75–94.

44. Kerns JG. 2006. Anterior cingulate and prefrontal cortex activity in an FMRI study of trial-to-trial adjustments on the Simon task. *Neuroimage* 33: 399–405.

45. Kerns JG, Cohen JD, MacDonald AW, 3rd, Cho RY, Stenger VA, Carter CS. 2004. Anterior cingulate conflict monitoring and adjustments in control. *Science* 303: 1023–1026.

46. Koechlin E, Ody C, Kouneiher F. 2003. The architecture of cognitive control in the human prefrontal cortex. *Science* 302: 1181–1185.

47. Koski L, Paus T. 2000. Functional connectivity of the anterior cingulate cortex within the human frontal lobe: a brain-mapping meta-analysis. *Exp Brain Res* 133: 55–65.

48. Kouneiher F, Charron S, Koechlin E. 2009. Motivation and cognitive control in the human prefrontal cortex. *Nat Neurosci* 12: 939–945.

49. Lewis DA, Melchitzky DS, Burgos GG. 2002. Specificity in the functional architecture of primate prefrontal cortex. *J Neurocytol* 31: 265–276.

50. Lu MT, Preston JB, Strick PL. 1994. Interconnections between the prefrontal cortex and the premotor areas in the frontal lobe. *J Comp Neurol* 341: 375–392.

51. Luppino G, Matelli M, Camarda RM, Gallese V, Rizzolatti G. 1991. Multiple representations of body movements in mesial area 6 and the adjacent cingulate cortex: an intracortical microstimulation study in the macaque monkey. *J Comp Neurol* 311: 463–482.

52. Margulies DS, Kelly AM, Uddin LQ, Biswal BB, Castellanos FX, Milham MP. 2007. Mapping the functional connectivity of anterior cingulate cortex. *Neuroimage* 37: 579–588.

53. Matelli M, Luppino G, Rizzolatti G. 1985. Patterns of cytochrome oxidase activity in the frontal agranular cortex of the macaque monkey. *Behav Brain Res* 18: 125–136.

54. Matelli M, Luppino G, Rizzolatti G. 1991. Architecture of superior and mesial area 6 and the adjacent cingulate cortex in the macaque monkey. *J Comp Neurol* 311: 445–462.

55. Matsumoto M, Hikosaka O. 2009. Two types of dopamine neuron distinctly convey positive and negative motivational signals. *Nature* 459: 837–841.

56. Medalla M, Barbas H. 2009. Synapses with inhibitory neurons differentiate anterior cingulate from dorsolateral prefrontal pathways associated with cognitive control. *Neuron* 61: 609–620.

57. Medalla M, Barbas H. 2010. Anterior cingulate synapses in prefrontal areas 10 and 46 suggest differential influence in cognitive control. *J Neurosci* 30: 16068–16081.

58. Miller EK, Cohen JD. 2001. An integrative theory of prefrontal cortex function. *Annu Rev Neurosci* 24: 167–202.

59. Morecraft RJ, Tanji J. 2009. Cingulofrontal interactions and the cingulate motor areas. In: Cingulate Neurobiology and Disease (Vogt B, ed), pp 113–144. Oxford: Oxford University Press.

60. Morris R, Pandya DN, Petrides M. 1999. Fiber system linking the mid-dorsolateral frontal cortex with the retrosplenial/presubicular region in the rhesus monkey. *J Comp Neurol* 407: 183–192.

61. Nimchinsky EA, Hof PR, Young WG, Morrison JH. 1996. Neurochemical, morphologic, and laminar characterization of cortical projection neurons in the cingulate motor areas of the macaque monkey. *J Comp Neurol* 374: 136–160.

62. Nishino H, Ono T, Muramoto K, Fukuda M, Sasaki K. 1987. Neuronal activity in the ventral tegmental area (VTA) during motivated bar press feeding in the monkey. *Brain Res* 413: 302–313.

63. Palomero-Gallagher N, Vogt BA, Schleicher A, Mayberg HS, Zilles K. 2009. Receptor architecture of human cingulate cortex: evaluation of the four-region neurobiological model. *Hum Brain Mapp* 30: 2336–2355.

64. Pandya DN, Yeterian EH. 1998. Comparison of prefrontal architecture and connections. In: The Prefrontal Cortex. Executive and Cognitive Functions (Roberts AC, Robbins TW, Weiskrantz L, eds), pp 51–66. New York: Oxford University Press.

65. Passingham RE, Stephan KE, Kotter R. 2002. The anatomical basis of functional localization in the cortex. *Nat Rev Neurosci* 3: 606–616.

66. Petrides M. 2002. The mid-ventrolateral prefrontal cortex and active mnemonic retrieval. *Neurobiol Learn Mem* 78: 528–538.

67. Petrides M. 2005. Lateral prefrontal cortex: architectonic and functional organization. *Philos Trans R Soc Lond B Biol Sci* 360: 781–795.

68. Petrides M, Pandya DN. 1994. Comparative architectonic analysis of the human and the macaque frontal cortex. In: Handbook of Neuropsychology (Boller F, Grafman J, eds), pp 17–58: Amsterdam: Elsevier Science.

69. Petrides M, Pandya DN. 1999. Dorsolateral prefrontal cortex: comparative cytoarchitectonic analysis in the human and the macaque brain and corticocortical connection patterns. *Eur J Neurosci* 11: 1011–1036.

70. Petrides M, Pandya DN. 2004. The frontal cortex. In: The Human Nervous System, 2nd ed. (Paxinos G, Mai JK, eds), pp 950–972: Amsterdam: Elsevier.

71. Petrides M, Pandya DN. 2006. Efferent association pathways originating in the caudal prefrontal cortex in the macaque monkey. *J Comp Neurol* 498: 227–251.

72. Petrides M, Pandya DN. 2007. Efferent association pathways from the rostral prefrontal cortex in the macaque monkey. *J Neurosci* 27: 11573–11586.

73. Picard N, Strick PL. 1996. Motor areas of the medial wall: a review of their location and functional activation. *Cereb Cortex* 6: 342–353.

74. Pucak ML, Levitt JB, Lund JS, Lewis DA. 1996. Patterns of intrinsic and associational circuitry in monkey prefrontal cortex. *J Comp Neurol* 376: 614–630.

75. Quilodran R, Rothe M, Procyk E. 2008. Behavioral shifts and action valuation in the anterior cingulate cortex. *Neuron* 57: 314–325.

76. Rushworth MF, Behrens TE. 2008. Choice, uncertainty and value in prefrontal and cingulate cortex. *Nat Neurosci* 11: 389–397.

77. Schmahmann JD, Pandya DN. 2006. Fiber Pathways of the Brain. Oxford: Oxford University Press.

78. Schmahmann JD, Pandya DN, Wang R, Dai G, D'Arceuil HE, de Crespigny AJ, Wedeen VJ. 2007. Association fibre pathways of the brain: parallel observations from diffusion spectrum imaging and autoradiography. *Brain* 130: 630–653.

79. Sporns O. 2009. The human connectome: linking structure and function in the human brain. In: Diffusion MRI (Johansen-Berg H, Behrens T, eds). London: Academic Press.

80. Takada M, Nambu A, Hatanaka N, Tachibana Y, Miyachi S, Taira M, Inase M. 2004. Organization of prefrontal outflow toward frontal motor-related areas in macaque monkeys. *Eur J Neurosci* 19: 3328–3342.

81. Tobler PN, Fiorillo CD, Schultz W. 2005. Adaptive coding of reward value by dopamine neurons. *Science* 307: 1642–1645.

82. Vezoli J, Falchier A, Jouve B, Knoblauch K, Young M, Kennedy H. 2004. Quantitative analysis of connectivity in the visual cortex: extracting function from structure. *Neuroscientist* 10: 476–482.

83. Vogt BA, ed. 2009. Cingulate Neurobiology and Disease. Oxford: Oxford University Press.

84. Vogt BA, Nimchinsky EA, Hof PR. 1995. Human cingulate cortex: surface features, flat maps, and cytoarchitecture. *J Comp Neurol* 359: 490–506.

85. Vogt BA, Pandya DN. 1987. Cingulate cortex of the rhesus monkey: II. Cortical afferents. *J Comp Neurol* 262: 271–289.

86. Vogt BA, Vogt L. 2003. Cytology of human dorsal midcingulate and supplementary motor cortices. *J Chem Neuroanat* 26: 301–309.

87. Vogt BA, Vogt L, Farber NB, Bush G. 2005. Architecture and neurocytology of monkey cingulate gyrus. *J Comp Neurol* 485: 218–239.

88. Volz HP, Rzanny R, May S, Hegewald H, Preussler B, Hajek M, Kaiser WA, Sauer H. 1997. 31P magnetic resonance spectroscopy in the dorsolateral prefrontal cortex of schizophrenics with a volume selective technique—preliminary findings. *Biol Psychiatry* 41: 644–648.

89. Wang Y, Shima K, Isoda M, Sawamura H, Tanji J. 2002. Spatial distribution and density of prefrontal cortical cells projecting to three sectors of the premotor cortex. *Neuroreport* 13: 1341–1344.

90. Williams SM, Goldman-Rakic PS. 1993. Characterization of the dopaminergic innervation of the primate frontal cortex using a dopamine-specific antibody. *Cereb Cortex* 3: 199–222.

91. Williams SM, Goldman-Rakic PS. 1998. Widespread origin of the primate mesofrontal dopamine system. *Cereb Cortex* 8: 321–345.

2 Neural Circuits of Reward and Decision Making: Integrative Networks across Corticobasal Ganglia Loops

Suzanne N. Haber

Anatomical connectivity studies provide a key element for understanding the neural networks involved in evaluating environmental stimuli that transform this information into actions, thus leading to expected outcomes. The reward circuit is a central component of the network that drives incentive-based learning, appropriate responses to stimuli, and good decision making. The idea that there is an anatomically identifiable reward circuit initially came from experiments that demonstrated rats would work for electrical stimulation in specific brain sites[51] and was later supported by pharmacological manipulation of those sites through intracranial injections of drugs of abuse.[8] Although this circuit included several brain regions, the orbital (OFC) and anterior cingulate cortices (ACC), the n. accumbens (NAcc), and the ventral tegmental area (VTA) dopamine neurons are central.[29,60,62,71] Recent studies extend the striatal and midbrain reward-related areas to include the entire ventral striatum (VS) and the dopamine neurons of the substantia nigra, pars compacta (SNc).* The VS receives its main cortical input from the OFC and ACC, and a massive dopaminergic input from the midbrain. The VS projects to the ventral pallidum (VP) and to the VTA-SN, which in turn project back to the prefrontal cortex (PFC), via the medial dorsal nucleus (MD) of the thalamus. These structures are part of the corticobasal ganglia system and are at the center of the reward circuit (figure 2.1).[25]

While the reward circuit is now considered part of the corticobasal ganglia network, historically, the basal ganglia was considered solely part of the sensory–motor control system.[47] The conceptual change from a purely sensory–motor function to a more complex set of functions can be traced to the demonstration that an additional (and separate) functional loop, the limbic loop, exists within the basal ganglia.[30] The idea of separate cortical loops in the basal ganglia was subsequently

---

* In addition, other structures, including the other prefrontal cortical areas, amygdala, hippocampus, hypothalamus, lateral habenular nucleus, and specific brainstem structures, such as the pedunculopontine nucleus, and the raphe nuclei, are also key components that regulate the reward circuit.

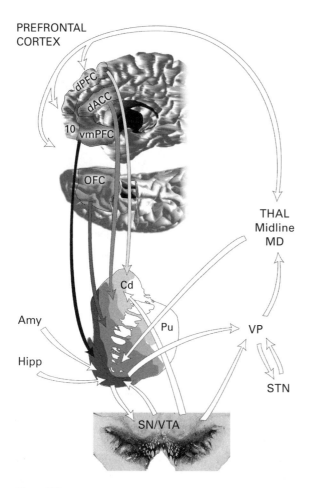

Figure 2.1
Schematic illustrating key structures and pathways of the reward circuit. Black arrow = input from the vmPFC; dark gray arrow = input from the OFC; light medium gray arrow = input from the dACC; light gray arrow = input from the dPFC; white arrows = other main connections of the reward circuit. Amy, amygdala; dACC, dorsal anterior cingulate cortex; dPFC, dorsal prefrontal cortex; Cd, caudate nucleus; Hipp, hippocampus; MD, medial dorsal nucleus of the thalamus; OFC, orbital frontal cortex; Pu, putamen; S, shell; SN, substantia nigra; STN, subthalamic n.; Thal, thalamus; VP, ventral pallidum; VTA, ventral tegmental area; vmPFC, ventral medial prefrontal cortex.

expanded to include several parallel and segregated functional loops (limbic, associative, and sensorimotor).[1] Although this concept has dominated the field for the past 20 years, several studies demonstrate integration across these circuits. Network crosstalk between limbic associative functions is consistent with the idea that adaptive behaviors require a combination of reward evaluation and associative learning to develop appropriate action plans and inhibit inappropriate choices. Not surprisingly, the idea of motivation-to-movement interface through basal ganglia circuits was developed soon after the discovery of the limbic component to the basal ganglia.[43,46] Thus, the ventral corticobasal ganglia network, while at the heart of reward processing, does not work in isolation.[3,5,12,23,24] In fact, within each station of the circuit there are interfaces between pathways that allow communication between different parts of the reward circuit and between the reward circuit and the associative circuit. In this chapter, we describe first the organization of the reward (and associative) circuit(s) and second, specific places in the network where crosstalk between circuits can occur.

Organization of the Reward Circuit

Prefrontal Cortex and Its Projections to the Striatum

The PFC comprises multifunctional regions involved in reinforcement-based learning and decision making. Different prefrontal cortical areas and corresponding striatal regions are involved in these various aspects of motivation and learning, and pathophysiology in the circuit is associated with sadness and depression, pathological risk taking, addictive behaviors, and obsessive-compulsive disorder.[15,38,41,50,69] The PFC is a complex and heterogenous region, but can broadly be divided into (1) the orbitofrontal cortex, or OFC (lateral OFC and part of insular cortex); (2) a ventral, medial prefrontal cortex, or vmPFC (medial OFC, subgenual ACC, and area 10); (3) the dorsal anterior cingulate cortex, or dACC (area 24); and (4) the dorsal prefrontal cortex, or dPFC (areas 9 and 46).[10,25,52] The vmPFC and OFC, collectively referred to as the ventral prefrontal cortex (vPFC), and the dACC, along with its basal ganglia components, mediate different aspects of reward-based behaviors, error prediction, and conflict detection.[6,15,49,61] In addition, the vmPFC has also been shown to be important for extinction and extinction recall.[42] In contrast, the dPFC is associated with cognitive processing and working memory, and provides cognitive control over motivational and emotional behaviors.[12,33] Overall, PFC regions work together in a complementary fashion to compare valued options and choose among them. The main subcortical outputs from the vPFC are to the VS and thalamus.

The VS includes the NAcc and the broad ventral continuity between the caudate nucleus and the putamen rostral to the anterior commissure.[24,31] This entire region has been a focus for the study of reinforcement, and the transition between drug use for a reward and as a habit.[16,56] However, neither cytoarchitectonic nor histochemistry distinctions mark a clear boundary between the VS and the dorsal striatum. The best way to define the VS, therefore, is to use its cortical afferent projections from areas that mediate different aspects of reward and emotional processing, that is, inputs from the vPFC, dACC, and the medial temporal lobe, including the amygdala. Using these projections as a guide, the VS occupies over 20% of the striatum in nonhuman primates.[24]

Corticostriatal projections form dense, focal patches that are organized in a functional topographic manner.[24,64] Inputs from the vmPFC, OFC, and dACC terminate within subregions of the VS (figure 2.1).[26] The focal projection field from the vmPFC is the most limited. It is concentrated within the most ventral and medial parts of the VS, including the shell. The vmPFC also projects to the medial wall of the caudate n., adjacent to the ventricle. The densest input from agranular insular cortex also terminates in the NAcc and at the medial wall of the caudate.[9] Fewer data are available concerning the projections of area 10 to the VS, particularly medial area 10. However, one might assume that the medial and ventral area 10 would also terminate in the ventral, medial VS, given the overall topography of other projections from the vPFC. Thus, this VS region receives convergent input from the olfactory and visceral-associated insula, from the vmPFC, and most likely from area 10.

The dorsal and lateral parts of the VS receive inputs from the OFC. These terminals also extend dorsally, along the medial caudate n., but lateral to those derived from the vmPFC. The medial to lateral and rostral to caudal topographic organization of the OFC terminal fields is consistent with the positions of OFC regions in the PFC. That is, inputs from lateral parts of the OFC (i.e., area 12) terminate lateral to those derived from more medial areas (area 13). Projections from the dACC terminate lateral to those from the OFC. Taken together, the vmPFC, OFC, and dACC project primarily to the rostral striatum, with the vmPFC projecting most medially, and the dACC most laterally, with the OFC terminal fields positioned in between.[24] In contrast, the dPFC projects throughout the rostrocaudal extent of the striatum, terminating primarily in the head of the caudate and in part of the rostral putamen, but continuing into the caudal caudate nucleus. Like vPFC projections, axons from areas 9 and 46 also occupy somewhat different territories that, at rostral levels, span across the internal capsule.[7] At more caudal levels, these inputs are primarily confined to the dorsal caudate n. The two other main afferent projections to the striatum are derived from the midbrain and thalamus. Additional inputs from the amygdala and hippocampus make the VS a unique striatal region, in that these two structures do not innervate the dorsal striatum.

Midbrain Dopamine Projections to the VS

The central role of the dopamine neurons in the reward circuit is well established, along with the fact that this role in not limited to the VTA, but includes cells of the SNc.[63,71] The midbrain dopamine striatal projection follows a general mediolateral and inverse dorsoventral topography.[34] Thus, the VTA and the dorsal tier of SNc neurons project to the VS, and the ventral SNc neurons project to the dorsolateral striatum. The shell receives the most limited midbrain input, primarily derived from the medial VTA. The rest of the VS receives input from the VTA and from the medial and dorsal part of the SNc. In contrast to the VS, the striatal area innervated by the dPFC receives input from a wider region of centrally located dopamine cells. The dorsolateral (motor-related) striatum receives the largest midbrain projection from cells throughout the ventral SNc. Thus, in addition to an inverse topography, there is also a differential ratio of dopamine projections to the different striatal areas,[23] with the VS receiving the most limited dopamine input and the dorsolateral striatum receiving the largest input. It's important to note, however, that despite the overall topographic organization, individual dopamine axons arborize extensively within the striatum and are therefore likely to cross regional striatal boundaries.[37]

Thalamic Projections to the VS

The midline, medial intralaminar and medial MD thalamic nuclei project to medial prefrontal areas, the VS, amygdala, and hippocampus, and are referred to as the limbic-related thalamic groups.[20,21,32,72] The shell receives the most limited input, derived almost exclusively from the midline nuclei. The medial wall of the caudate n. receives projections, not only from the midline and the medial intralaminar nuclei, but also from the central superior lateral nucleus. In contrast, the lateral part of the VS receives a limited projection from the midline thalamic nuclei. Its input is derived from the intralaminar nuclei (the parafascicular nucleus and the central superior lateral nucleus). In addition to the midline and intralaminar thalamostriatal projections, there is a large input from the "specific" thalamic basal ganglia relay nuclei: the MD, ventral anterior, and ventral lateral nuclei.[39] The VS receives this input from the MD and a limited projection from the magnocellular subdivision of the ventral anterior nucleus. Thalamic input to the striatum is glutamatergic and can be distinguished from cortical synapses. Recent studies show that the thalamic and cortical synapses associated with dopaminergic terminals are similar.[44]

The amygdala is a prominent limbic structure that plays a key role in emotional coding of environmental stimuli.[45,58] Overall, the basal nucleus and the magnocellular division of the accessory basal nucleus are the main sources of inputs to the VS.[19] The amygdala has few inputs to the dorsal striatum in primates. The shell is set apart from the rest of the VS by a specific set of connections derived from the medial part of the central nucleus (CeM), periamygdaloid cortex, and the medial nucleus of the amygdala. In contrast to the amygdala, the hippocampal formation projection is essentially confined to the shell.[18] Taken together, the existence of convergent fibers from cortex within the VS, along with hippocampal and amygda-lostriatal projections along with broad dopamine modulation, places the VS as a key entry port for processing emotional and motivational information.

Efferent Projections of the VS

The VS, like the dorsal striatum, primarily projects to the pallidum and midbrain.[28] The VP is an important component of the reward circuit in that cells in this forebrain region respond specifically during the learning and performance of reward-incentive behaviors and play a central role in addictive behaviors.[65,68] The VP is best described as the pallidal region that receives its input from the VS. VS fibers terminate topo-graphically in the subcommissural VP, the rostral pole of the external segment, and the rostromedial portion of the internal segment. For example, the shell projects to the border areas between the VP and the bed nucleus of the stria terminalis, and more lateral VS areas project to the lateral VP.[28] The topography created by vPFC and dACC projections to the VS, is reflected in the VS output to the VP.[26] Like the dorsal pallidum, components of the VP project topographically to the subthalamic nucleus (STN), SN, and thalamus.

Striatal projections to the midbrain terminate in both the pars reticulata and the pars compacta. In fact, the striatonigral projection provides a massive projection to the midbrain dopamine cells, terminating in both the VTA and SNc. These projec-tion fields are not as topographically organized as those projecting to the pallidum. As seen with the nigrostriatal projection, these projections have a medial-lateral and an inverse ventral-dorsal topography. In other words, the VS projects to the dorsal midbrain and the dorsal striatum terminates in the ventral midbrain.[23,35,67] The largest terminal fields are derived from the VS and the associative striatum. In contrast, the dorsolateral striatal projection to the SN is confined to a relatively small ventrolateral position. The output from the medial SNr and VP are primarily to the MD nucleus, which, in turn, projects to the frontal cortex, and is the final link in the reward circuit.[27,59]

Crosstalk between Functional Circuits

Integration between Corticostriatal Projections

Although the topographic organization of corticostriatal projections is well docu-mented, there is increasing evidence of regions of interface between terminals from different cortical areas, suggesting functional integration. For example, early studies showed that corticostriatal terminals from sensory and motor cortex converge within the striatum.[17] Here, axons from each area synapse onto single fast-spiking GABAergic interneurons. Interestingly, these interneurons are more responsive to cortical input than the medium spiny cells, suggesting a potentially critical role for interneurons to integrate information from different cortical areas before passing that information on to the medium spiny projection cells.[36,57]

Projections from the OFC, vmPFC, and dACC also converge in specific regions within the VS. Thus, focal terminal fields from the vmPFC, OFC, and dACC show a complex interweaving and convergence[24] (figure 2.2a). For example, axons from the dACC and OFC regions do not occupy completely separate territories in any part

a)
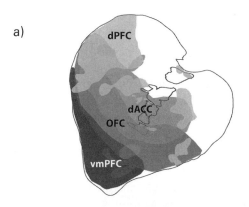

b)
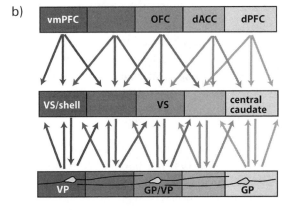

Figure 2.2
Schematics illustrating integrative connections through convergence of terminals from different functional regions. (a) A mediofrontal view of a three-dimensional reconstruction illustrating convergence of inputs from PFC inputs. (b) Schematic illustrating convergence at the PFC-striatal and the striato-pallidostriatal levels.

of the striatum. They converge most extensively at rostral levels, providing an anatomical substrate for modulation between these circuits. In addition, projections
from dACC and OFC also converge with inputs from the dPFC, particularly at the
most rostral striatal levels. A similar pattern of both topographic and integrative
connectivity of corticostriatal projections has recently been demonstrated in the
human brain using diffusion tensor imaging (DTI). These data show a similar overall
organization of the different cortical regions and the striatum, and provide a strong
correlation between monkey anatomical tracing studies and human DTI studies.[14]
Taken together, a coordinated activation of dPFC, dACC, and/or OFC terminals in
these subregions could produce a unique combinatorial activation at the specific
sites for channeling reward-based incentive drive in selecting among different
valued options. The existence of these areas may help explain complex activation
patterns following different reward-related paradigms or the interface between
reward and cognitive feedback.[12]

Ventral Pallidal Connections

Pallidal dendrites are long, stretching across multiple functional regions, and are
oriented perpendicular to incoming striatal fibers. Thus, each pallidal dendrite is in
a position to intercept efferents originating from more than one functional striatal
district[54] (figure 2.2b). In addition, descending projections from the VP converge
with those from the dorsal pallidum on single dopaminergic neurons.[5] Therefore,
individual SN cells receive both limbic and nonlimbic input. This convergence has
important implications for the role of the dopamine cells in processing diverse
information, which in turn is sent back to the striatum. Moreover, VP and dorsal
pallidal projections also converge at the interface between the projection fields in
the STN.[4] An additional unique projection of the VP is to both the internal and
external segments of the dorsal pallidum. The dorsal pallidum does not seem to
project ventrally.[27] Finally, part of the VP (as with the external segment of the pallidum) also projects to the striatum.[66] This pallidostriatal pathway is extensive
and more widespread than reciprocal striatopallidal projection, providing a broad
feedback signal (figure 2.2b).

The Striatonigrostriatal Network

VS (limbic) influence on the dorsal striatum (motor) through the midbrain dopamine cells was originally shown in rats.[48] The concept of transferring information
through different striatal regions via the midbrain was expanded on, taking into
account the functionally more complex and diverse primate striatum.[23] The VTA
and medial SN are associated with limbic regions, and the central and ventral SN
are associated with the associative and motor striatal regions, respectively. However,
as described previously, each functional region differs in its proportional projections.
The VS receives a limited midbrain input, but projects to a large region. In contrast,

the dorsolateral striatum receives a wide input, but projects to a limited region. In other words, the VS influences a wide range of dopamine neurons, but is itself influenced by a relatively limited group of dopamine cells. On the other hand, the dorsolateral striatum influences a limited midbrain region, but is affected by a relatively large midbrain region.

Thus, while the main efferent projection from the VS to the midbrain is to the dorsal tier of dopamine cells, this projection field extends beyond the tight VS–dorsal tier–VS circuit. Indeed, the VS also terminates more ventrally, in a position to influence more dorsal striatal regions, particularly those that receive input from associative cortical regions (e.g., dPFC). This part of the ventral tier is reciprocally connected to the central (or associative) striatum. The central striatum also projects to a more ventral region than it receives input from. This region, in turn, projects to the dorsolateral (or motor) striatum. Taken together, the interface between different striatal regions via the midbrain DA cells is organized in an ascending spiral that interconnects different functional regions of the striatum and creates a feedforward organization, from reward-related regions of the striatum to cognitive and motor areas (figure 2.3a).

Although the short latency burst-firing activity of dopamine that signals immediate reinforcement is likely to be triggered from brainstem nuclei,[13] the corticostriato-midbrain pathway is in the position to influence dopamine cells to distinguish rewards and modify responses to incoming salient stimuli over time, placing the striatonigrostriatal pathway in a pivotal position for transferring information from the VS to the dorsal striatum during learning and habit formation. Indeed, cells in the dorsal striatum are progressively recruited during different types of learning and habit formation.[3,53,55,70]

Additional VS Connections

The VS also terminates in non–basal ganglia regions.[28] The shell sends fibers caudally and medially into the lateral hypothalamus and, to some extent, into the periaqueductal gray. Axons from the medial VS also terminate in the bed nucleus of the stria terminalis, indicating a direct striatal influence on the extended amygdala. Finally, fibers from ventral regions of the VS terminate in the nucleus basalis.[2,22,73] The n. basalis is the main source of cholinergic fibers to the cerebral cortex and the amygdala. Thus, the VS can influence cortex directly through a connection that does not pass through the pallidal thalamic circuit, providing a route through which the reward circuit has wide access to multiple regions of frontal cortex.

Thalamocorticothalamic Connection

Thalamocortical connections are bidirectional. However, the corticothalamic projections are more extensive than the thalamocortical projections.[11,40] Moreover,

a)

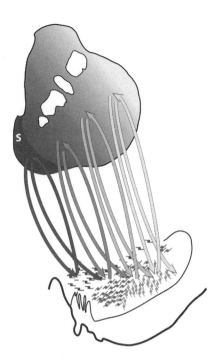

S

b)

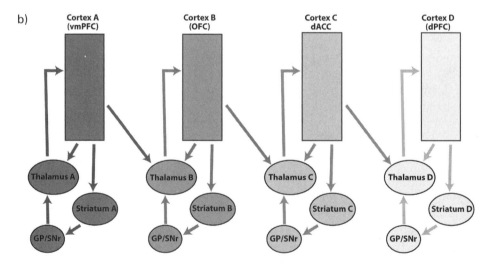

Figure 2.3
Schematics illustrating integrative connections through reciprocal and nonreciprocal connections.
(a) Connections between the striatum and substantia nigra. The arrows indicated illustrate how the
ventral striatum can influence the dorsal striatum through the midbrain dopamine cells. Shades of gray
indicate functional regions of the striatum, based on cortical inputs (figure 2.1). Midbrain projections
from the shell target both the VTA and ventromedial SNc. Projections from the VTA to the shell form
a "closed," reciprocal loop, but also project more laterally to impact on dopamine cells projecting the
rest of the ventral striatum forming the first part of a feed forward loop (or spiral). The spiral continues
through the striatonigrostriatal projections through which the ventral striatum impacts on cognitive and
motor striatal areas (not illustrated) via the midbrain dopamine cells. (b) Connections between the cortex
and thalamus. Arrows illustrate how the nonreciprocal component of the corticothalamic projection can
influence another cortico–basal ganglia function loop through the thalamus. Black arrows = inputs from
the vmPFC; dark gray arrows = inputs form the OFC and dACC; light arrows = inputs from the dPFC.

in addition to the reciprocal thalamocorticothalamic connection, there is also a nonreciprocal corticothalamic component. Thus, while the MD completes the reward circuit back to cortex, a nonreciprocal cortical input to the MD is derived from functionally distinct frontal cortical areas. For example, the central MD has not only reciprocal projections with the OFC, but also a nonreciprocal input from vmPFC. Similarly, more lateral MD areas are reciprocally connected to the dPFC, but also have a nonreciprocal input from the OFC.[40] Therefore, similar to the striatonigrostriatal projection system, the thalamic relay nuclei from the basal ganglia also appear to integrate information flow from reward and higher cortical "association" areas of the prefrontal cortex (figure 2.3b). A recent DTI study indicates that integration between these cortical areas in the thalamus is also likely to exist in humans.[14]

Summary

Although the reward network comprises a specific set of connections, it does not work in isolation, but also interfaces with circuits that mediate cognitive function and motor planning. Integration across cortico–basal ganglia circuits occurs through convergence zones, for example, between corticostriatal projections or pallidal-nigral connections, that can link areas associated with different functions to permit dissemination of cortical information across multiple functional regions. It also occurs via reciprocal-nonreciprocal networks (through the striatonigrostriatal pathway and thalamocorticothalamic circuit). Through these interactive networks, information about reward can be channeled through cognitive and motor control circuits to mediate the development of adaptive action plans. Thus, whereas reward anticipation tends to coactivate the VS and midbrain, reward outcomes subsequently recruit the medial caudate and putamen, followed by the dorsal caudate. This recruitment likely involves the dopamine pathways, through the striatonigrostriatal spiral.[3,55] Thus, knowledge gained from anatomical connectivity studies, including areas of potential network interfaces, will increase our understanding and ability to predict how and when seemingly unconnected structures might be activated or coactivated.

Outstanding Questions

• Prefrontal cortex receives dopamine connections, but there is only a limited cortical projection to the dopamine cells (see Frankle et al. in Further Reading). How does the cortex influence the dopamine neurons?

• The striatum has been described as being composed of striosomes and matrisomes, with prefrontal cortex projecting only to the striosomes. Could this concept be included in the description proposed in this chapter? If so, what would be the functional impact of such implementation?

• Do the different DA populations have different roles?

Further Reading

Haber SN, Knutson B. 2010. The reward circuit: linking primate anatomy and human imaging. *Neuropsychopharmacology* 35: 4–26. A nice review linking data regarding anatomy in monkeys and imaging data in humans.

Frankle WG, Laruelle M, Haber SN. 2006. Prefrontal cortical projections to the midbrain in primates: evidence for a sparse connection. *Neuropsychopharmacology* 31:1627–1636. This paper describes anatomical evidence that the prefrontal cortex could influence DA midbrain activity.

Graybiel AM. 2008. Habits, rituals, and the evaluative brain. *Annu Rev Neurosci* 31:359–387. A review of how habitual behaviors emerge as a result experience-dependent plasticity in basal ganglia–based networks.

References

1. Alexander GE, Crutcher MD, DeLong MR. 1990. Basal ganglia-thalamocortical circuits: parallel substrates for motor, oculomotor, "prefrontal" and "limbic" functions. *Prog Brain Res* 85: 119–146.

2. Beach TG, Tago H, McGeer EG. 1987. Light microscopic evidence for a substance P-containing innervation of the human nucleus basalis of Meynert. *Brain Res* 408: 251–257.

3. Belin D, Everitt BJ. 2008. Cocaine seeking habits depend upon dopamine-dependent serial connectivity linking the ventral with the dorsal striatum. *Neuron* 57: 432–441.

4. Bevan MD, Clarke NP, Bolam JP. 1997. Synaptic integration of functionally diverse pallidal information in the entopeduncular nucleus and subthalamic nucleus in the rat. *J Neurosci* 17: 308–324.

5. Bevan MD, Smith AD, Bolam JP. 1996. The substantia nigra as a site of synaptic integration of functionally diverse information arising from the ventral pallidum and the globus pallidus in the rat. *Neuroscience* 75: 5–12.

6. Botvinick M, Nystrom LE, Fissell K, Carter CS, Cohen JD. 1999. Conflict monitoring versus selection-for-action in anterior cingulate cortex. *Nature* 402: 179–181.

7. Calzavara R, Mailly P, Haber SN. 2007. Relationship between the corticostriatal terminals from areas 9 and 46, and those from area 8A, dorsal and rostral premotor cortex and area 24c: an anatomical substrate for cognition to action. *Eur J Neurosci* 26: 2005–2024.

8. Carlezon WA, Wise RA. 1996. Rewarding actions of phencyclidine and related drugs in nucleus accumbens shell and frontal cortex. *J Neurosci* 16: 3112–3122.

9. Chikama M, McFarland N, Amaral DG, Haber SN. 1997. Insular cortical projections to functional regions of the striatum correlate with cortical cytoarchitectonic organization in the primate. *J Neurosci* 17: 9686–9705.

10. Croxson PL, Johansen-Berg H, Behrens TE, Robson MD, Pinsk MA, Gross CG, Richter W, Richter MC, Kastner S, Rushworth MF. 2005. Quantitative investigation of connections of the prefrontal cortex in the human and macaque using probabilistic diffusion tractography. *J Neurosci* 25: 8854–8866.

11. Darian-Smith C, Tan A, Edwards S. 1999. Comparing thalamocortical and corticothalamic microstructure and spatial reciprocity in the macaque ventral posterolateral nucleus (VPLc) and medial pulvinar. *J Comp Neurol* 410: 211–234.

12. Delgado MR, Gillis MM, Phelps EA. 2008. Regulating the expectation of reward via cognitive strategies. *Nat Neurosci* 11: 880–881.

13. Dommett E, Coizet V, Blaha CD, Martindale J, Lefebvre V, Walton N, Mayhew JE, Overton PG, Redgrave P. 2005. How visual stimuli activate dopaminergic neurons at short latency. *Science* 307: 1476–1479.

14. Draganski B, Kherif F, Kloppel S, Cook PA, Alexander DC, Parker GJ, Deichmann R, Ashburner J, Frackowiak RS. 2008. Evidence for segregated and integrative connectivity patterns in the human basal ganglia. *J Neurosci* 28: 7143–7152.

15. Elliott R, Newman JL, Longe OA, Deakin JF. 2003. Differential response patterns in the striatum and orbitofrontal cortex to financial reward in humans: a parametric functional magnetic resonance imaging study. *J Neurosci* 23: 303–307.

16. Everitt BJ, Robbins TW. 2005. Neural systems of reinforcement for drug addiction: from actions to habits to compulsion. *Nat Neurosci* 8: 1481–1489.

17. Flaherty AW, Graybiel AM. 1993. Two input systems for body representations in the primate striatal matrix: experimental evidence in the squirrel monkey. *J Neurosci* 13: 1120–1137.

18. Friedman DP, Aggleton JP, Saunders RC. 2002. Comparison of hippocampal, amygdala, and perirhinal projections to the nucleus accumbens: combined anterograde and retrograde tracing study in the macaque brain. *J Comp Neurol* 450: 345–365.

19. Fudge JL, Kunishio K, Walsh C, Richard D, Haber SN. 2002. Amygdaloid projections to ventromedial striatal subterritories in the primate. *Neuroscience* 110: 257–275.

20. Gaffan D, Murray EA. 1990. Amygdalar interaction with the mediodorsal nucleus of the thalamus and the ventromedial prefrontal cortex in stimulus reward associative learning in the monkey. *J Neurosci* 10: 3479–3493.

21. Giménez-Amaya JM, McFarland NR, de las Heras S, Haber SN. 1995. Organization of thalamic projections to the ventral striatum in the primate. *J Comp Neurol* 354: 127–149.

22. Haber SN. 1987. Anatomical relationship between the basal ganglia and the basal nucleus of Maynert in human and monkey forebrain. *Proc Natl Acad Sci USA* 84: 1408–1412.

23. Haber SN, Fudge JL, McFarland NR. 2000. Striatonigrostriatal pathways in primates form an ascending spiral from the shell to the dorsolateral striatum. *J Neurosci* 20: 2369–2382.

24. Haber SN, Kim KS, Mailly P, Calzavara R. 2006. Reward-related cortical inputs define a large striatal region in primates that interface with associative cortical inputs, providing a substrate for incentive-based learning. *J Neurosci* 26: 8368–8376.

25. Haber SN, Knutson B. 2010. The reward circuit: linking primate anatomy and human imaging. *Neuropsychopharmacology* 35: 4–26.

26. Haber SN, Kunishio K, Mizobuchi M, Lynd-Balta E. 1995. The orbital and medial prefrontal circuit through the primate basal ganglia. *J Neurosci* 15: 4851–4867.

27. Haber SN, Lynd-Balta E, Mitchell SJ. 1993. The organization of the descending ventral pallidal projections in the monkey. *J Comp Neurol* 329: 111–129.

28. Haber SN, Lynd E, Klein C, Groenewegen HJ. 1990. Topographic organization of the ventral striatal efferent projections in the rhesus monkey: an anterograde tracing study. *J Comp Neurol* 293: 282–298.

29. Hayden BY, Platt ML. 2010. Neurons in anterior cingulate cortex multiplex information about reward and action. *J Neurosci* 30: 3339–3346.

30. Heimer L. 1978. The olfactory cortex and the ventral striatum. In: Limbic Mechanisms (Livingston KE, Hornykiewicz O, eds), pp 95–187. New York: Plenum Press.

31. Heimer L, De Olmos JS, Alheid GF, Person J, Sakamoto N, Shinoda K, Marksteiner J, Switzer RC. 1999. The human basal forebrain. Part II. In: Handbook of Chemical Neuroanatomy (Bloom FE, Bjorkland A, Hokfelt T, eds), pp 57–226. Amsterdam: Elsevier.

32. Hsu DT, Price JL. 2007. Midline and intralaminar thalamic connections with the orbital and medial prefrontal networks in macaque monkeys. *J Comp Neurol* 504: 89–111.

33. Levy R, Goldman-Rakic PS. 2000. Segregation of working memory functions within the dorsolateral prefrontal cortex. *Exp Brain Res* 133: 23–32.

34. Lynd-Balta E, Haber SN. 1994. The organization of midbrain projections to the striatum in the primate: sensorimotor-related striatum versus ventral striatum. *Neuroscience* 59: 625–640.

35. Lynd-Balta E, Haber SN. 1994. Primate striatonigral projections: a comparison of the sensorimotor-related striatum and the ventral striatum. *J Comp Neurol* 345: 562–578.

36. Mallet N, Le Moine C, Charpier S, Gonon F. 2005. Feedforward inhibition of projection neurons by fast-spiking GABA interneurons in the rat striatum in vivo. *J Neurosci* 25: 3857–3869.

37. Matsuda W, Furuta T, Nakamura KC, Hioki H, Fujiyama F, Arai R, Kaneko T. 2009. Single nigrostriatal dopaminergic neurons form widely spread and highly dense axonal arborizations in the neostriatum. *J Neurosci* 29: 444–453.

38. Mayberg HS, Brannan SK, Tekell JL, Silva JA, Mahurin RK, McGinnis S, Jerabek PA. 2000. Regional metabolic effects of fluoxetine in major depression: serial changes and relationship to clinical response. *Biol Psychiatry* 48: 830–843.

39. McFarland NR, Haber SN. 2001. Organization of thalamostriatal terminals from the ventral motor nuclei in the macaque. *J Comp Neurol* 429: 321–336.

40. McFarland NR, Haber SN. 2002. Thalamic relay nuclei of the basal ganglia form both reciprocal and nonreciprocal cortical connections, linking multiple frontal cortical areas. *J Neurosci* 22: 8117–8132.

41. Menzies L, Chamberlain SR, Laird AR, Thelen SM, Sahakian BJ, Bullmore ET. 2008. Integrating evidence from neuroimaging and neuropsychological studies of obsessive-compulsive disorder: the orbitofronto-striatal model revisited. *Neurosci Biobehav Rev* 32: 525–549.

42. Milad MR, Wright CI, Orr SP, Pitman RK, Quirk GJ, Rauch SL. 2007. Recall of fear extinction in humans activates the ventromedial prefrontal cortex and hippocampus in concert. *Biol Psychiatry* 62: 446–454.

43. Mogenson GJ, Jones DL, Yim CY. 1980. From motivation to action: functional interface between the limbic system and the motor system. *Prog Neurobiol* 14: 69–97.

44. Moss J, Bolam JP. 2008. A dopaminergic axon lattice in the striatum and its relationship with cortical and thalamic terminals. *J Neurosci* 28: 11221–11230.

45. Murray EA. 2007. The amygdala, reward and emotion. *Trends Cogn Sci* 11: 489–497.

46. Nauta HJW. 1986. The relationship of the basal ganglia to the limbic system. In: Handbook of Clinical Neurology: Extrapyramidal Disorders (Vinken PJ, Bruyn GW, Klawans JJ, eds), pp 19–31. Amsterdam: Elsevier.

47. Nauta WJ, Mehler WR. 1966. Projections of the lentiform nucleus in the monkey. *Brain Res* 1: 3–42.

48. Nauta WJH, Smith GP, Faull RLM, Domesick VB. 1978. Efferent connections and nigral afferents of the nucleus accumbens septi in the rat. *Neuroscience* 3: 385–401.

49. O'Doherty J, Critchley H, Deichmann R, Dolan RJ. 2003. Dissociating valence of outcome from behavioral control in human orbital and ventral prefrontal cortices. *J Neurosci* 23: 7931–7939.

50. O'Doherty J, Dayan P, Schultz J, Deichmann R, Friston K, Dolan RJ. 2004. Dissociable roles of ventral and dorsal striatum in instrumental conditioning. *Science* 304: 452–454.

51. Olds J, Milner P. 1954. Positive reinforcement produced by electrical stimulation of septal area and other regions of rat brain. *J Comp Physiol Psychol* 47: 419–427.

52. Passingham RE, Stephan KE, Kotter R. 2002. The anatomical basis of functional localization in the cortex. *Nat Rev Neurosci* 3: 606–616.

53. Pasupathy A, Miller EK. 2005. Different time courses of learning-related activity in the prefrontal cortex and striatum. *Nature* 433: 873–876.

54. Percheron G, Yelnik J, Francois C. 1984. The primate striato-pallido-nigral system: an integrative system for cortical information. In: The Basal Ganglia: Structure and Function (McKenzie JS, Kemm RE, Wilcock LN, eds), pp 87–105. London: Plenum Press.

55. Porrino LJ, Lyons D, Smith HR, Daunais JB, Nader MA. 2004. Cocaine self-administration produces a progressive involvement of limbic, association, and sensorimotor striatal domains. *J Neurosci* 24: 3554–3562.

56. Porrino LJ, Smith HR, Nader MA, Beveridge TJ. 2007. The effects of cocaine: a shifting target over the course of addiction. *Prog Neuropsychopharmacol Biol Psychiatry* 31: 1593–1600.

57. Ramanathan S, Hanley JJ, Deniau JM, Bolam JP. 2002. Synaptic convergence of motor and somatosensory cortical afferents onto GABAergic interneurons in the rat striatum. *J Neurosci* 22: 8158–8169.

58. Ramirez DR, Savage LM. 2007. Differential involvement of the basolateral amygdala, orbitofrontal cortex, and nucleus accumbens core in the acquisition and use of reward expectancies. *Behav Neurosci* 121: 896–906.

59. Ray JP, Price JL. 1993. The organization of projections from the mediodorsal nucleus of the thalamus to orbital and medial prefrontal cortex in macaque monkeys. *J Comp Neurol* 337: 1–31.

60. Rolls ET. 2000. The orbitofrontal cortex and reward. *Cereb Cortex* 10: 284–294.

61. Rushworth MF, Behrens TE. 2008. Choice, uncertainty and value in prefrontal and cingulate cortex. *Nat Neurosci* 11: 389–397.

62. Schultz W. 2000. Multiple reward signals in the brain. *Nat Rev Neurosci* 1: 199–207.

63. Schultz W. 2002. Getting formal with dopamine and reward. *Neuron* 36: 241–263.

64. Selemon LD, Goldman-Rakic PS. 1985. Longitudinal topography and interdigitation of corticostriatal projections in the rhesus monkey. *J Neurosci* 5: 776–794.

65. Smith KS, Tindell AJ, Aldridge JW, Berridge KC. 2009. Ventral pallidum roles in reward and motivation. *Behav Brain Res* 196: 155–167.

66. Spooren WPJM, Lynd-Balta E, Mitchell S, Haber SN. 1996. Ventral pallidostriatal pathway in the monkey: evidence for modulation of basal ganglia circuits. *J Comp Neurol* 370: 295–312.

67. Szabo J. 1979. Strionigral and nigrostriatal connections. Anatomical studies. *Appl Neurophysiol* 42: 9–12.

68. Tindell AJ, Smith KS, Pecina S, Berridge KC, Aldridge JW. 2006. Ventral pallidum firing codes hedonic reward: when a bad taste turns good. *J Neurophysiol* 96: 2399–2409.

69. Volkow ND, Wang GJ, Ma Y, Fowler JS, Wong C, Ding YS, Hitzemann R, Swanson JM, Kalivas P. 2005. Activation of orbital and medial prefrontal cortex by methylphenidate in cocaine-addicted subjects but not in controls: relevance to addiction. *J Neurosci* 25: 3932–3939.

70. Volkow ND, Wang GJ, Telang F, Fowler JS, Logan J, Childress AR, Jayne M, Ma Y, Wong C. 2006. Cocaine cues and dopamine in dorsal striatum: mechanism of craving in cocaine addiction. *J Neurosci* 26:6583–6588.

71. Wise RA. 2002. Brain reward circuitry: insights from unsensed incentives. *Neuron* 36: 229–240.

72. Yakovlev PI, Locke S, Koskoff DY, Patton RA. 1960. Limbic nuclei of thalamus and connections of limbic cortex. I. Organization of the projections of the anterior group of nuclei and of the midline nuclei of the thalamus to the anterior cingulate gyrus and hippocampal rudiment in the monkey. *Arch Neurol* 3: 620–641.

73. Zaborszky L, Cullinan WE. 1992. Projections from the nucleus accumbens to cholinergic neurons of the ventral pallidum: a correlated light and electron microscopic double-immunolabeling study in rat. *Brain Res* 570: 92–101.

3 Neurochemistry of Performance Monitoring

Markus Ullsperger

To survive in a changeable environment, it is essential to monitor for deviations of action outcomes from the intended goals and detect situations requiring behavioral adjustments. If outcomes are worse than intended or an expected outcome is at risk, the performance-monitoring system interacts with other brain regions to initiate the appropriate remedial actions. The posterior medial frontal cortex (pMFC) appears to play a key role in performance monitoring, as reflected in consistent activity increases in neuroimaging on errors, negative feedback, response and decision conflict. and increased error likelihood.[7,9,77,78] Electroencephalographic (EEG) correlates of performance monitoring are the error-related negativity (ERN)[30,38] on self-detected errors, the feedback-related negativity (FRN)[61] on feedback indicating a negative action outcome and the need to adjust behavior, and modulations of the N2 component that seem to reflect the effort recruited for the task at hand.[25,95] The ERN has a rather high test-retest reliability[62,86] and shows a substantial heritability,[2] such that it might be well-suited as an endophenotype in genetic studies. Consistent with these EEG findings, the heritability of hemodynamic signal changes in the pMFC related to response conflict was moderate.[59] Based on these findings, a number of approaches can be chosen to investigate the neurochemistry of performance monitoring: (1) pharmacological challenges affecting the release and/or elimination of a neurotransmitter or influencing receptor activity directly, (2) imaging genetics[58,60] making use of polymorphisms in candidate genes specifically affecting neurotransmission, (3) positron emission tomography (PET) with tracers tapping into neurotransmission, and (4) studies in patients with diseases specifically affecting the function of a neurotransmitter system (e.g., dopamine, DA, in Parkinson's disease).

This chapter discusses the neurochemical bases of performance monitoring and gives an overview of the knowledge gathered in humans, mostly using pharmacological challenges and imaging genetics. Results from patient studies are discussed in chapter 15 of this volume. The main focus will be on neuromodulators such as dopamine (DA), serotonin (5-hydroxytryptamine, 5-HT), and norepinephrine (noradrenaline, NE), which, according to theoretical accounts and animal models, are hypothesized to play major roles in performance monitoring and resulting adaptations.

Dopamine

Research in nonhuman primates has revealed that phasic changes in the firing rate of mesencephalic dopaminergic neurons encode a reward prediction error (RPE).[81–83] Unexpected reward or correct responses are associated with burst firing—that is, a phasic increase in firing rate—whereas unexpected loss, errors, or omissions of expected rewards are associated with a short-lived reduction or cessation of firing. After conditioning and learning, the phasic dopamine response occurs at the first event that predicts the outcome with high certainty, which is highly reminiscent of temporal difference learning in artificial intelligence.[83] Moreover, the phasic change in firing rate of DA neurons scales with reward magnitude and probability (i.e., expected value).[32,90] At the terminals of the mesostriatal, mesolimbic, and mesocortical DA systems, this RPE-related change in firing rate is assumed to lead to strong changes in DA release that in turn may serve as a teaching signal for reinforcement learning and the selection of appropriate actions. The first to transfer these findings to human performance monitoring were Holroyd and Coles, whose reinforcement learning theory of error detection has had a great impact.[40] Briefly, they propose an adaptive actor-critic model in which the basal ganglia constitute the critic evaluating each event whether it indicates a better or worse than expected action outcome. This prediction error information is then conveyed via the mesencephalic DA system back to the striatum, where it improves the outcome prediction, and to the frontal cortex, in particular a putative action control filter in the pMFC, selecting the appropriate remedial action when necessary. Predictions of this mathematically formalized model have been tested using EEG and functional magnetic resonance imaging (fMRI).[40–42,57,65] A specific assumption of the theory, however, has recently been challenged. The theory suggests that the phasic change in DA release in the pMFC leads to a change in activity at the apical dendrites of pyramidal cells that sums up and is reflected in the ERN and FRN.[40] Comparing the timing and the transient nature of these components with findings from animal and in vitro research indicating a slower and more sustained effect of reductions in DA release in the cortex,[55,63] which in contrast to the striatum is practically devoid of DA transporters,[87] calls this account into question.[46,54] Notably, this does not speak against a role of DA in the pMFC for performance monitoring and subsequent flexible adjustments, but the presence and direction of causality between ERN and phasic change in DA release remain unclear.

Further, it should be noted that several other recent theories of decision making and feedback-based learning capitalize on the phasic RPE signal of the DA system.[67,68] A rather successful neurobiologically informed computational model of decision making focuses on the differential roles of DA D1 and D2 receptors and the direct and indirect pathways in the basal ganglia circuits[33,36] (see also chapter 17, this volume). It predicts differential effects of changes in DA transmission on learning to choose positive actions and to avoid negative actions. Moreover, DA has general effects on other stages of human cognitive control beyond reinforcement learning, such as working memory and flexibility, distractibility and impulsivity versus stability, and inflexibility in trial-to-trial adaptations.[6,8,15,16,85] These functions appear to depend on a balance of DA transmission between the frontal cortex and the striatum (as well as between different striatal compartments). Finally, DA in the striatum as well as the medial frontal cortex seems to influence value-based decision making as reflected in effort-discounting.[79,84] In sum, the role of DA in adaptive behavior is the result of complex interactions in various brain regions.

Despite the limitations that noninvasive research in humans poses for interpretation on regionally, temporally, and receptor-specific neuromodulator functions, a large body of evidence favoring a prominent role of DA in performance monitoring has been accumulated.[46] De Bruijn and colleagues found that the catecholamine (DA, NE) releasing drug amphetamine increased the amplitude of the ERN in the absence of effects on performance.[21] In line with this result, they also found that the DA D2 receptor antagonists haloperidol and olanzapine decreased the ERN amplitude.[23] A further study showed a reduction of the ERN and a concomitant increase in error rate with a similar dose of haloperidol.[96] Neuroimaging studies with pharmacological challenges also demonstrated a role of DA in feedback processing. However, drug effects in the pMFC were seen rarely, in contrast to clear changes in the (ventral) striatum induced by DA agonists and antagonists.[17,24,45,71,73] This is contrasts with a recent PET study on the DA D2 receptor-specific ligand [$_{11}$C]FLB 457, which suggests an increase of DA release in the pMFC during a sorting task in which choices had to be updated on the basis of external feedback.[52] Finally, it should be noted that low-dose DA D2 receptor antagonism with amisulpride resulted in enhanced tracking of action values in the ventromedial prefrontal cortex and enhanced discrimination of choices of similarly high value.[45]

A number of imaging genetics studies have addressed the impact of polymorphisms affecting DA transmission on performance monitoring and decision making.[91] Surprisingly, the findings on modulations of the ERN in speeded forced-choice reaction time tasks are sparse and inconsistent. In contrast, studies on feedback processing seem to yield a clearer picture. The FRN amplitude as well as feedback-related pMFC activity have been shown to be influenced by the catecholamine-O-methyltransferase (COMT) Val[158]Met polymorphism.[10,56] In addition, this COMT gene polymorphism affecting the efficiency of DA degradation has been associated with differences in feedback processing and reward-based learning in the striatum.[10,53,94] So far, the most consistent findings have been made regarding polymorphisms of the DA D2 receptor gene (DRD2). Polymorphisms associated with reduced striatal D2 receptor density[48] have been found to be associated with reduced striatal reward- and (positive) RPE-related signals[13,14,50,51] and in the pMFC.[51] At the behavioral level, genetic variants linked to lower D2 receptor density were associated with reduced learning to avoid negative actions.[34,35,51] In a probabilistic response reversal task, carriers of the low-receptor-density variant showed reduced shift-related activity in the ventral striatum and lateral orbitofrontal cortex and a slower increase in pMFC activity in sequence negative feedback and accumulating evidence for the necessity of a behavioral shift.[44]

In sum, there is increasing evidence for an essential role of DA in performance monitoring, feedback-based decision making, and reinforcement learning. The action of DA seems to affect different cortical as well as subcortical areas, although systemic administration of DA and genetic approaches combined with neuroimaging can hardly discriminate between direct and remote effects. The role of DA is thus not confined to providing a phasic teaching signal coding the RPE and allowing reinforcement learning in the striatum (see also chapter 10, this volume). DA release at different time scales seems to set the stage for cortical learning processes, flexible selection of appropriate (remedial, adaptive) actions, and value representations. For a better understanding of the role of DA studies making use of model-based approaches, selective tracers and combinations of different methods are needed. Furthermore, an integration of models explaining the role of DA at different levels of processing and in different contexts, such as the reinforcement learning models for the basal ganglia[33,67] and neuronal mass models of net activity changes in the prefrontal cortex,[85] need to be integrated. In addition, invasive studies in animals allowing study of catecholamine release at high temporal resolution provide a highly promising research avenue.[37]

Serotonin

Serotonergic neurons originate in the dorsal and median raphé nuclei and innervate virtually the entire forebrain. 5-HT is involved in affective regulation, motivational processes, cognitive flexibility, and impulse control.[12,18,19] Therefore, it is conceivable that 5-HT is essential in regulating performance monitoring. In addition to pharmacological studies, central 5-HT activity can also be modulated by dietary means. Acute dietary tryptophan depletion (ATD) results in a rapid decrease in the synthesis and, presumably, release of 5-HT.[66]

Studies on the involvement of 5-HT in performance monitoring have yielded mixed results depending on the used task and the way serotonergic activity was modulated. With the Stroop task, a decreased pMFC signal-to-response conflict was found in ATD.[28,43] Furthermore, performance-monitoring-related pMFC activity in a Go/NoGo task was reduced in ATD.[29] This contrasts with the finding of increased error-related pMFC activity in a probabilistic reversal learning task in ATD.[27] Specific deficits in reversal learning, but not in response inhibition, were found in subjects treated with a selective serotonin reuptake inhibitor (SSRI),[11] providing further evidence for a role of 5-HT in reversal learning as suggested from animal research.[12]

Also studies of 5-HT effects on the ERN are inconclusive. De Bruijn et al. found no effect of mirtazapine (a drug acting on 5-HT, α_1, α_2, and H1 receptors) and the SSRI paroxetine on the ERN.[21,23] In contrast, some studies on the variable number of tandem repeats polymorphism in the promotor region of the 5-HT transporter gene (5-HTTLPR) found that carriers of the short (S) allele, associated with lower expression of the transporter and presumably higher 5-HT levels, had a larger ERN amplitude,[1,31] whereas others failed to replicate this finding in a relatively large sample.[69] A recent study in our own lab comparing 16 homozygotes of the long (L) allele with 15 homozygotes of the S allele with and without treatment with the SSRI citalopram (10 mg iv) did not reveal any genetic or drug effects on the ERN in a flanker task (Fischer and Ullsperger, unpublished observations). Finally, even prolonged therapy of obsessive-compulsive disorder with SSRI did not lead to a change of the (elevated) ERN amplitude, despite clinical effects of treatment.[89]

Thus, the role of 5-HT in performance monitoring, although highly reasonable to assume, is still unclear. It may be speculated that 5-HT influences the adjustments resulting from monitoring rather than the monitoring process itself.

Norepinephrine

As in the 5-HT system, norepinephinergic terminals supply almost the entire forebrain. The most important nucleus with NE neurons is the locus coeruleus (LC) in the brainstem. Fluctuations in tonic and phasic LC firing modes have been found to index variability in performance efficiency that can be linked to lapses of task engagement in rodents.[72,93] Thus, in their adaptive gain theory, Aston-Jones and Cohen recently hypothesized that the LC-NE plays a role in higher-order cognitive functioning and task engagement.[4] Phasic LC activity, via increased NE release, is suggested to modulate the gain of target neurons, thereby facilitating the execution of the appropriate behavioral response. In contrast, at high levels of tonic LC activity, generally increased NE levels do not facilitate a particular behavior but make actions more random and, therefore, seem to facilitate exploration at the cost of exploitation. Most likely, the transition between phasic and tonic firing modes is signaled to the LC by orbitofrontal cortex–anterior insula and anterior cingulate cortex.[4,64] Thus, it can be hypothesized that NE influences the adaptations and decision-making processes that result from performance monitoring rather than the detection of the performance problem itself. For example, we recently hypothesized that the general increase in arousal, that is, the orienting response,[88] associated with errors and accompanied by posterror slowing, autonomic responses, and conscious perception of the error are substantially driven by phasic NE release.[92] Moreover, it is likely that maladaptive disengagement from task that may result in errors[26] is associated with (tonic) changes in LC activity.

Despite the impressive theoretical framework, to date only a single study has investigated the role of NE in performance monitoring by pharmacological manipulation. Yohimbine, an antagonist of α_2-adrenergic receptors present as autoreceptors on LC neurons, increases the firing rate of LC neurons and thus the release of NE. Administration of yohimbine increased the amplitude of the ERN parallel to a reduction in error rates.[74] This is in line with the adaptive gain theory by Aston-Jones and Cohen[4]: by antagonizing autoreceptors, yohimbine might have enhanced LC phasic activity to the stimulus, thereby facilitating execution of the appropriate action, which, in turn, is reflected in a net decrease in error rate. Similarly, the enhanced ERN might result from an increased gain, that is, enhanced responsiveness of cortical neurons induced by phasic NE release to the target stimulus. The error event itself is salient and rare and therefore likely to elicit a phasic NE release that should, according to a recent account[64] (see also chapter 12, this volume), modulate the error positivity (Pe, a P300-like component associated with erroneous responses[70]). However, though not directly investigated statistically, the figures in the yohimbine study seem not to suggest any modulation of the Pe.[74]

Amphetamine leads to an increase in extracellular DA as well as NE[5]; therefore, the ERN increase associated with administration of this drug[21] can also be explained in the context of the adaptive gain theory. Again, the Pe seemed unaffected by amphetamine,[21] while the P2 deflection elicited by feedback was increased by the same treatment.[22] Selective NE reuptake inhibitors such as reboxetine and atomoxetine might be useful tools to further follow up on these questions and to confirm the specific role of NE in performance monitoring.

Further Transmitter Systems

Specific performance monitoring functions of the transmitter systems that are most abundant in the human brain, such as glutamate and endocannabinoids are very difficult to test noninvasively in humans as systemic pharmacological challenges would have broad and often nonspecific effects. GABA is also widely distributed in the human brain and is responsible for most of the fast inhibitory transmission. A number of studies addressed the effects of benzodiazepines (BDZ) and alcohol, both acting on $GABA_A$ receptors, on performance monitoring. Acute administration of BDZ and alcohol, respectively, was consistently associated with reduced ERN amplitudes and impairments of posterror adjustments reflected in lower correction rates and the abolition of posterror slowing and posterror reduction of interference.[21,47,75,76]

Further, neurotransmitter and neuromodulator systems are likely to be involved in performance monitoring. For example, acetylcholine (ACh) plays a major role in cortical excitability, attention, and arousal, in addition to modulating DA transmission in the striatum. It has been suggested that ACh could mediate the top-down control of attentional processing after detecting an error or performance decrement.[80] It has been argued that processing of the task-relevant stimulus feature can be enhanced by prefrontal projections to the basal cholinergic forebrain. Although the cholinergic nucleus basalis of Meynert supplies the entire neocortex with ACh, the projections are not extensively collateralized. This suggests that the basal forebrain can be conceived as a modular system with specific regions in the nucleus basalis innervating restricted cortical areas. Thus, it seems conceivable that cholinergic transmission can be modulated in a region- and thus modality-specific fashion. This would enable top-down control by enhancing cholinergic transmission in the cortical region processing the relevant stimulus feature. Recently, such posterior top-down enhancement of perceptual processing has been demonstrated,[49] but the neurochemistry underlying this effect remains to be elucidated. Moreover, it has been demonstrated that stimulation of the nucleus basalis improved perceptual representations in visual cortex via muscarinic ACh receptors.[39]

Outlook

In sum, the investigation of the specific neurochemistry of performance monitoring is only at its infancy. While DA appears to be essential for this function, its complex actions at different brain regions, time scales, and stages of information processing are still only partly understood and require integration in an overarching model. Theoretical considerations clearly predict key roles for 5-HT, NE, and ACh in performance monitoring, but the evidence gathered in humans is still rather sparse and sometimes mixed.

The brain as a dynamic system responds to pharmacological challenges of one transmitter system by complex adaptations in other systems. This clearly calls for models that try to integrate more than one neuromodulator. For example, DA and 5-HT have been suggested to interact in a partly opponent way.[20] Pharmacological challenge studies should investigate the interactions of several drugs to address these questions. Great hope lies in the increased use of PET with specific radioligands in the field of cognitive neuroscience. Furthermore, baseline activity of the neurotransmitter systems need to be taken into account, as dose-effect dependencies are often nonlinear and may follow a inverted u-shaped curve, as repeatedly demonstrated for DA.[3,94] Finally, genetic approaches, particularly in combination with pharmacological challenges have a great potential in testing hypotheses on the neurochemistry of performance monitoring. Genomewide association studies with endophenotypes related to performance monitoring will provide new hypotheses and reveal novel insights that go far beyond the current theories of adaptive behavior.

The neurochemistry of the brain is complex, but it must not be neglected in cognitive neuroscience. Only a better understanding of neurotransmitter action in healthy performance monitoring can be the basis to understand pathological changes in neurological and psychiatric diseases.

Outstanding Questions

• How can the actions of dopamine on different stages of performance monitoring, ranging from error detection via immediate flexible adjustments to learning and updates in value representations, be integrated into a single framework?

• What is the nature of the interactions between the monoaminergic neuromodulators dopamine, norepinephrine, and serotonin in cognitive control, and how are their interactions regulated?

• Can neurochemistry and its pathological changes explain specific performance monitoring deficits in neuropsychiatric disorders? Are there ways of therapeutical modulation?

Further Reading

Jocham G, Ullsperger M. 2009. Neuropharmacology of performance monitoring. *Neurosci Biobehav Rev* 33: 48–60. Comprehensive overview of neuropsychopharmacological studies of performance monitoring in humans. Discusses current theories and their limitations in detail.

Cools R. 2008. Role of dopamine in the motivational and cognitive control of behavior. *Neuroscientist* 14: 381–395. Article focusing on the seemingly paradoxical effects of dopamine in different cortical and striatal compartments with respect to stability and inflexibility versus flexibility and distractibility in cognitive control. Discusses reward-based learning as well as fast cognitive adjustments.

Schultz W. 2007. Multiple dopamine functions at different time courses. *Annu Rev Neurosci* 30: 259–288. Review of animal research and theoretical considerations on how dopamine is involved in mediating the reactivity of the organism to the environment at different time scales, from fast impulse responses related to reward via slower changes with uncertainty, punishment, and possibly movement to the tonic enabling of postsynaptic motor, cognitive, and motivational systems.

References

1. Althaus M, Groen Y, Wijers AA, Mulder LJ, Minderaa RB, Kema IP, Dijck JD, Hartman CA, Hoekstra PJ. 2009. Differential effects of 5-HTTLPR and DRD2/ANKK1 polymorphisms on electrocortical measures of error and feedback processing in children. *Clin Neurophysiol* 120: 93–107.

2. Anokhin AP, Golosheykin S, Heath AC. 2008. Heritability of frontal brain function related to action monitoring. *Psychophysiology* 45: 524–534.

3. Arnsten AF. 1997. Catecholamine regulation of the prefrontal cortex. *J Psychopharmacol* 11: 151–162.

4. Aston-Jones G, Cohen JD. 2005. An integrative theory of locus coeruleus-norepinephrine function: adaptive gain and optimal performance. *Annu Rev Neurosci* 28: 403–450.

5. Berridge CW, Stalnaker TA. 2002. Relationship between low-dose amphetamine-induced arousal and extracellular norepinephrine and dopamine levels within prefrontal cortex. *Synapse* 46: 140–149.

6. Bilder RM, Volavka J, Lachman HM, Grace AA. 2004. The catechol-O-methyltransferase polymorphism: relations to the tonic-phasic dopamine hypothesis and neuropsychiatric phenotypes. *Neuropsychopharmacology* 29: 1943–1961.

7. Botvinick MM. 2007. Conflict monitoring and decision making: reconciling two perspectives on anterior cingulate function. *Cogn Affect Behav Neurosci* 7: 356–366.

8. Braver TS, Cohen JD. 2000. On the control of control: The role of dopamine in regulating prefrontal function and working memory. In: Attention and Performance XVIII: Control of Cognitive Processes (Monsell S, Driver J, eds), pp 713–737. Cambridge, MA: MIT Press.

9. Brown JW, Braver TS. 2005. Learned predictions of error likelihood in the anterior cingulate cortex. *Science* 307: 1118–1121.

10. Camara E, Kramer UM, Cunillera T, Marco-Pallares J, Cucurell D, Nager W, Mestres-Misse A, et al. 2010. The effects of COMT (Val108/158Met) and DRD4 (SNP -521) dopamine genotypes on brain activations related to valence and magnitude of rewards. *Cereb Cortex* 20: 1985–1996.

11. Chamberlain SR, Muller U, Blackwell AD, Clark L, Robbins TW, Sahakian BJ. 2006. Neurochemical modulation of response inhibition and probabilistic learning in humans. *Science* 311: 861–863.

12. Clarke HF, Walker SC, Crofts HS, Dalley JW, Robbins TW, Roberts AC. 2005. Prefrontal serotonin depletion affects reversal learning but not attentional set shifting. *J Neurosci* 25: 532–538.

13. Cohen MX, Krohn-Grimberghe A, Elger CE, Weber B. 2007. Dopamine gene predicts the brain's response to dopaminergic drug. *Eur J Neurosci* 26: 3652–3660.

14. Cohen MX, Young J, Baek JM, Kessler C, Ranganath C. 2005. Individual differences in extraversion and dopamine genetics predict neural reward responses. *Brain Res Cogn Brain Res* 25: 851–861.

15. Cools R. 2008. Role of dopamine in the motivational and cognitive control of behavior. *Neuroscientist* 14: 381–395.

16. Cools R, Gibbs SE, Miyakawa A, Jagust W, D'Esposito M. 2008. Working memory capacity predicts dopamine synthesis capacity in the human striatum. *J Neurosci* 28: 1208–1212.

17. Cools R, Lewis SJ, Clark L, Barker RA, Robbins TW. 2007. L-DOPA disrupts activity in the nucleus accumbens during reversal learning in Parkinson's disease. *Neuropsychopharmacology* 32: 180–189.

18. Cools R, Roberts AC, Robbins TW. 2008. Serotoninergic regulation of emotional and behavioural control processes. *Trends Cogn Sci* 12: 31–40.

19. Crockett MJ, Clark L, Robbins TW. 2009. Reconciling the role of serotonin in behavioral inhibition and aversion: acute tryptophan depletion abolishes punishment-induced inhibition in humans. *J Neurosci* 29: 11993–11999.

20. Daw ND, Kakade S, Dayan P. 2002. Opponent interactions between serotonin and dopamine. *Neural Netw* 15: 603–616.

21. De Bruijn ERA, Hulstijn W, Verkes RJ, Ruigt GS, Sabbe BG. 2004. Drug-induced stimulation and suppression of action monitoring in healthy volunteers. *Psychopharmacology (Berl)* 177: 151–160.

22. De Bruijn ERA, Hulstijn W, Verkes RJ, Ruigt GS, Sabbe BG. 2005. Altered response evaluation. monitoring of late responses after administration of D-Amphetamine. *J Psychophysiol* 19: 311–318.

23. De Bruijn ERA, Sabbe BG, Hulstijn W, Ruigt GS, Verkes RJ. 2006. Effects of antipsychotic and antidepressant drugs on action monitoring in healthy volunteers. *Brain Res* 1105: 122–129.

24. Dodds CM, Muller U, Clark L, van Loon A, Cools R, Robbins TW. 2008. Methylphenidate has differential effects on blood oxygenation level-dependent signal related to cognitive subprocesses of reversal learning. *J Neurosci* 28: 5976–5982.

25. Eichele H, Juvodden HT, Ullsperger M, Eichele T. 2010. Mal-adaptation of event-related EEG responses preceding performance errors. *Front Hum Neurosci* 4: 65.

26. Eichele T, Debener S, Calhoun VD, Specht K, Engel AK, Hugdahl K, von Cramon DY, Ullsperger M. 2008. Prediction of human errors by maladaptive changes in event-related brain networks. *Proc Natl Acad Sci USA* 105: 6173–6178.

27. Evers EA, Cools R, Clark L, van der Veen FM, Jolles J, Sahakian BJ, Robbins TW. 2005. Serotonergic modulation of prefrontal cortex during negative feedback in probabilistic reversal learning. *Neuropsychopharmacology* 30: 1138–1147.

28. Evers EA, van der Veen FM, Jolles J, Deutz NE, Schmitt JA. 2006. Acute tryptophan depletion improves performance and modulates the BOLD response during a Stroop task in healthy females. *Neuroimage* 32: 248–255.

29. Evers EA, van der Veen FM, van Deursen JA, Schmitt JA, Deutz NE, Jolles J. 2006. The effect of acute tryptophan depletion on the BOLD response during performance monitoring and response inhibition in healthy male volunteers. *Psychopharmacology (Berl)* 187: 200–208.

30. Falkenstein M, Hohnsbein J, Hoormann J, Blanke L. 1990. Effects of errors in choice reaction tasks on the ERP under focused and divided attention. In: Psychophysiological Brain Research (Brunia CHM, Gaillard AWK, Kok A, eds), pp 192–195. Tilburg: Tilburg University Press.

31. Fallgatter AJ, Herrmann MJ, Roemmler J, Ehlis AC, Wagener A, Heidrich A, Ortega G, Zeng Y, Lesch KP. 2004. Allelic variation of serotonin transporter function modulates the brain electrical response for error processing. *Neuropsychopharmacology* 29: 1506–1511.

32. Fiorillo CD, Tobler PN, Schultz W. 2003. Discrete coding of reward probability and uncertainty by dopamine neurons. *Science* 299: 1898–1902.

33. Frank MJ. 2005. Dynamic dopamine modulation in the basal ganglia: a neurocomputational account of cognitive deficits in medicated and nonmedicated Parkinsonism. *J Cogn Neurosci* 17: 51–72.

34. Frank MJ, Hutchison K. 2009. Genetic contributions to avoidance-based decisions: striatal D2 receptor polymorphisms. *Neuroscience* 164: 131–140.

35. Frank MJ, Moustafa AA, Haughey HM, Curran T, Hutchison KE. 2007. Genetic triple dissociation reveals multiple roles for dopamine in reinforcement learning. *Proc Natl Acad Sci USA* 104: 16311–16316.

36. Frank MJ, Seeberger LC, RC. 2004. By carrot or by stick: cognitive reinforcement learning in Parkinsonism. *Science* 306: 1940–1943.

37. Gan JO, Walton ME, Phillips PE. 2010. Dissociable cost and benefit encoding of future rewards by mesolimbic dopamine. *Nat Neurosci* 13: 25–27.

38. Gehring WJ, Goss B, Coles MG, Meyer DE, Donchin E. 1993. A neural system for error detection and compensation. *Psychol Sci* 4: 385–390.

39. Goard M, Dan Y. 2009. Basal forebrain activation enhances cortical coding of natural scenes. *Nat Neurosci* 12: 1444–1449.

40. Holroyd CB, Coles MG. 2002. The neural basis of human error processing: reinforcement learning, dopamine, and the error-related negativity. *Psychol Rev* 109: 679–709.

41. Holroyd CB, Krigolson OE. 2007. Reward prediction error signals associated with a modified time estimation task. *Psychophysiology* 44: 913–917.

42. Holroyd CB, Krigolson OE, Baker R, Lee S, Gibson J. 2009. When is an error not a prediction error? An electrophysiological investigation. *Cogn Affect Behav Neurosci* 9: 59–70.

43. Horacek J, Zavesicka L, Tintera J, Dockery C, Platilova V, Kopecek M, Spaniel F, Bubenikova V, Hoschl C. 2005. The effect of tryptophan depletion on brain activation measured by functional magnetic resonance imaging during the Stroop test in healthy subjects. *Physiol Res* 54: 235–244.

44. Jocham G, Klein TA, Neumann J, von Cramon DY, Reuter M, Ullsperger M. 2009. Dopamine DRD2 polymorphism alters reversal learning and associated neural activity. *J Neurosci* 29: 3695–3704.

45. Jocham G, Klein TA, Ullsperger M. 2010. Dopamine-mediated reinforcement learning signals in the striatum and ventromedial prefrontal cortex underlie value-based choices. *J Neurosci* 31: 1606–1613.

46. Jocham G, Ullsperger M. 2009. Neuropharmacology of performance monitoring. *Neurosci Biobehav Rev* 33: 48–60.

47. Johannes S, Wieringa BM, Nager W, Dengler R, Munte TF. 2001. Oxazepam alters action monitoring. *Psychopharmacology (Berl)* 155: 100–106.

48. Jönsson EG, Nothen MM, Grunhage F, Farde L, Nakashima Y, Propping P, Sedvall GC. 1999. Polymorphisms in the dopamine D2 receptor gene and their relationships to striatal dopamine receptor density of healthy volunteers. *Mol Psychiatry* 4: 290–296.

49. King JA, Korb FM, Von Cramon DY, Ullsperger M. 2010. Post-error behavioral adjustments are facilitated by activation and suppression of task-relevant and task-irrelevant information processing. *J Neurosci* 30: 12759–12769.

50. Kirsch P, Reuter M, Mier D, Lonsdorf T, Stark R, Gallhofer B, Vaitl D, Hennig J. 2006. Imaging gene-substance interactions: the effect of the DRD2 TaqIA polymorphism and the dopamine agonist bromocriptine on the brain activation during the anticipation of reward. *Neurosci Lett* 405: 196–201.

51. Klein TA, Neumann J, Reuter M, Hennig J, von Cramon DY, Ullsperger M. 2007. Genetically determined differences in learning from errors. *Science* 318: 1642–1645.

52. Ko JH, Ptito A, Monchi O, Cho SS, Van Eimeren T, Pellecchia G, Ballanger B, Rusjan P, Houle S, Strafella AP. 2009. Increased dopamine release in the right anterior cingulate cortex during the performance of a sorting task: a [11C]FLB 457 PET study. *Neuroimage* 46: 516–521.

53. Krugel LK, Biele G, Mohr PN, Li SC, Heekeren HR. 2009. Genetic variation in dopaminergic neuromodulation influences the ability to rapidly and flexibly adapt decisions. *Proc Natl Acad Sci USA* 106: 17951–17956.

54. Lapish CC, Kroener S, Durstewitz D, Lavin A, Seamans JK. 2007. The ability of the mesocortical dopamine system to operate in distinct temporal modes. *Psychopharmacology (Berl)* 191: 609–625.

55. Lavin A, Nogueira L, Lapish CC, Wightman RM, Phillips PE, Seamans JK. 2005. Mesocortical dopamine neurons operate in distinct temporal domains using multimodal signaling. *J Neurosci* 25: 5013–5023.

56. Marco-Pallares J, Cucurell D, Cunillera T, Kramer UM, Camara E, Nager W, Bauer P, Schule R, Schols L, Munte TF, Rodriguez-Fornells A. 2009. Genetic variability in the dopamine system (dopamine receptor D4, catechol-*O*-methyltransferase) modulates neurophysiological responses to gains and losses. *Biol Psychiatry* 66: 154–161.

57. Mars RB, Coles MG, Grol MJ, Holroyd CB, Nieuwenhuis S, Hulstijn W, Toni I. 2005. Neural dynamics of error processing in medial frontal cortex. *Neuroimage* 28: 1007–1013.

58. Mattay VS, Goldberg TE. 2004. Imaging genetic influences in human brain function. *Curr Opin Neurobiol* 14: 239–247.

59. Matthews SC, Simmons AN, Strigo I, Jang K, Stein MB, Paulus MP. 2007. Heritability of anterior cingulate response to conflict: an fMRI study in female twins. *Neuroimage* 38: 223–227.

60. Meyer-Lindenberg A, Weinberger DR. 2006. Intermediate phenotypes and genetic mechanisms of psychiatric disorders. *Nat Rev Neurosci* 7: 818–827.

61. Miltner WHR, Braun CH, Coles MGH. 1997. Event-related brain potentials following incorrect feedback in a time-estimation task: evidence for a "generic" neural system for error detection. *J Cogn Neurosci* 9: 788–798.

62. Morris SE, Mann-Wrobel MC. 2008. A naturalistic study of the test-retest reliability of ERN amplitude in healthy adults. *Psychophysiology* 45: S80.

63. Mundorf ML, Joseph JD, Austin CM, Caron MG, Wightman RM. 2001. Catecholamine release and uptake in the mouse prefrontal cortex. *J Neurochem* 79: 130–142.

64. Nieuwenhuis S, Aston-Jones G, Cohen JD. 2005. Decision making, the P3, and the locus coeruleus-norepinephrine system. *Psychol Bull* 131: 510–532.

65. Nieuwenhuis S, Holroyd CB, Mol N, Coles MG. 2004. Reinforcement-related brain potentials from medial frontal cortex: origins and functional significance. *Neurosci Biobehav Rev* 28: 441–448.

66. Nishizawa S, Benkelfat C, Young SN, Leyton M, Mzengeza S, de Montigny C, Blier P, Diksic M. 1997. Differences between males and females in rates of serotonin synthesis in human brain. *Proc Natl Acad Sci USA* 94: 5308–5313.

67. O'Doherty JP, Dayan P, Friston K, Critchley H, Dolan RJ. 2003. Temporal difference models and reward-related learning in the human brain. *Neuron* 38: 329–337.

68. O'Doherty JP, Hampton A, Kim H. 2007. Model-based fMRI and its application to reward learning and decision making. *Ann N Y Acad Sci* 1104: 35–53.

69. Olvet DM, Hatchwell E, Hajcak G. 2010. Lack of association between the 5-HTTLPR and the error-related negativity (ERN). *Biol Psychol* 85: 504–508.

70. Overbeek TJM, Nieuwenhuis S, Ridderinkhof KR. 2005. Dissociable components of error processing: on the functional significance of the Pe vis-à-vis the ERN/Ne. *J Psychophysiol* 19: 319–329.

71. Pessiglione M, Seymour B, Flandin G, Dolan RJ, Frith CD. 2006. Dopamine-dependent prediction errors underpin reward-seeking behaviour in humans. *Nature* 442: 1042–1045.

72. Rajkowski J, Majczynski H, Clayton E, Aston-Jones G. 2004. Activation of monkey locus coeruleus neurons varies with difficulty and performance in a target detection task. *J Neurophysiol* 92: 361–371.

73. Riba J, Kramer UM, Heldmann M, Richter S, Munte TF. 2008. Dopamine agonist increases risk taking but blunts reward-related brain activity. *PLoS ONE* 3: e2479.

74. Riba J, Rodriguez-Fornells A, Morte A, Munte TF, Barbanoj MJ. 2005. Noradrenergic stimulation enhances human action monitoring. *J Neurosci* 25: 4370–4374.

75. Riba J, Rodriguez-Fornells A, Munte TF, Barbanoj MJ. 2005. A neurophysiological study of the detrimental effects of alprazolam on human action monitoring. *Brain Res Cogn Brain Res* 25: 554–565.

76. Ridderinkhof KR, de Vlugt Y, Bramlage A, Spaan M, Elton M, Snel J, Band GP. 2002. Alcohol consumption impairs detection of performance errors in mediofrontal cortex. *Science* 298: 2209–2211.

77. Ridderinkhof KR, Ullsperger M, Crone EA, Nieuwenhuis S. 2004. The role of the medial frontal cortex in cognitive control. *Science* 306: 443–447.

78. Rushworth MF, Behrens TE. 2008. Choice, uncertainty and value in prefrontal and cingulate cortex. *Nat Neurosci* 11: 389–397.

79. Salamone JD, Correa M, Farrar AM, Nunes EJ, Pardo M. 2009. Dopamine, behavioral economics, and effort. *Front Behav Neurosci* 3: 13.

80. Sarter M, Gehring WJ, Kozak R. 2006. More attention must be paid: the neurobiology of attentional effort. *Brain Res Brain Res Rev* 51: 145–160.

81. Satoh T, Nakai S, Sato T, Kimura M. 2003. Correlated coding of motivation and outcome of decision by dopamine neurons. *J Neurosci* 23: 9913–9923.

82. Schultz W. 2007. Multiple dopamine functions at different time courses. *Annu Rev Neurosci* 30: 259–288.

83. Schultz W, Dayan P, Montague P. 1997. A neural substrate of prediction and reward. *Science* 275: 1593.

84. Schweimer J, Hauber W. 2006. Dopamine D1 receptors in the anterior cingulate cortex regulate effort-based decision making. *Learn Mem* 13: 777–782.

85. Seamans JK, Yang CR. 2004. The principal features and mechanisms of dopamine modulation in the prefrontal cortex. *Prog Neurobiol* 74: 1–58.

86. Segalowitz SJ, Santesso DL, Murphy TI, Homan D, Chantziantoniou DK, Khan S. 2010. Retest reliability of medial frontal negativities during performance monitoring. *Psychophysiology* 47: 260–270.

87. Sesack SR, Hawrylak VA, Guido MA, Levey AI. 1998. Cellular and subcellular localization of the dopamine transporter in rat cortex. *Adv Pharmacol* 42: 171–174.

88. Sokolov EN. 1963. Higher nervous functions; the orienting reflex. *Annu Rev Physiol* 25: 545–580.

89. Stern ER, Liu Y, Gehring WJ, Lister JJ, Yin G, Zhang J, Fitzgerald KD, Himle JA, Abelson JL, Taylor SF. 2010. Chronic medication does not affect hyperactive error responses in obsessive-compulsive disorder. *Psychophysiology* 47: 913–920.

90. Tobler PN, Fiorillo CD, Schultz W. 2005. Adaptive coding of reward value by dopamine neurons. *Science* 307: 1642–1645.

91. Ullsperger M. 2010. Genetic association studies of performance monitoring and learning from feedback: the role of dopamine and serotonin. *Neurosci Biobehav Rev* 34: 649–659.

92. Ullsperger M, Harsay HA, Wessel JR, Ridderinkhof KR. 2010. Conscious perception of errors and its relation to the anterior insula. *Brain Struct Funct* 214: 629–643.

93. Usher M, Cohen JD, Servan-Schreiber D, Rajkowski J, Aston-Jones G. 1999. The role of locus coeruleus in the regulation of cognitive performance. *Science* 283: 549–554.

94. Yacubian J, Sommer T, Schroeder K, Glascher J, Kalisch R, Leuenberger B, Braus DF, Buchel C. 2007. Gene-gene interaction associated with neural reward sensitivity. *Proc Natl Acad Sci USA* 104: 8125–8130.

95. Yeung N, Botvinick MM, Cohen JD. 2004. The neural basis of error detection: conflict monitoring and the error-related negativity. *Psychol Rev* 111: 931–959.

96. Zirnheld PJ, Carroll CA, Kieffaber PD, O'Donnell BF, Shekhar A, Hetrick WP. 2004. Haloperidol impairs learning and error-related negativity in humans. *J Cogn Neurosci* 16: 1098–1112.

II A CORTICAL PERSPECTIVE ON THE FUNCTIONAL BASIS OF CONTROL

The following chapters examine the function of various cortical areas in motivational and cognitive control. The majority of the chapters deal with the prefrontal cortex (PFC), in line with the prevailing view that executive control is primarily the prerogative of this part of the cortex. This approach is consistent with the marked expansion of this part of the brain in humans compared to other species, including the nonhuman primates on which much of our knowledge about PFC is based.

Simple functional dissociations between subdivisions of PFC have proven difficult to establish, with activity in the same parts of PFC evident in studies that have used quite different paradigms, and with single neurons seemingly having highly flexible tuning properties that adapt according to task demands.[3,7] Indeed, it has been argued that this "adaptive coding" is one of the hallmarks of cognitive control.[10] In this view, cognitive control is not a preset function, but the emergent property of the reconfiguration of more elementary information processing in posterior brain areas. This view is highly consistent with one dominant description of PFC as being involved in biasing the flow of neural activity along neural pathways from perception to action.[8] The chapter by Mars and colleagues illustrates this point, showing how parts of the frontal lobes influence the motor cortex during action reprogramming. Furthermore, as discussed by Laubach, similar functional properties are evident in the rat PFC.

The question then is whether there is an overarching principle of functional organization for the PFC. A number of schemes have been proposed of which a hierarchy of action control along the causal-rostral axis is seen as particularly influential. One of the first prominent theories proposing such a hierarchy is Fuster's perception-action cycle.[4] According to this model, PFC sits on top of the cortical hierarchy, being critically involved in the temporal organization of information in posterior brain areas. Recent models have extended this reasoning to areas within the frontal lobe itself, proposing that increasingly abstract information is processed or represented as one moves more and more rostrally within PFC.[1] For example, Koechlin and colleagues have formalized this hypothesis using information theory to model the different levels of abstraction of information,[5] and neuroimaging to map the neural basis of levels of representational abstraction along the caudal-rostral axis. This approach was recently extended to suggest parallel hierarchies in medial and lateral PFC, with medial areas conveying motivational information to the lateral PFC at each level of abstract and lateral PFC exerting the top-down control.[6]

The chapters by Kennerley and Tobler and by Boorman and Noonan illustrate recent advances in our understanding of the roles of different parts of the PFC. Consistent with the adaptive coding theory, PFC has been implicated in the representation of abstract decision variables. These two chapters illustrate the increasing theoretical and methodological convergence between studies of motivational or reward-based decision making on the one hand, and what has traditionally been labeled cognitive control on the other; they provide a useful framework for conceptualizing the role of the frontal cortex in the guidance of decisions.

Regions within parietal cortex are commonly coactivated with those in PFC during the performance of cognitive control paradigms and the role of these regions in motivational and cognitive control is increasingly appreciated. A recent study shows remarkable behavioral changes in a standard response conflict paradigm in patients with inferior parietal lesions, which are markedly different from the results commonly obtained in patients with lesions confined to PFC.[2] Parts of the posterior parietal cortex and intraparietal sulcus have long been known to encode visual and motor information in various coordinate systems. Moreover, neurons in parietal cortex have been shown to be sensitive to motivation and reward. In a seminal study, Platt and Glimcher[9] demonstrated that neurons in the lateral intraparietal area, a region previously suggested to be mainly related to eye movement control, modulate their activity as a function of the gain a monkey can expect to realize and the probability that it will realize this gain. The authors suggested that a decision-theoretic model can provide an overarching framework for many of the processes in parietal cortex. In their chapter, Pearson, Hayden, and Platt turn their attention to another region outside the frontal lobes that is often reported but ignored in studies on control, the posterior cingulate, illustrating its role in switching between response strategies.

For all this wealth of data on the cortex, one would have only a very limited view on the neural basis of motivational and cognitive control if one ignored the contributions of subcortical systems, which are the focus of the four chapters in section III.

References

1. Badre D, D'Esposito M. 2009. Is the rostro-caudal axis of the frontal lobe hierarchical? *Nat Rev Neurosci* 10: 659–669.

2. Coulthard EJ, Nachev P, Husain M. 2008. Control over conflict during movement preparation: role of posterior parietal cortex. *Neuron* 58: 144–157.

3. Freedman DJ, Reisenhuber M, Poggio T, Miller EK. 2001. Categorical representation of visual stimuli in the primate prefrontal cortex. *Science* 291: 312–316.

4. Fuster JM. 1997. The Prefrontal Cortex: Anatomy, Physiology, and Neuropsychology of the Frontal Lobe. Philadelphia: Lippincott-Raven.

5. Koechlin E, Summerfield C. 2007. An information theoretical approach to prefrontal executive function. *Trends Cogn Sci* 11: 229–235.

6. Kouneiher F, Charron S, Koechlin E. 2009. Motivation and cognitive control in the human prefrontal cortex. *Nat Neurosci* 12: 939–945.

7. Machens CK, Romo R, Brody CD. 2005. Flexible control of mutual inhibition: a neural model of two-interval discrimination. *Science* 307: 1121–1124.

8. Miller EK, Cohen JD. 2001. An integrative theory of prefrontal cortex function. *Annu Rev Neurosci* 24: 167–202.

9. Platt ML, Glimcher PW. 1999. Neural correlates of decision variables in parietal cortex. *Nature* 400: 233–238.

10. Ridderinkhof KR, Van den Wildenberg WPM. 2005. Adaptive coding. *Science* 307: 1059–1060.

4 Contributions of Ventromedial Prefrontal and Frontal Polar Cortex to Reinforcement Learning and Value-Based Choice

Erie D. Boorman and MaryAnn P. Noonan

A central question crossing a range of disciplines, from neuroscience, psychology, and behavioral ecology to economics and computer science, concerns how agents select among options on the basis of their reinforcing value. The diversity of fields interested in reinforcement learning (RL) and value-based choice highlights the considerable impact of the topic. Research on the neural mechanisms that underpin value-based choice has witnessed a fruitful convergence of approaches across these disciplines. Complementing the extensive knowledge of animal behavior and brain function developed in psychology, behavioral ecology, and neuroscience, behavioral models developed in economics provide a richer model of decision-making behavior that can be tested directly with neural data. Meanwhile, machine learning has provided quantitative predictions of the critical parameters theorized to underpin components of value-based choice, thereby enabling neural data to be linked to unobservable computational processes. This synergy has led to basic insights into the neural underpinnings of RL and value-guided choice, much of which is discussed in this chapter.

Values must frequently be learned. Once values are acquired, choices can be made among explicitly presented options, such as between a glass of mulled wine and a cup of tea. Here, we will consider both interference and recording evidence concerning the functional contributions of the ventromedial prefrontal cortex (VMPFC), adjacent lateral orbital frontal cortex (OFC), and frontal polar cortex (FPC) to both the acquisition of values and the selection of options whose values were previously learned (see chapter 5, this volume, for a comprehensive treatment of the role of other frontal cortex regions in value-based choice).

Nonhuman Studies

Orbital Frontal Cortex

Lesion studies in monkeys and rats have consistently implicated the OFC in the guidance of flexible behavior. This role has been attributed to the OFC partly on the basis of two consistent impairments in lesion studies: perseveration of previously rewarded choices following reversals of deterministic stimulus-outcome associations[14,19,37,38] and insensitivity to outcome devaluation.[3,26,37] It has been proposed that the core deficit mediating these effects is an insensitivity to negative reinforcement (or errors)[20,47] or an inability to inhibit previously chosen actions.[14,15,19,38] More recent work,[78,82,95] however, indicates that such accounts are unlikely. For example, monkeys with OFC lesions performing three-alternative stimulus-based choice tasks actually switch as frequently as or more frequently than controls and are equally capable of responding to *local* changes in reward likelihood. Taken together, these studies demonstrate that, since OFC animals switch responses at least as frequently as control animals, their deficit cannot be explained by an inability to inhibit previously rewarded responses. Furthermore, because OFC animals were able to respond to local changes in reward rate following both rewarded and unrewarded outcomes, insensitivity to negative outcomes alone also cannot explain the pattern of impairment induced by OFC lesions.

An alternative proposal is that the OFC's contribution to adaptive behavior stems from its ability to represent outcome expectations predicted by cues in the environment.[80,82,83] In outcome-specific devaluation studies, an animal is trained to associate a particular cue with a particular reward. The value of the reward is then reduced by pairing it with satiety or illness. Animals normally show a reduction in response only to the specific cue with which the devalued reward has been paired. Following OFC lesions, both rats and monkeys fail to reduce responses to the devalued cue.[26,37] This selective effect suggests that the OFC contains information about the subjective value of the specific outcomes with which the cues have been paired.[80,82] In a simple reward discrimination task, where cues deterministically predict either a rewarding or nonrewarding outcome, rats begin to approach a food well faster after sampling the positively predictive cue. This effect, believed to be caused by the differential expectation of a rewarding compared to a nonrewarding outcome, is also abolished by OFC lesions.[84] Additional evidence supporting the hypothesis that the OFC is necessary for representing specific rewarding outcomes triggered by environmental cues comes from Pavlovian-to-instrumental transfer (PIT) experiments. In these experiments, animals learn to independently associate a cue (such as a tone) and a response (such as a lever press) with a specific reward (such as sucrose). The response will subsequently be increased in the presence of the cue during extinction, an effect that is outcome-specific. It has been shown that such outcome-specific PIT effects are abolished by OFC lesions made post-training.[62] Taken together, these studies demonstrate that OFC is critical for value-based decision making even in scenarios where contingencies do not change, suggesting a role in encoding specific outcome expectations.

It was posited that OFC representation of expected reward plays a role in reversal learning, and learning in general, by contributing to the computation of reward prediction errors—the discrepancy between experienced and expected reward outcomes.[83] In one cunning study,[87] this hypothesis was tested using an overexpectation task. In this task, two independent predictors of reward are presented simultaneously, followed by the same reward as when they were each presented in isolation. Healthy rats show an immediate reduction in their conditioned response when either of these cues is then subsequently presented alone. This response reduction is thought to result from negative prediction errors generated when the experienced outcome is worse than the combined expectation evoked by the simultaneous cue presentation. Takahashi and colleagues demonstrated that reversible inactivation of the rat OFC during compound training prevents this response reduction to the individual cues because, they argue, it prevents expectation summation during compound training.[82] This study suggests that the role of the OFC in learning relates to encoding predicted outcome values, which contribute to signaling when experienced outcomes deviate from expectations. Additional work in primates, however, demonstrates that any such role appears to be crucial for learning about, and/or choosing between stimuli, but not actions.[37,78] Rudebeck and colleagues[78] demonstrated that OFC lesions in monkeys do not impair action-outcome reversals or action-outcome matching, whereas they do impair stimulus-outcome reversals[37] and stimulus-outcome matching.[78] The OFC may therefore preferentially represent the expected rewarding value of stimuli associated with specific outcomes.[80]

A recent parallel line of research implicates the OFC in encoding the contingency between environmental stimuli and rewarding outcomes, a role that could also theoretically explain the involvement of the OFC in value-guided learning. Work in rats demonstrates that, although OFC lesions abolish outcome-specific devaluation effects, they do not appear to affect instrumental performance to outcome devaluation,[62] adding to the evidence that the OFC is especially concerned with stimulus-outcome learning. It has been proposed that the function of the OFC that underlies the effects in outcome-specific devaluation and PIT tasks is not in encoding the incentive value of stimuli, but instead in encoding the contingent relationship between specific cues and specific outcomes in a way that biases action selection.[61] This account is supported by an experiment that assessed the effect of OFC lesions on Pavlovian contingency degradation learning.[62] Rats were trained to asymptote on two distinct stimulus-outcome relationships (e.g., noise → grain and tone → sucrose) before receiving OFC or sham surgery. The relationship of one of the two stimulus-outcome contingencies was then degraded by presenting the outcome with a fixed probability independently of whether or not the stimulus was presented. Whereas the sham group decreased responses to the degraded but not the nondegraded stimulus, the OFC group reduced responding to both stimuli. This suggests that the OFC is important for encoding and updating predictive stimulus-outcome relationships.[61]

A very recent experiment in monkeys also suggests that the OFC is necessary for encoding contingency, but further posits that it is critical for *credit assignment*—the assigning of causal responsibility for a particular reward to a particular choice.[95] As discussed earlier, Walton, Behrens, and colleagues tested OFC-lesioned monkeys on different versions of three-armed-bandit tasks. Multiple logistic regression analyses were conducted to assess the influence of three variables: the recency-weighted history of choices, the recency-weighted history of reward, and the precise conjoint choice-reward relationships between particular choices and particular rewards in the past. Preoperatively, monkeys showed modest but significant effects of the recency-weighted history of both choices and rewards from the most recent trials in the past on current choices. Thus, there was a small tendency to associate outcomes with unrelated choices made near in time—a phenomenon termed "Spread-of-Effect." As expected, animals also showed very strong effects of the specific choice-by-reward history for many trials into the past, an effect that diminished with distance from the current trial. Thus, healthy monkeys were able to associate specific choices with their correct outcomes. Postoperatively, monkeys continued to exhibit Spread-of-Effect. However, OFC-lesioned animals were no longer able to use the direct association between a specific choice and its resulting outcome to guide choices. These data indicate that OFC monkeys are able to form an association between the overall integrated history of choices and an overall integrated history of outcomes but are no longer able to associate these outcomes with the preceding choice on which they were contingent.[95] Thus, there is also strong evidence from lesion studies that OFC is important for encoding contingency and, specifically, credit assignment.

Uncertainty about the function of OFC in guiding decision making may be due to its medial and lateral divisions having distinct functions. Although the OFC itself is often treated as one homogenous region, a recent series of detailed anatomical studies have demonstrated that this is far from the case, and it is instead composed of a mosaic of areas.[2,59,80] Based on differential corticocortical and corticosubcortical connections, these subregions have been broadly divided into two connectional networks: the medial and the more lateral orbital prefrontal network. Cytoarchitectonic areas 11, 12, and 13 in central and lateral OFC (lOFC, unless otherwise specified) are preferentially interconnected with higher-order sensory areas, such as the inferior temporal lobe, somatosensory, gustatory, and olfactory cortex, that process stimuli. In contrast, area 14 of medial OFC (mOFC) has stronger connections with the rest of the medial network including cingulate areas 24, 25, and 32 and medial frontal polar area 10.[12,60] Although both the medial and lateral OFC are connected with the amygdala and ventral striatum, the regions of projection and termination in these subcortical structures again distinguish the two frontal regions, suggesting dissociable information processing.[11,24,31]

Claims of functional differentiation based on cytoarchitecture and connective patterns must be tested directly with behavioral experiments. In a recent experiment, we hypothesized that mOFC was more concerned with reward-guided decision making, in contrast with the lOFCs role in reward-guided learning.[53] Macaques performed three-armed-bandit tasks designed to probe different aspects of learning and choice behavior, and the effects of selective mOFC lesions were contrasted with lOFC lesions. We found that, though lOFC was required for appropriate credit assignment, mOFC was critical for comparison of the cues' values during decision making. In unchanging probabilistic environments, mOFC lesions induced decision-making impairments when value comparison was difficult without affecting credit assignment and associative learning. By contrast, lOFC lesions caused the opposite pattern of impairment. Furthermore, the results suggested that contrary to axiomatic assumptions of decision theory, the mOFC-lesioned animals' value comparisons were no longer independent of context, or the presence of alternative options (figure 4.1). mOFC-lesioned animals were beguiled into choosing the second best option partly as a function of a large difference in value between it and the worst option.

Electrophysiological investigations into OFC function have almost exclusively focused on areas 11 and 13 in lateral OFC. These studies have provided complementary evidence in support of the proposals that lateral OFC encodes stimulus-based outcome value expectations and stimulus-outcome contingencies. Although there appears to be little information in monkey OFC related to actions,[64,65,91,92] OFC contains a representation of the sensorial properties of specific rewards.[73,74,79] In addition to representing sensorial features and identities of specific rewards, the OFC encodes both the experienced and expected value of specific rewards.[59] For instance, caudolateral OFC neurons decrease their firing rate following receipt of a specific outcome that has been fed to satiety but not following outcomes that were not devalued,[76] indicating that the OFC encodes the experienced subjective value of specific rewards according to internal states such as hunger. Moreover, OFC neurons encode reward probability,[41] reward magnitude,[94] and reward identity[64] during choice or in anticipation of reward receipt. Earlier work also suggested that OFC encodes the reward preference of the animal.[91] In a delayed-response task, OFC neurons exhibited selectivity for the preferred reward during the presentation of a predictive cue during a block of trials in which either of two rewards was presented repeatedly. OFC neurons responded in a context-dependent manner in this task; the activity in response to the same cue-reward pair depended on whether it was the preferred pair in a given block of trials.

Two recent experiments, however, have challenged this finding.[63,65] In the task employed in these experiments, any two of three color cues symbolizing specific juices were randomly offered to monkeys in a given trial. By varying the amount of each juice offered (represented by the number of colored squares) and measuring

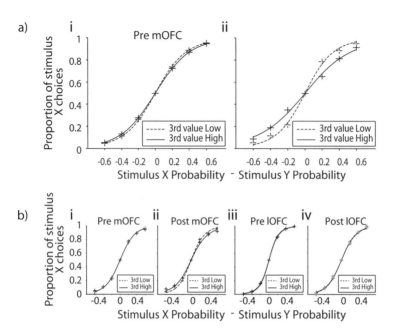

Figure 4.1
Irrelevant third alternatives impede mOFC-lesioned but not lOFC-lesioned animals' choices. (a) Proportion of trials in which monkeys chose options as a function of the value difference with respect to one other option in the context of a high (solid line) or low (dashed line) value-irrelevant third option before (i) and after (ii) mOFC lesion. (b) The same effect remained statistically significant in the mOFC lesion group, even if small in absolute terms, when the analysis focused on just the first halves of each testing session and performance tended to be strong even postoperatively (bi and bii), but no such effect was seen after lOFC lesions (biii and biv). Adapted from Noonan et al.,[53] with permission.

monkeys' choices, indifference points between any two juices could be computed and subjective values derived. In this context, OFC neurons in area 13 encode subjective value expectations in two ways. First, they encode the absolute value of the reward that has been chosen and is therefore expected. Second, they encode the absolute value (or absolute quantity) of the reward type on offer. This second type of signal may serve as an input into a decision-making mechanism between goods and is notably distinct from value encoding in other regions such as lateral intraparietal sulcus, where value is encoded in terms of the evidence in favor of a neurons' preferred response direction *relative* to the alternatives.[40] Taken together, these data indicate that OFC neurons can encode value in a menu-invariant manner: The coding of the subjective value of one item is independent of the other item against which it is offered and therefore whether or not it is preferred. Although these findings seem to contradict the results from Tremblay and Schultz,[91] it may be the case that absolute value is encoded by OFC over the short term (when decisions have to be made between different items on each trial), whereas relative value is encoded over the long term (when items are paired repeatedly over many trials).[65,79]

Finally, two very recent experiments have demonstrated that, although OFC encoding can be invariant to menu, it can also be range dependent.[43,63] Using the task described previously, Padoa-Schioppa found that both chosen and offer value neurons adapt to the range of rewards in a given condition.[63] Specifically, the mean slope of the relationship between firing rate and subjective value across the population of OFC neurons (either averaged across or within individual task-related trial events) is linearly related to the inverse of the range of rewards. The *range* of the firing rate, however, did not depend on the range of rewards. Kobayashi and colleagues[43] similarly found that a subset of OFC neurons adapted to the range of rewards expected from a cue that instructed a saccade and during a delay preceding the saccade. The proportion of the overall population reported to be range adaptive, however, was notably smaller than in the study by Padoa-Schioppa. It was also shown that the proportion of adaptive neurons depended on the length of a block; adaptive neurons were far more prevalent during longer than shorter blocks. Since the range of rewards in the study by Padoa-Schioppa did not change for many trials at a time, the discrepancy between studies may reflect the length of trial blocks before ranges changed. Alternatively, there may be differences in adaptive coding between decision-making and stimulus-response tasks. Collectively, these studies demonstrate that OFC neurons can encode the subjective value of both the expectation and experience of specific rewards in a transitive and computationally efficient manner during value-based choice. Such adaptation is reminiscent of the adaptive coding exhibited by dopamine neurons during prediction error coding.[89]

There is also some evidence that the OFC encodes signals that would be useful for solving the credit assignment problem.[95] As reviewed previously, a subset of OFC neurons encode the identity and sensory properties of specific reward outcomes before and after they are received. Recent work shows that OFC neurons encode and maintain information about specific rewards of current relevance to behavior rather than distracting outcomes.[48] Finally, some OFC neurons encode choices and stimuli across time or reactivate them at the time of feedback,[8,50,92,94] a prerequisite for credit assignment.[95] It might be the case that such information is encoded by OFC even more strongly during reinforcement learning tasks.

Given the evidence of specialization of value processing within the subdivisions of the OFC,[53] is there evidence for a similar dissociation at the neuronal level? Bouret and Richmond[8] examined neurons in the lOFC and VMPFC (including mOFC) during a task that manipulated both actions (release of a bar) and reward size (1, 2, or 4 drops of juice) in "cued active" trials, or just reward size in "cued passive" trials. Self-initiated trials were included in which the monkey released the bar at will and received different sizes of reward depending on the block. Neurons in both regions were found to encode the perceived value of task events. In cued active trials, while neurons in both regions were more sensitive to reward size at cue onset and action at the feedback, the response patterns in lOFC and VMPFC were different. Specifically, at the onset of the cue reward size was more prominent and arose earlier in lOFC than VMPFC. In contrast, around the time of feedback, neurons became more sensitive to the action, and this occurred earlier in VMPFC (before feedback) than in lOFC (after feedback). Furthermore, neurons in the VMPFC encoded reward size predominantly during self-initiated trials, while lOFC neurons encoded reward size mostly during cued trials. It will be interesting to examine whether lOFC and VMPFC neurons are similarly dissociable by other environmental-centered and subject-centered motivational factors, respectably.

Frontal Polar Cortex

Experiments investigating FPC function in macaque monkeys have been lacking due to an overlying bony sinus, which limited access to this area of cortex. This technical challenge has only recently been overcome.[51] Although the function of the monkey FPC has yet to be examined during value-based choice, a very recent study[92] recorded from FPC neurons during both an abstract rule task and delayed response task. The researchers found that FPC encoded the decision (left or right) at the time of feedback, a response that was stronger during correct than error trials. When an extended delay was introduced between saccade and feedback, the FPC maintained its representation of the decision across this delay during the abstract rule task, during which the response was necessary to identify the correct response at the upcoming trial, but not in the delayed response task, during which the response was irrelevant. The authors conclude that the monkey FPC plays a role in evaluating self-generated decisions.

Human Studies

On the whole, there has been a surprising degree of concordance between the monkey work reviewed here and human research, in particular from studies using functional magnetic resonance imaging (fMRI), on RL and value-based choice. Nevertheless, human experiments do highlight some novel predictions, subregional functional dissociations, and potential interspecies differences not yet directly tested by animal studies.

Ventromedial Prefrontal Cortex

Lesions centered on human OFC and adjacent regions of medial prefrontal cortex due to stroke, aneurysm rupture, or traumatic brain injury have also underscored its importance in RL and value-based choice. Important early studies demonstrated profound deficits in these patients on the Iowa gambling task (IGT) that were attributed to impairments in decision making.[4] Successful performance in the IGT requires the deployment of several cognitive functions including both learning from negative and positive feedback and decision making under uncertainty. It has subsequently been shown that VMPFC patients are impaired following a change in deterministic contingencies in a simple reversal learning task[21] and that bilateral but not unilateral lesions centered on OFC led to deficits in a probabilistic reversal learning task.[35] Moreover, VMPFC patients were unimpaired on a reshuffled version of the IGT that did not contain any reversals in the identity of the most valuable deck.[22] More recent work has suggested that this deficit might stem from difficulty learning from negative rather than positive feedback,[97] in contrast to the results in monkeys[78,95] reported in the previous section. Further human lesion work using three-option choice tasks with stochastic and dynamically changing rewards could help to clarify such discrepancies.

In addition to deficits in learning, additional work has shown that VMPFC patients are indeed impaired in decision-making tests even in the absence of learning requirements. For instance, patients with damage focused on the OFC chose suboptimally and deliberated for longer during a risky decision-making task compared to patients with dorsolateral or medial PFC damage and healthy controls.[72] More recent research has shown that VMPFC patients are insensitive to the degree of uncertainty and risk during decision making,[36] raising the following question: Is it the intact processing of uncertainty, rather than decision making per se that is compromised in such patient groups? One study[23] addressed this question in a group of VMPFC patients by simply examining preferences in the absence of uncertainty between pairs of items in one of three categories: foods, famous people, or colors. VMPFC patients made significantly fewer internally consistent preference judgments than either patients with frontal cortex damage sparing VMPFC or healthy controls, consistent with a role in computing relative value. Furthermore, the deficits in relative value judgment did not correlate with deficits in reversal learning in these patients, suggesting two potentially dissociable functions of the VMPFC.[20] An important avenue for future research would be to attempt to dissociate these functions anatomically using larger samples of patients or other methods.

Neuroimaging studies have been vital in both extending the animal findings reviewed in the previous section to humans and further revealing potential functional distinctions between anatomical subregions of VMPFC and adjacent lateral OFC. Several studies have demonstrated that the blood oxygen level–dependent (BOLD) response in regions of VMPFC correlates with the subjective value of both expected and experienced rewards of a variety of types. Confirming findings from monkeys, sensory-specific satiety effects in human central OFC have been reported for both olfactory and visual stimulus cues predicting a specific food or the odor of a specific food with which participants were fed to satiety.[29,57] Furthermore, activity recorded in the VMPFC—often incorporating a medial portion of OFC, the pregenual cingulate cortex, and a posterior subregion of medial FPC[5]—has been consistently shown to correlate with expected value across a variety of contexts.[5,6,17,33,34,39,42,68] VMPFC activity has been shown to correlate with the expected monetary value (reward probability × reward magnitude) associated with a stimulus even in the absence of choice.[42] Further evidence that this region plays a role in valuation comes from studies showing that VMPFC activity correlates with an individual's willingness to pay for a food item.[68] Extensive evidence also indicates that VMPFC activity scales with the value of the chosen option during *decision making*. For instance, VMPFC activity encodes the chosen expected value in a way that incorporates the abstract structure of a probabilistic reversal task,[33] the extent to which people trust a confederate's advice relative to their own experience[5] and idiosyncratic temporal discount functions.[39,69] More recent work has demonstrated that such value coding extends to choices between actions[27,98] and goods of various type.[13] It has been proposed that the VMPFC therefore encodes a common currency enabling consistent economic choices.[13,65] However, it remains possible that only attributes associated with an outcome such as delay, probability, and size are encoded by VMPFC, whereas those associated with the action required to obtain the outcome, such as the effort cost, are encoded in dorsal ACC.[71] This proposal is consistent with the findings that individual neurons and BOLD activity in dorsal ACC encode value in a way that incorporates effort cost, a coding not as evident in OFC or lateral prefrontal cortex (see chapter 5, this volume).[16,41,69] Because the values of the decision options are not varied independently in many studies, however, another unresolved question was whether such subjective value signals measured in VMPFC during choice reflect the absolute or *relative* value.

We set out to address this question in an fMRI experiment in which the reward probabilities associated with two stimuli were varied independently from trial-to-trial according to a fixed volatility.[7] Unlike reward probability, which subjects could learn from the outcomes of their choices, random reward magnitudes from 0 to 100 were explicitly presented on each trial for the subjects to see. This manipulation forced subjects to evaluate both options following trial onset when making decisions. We found that the VMPFC encoded the *relative* chosen value: the chosen expected value relative to the unchosen expected value (figure 4.2). Moreover, the signal scaled linearly with both the relative chosen reward probability and relative chosen reward magnitude (figure 4.2c). This finding has since been corroborated by two studies that examined decision making in very distinct contexts. One study[25] showed that VMPFC activity reflected the difference in subjective value between

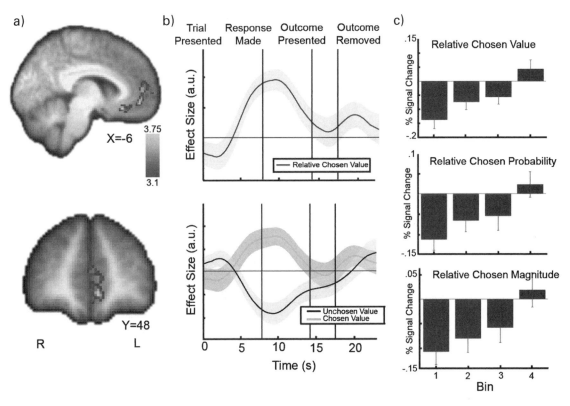

Figure 4.2
The VMPFC encodes the relative chosen value during decision making. (a) Sagittal and coronal slices through Z-statistic maps relating to the relative chosen value (chosen-unchosen expected value). Z-statistic maps are corrected for multiple comparisons across the whole brain by means of cluster-based Gaussian random-field correction at $p < 0.05$. Color bar indicates Z-score. (b) Top panel: Time course for the effect size of the relative chosen value in the VMPFC is shown throughout the duration of the trial. Bottom panel: The same time course is shown with the signal decomposed into chosen and unchosen values. Thick lines = mean effect sizes; shadows = standard error of the mean. (c) Bar plots showing mean VMPFC responses, binned according to relative chosen value (top), relative chosen probability (middle), and relative chosen magnitude (bottom). Adapted from Boorman et al.,[7] with permission.

incommensurable goods under conditions of both gain and loss. In a second study,[66] VMPFC activity reflected the difference between the integrated probabilistic evidence that a face or a house choice would yield a reward. Such signals are consistent with the proposal that during decision making the VMPFC may actively compare the available options competing for choice. It is possible that these relative value signals reflect the net result of a competitive interaction between populations of VMPFC neurons competing for choice or a local comparison that serves as an input to an evidence accumulation process elsewhere in the brain such as the posterior parietal cortex. Another interpretation of the relative value signal is that VMPFC activity reflects both the chosen option's value and the opportunity cost associated with forgoing the alternative.

It has been suggested that rather than relative value, VMPFC activity could reflect the level of attentional engagement, a claim based on studies implicating the VMPFC in the default-mode network.[90] The argument is as follows: As attention is further engaged, VMPFC activity becomes further *deactivated*. Thus, when the relative decision value is high (and decisions are easier), VMPFC is less deactivated; when the relative decision value is low (and decisions become more difficult), VMPFC will deactivate more. The net result therefore produces a positive correlation with relative value. However, a recent study[49] has shown that, across appetitive and aversive foods, VMPFC activity encodes the value of the offered item rather than its salience, arguing against an attention-based account of VMPFC activity.

In addition to encoding expected and relative value during valuation and choice, activity in parts of VMPFC respond to the subjective value of experienced rewards. This has been shown not only for gustatory stimuli and its properties, but also for olfactory, somatosensory, auditory, and visual stimuli,[1,28,30,56,57,59,75,77] and for abstract stimuli such as money and social praise.[55,58] Furthermore, such responses are modulated by cognitive expectancy.[18,69] These responses were predominately observed in central and/or medial parts of OFC.

There is also some evidence that the choice itself is reflected in VMPFC activity. Three studies have shown that the VMPFC signal following presentation of feedback predicts whether the subject will go on to repeat or change their choice on the following trial.[27,32,54] VMPFC activity is higher before the subject repeats the current choice than before they switch choices at subsequent decisions.

It has also been suggested that medial portions of OFC may be selectively involved in the goal-directed component of instrumental learning by computing goal values, while central OFC may be preferentially involved in Pavlovian stimulus-outcome learning by computing Pavlovian or stimulus values.[2,59] This interpretation is partly based on the finding that medial OFC is sensitive to devaluation effects in a task that included both instrumental and Pavlovian components but not in a task with no instrumental component, whereas central OFC was sensitive to devaluation effects in both tasks.[29,92]

Many goal-directed tasks inadvertently confound learning and decision making. During some tasks designed to investigate decision making, once a choice is made the outcome is used to update reward expectancies. Similarly, during some tasks designed to investigate learning, subjects are choosing between stimuli and actions. For example, a devaluation test using extinction, which aims to assess choice in the absence of the confound of rewarding outcome, is alternatively confounded by violations of learned expectations: negative prediction errors. Even though this effect can be observed on the first trial, it is still the case that subsequent trials will lead to negative prediction errors.[82]

Given the recent animal research on the role of the OFC in contingency,[61,95] is there any evidence that OFC plays a role in calculating contingency in humans? One study investigated this question by manipulating the degree of contingency between actions (button presses) and outcomes (monetary reward).[88] In general accordance with findings from rat lesion studies, enhanced activity was found in dorsomedial striatum and VMPFC during blocks with greater contingency between actions and outcomes.[61] Moreover, activity in VMPFC tracked local changes in contingency within blocks. We investigated outcome-specific contingency learning with a novel version of the differential outcomes procedure, which combined initial preconditioning stimulus-outcome and response-outcome learning phases with a final stimulus-response learning phase.[52] During each phase, we manipulated the consistency of the specific outcomes that followed stimuli and actions. Behaviorally, subjects who could form stimulus and response outcome-specific associations were more accurate in tests of speed of learning and memory recall. Functional magnetic resonance imaging was used to investigate the neural systems underlying the behavioral accuracy advantage in subjects exposed to consistent outcomes. The results indicated that three areas commonly involved in reward-guided learning, the lateral OFC, medial OFC, and ACC were activated by the task. We show that each area's contribution can be dissociated, with only the lOFC and ACC more active in subjects with knowledge of reward consistency. In the absence of choice confounds, this experiment mirrors the findings of Walton and colleagues.[96]

Frontal Polar Cortex

Only a few studies have examined the role of the FPC in value-based choice. In a decision-making task that required subjects to integrate past actions and outcomes over varying temporal windows, right FPC, and DLPFC activity was found to increase with increased temporal integration demands.[99] In another decision-making study,[86] it was shown using multivariate statistical decoding techniques that medial and lateral FPC predicted an upcoming left/right decision seconds before subjects indicated that they were aware of their choice. Furthermore, in a study[17] in which subjects selected between four slot machines whose mean payoff rates varied independently, lateral FPC activity increased during exploratory choices compared to exploitative choices. It was suggested that such activity reflected a mechanism for gathering new information in a changing environment. A parallel set of experiments on task control has implicated the FPC in juggling mnemonic demands in the service of future behavior.[10,44,45,81] In particular, FPC activity has been shown when subjects switch between task sets, especially when information must be maintained in working memory when switching to the alternative.[9,44,46,70] One intriguing theory postulates that the FPC maintains the pending task set during an ongoing behavior in order to switch to the pending task set once the current behavior is completed.[45] It was unclear whether such functions extend to value-based choice and to switching between simple choices rather than complex task sets. In light of this work on task control, it seemed possible that at least part of the FPC's role in exploratory decision making may be related to the representation of variables related to pending or unchosen options.

In an fMRI study,[7] we aimed to help bridge the gap in understanding between the role of the FPC in task control on the one hand and value-based choice on the other hand. We examined decision variables associated with unchosen options in the two-arm-bandit fMRI task described earlier with tractable reward probabilities and random reward magnitudes.[7] Lateral FPC encoded the log likelihood ratio favoring the unchosen option over the chosen option (figure 4.3). This is consistent with a region that tracks the reward expectation associated with the pending option, a metric that would be useful for determining when to switch choices to that option in the future. Unlike the VMPFC, where activity reflected the relative chosen *expected value* during the decision period (see figure 4.2), the FPC effect was independent of reward magnitude and extended temporally across the decision and outcome periods. Across the population of participants, the greater the effect in the FPC, the more effectively people switched choices to the formerly unchosen option. Taken together, these findings suggest that, during decision making in dynamic and stochastic environments, FPC tracks the reward-based evidence promoting future choice adaptation. It would be interesting to examine FPC coding during decision making among multiple alternatives.

Summary

The abundant research on value-based choice over the past decade has begun to reveal the distinct but complementary systems-level computations performed by not only subcortical structures and parietal cortex but also subregions of frontal cortex. The OFC can be functionally partitioned into at least two subregions. Evidence from rats, monkeys, and humans implicate more lateral OFC regions in encoding the subjective expected value of environmental stimuli and playing an important role in contingent learning, potentially by helping to solve the credit assignment problem. The medial OFC regions of the macaque meanwhile appear to be involved in value comparison. Human work further indicates that the VMPFC encodes a subjective expected value signal during valuation and a value comparison signal during choice.

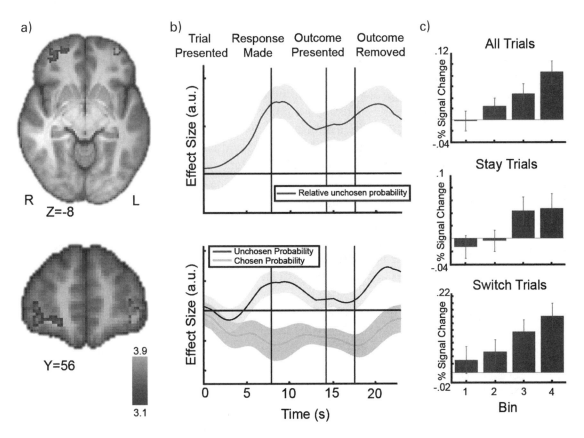

Figure 4.3
The lateral FPC tracks the relative unchosen probability. (a) Axial and coronal slices through z-statistic maps relating to the relative unchosen probability [log (unchosen probability/chosen probability)]. (b) Top panel: Time course for the effect size of the relative unchosen probability is shown throughout the trial. Bottom panel: The time course is separated into log unchosen and log chosen probabilities. (c) The bar plots show the mean BOLD percent signal change in the FPC, with trials binned by the relative unchosen probability for all trials (top), stay trials (middle), and switch trials (bottom). Adapted from Boorman et al.,[7] with permission.

Although there may be differences between medial and lateral subdivisions of human FPC, the research to date on the FPC during value-based choice suggests potential differences across species, a possibility supported by evidence of dramatic enlargement and specialization of human FPC relative to other great apes.[85] The one published study to examine the FPC in macaque monkeys suggests a role in evaluating or monitoring self-generated decisions at the time of feedback. By contrast, human studies point to a possible mnemonic role for lateral FPC in tracking the evidence favoring alternative options for future consideration and in exploration.

Outstanding Questions

• What precise computational role does VMPFC play during RL and value-based choice? Four non–mutually exclusive proposals are emerging: VMPFC (a) compares evidence between competing options during goal-based decision making; (b) provides the input to a decision-making integrator elsewhere in the brain; (c) encodes the subjective value of the chosen option in a way that incorporates the opportunity cost of the alternative option; and (d) transmits chosen value predictions to DA neurons (and elsewhere) for prediction error computation.

• Under what precise circumstances is FPC recruited during value-based choice? A related question concerns how and when FPC and VMPFC interact if at all during value-based choice?

• In what other ways do the fine-grained anatomical subdivisions of the VMPFC, OFC, and FPC indicate specialization of function? Can more sophisticated lesion and imaging techniques confine function to increasingly more precise foci?

Further Reading

Rushworth MFS and Behrens TEJ. 2008. Choice, uncertainty and value in prefrontal and cingulate cortex. *Nat Neurosci* 11: 389–397. Comprehensive overview of value-based decision making, taking into account not just the effects of reward estimates, but also the uncertainty in these estimates.

Rangel A and Hare T. 2010. Neural computations associated with goal-directed choice. *Curr Opin Neurobiol* 20: 262–270. A review of the neural mechanisms underlying goal-directed choice, with an emphasis on how action values and action costs are computed.

Kabel JW and Glimcher PW. 2009. The neurobiology of decision: Consensus and controversy. *Neuron* 63: 733–745. This synthesis of data on the neural basis of decision making focuses on frontal, but also parietal and subcortical structures.

References

1. Anderson AK, Christoff K, Stappen I, Panitz D, Ghahremani DG, Glover G, Gabrieli JD, Sobel N. 2003. Dissociated neural representations of intensity and valence in human olfaction. *Nat Neurosci* 6: 196–202.

2. Balleine BW, Daw ND, O'Doherty JP. 2009. Multiple forms of value learning and the function of dopamine. In: Neuroeconomics: Decision Making and the Brain (Glimcher PW, Camerer CF, Fehr E, Poldrack RA, eds), pp. 367–387. Amsterdam: Elsevier.

3. Baxter MG, Parker A, Lindner CC, Izquierdo AD, Murray EA. 2000. Control of response selection by reinforcer value requires interaction of amygdala and orbital prefrontal cortex. *J Neurosci* 20: 4311–4319.

4. Bechara A, Damasio H, Damasio AR. 2000. Emotion, decision making and the orbitofrontal cortex. *Cereb Cortex* 10: 295–307.

5. Behrens TE, Hunt LT, Woolrich MW, Rushworth MF. 2008. Associative learning of social value. *Nature* 456: 245–249.

6. Behrens TE, Woolrich MW, Walton ME, Rushworth MF. 2007. Learning the value of information in an uncertain world. *Nat Neurosci* 10: 1214–1221.

7. Boorman ED, Behrens TE, Woolrich MW, Rushworth MF. 2009. How green is the grass on the other side? Frontopolar cortex and the evidence in favor of alternative courses of action. *Neuron* 62: 733–743.

8. Bouret S, Richmond BJ. 2010. Ventromedial and orbital prefrontal neurons differentially encode internally and externally driven motivational values in monkeys. *J Neurosci* 30: 8591–8601.

9. Braver TS, Reynolds JR, Donaldson DI. 2003. Neural mechanisms of transient and sustained cognitive control during task switching. *Neuron* 39: 713–726.

10. Burgess PW, Scott SK, Frith CD. 2003. The role of the rostral frontal cortex (area 10) in prospective memory: a lateral versus medial dissociation. *Neuropsychologia* 41: 906–918.

11. Carmichael ST, Price JL. 1995. Sensory and premotor connections of the orbital and medial prefrontal cortex of macaque monkeys. *J Comp Neurol* 363: 642–664.

12. Carmichael ST, Price JL. 1996. Connectional networks within the orbital and medial prefrontal cortex of macaque monkeys. *J Comp Neurol* 371: 179–207.

13. Chib VS, Rangel A, Shimojo S, O'Doherty JP. 2009. Evidence for a common representation of decision values for dissimilar goods in human ventromedial prefrontal cortex. *J Neurosci* 29: 12315–12320.

14. Chudasama Y, Robbins TW. 2003. Dissociable contributions of the orbitofrontal and infralimbic cortex to pavlovian autoshaping and discrimination reversal learning: further evidence for the functional heterogeneity of the rodent frontal cortex. *J Neurosci* 23: 8771–8780.

15. Clarke HF, Robbins TW, Roberts AC. 2008. Lesions of the medial striatum in monkeys produce perseverative impairments during reversal learning similar to those produced by lesions of the orbitofrontal cortex. *J Neurosci* 28: 10972–10982.

16. Croxson PL, Walton ME, O'Reilly JX, Behrens TE, Rushworth MF. 2009. Effort-based cost-benefit valuation and the human brain. *J Neurosci* 29: 4531–4541.

17. Daw ND, O'Doherty JP, Dayan P, Seymour B, Dolan RJ. 2006. Cortical substrates for exploratory decisions in humans. *Nature* 441: 876–879.

18. De Araujo IE, Rolls ET, Velazco MI, Margot C, Cayeux I. 2005. Cognitive modulation of olfactory processing. *Neuron* 46: 671–679.

19. Dias R, Robbins TW, Roberts AC. 1996. Dissociation in prefrontal cortex of affective and attentional shifts. *Nature* 380: 69–72.

20. Fellows LK. 2007. The role of orbitofrontal cortex in decision making: a component process account. *Ann N Y Acad Sci* 1121: 421–430.

21. Fellows LK, Farah MJ. 2003. Ventromedial frontal cortex mediates affective shifting in humans: evidence from a reversal learning paradigm. *Brain* 126: 1830–1837.

22. Fellows LK, Farah MJ. 2005. Different underlying impairments in decision-making following ventromedial and dorsolateral frontal lobe damage in humans. *Cereb Cortex* 15: 58–63.

23. Fellows LK, Farah MJ. 2007. The role of ventromedial prefrontal cortex in decision making: judgment under uncertainty or judgment per se? *Cereb Cortex* 17: 2669–2674.

24. Ferry AT, Ongur D, An X, Price JL. 2000. Prefrontal cortical projections to the striatum in macaque monkeys: evidence for an organization related to prefrontal networks. *J Comp Neurol* 425: 447–470.

25. FitzGerald TH, Seymour B, Dolan RJ. 2009. The role of human orbitofrontal cortex in value comparison for incommensurable objects. *J Neurosci* 29: 8388–8395.

26. Gallagher M, McMahan RW, Schoenbaum G. 1999. Orbitofrontal cortex and representation of incentive value in associative learning. *J Neurosci* 19: 6610–6614.

27. Glascher J, Hampton AN, O'Doherty JP. 2009. Determining a role for ventromedial prefrontal cortex in encoding action-based value signals during reward-related decision making. *Cereb Cortex* 19: 483–495.

28. Gottfried JA, O'Doherty J, Dolan RJ. 2002. Appetitive and aversive olfactory learning in humans studied using event-related functional magnetic resonance imaging. *J Neurosci* 22: 10829–10837.

29. Gottfried JA, O'Doherty J, Dolan RJ. 2003. Encoding predictive reward value in human amygdala and orbitofrontal cortex. *Science* 301: 1104–1107.

30. Grabenhorst F, Rolls ET, Parris BA, d'Souza AA. 2010. How the brain represents the reward value of fat in the mouth. *Cereb Cortex* 20: 1082–1091.

31. Haber SN, Kim KS, Mailly P, Calzavara R. 2006. Reward-related cortical inputs define a large striatal region in primates that interface with associative cortical connections, providing a substrate for incentive-based learning. *J Neurosci* 26: 8368–8376.

32. Hampton AN, Adolphs R, Tyszka MJ, O'Doherty JP. 2007. Contributions of the amygdala to reward expectancy and choice signals in human prefrontal cortex. *Neuron* 55: 545–555.

33. Hampton AN, Bossaerts P, O'Doherty JP. 2006. The role of the ventromedial prefrontal cortex in abstract state-based inference during decision making in humans. *J Neurosci* 26: 8360–8367.

34. Hare TA, O'Doherty J, Camerer CF, Schultz W, Rangel A. 2008. Dissociating the role of the orbitof-rontal cortex and the striatum in the computation of goal values and prediction errors. *J Neurosci* 28: 5623–5630.

35. Hornak J, O'Doherty J, Bramham J, Rolls ET, Morris RG, Bullock PR, Polkey CE. 2004. Reward-related reversal learning after surgical excisions in orbito-frontal or dorsolateral prefrontal cortex in humans. *J Cogn Neurosci* 16: 463–478.

36. Hsu M, Bhatt M, Adolphs R, Tranel D, Camerer CF. 2005. Neural systems responding to degrees of uncertainty in human decision-making. *Science* 310: 1680–1683.

37. Izquierdo A, Suda RK, Murray EA. 2004. Bilateral orbital prefrontal cortex lesions in rhesus monkeys disrupt choices guided by both reward value and reward contingency. *J Neurosci* 24: 7540–7548.

38. Jones B, Mishkin M. 1972. Limbic lesions and the problem of stimulus—reinforcement associations. *Exp Neurol* 36: 362–377.

39. Kable JW, Glimcher PW. 2007. The neural correlates of subjective value during intertemporal choice. *Nat Neurosci* 10: 1625–1633.

40. Kable JW, Glimcher PW. 2009. The neurobiology of decision: consensus and controversy. *Neuron* 63: 733–745.

41. Kennerley SW, Wallis JD. 2009. Evaluating choices by single neurons in the frontal lobe: outcome value encoded across multiple decision variables. *Eur J Neurosci* 29: 2061–2073.

42. Knutson B, Taylor J, Kaufman M, Peterson R, Glover G. 2005. Distributed neural representation of expected value. *J Neurosci* 25: 4806–4812.

43. Kobayashi S, Pinto de Carvalho O, Schultz W. 2010. Adaptation of reward sensitivity in orbitofrontal neurons. *J Neurosci* 30: 534–544.

44. Koechlin E, Basso G, Pietrini P, Panzer S, Grafman J. 1999. The role of the anterior prefrontal cortex in human cognition. *Nature* 399: 148–151.

45. Koechlin E, Hyafil A. 2007. Anterior prefrontal function and the limits of human decision-making. *Science* 318: 594–598.

46. Koechlin E, Summerfield C. 2007. An information theoretical approach to prefrontal executive function. *Trends Cogn Sci* 11: 229–235.

47. Kringelbach ML, Rolls ET. 2004. The functional neuroanatomy of the human orbitofrontal cortex: evidence from neuroimaging and neuropsychology. *Prog Neurobiol* 72: 341–372.

48. Lara AH, Kennerley SW, Wallis JD. 2009. Encoding of gustatory working memory by orbitofrontal neurons. *J Neurosci* 29: 765–774.

49. Litt A, Plassmann H, Shiv B, Rangel A. 2011. Dissociating valuation and saliency signals during decision-making. *Cereb Cortex* 21: 95–102.

50. Meunier M, Bachevalier J, Mishkin M. 1997. Effects of orbital frontal and anterior cingulate lesions on object and spatial memory in rhesus monkeys. *Neuropsychologia* 35: 999–1015.

51. Mitz AR, Tsujimoto S, Maclarty AJ, Wise SP. 2009. A method for recording single-cell activity in the frontal-pole cortex of macaque monkeys. *J Neurosci Methods* 177: 60–66.

52. Noonan MP, Mars RB, Rushworth MF. submitted. Distinct roles of three frontal cortical areas in reward-guided decision making.

53. Noonan MP, Walton ME, Behrens TE, Sallet J, Buckley MJ, Rushworth M. 2010. Separate value comparison and learning mechanisms in macaque medial and lateral orbitofrontal cortex. *Proc Natl Acad Sci USA* 107: 20547–20552.

54. O'Doherty J, Critchley H, Deichmann R, Dolan RJ. 2003. Dissociating valence of outcome from behavioral control in human orbital and ventral prefrontal cortices. *J Neurosci* 23: 7931–7939.

55. O'Doherty J, Kringelbach ML, Rolls ET, Hornak J, Andrews C. 2001. Abstract reward and punishment representations in the human orbitofrontal cortex. *Nat Neurosci* 4: 95–102.

56. O'Doherty J, Rolls ET, Francis S, Bowtell R, McGlone F. 2001. Representation of pleasant and aversive taste in the human brain. *J Neurophysiol* 85: 1315–1321.

57. O'Doherty J, Rolls ET, Francis S, Bowtell R, McGlone F, Kobal G, Renner B, Ahne G. 2000. Sensory-specific satiety-related olfactory activation of the human orbitofrontal cortex. *Neuroreport* 11: 893–897.

58. O'Doherty J, Winston J, Critchley H, Perrett D, Burt DM, Dolan RJ. 2003. Beauty in a smile: the role of medial orbitofrontal cortex in facial attractiveness. *Neuropsychologia* 41: 147–155.

59. O'Doherty JP. 2007. Lights, camembert, action! The role of human orbitofrontal cortex in encoding stimuli, rewards, and choices. *Ann N Y Acad Sci* 1121: 254–272.

60. Ongur D, Price JL. 2000. The organization of networks within the orbital and medial prefrontal cortex of rats, monkeys and humans. *Cereb Cortex* 10: 206–219.

61. Ostlund SB, Balleine BW. 2007. The contribution of orbitofrontal cortex to action selection. *Ann N Y Acad Sci* 1121: 174–192.

62. Ostlund SB, Balleine BW. 2007. Orbitofrontal cortex mediates outcome encoding in Pavlovian but not instrumental conditioning. *J Neurosci* 27: 4819–4825.

63. Padoa-Schioppa C. 2009. Range-adapting representation of economic value in the orbitofrontal cortex. *J Neurosci* 29: 14004–14014.

64. Padoa-Schioppa C, Assad JA. 2006. Neurons in the orbitofrontal cortex encode economic value. *Nature* 441: 223–226.

65. Padoa-Schioppa C, Assad JA. 2008. The representation of economic value in the orbitofrontal cortex is invariant for changes of menu. *Nat Neurosci* 11: 95–102.

66. Philiastides MG, Biele G, Heekeren HR. 2010. A mechanistic account of value computation in the human brain. *Proc Natl Acad Sci USA* 107: 9430–9435.

67. Plassmann H, O'Doherty J, Rangel A. 2007. Orbitofrontal cortex encodes willingness to pay in everyday economic transactions. *J Neurosci* 27: 9984–9988.

68. Plassmann H, O'Doherty J, Shiv B, Rangel A. 2008. Marketing actions can modulate neural representations of experienced pleasantness. *Proc Natl Acad Sci USA* 105: 1050–1054.

69. Prévost C, Pessiglione M, Météreau E, Cléry-Melin ML, Dreher JC. 2010. Separate valuation subsystems for delay and effort decision costs. *J Neurosci* 30: 14080–14090.

70. Ramnani N, Owen AM. 2004. Anterior prefrontal cortex: insights into function from anatomy and neuroimaging. *Nat Rev Neurosci* 5: 184–194.

71. Rangel A, Hare T. 2010. Neural computations associated with goal-directed choice. *Curr Opin Neurobiol* 20: 262–270.

72. Rogers RD, Everitt BJ, Baldacchino A, Blackshaw AJ, Swainson R, Wynne K, Baker NB, et al. 1999. Dissociable deficits in the decision-making cognition of chronic amphetamine abusers, opiate abusers, patients with focal damage to prefrontal cortex, and tryptophan-depleted normal volunteers: evidence for monoaminergic mechanisms. *Neuropsychopharmacology* 20: 322–339.

73. Rolls ET, Baylis LL. 1994. Gustatory, olfactory, and visual convergence within the primate orbitofrontal cortex. *J Neurosci* 14: 5437–5452.

74. Rolls ET, Critchley HD, Browning AS, Hernadi I, Lenard L. 1999. Responses to the sensory properties of fat of neurons in the primate orbitofrontal cortex. *J Neurosci* 19: 1532–1540.

75. Rolls ET, Grabenhorst F, Parris BA. 2008. Warm pleasant feelings in the brain. *Neuroimage* 41: 1504–1513.

76. Rolls ET, Sienkiewicz ZJ, Yaxley S. 1989. Hunger modulates the responses to gustatory stimuli of single neurons in the caudolateral orbitofrontal cortex of the macaque monkey. *Eur J Neurosci* 1: 53–60.

77. Rolls ET, Verhagen JV, Kadohisa M. 2003. Representations of the texture of food in the primate orbitofrontal cortex: neurons responding to viscosity, grittiness, and capsaicin. *J Neurophysiol* 90: 3711–3724.

78. Rudebeck PH, Behrens TE, Kennerley SW, Baxter MG, Buckley MJ, Walton ME, Rushworth MF. 2008. Frontal cortex subregions play distinct roles in choices between actions and stimuli. *J Neurosci* 28: 13775–13785.

79. Rushworth MF, Behrens TE. 2008. Choice, uncertainty and value in prefrontal and cingulate cortex. *Nat Neurosci* 11: 389–397.

80. Rushworth MF, Behrens TE, Rudebeck PH, Walton ME. 2007. Contrasting roles for cingulate and orbitofrontal cortex in decisions and social behaviour. *Trends Cogn Sci* 11: 168–176.

81. Sakai K, Passingham RE. 2006. Prefrontal set activity predicts rule-specific neural processing during subsequent cognitive performance. *J Neurosci* 26: 1211–1218.

82. Schoenbaum G, Roesch MR, Stalnaker TA, Takahashi YK. 2009. A new perspective on the role of the orbitofrontal cortex in adaptive behaviour. *Nat Rev Neurosci* 10: 885–892.

83. Schoenbaum G, Saddoris MP, Stalnaker TA. 2007. Reconciling the roles of orbitofrontal cortex in reversal learning and the encoding of outcome expectancies. *Ann N Y Acad Sci* 1121: 320–335.

84. Schoenbaum G, Setlow B, Nugent SL, Saddoris MP, Gallagher M. 2003. Lesions of orbitofrontal cortex and basolateral amygdala complex disrupt acquisition of odor-guided discriminations and reversals. *Learn Mem* 10: 129–140.

85. Semendeferi K, Armstrong E, Schleicher A, Zilles K, Van Hoesen GW. 2001. Prefrontal cortex in humans and apes: a comparative study of area 10. *Am J Phys Anthropol* 114: 224–241.

86. Soon CS, Brass M, Heinze HJ, Haynes JD. 2008. Unconscious determinants of free decisions in the human brain. *Nat Neurosci* 11: 543–545.

87. Takahashi YK, Roesch MR, Stalnaker TA, Haney RZ, Calu DJ, Taylor AR, Burke KA, Schoenbaum G. 2009. The orbitofrontal cortex and ventral tegmental area are necessary for learning from unexpected outcomes. *Neuron* 62: 269–280.

88. Tanaka SC, Balleine BW, O'Doherty JP. 2008. Calculating consequences: brain systems that encode the causal effects of actions. *J Neurosci* 28: 6750–6755.

89. Tobler PN, Fiorillo CD, Schultz W. 2005. Adaptive coding of reward value by dopamine neurons. *Science* 307: 1642–1645.

90. Tosoni A, Galati G, Romani GL, Corbetta M. 2008. Sensory-motor mechanisms in human parietal cortex underlie arbitrary visual decisions. *Nat Neurosci* 11: 1446–1453.

91. Tremblay L, Schultz W. 1999. Relative reward preference in primate orbitofrontal cortex. *Nature* 398: 704–708.

92. Tsujimoto S, Genovesio A, Wise SP. 2009. Monkey orbitofrontal cortex encodes response choices near feedback time. *J Neurosci* 29: 2569–2574.

93. Valentin VV, Dickinson A, O'Doherty JP. 2007. Determining the neural substrates of goal-directed learning in the human brain. *J Neurosci* 27: 4019–4026.

94. Wallis JD, Miller EK. 2003. Neuronal activity in primate dorsolateral and orbital prefrontal cortex during performance of a reward preference task. *Eur J Neurosci* 18: 2069–2081.

95. Walton ME, Behrens TE, Buckley MJ, Rudebeck PH, Rushworth MF. 2010. Separable learning systems in the macaque brain and the role of orbitofrontal cortex in contingent learning. *Neuron* 65: 927–939.

96. Walton ME, Devlin JT, Rushworth MF. 2004. Interactions between decision making and performance monitoring within prefrontal cortex. *Nat Neurosci* 7: 1259–1265.

97. Wheeler EZ, Fellows LK. 2008. The human ventromedial frontal lobe is critical for learning from negative feedback. *Brain* 131: 1323–1331.

98. Wunderlich K, Rangel A, O'Doherty JP. 2009. Neural computations underlying action-based decision making in the human brain. *Proc Natl Acad Sci USA* 106: 17199–17204.

99. Yarkoni T, Gray JR, Chrastil ER, Barch DM, Green L, Braver TS. 2005. Sustained neural activity associated with cognitive control during temporally extended decision making. *Brain Res Cogn Brain Res* 23: 71–84.

5 Decision Making in Frontal Cortex: From Single Units to fMRI

Steven W. Kennerley and Philippe N. Tobler

A glass of Riesling or a bottle of Pinot Noir? Cycle to work or take public transport? Continue foraging in the current patch or explore a new area in hopes of more plentiful food? Many of the decisions that humans and animals face on a daily basis require consideration of multiple decision variables. Even the routine decision of what and where to eat is likely to be influenced by a number of very disparate variables. First, you have to evaluate your current internal state (thirst/appetite); if your current needs are satisfied you can eat later. Assuming food is currently desired, you might be influenced by how hungry you are (how much should I eat?), what type of food you currently prefer (which is likely to be influenced by your recent history of food choices), what your goals are (save money, eat less/healthy), nonphysical costs associated with each food option (e.g., uncertainty of how palatable the food may be, delay before food will be obtained), and physical costs, such as the energy that must be expended to obtain food.

Despite the variety of decision alternatives available in any given moment, the brain must somehow determine which option best meets our current needs and goals. One influential idea is that the brain assigns values to all relevant decision variables and then integrates across these variables to generate a single value estimate for each decision alternative, a type of neuronal currency that can be used to compare very disparate outcomes.[80] Yet, how and where different decision variables are represented in the brain and where this information is integrated (if at all) is a topic of great interest. Mounting evidence from multiple methodologies emphasizes the role of the frontal cortex in some aspect of this type of multivariate decision process,[112] as damage here causes dramatic decision-making impairments, especially on multivariate decisions.[31,32,109,110]

Here we summarize recent findings from both single neuron electrophysiology and functional neuroimaging with respect to the role of the frontal cortex—especially anterior cingulate cortex (ACC), lateral prefrontal cortex (LPFC), orbitofrontal cortex (OFC), and ventromedial prefrontal cortex (VMPFC)—in the representation of key processes underlying optimal choice. To capture the behavioral and neural processes involved in decision making, a computational framework may be useful.[9,100,127,151] Our review is broadly based on recent decision-making frameworks that highlight several cognitive processes necessary for optimal goal-directed choice, including representation of internal states, representation of external variables that will influence the value of the outcome (e.g., risk, probability, delay), assigning values to actions based on expected outcomes minus action costs (e.g., effort), and optimal selection based on comparison of action values.[100,101]

The Influence of Internal States

Humans and animals will typically work more when they are hungry or thirsty, thus a critical component driving decision making and goal-directed behavior is one's current internal state. Models of decision making incorporate a value system that monitors one's internal needs, such as metabolic state.[100.] Several studies have shown that neuronal activity in OFC[82,108] and VMPFC[15] changes as subjects become sated, although the lateral hypothalamus may have a more prominent role in signaling changes in internal state.[26] In humans, OFC activity to tastes such as sucrose is elevated when participants are hungry rather than sated.[43] Posterior lateral OFC, LPFC, and ACC show activation increases after the infusion of the satiety signaling peptide PYY compared to saline infusion.[5] Water elicits activation in caudal OFC only when participants are thirsty, not when they are sated.[27]

One procedure used to assess how internal reward representations guide behavior is reinforcer devaluation. Subjects learn that particular rewards are associated with neutral objects, and then one of the rewards is devalued, by either feeding the reward to satiety or pairing the reward with chemically induced illness. When subsequently tested in a choice context, normal animals avoid the stimulus associated with the devalued food, but animals with damage to OFC (but not LPFC or ventrolateral PFC) continue selecting the stimulus associated with the devalued reward.[6,7] Importantly, this impairment is present only when selecting between objects associated with the devalued reward, rather than between the two foods directly.[55] It has been suggested that this type of decision may not simply be guided by a change in the incentive value of the outcome, but is influenced by the contingent link between a stimulus and a particular outcome type.[87] These findings suggest OFC, in conjunction with the amygdala,[8] has an important role in updating stimulus-outcome associations based on current internal state. An avenue for future research is to explore whether stimulus- and action-based devaluation effects depend on different neural structures. So far, the two forms have typically been studied separately. In an action-based devaluation study, medial, central, and lateral OFC showed reduced activation at the time of action selection for a juice that had been sated in a sensory-specific manner.[145] Conversely, in a stimulus-based devaluation study, central OFC and ACC showed reduced activation at the time of a stimulus predicting devalued reward.[41] The implied regional distinction maps well onto OFC anatomy, as lateral and central areas of OFC are primarily innervated by sensory areas (which could form the basis of stimulus-based devaluation) while medial OFC is innervated by regions with a stronger motor function[86] such as medial PFC and ACC (which could form the basis of action-based devaluation). Thus, a critical challenge for future studies is to better understand how the brain utilizes information about internal state in updating both stimulus and action values to influence optimal action selection.

The Determination of Outcome Value

Single neurons across most of the brain—but especially within ACC, LPFC, and OFC—are modulated by almost every decision variable investigators have used to manipulate the value of an outcome. Neurons in these frontal areas are sensitive to the size and/or probability of a positive or negative outcome,[2,58,59,61,66,67,81,99,103,104,116,123,146] size and temporal proximity to reward,[64,105,107] reward preference,[50,74,90,91,143] effort required to harvest reward,[51,58] and one's confidence in the choice outcome.[63]

The shear overlap of these signals across frontal areas highlights the difficulty in inferring functional specialization by comparing across studies, especially from studies that manipulate the value of an outcome using a single decision variable (e.g., reward magnitude) and record activity from a single brain area. We approached this issue in two different ways. First, we designed an experiment with the precise goal of determining whether neurons in different frontal areas exhibit preferences for encoding different variables related to a decision's value. We trained monkeys to make choices between different behavioral outcomes that varied in terms of either reward probability, reward magnitude, or effort (number of lever presses necessary to earn reward).[58] We recorded from OFC, ACC, and LPFC simultaneously, thus allowing us to directly pit these three frontal areas against each other in animals in the same behavioral state using the same analytical methods. We found that neurons encoded value across the different decision variables in diverse ways. For example, some neurons encoded the value of just a single decision variable, others encoded the value of choices for two of the variables but not the third, while still others encoded value across all three decision variables (figure 5.1). We found no evidence that any of the three frontal areas were specialized for encoding any particular decision variable (figure 5.1C); instead, we found that a single area,

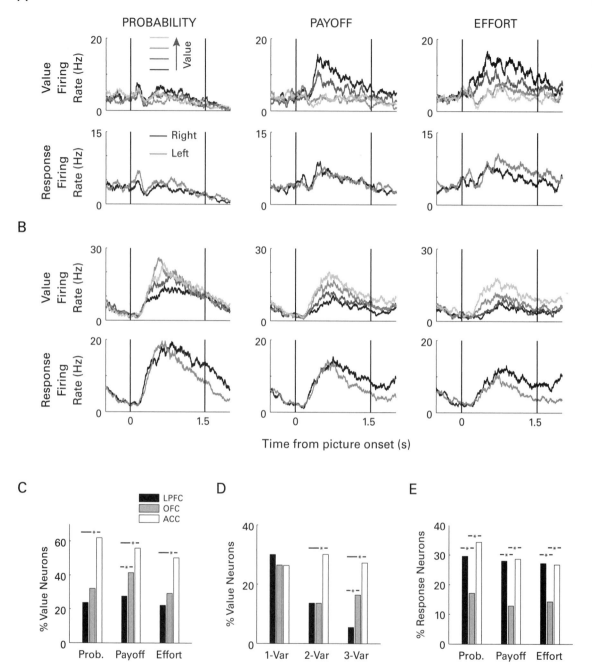

ACC, was specialized for encoding two or three decision variables (figure 5.1D). Thus, single ACC neurons are capable of encoding the value of multiple decision variables across trials, a type of multiplexed value representation that may allow the integration of the individual components of a decision and underlie ACC's critical contribution to decision making.

Human functional neuroimaging offers a clear advantage over animal electrophysiology studies; it is a whole-brain technique that affords the opportunity to compare activity across areas in the same testing session. We performed a second series of experiments exploring how different parts of the human frontal cortex process a variety of decision variables that we varied independently. We found that the same three regions (OFC, ACC, and LPFC) are also activated consistently in human studies of value processing, thus complementing animal studies. In an operant design, humans performed an action on presentation of different stimuli that predicted different magnitudes of reward with different probability.[136,137,140] All measurements occurred after learning and at the time of stimulus presentation. Activation in LPFC (figure 5.2) increased with reward probability, magnitude and their combination of expected value,[140] underweighted small but overweighted large reward probabilities,[136] and integrated value and risk (independent and dissociable from probability) such that activation related to reward value increased further with the addition of risk if participants were risk seeking but decreased if they were risk averse.[137] Activation in medial prefrontal cortex, partly extending into ACC processed reward magnitude and expected value, whereas distinct regions in OFC processed reward probability (medial OFC) and risk (lateral OFC).[140] A second mediolateral dissociation occurred in OFC such that risk-related activations increased in medial regions the more risk seeking participants were and in lateral regions the more risk averse participants were.[140] These data confirm and extend human imaging data that have revealed a role of LPFC, ACC, and OFC in the processing of economic value,[34,40,46,47,65,96] temporal proximity to reward,[4,56,72] as well as risk, uncertainty, volatility and ambiguity.[11,20,35,53,54,98,137]

Figure 5.1
Single neurons encode value and actions. (A, B) Spike density histograms illustrating the activity recorded from single neurons under three different types of value manipulation (probability, payoff, or effort). The vertical lines indicate the onset of the pictures showing the value of the choice (left) and the time at which the animal was able to make his choice (right). The different colored lines indicate the value of the choice under consideration or which action the subject would select. (A) ACC neuron encodes payoff and effort but not probability. (B) ACC neuron encodes the value and action of all three decision variables. (C) Percentage of all neurons selective for value for each decision variable. All variables are predominately coded in ACC. (D) Percentage of all neurons selective for value as a function of number of decision variables encoded. ACC neurons tend to multiplex decision value across two (as in A) and three (as in B) decision variables. (E) Percentage of all neurons selective for action for each decision variable. OFC neurons are less likely to encode action information relative to LPFC and ACC. *, χ^2 test, $P < 0.05$.

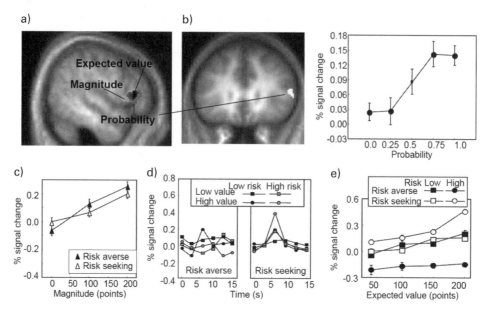

Figure 5.2
Activation in LPFC reflecting integrated reward value parameters. (a) Location of LPFC showing activation increases with stimuli predicting reward of larger magnitude, higher probability, and the combination of these two variables.[140] (b) Location (left) in LPFC region with activity (right) underweighting small and overweighting large predicted reward probability on presentation of reward predicting stimuli.[136] (c) Activation in LPFC increasing with stimuli predicting larger risk-free reward magnitudes, irrespective of risk attitude. (d) Time courses of activations to stimuli predicting low or high value and low or high risk, shown separately for risk-averse (left) and risk-seeking (right) participants. (e) With risk, value signals are further enhanced in risk-seeking participants but suppressed in risk-averse participants.[137]

Adaptive Coding of Outcome Value

Neurons have a limited firing rate range (typically < 50 Hz) with which to represent a seemingly infinite number of possible outcomes. However, some OFC neurons—particularly in area 13—solve this limitation by adjusting their firing rate to the range of values available.[67,89,143] Such adaptive coding is efficient because it allows for maximum discrimination between each distribution of possible outcomes, and it allows flexibility to encode values across decision contexts that may differ substantially in value (e.g., a choice of what type of food to buy versus a choice of what type of car to buy). However, the majority of outcome-sensitive OFC neurons do not adapt their firing rates to the range (or type) of outcomes available, thus encoding value on a fixed scale.[67,91] The fact that some OFC neurons are not range adaptive and thus are invariant to the set of offers available indicates value transitivity, a key trait of economic choice.[91] Thus, as a population, OFC expresses both range adaptation and value transitivity, indicating two fundamental traits necessary for optimal choice. Unfortunately, these studies did not examine activity of neurons in other frontal cortical regions. Although some evidence suggests that ACC neurons may adapt their firing rate depending on the distribution of values available,[51,116] reports of range adaptation in single neurons typically focus on OFC or areas outside of frontal cortex, such as striatal and dopamine neurons.[23,139] It therefore remains an open question whether range adaptation in frontal cortex is a unique trait of OFC neurons.

By adjusting neuronal activity based on the distribution of outcome values, adaptive coding provides an example of relative value processing, which is an integral part of modern economic theories such as prospect theory.[57] Human imaging data reveal adaptive as well as relative outcome coding in OFC[21,30,42] but also in ACC,[21,36] LPFC,[21,36,72] middorsal frontal cortex,[73,83] and regions outside frontal cortex such as posterior cingulate cortex,[83] parietal cortex,[73,83] striatum,[16,30,73,83] and amygdala.[16,30] Taken together, the data suggest that adaptive or relative value processing may not be only a cornerstone of economic theory but also a pervasive feature of the brain (see also Seymour and McClure[124]).

The Determination of Action Costs

Most studies of decision making tend to focus on variables that influence the value of an outcome, such as variables like risk, probability, and delay as discussed earlier. In natural environments, however, the distance and terrain that one might encounter in obtaining food (or traveling to work) produce energetic costs (e.g., effort), which is a critical component in optimal choice.[131,132] Growing evidence suggests that ACC may have a specialized role in influencing effort-based decision making. Damage to ACC biases animals toward actions that are associated with less effort even when a more rewarding option is available.[147] In contrast, OFC lesions impair delay-based decision making, but not effort-based decision making.[111] Several fMRI studies have also emphasized the role of the ACC and striatum in representing the effort costs necessary to obtain an outcome.[14,25,68,135]

Direct manipulations of physical effort during single-neuron electrophysiology of frontal cortex are sparse. Neurons in ACC increase their activity as monkeys work through multiple actions toward reward.[125] Although neurons in ACC are significantly more likely to encode effort than neurons in LPFC or OFC, this is also true for the reward variables.[58,60] Thus, while ACC may have a specialized role in encoding effort costs, this may be part of its broader role in integrating the costs and benefits of a choice option in the determination of which action is optimal (see below). Consistent with this proposal, a recent study using the t-maze barrier task known to require ACC[111,147] showed that ACC neurons adapt their firing rate based on the cost-benefit ratio, suggesting ACC may encode a net value (reward-cost) signal.[51]

Interestingly, although ACC and OFC activity changes with satiety state and OFC lesions impair performance following reinforcer devaluation, damage to either OFC or ACC has no effect on an animal's willingness to work for reward, as shown in tests requiring animals to work progressively harder for reward.[8,55,94] Yet, in choice contexts where the amount of work is varied, ACC (but not OFC) lesions induce a preference for less work.[111,147] This implies that neither ACC nor OFC encodes a generalized motivational signal that drives behavior in all contexts. Rather, OFC maintains and updates expectancies about the specific outcomes associated with sensory stimuli that may be influenced by internal states,[17,119,134,143] while ACC appears to represent and update action-value associations,[62,112] a dissociation that is directly supported by lesion evidence.[109]

Although there has been considerable interest in the role of dopamine in cost-benefit calculation and its influence on the exertion of effort to obtain an outcome,[84,95,114,150] the way in which dopamine might functionally interact with frontal cortex in this process is far from clear. Dopamine antagonists or dopamine depletions within the nucleus accumbens (NAc) induce rats to prefer less effortful options.[22,28,115] Given that ACC lesions produce shifts toward less effortful options[111,147] and ACC receives a large dopamine input,[12,153] it is tempting to speculate that dopamine might influence ACC directly in effort-based decision making. Yet, while systemic and NAc dopamine depletion alters effort-based choice, direct dopamine depletion or blockade within ACC has had inconsistent effects.[28,120,121,148,149] Moreover, although dopamine release in the NAc reflects the rewarding value of an outcome, it encodes little information about the physical effort necessary to obtain the outcome.[38]

Linking Value to Action

Although neurons throughout the frontal cortex encode information about the value of an outcome, how these neurons influence action selection clearly differentiates frontal areas. Both ACC and LPFC send projections to the premotor areas, whereas OFC receives strong sensory input but weakly connects with motor areas.[18,19,24,29,152] Consistent with this anatomy, neurophysiological studies have consistently reported that ACC neurons tend to encode the value of the outcome and the action that led to the outcome.[49,58,74,75] LPFC neurons also encode information about actions, but neurons here tend to encode associations between the stimulus and action, whereas ACC neurons preferentially encode information about the action and outcome.[74,75,146] In contrast, OFC neurons encode the value of sensory stimuli with little encoding of motor responses.[58,60,81,90,91,146] Some recent reports suggest that OFC neurons may encode action information but typically after the action has been performed and the outcome is experienced.[15,144] Furthermore, OFC lesions impair choices between stimuli (but not actions) associated with different values, while ACC dysfunction impairs choices based on action-outcome associations.[44,62,109,126] Although the stimulus-outcome and action-outcome dissociation have been proposed of OFC and ACC function, respectively,[109] it is noteworthy that inactivation of ACC disrupts learning about stimulus-outcome associations,[2] whereas signal changes in VMPFC correlate with both stimulus-outcome and action-outcome associations.[40]

ACC may have an additional role in monitoring the outcome of the selected action to guide behavioral adjustment and reinforcement learning, as ACC activity is sensitive to errors or deviations in reward expectancy,[1,52,76] reflects the history of reward associated with different actions,[62,122,123,133] tracks volatility in reward rate of different actions,[11] and encodes counterfactual information about unchosen outcomes.[21,36,48] Moreover, ACC neurons detect changes in action value—or how preferable one action is relative to another—to directly influence adaptive action selection.[74,126,154] This suggests ACC—perhaps owing to its role in representing the effort costs of a decision—calculates the value of the action producing the outcome and monitors the success of behavioral outcomes over time to guide adaptive behavior. The representation of action value in ACC is likely influenced by interactions with the striatum, an area also known to encode action values.[70,117]

An additional action selection issue arises when different limbs/effectors can be used to make a response and therefore must be assigned a value. Recent research has explored whether different effectors, such as the left and the right hand, or the hand and the eye, use separate or shared value signals[39,92] (but see also Boorman and Glascher et al.[13,40]). While value signals in parietal cortex[39] and supplementary motor area[155] appear to be lateralized and effector-specific, results conflict as to whether VMPFC emits a net, nonlateralized chosen value signal,[39] a lateralized, effector-specific one emitted irrespective of choice[92] or both effector-specific and effector-unspecific value signals for chosen actions only.[155] Similarly, results conflict as to whether the striatum emits a lateralized, effector-specific[39] or a general, nonspecific prediction error signal.[92]

Integration or Specialization of Decision Variable Representations

Formal decision models suggest that the determination of an action's overall value rests on the integration of both the costs and benefits of a decision, akin to a neural currency.[80,101] Whether single neurons are capable of integrating across decision variables is a topic of great interest. Unfortunately, few electrophysiology studies have manipulated multiple decision variables in the same trial, a necessary component to examine the integration of decision variables into a net value signal. It is therefore important to draw distinctions between a neuron that encodes two decision variables when tested independently (or across studies) and a neuron that encodes the sum or difference of the two variables when they are assessed conjointly in the same testing session (integration).

There is some evidence to suggest that frontal areas might play an important role in this integration process. In ACC, neurons integrate both size and probability of reward,[2,116] multiplex reward size and probability with effort cost,[58] and encodes a signal indicative of net value.[51] Neurons in LPFC encode both positive and negative events[66] and integrate reward and delay information to form a temporally discounted value signal.[64] Neurons in OFC integrate preference and magnitude of reward,[90,91] and are sensitive to both reward size and delay[105] or positive and negative events[81,104] as if coding value on a common scale. However, for other OFC neurons, variables such as reward size and delay,[107] size and risk of reward,[85] or rewarding and aversive events[81] are encoded by largely separate populations of neurons.

A possible explanation for these discrepancies in OFC is that the studies by Roesch and colleagues[105,107] manipulated delay and reward size independently, just as we manipulated reward probability, magnitude, and effort independently.[58] Even though OFC and ACC neurons encode the value of multiple variables in these tasks as if they are multiplexing value parameters (figure 5.1), integrating these variables onto a common value scale was not necessary for optimal performance. Thus, differences in the degree to which neurons encode multiple decision variables or integrate across variables might depend on the task design or the strategy the subject uses to solve the task. When tasks specifically require integration across decision variables, neurons in OFC,[90] LPFC,[64] and ACC[2,51] each encode value as a common currency. In each case however, only a single brain area was examined, thus a systematic examination of neurons from different brain areas in a multivariable decision-making task is necessary to determine the functional specialization of these areas with respect to encoding an integrated value representation.

Although functional neuroimaging can identify only population (rather than single neuron) activity, several neuroimaging studies have also suggested that OFC and LPFC activity reflects an integrated value signal.[69,141] On the basis of neuroimaging and functional connectivity analyses,[45,46] Rangel and colleagues argue that though some brain regions may be functionally specialized for encoding particular decision variables, ultimately OFC (together with LPFC) integrates information about separate decision variables into a stimulus value that is used to guide choice.[101] We have shown that LPFC activity integrates reward probability and magnitude into expected value as well as reward value and risk (distinct from probability) into a risk-sensitive value signal.[137,140] A number of studies have also implicated areas of the striatum in the process of integrating across decision variables, including the representation of net value.[14,25,140]

At the same time, functional neuroimaging also suggests some apparent functional specialization with respect to valuation processes. For example, VMPFC appears to process preferentially reward magnitude rather than probability.[65,140] Moreover, ACC as well as posterior cingulate cortex process primarily the appetitive value of decision outcomes, whereas midcingulate regions process primarily aversive outcomes,[37] a regional specialization that coincides with many findings on positive and negative emotion. More dorsally adjacent regions encode the whole spectrum from aversive to appetitive outcomes.[37] Several studies have emphasized the role of ACC in social decision making.[9,10,110,113,142] More anterior frontal regions track the value, and thus the advantage, of switching to alternative courses of action.[13] Finally, experienced value appears to activate more anterior regions of medial OFC than decision value.[130]

Valence versus Saliency: The Evil Confound

An important issue potentially confounding the interpretation of value computations in the brain is the degree to which value signals can be independently interpreted from saliency signals.[77,103,106,138] Humans and animals are naturally more motivated by more valuable outcomes, thus processes like attention, arousal, motivation, or motor preparation all strongly correlate with value. One study highlighted this issue by recording from six different frontal areas and found that neurons encoding reward magnitude were most prevalent in premotor (rather than PFC) areas, which could reflect the way in which increasing value motivates the motor system to facilitate behavior.[103] Thus, even if we identify neurons that apparently encode a signal reflecting the subjective value of an outcome, these neurons could simply be encoding a saliency signal.

One approach to resolving this issue examines neuronal responses to both appetitive and aversive outcomes. Value signals incorporate both rewarding and aversive events on a linear scale, typically being positive for appetitive stimuli and negative for aversive stimuli. In contrast, saliency signals increase as a function of behavioral importance irrespective of its valence, and thus typically follow a v-shaped curve with increasing activation for both increasingly rewarding and increasingly aversive stimuli. LPFC, OFC, and premotor cortex each contain neurons that exhibit preferences for aversive or rewarding valence. However, for neurons that encode both types of valence, OFC neurons encode valence along a common value scale whereas premotor and PFC neurons tend to be modulated by both large rewards and large punishments indicative of a salience signal.[66,81,104] Recent functional neuroimaging and electrophysiology studies provide further support that saliency and value are dissociated; OFC, LPFC, and rostral ACC encode a value signal, while the amygdala and medial and lateral premotor areas encode a salience signal.[3,71,118,129,141]

Value signals are quickly becoming ubiquitous, evident not just in PFC areas as described thus far, but also in amygdala, premotor, parietal, posterior cingulate, and visual areas to name a few.[78,93,97,103,128] Although this emphasizes the importance the brain places on value representations—possibly to promote reinforcement learning and eventually inclusive fitness—it is unlikely these signals all serve the same function, especially given that damage to different brain areas does not always impair decision making. In fact, impairments in decision making and goal-directed behavior are typically present only after damage to frontal cortex and/or basal ganglia.[31–33,88,109,110,154] Thus, disambiguating the initial abstraction of an option's value from the associated cognitive processes that arise from the recognition that an option is valuable (e.g., attention, arousal, motivation) is paramount to advancing our understanding of how the brain facilitates optimal choice behavior.

Conclusion

Over the past two decades it has become clear that value signals are ubiquitous in the brain. Yet, evidence from neuropsychological studies emphasizes the importance of frontal cortex in decision making and goal-directed behavior. Mounting evidence points to a fundamental role of OFC in determining the current expected value of a behavioral outcome. ACC may integrate information about a decision's expected outcome (potentially from signals in OFC and amygdala) with information about an action's value to determine which course of behavior is optimal. LPFC may have a more indirect role in valuation, such as in allocating attentional resources or cognitive control to encode behaviorally relevant information.[46,61,79,102] Although we have highlighted a number of important computations necessary for optimal choice, disambiguating these computations to infer functional specialization in value computation continues to be a challenge.[11,47] Moreover, the ubiquity of these representations across multiple brain areas emphasizes the importance of direct comparison of different brain areas to determine the functional order and hierarchy in which these value computations are being performed.[58,59,103,146]

Acknowledgments

The preparation of this manuscript was supported by a Wellcome Trust VIP Award to SWK, and a University Research Fellowship of the Royal Society to PNT. The authors have no competing interests.

Outstanding Questions

• What are the mechanisms by which internal states (hunger/thirst) influence and update action values in the determination of whether a course of action is worth pursuing?

• How do dopamine and other neurotransmitters functionally interact with the striatum and cortex in the process by which the costs and benefits of an action are learned to influence optimal decision making?

• Value signals are ubiquitous in the brain. Does neuronal activity that correlates with value in different brain areas reflect essential value computations, or does it reflect associated cognitive processes (e.g., attention, arousal, motivation) that arise from the recognition that an option is valuable?

Further Reading

Glimcher PW, Camerer CF, Fehr E, Poldrach RA, eds. 2009. Neuroeconomics: Decision Making and the Brain. Amsterdam: Academic Press. An edited volume that provides an overview and history of the field of neuroeconomics.

Rushworth MFS, Behrens TEJ. 2008. Choice, uncertainty and value in prefrontal and cingulate cortex. *Nat Neurosci* 11: 389–397. An in-depth review of the roles of the prefrontal and cingulate cortex in reward processing, showing that it is not only the magnitude of the expected reward that modulates activity in these regions, but also the uncertainty in the estimate of the reward expectations, the value of the information to be gained, and the action costs.

Rangel A, Camerer C, and Montague PR. 2008. A framework for studying the neurobiology of value-based decision making. An attempt to bring together different aspects of decision making and reward processing into a single framework.

References

1. Amiez C, Joseph JP, Procyk E. 2005. Anterior cingulate error-related activity is modulated by predicted reward. *Eur J Neurosci* 21: 3447–3452.

2. Amiez C, Joseph JP, Procyk E. 2006. Reward encoding in the monkey anterior cingulate cortex. *Cereb Cortex* 16: 1040–1055.

3. Anderson AK, Christoff K, Stappen I, Panitz D, Ghahremani DG, Glover G, Gabrieli JD, Sobel N. 2003. Dissociated neural representations of intensity and valence in human olfaction. *Nat Neurosci* 6: 196–202.

4. Ballard K, Knutson B. 2009. Dissociable neural representations of future reward magnitude and delay during temporal discounting. *Neuroimage* 45: 143–150.

5. Batterham RL, ffytche DH, Rosenthal JM, Zelaya FO, Barker GJ, Withers DJ, Williams SC. 2007. PYY modulation of cortical and hypothalamic brain areas predicts feeding behaviour in humans. *Nature* 450: 106–109.

6. Baxter MG, Gaffan D, Kyriazis DA, Mitchell AS. 2008. Dorsolateral prefrontal lesions do not impair tests of scene learning and decision-making that require frontal-temporal interaction. *Eur J Neurosci* 28: 491–499.

7. Baxter MG, Gaffan D, Kyriazis DA, Mitchell AS. 2009. Ventrolateral prefrontal cortex is required for performance of a strategy implementation task but not reinforcer devaluation effects in rhesus monkeys. *Eur J Neurosci* 29: 2049–2059.

8. Baxter MG, Parker A, Lindner CC, Izquierdo AD, Murray EA. 2000. Control of response selection by reinforcer value requires interaction of amygdala and orbital prefrontal cortex. *J Neurosci* 20: 4311–4319.

9. Behrens TE, Hunt LT, Rushworth MF. 2009. The computation of social behavior. *Science* 324: 1160–1164.

10. Behrens TE, Hunt LT, Woolrich MW, Rushworth MF. 2008. Associative learning of social value. *Nature* 456: 245–249.

11. Behrens TE, Woolrich MW, Walton ME, Rushworth MF. 2007. Learning the value of information in an uncertain world. *Nat Neurosci* 10: 1214–1221.

12. Berger B. 1992. Dopaminergic innervation of the frontal cerebral cortex. Evolutionary trends and functional implications. *Adv Neurol* 57: 525–544.

13. Boorman ED, Behrens TE, Woolrich MW, Rushworth MF. 2009. How green is the grass on the other side? Frontopolar cortex and the evidence in favor of alternative courses of action. *Neuron* 62: 733–743.

14. Botvinick MM, Huffstetler S, McGuire JT. 2009. Effort discounting in human nucleus accumbens. *Cogn Affect Behav Neurosci* 9: 16–27.

15. Bouret S, Richmond BJ. 2010. Ventromedial and orbital prefrontal neurons differentially encode internally and externally driven motivational values in monkeys. *J Neurosci* 30: 8591–8601.

16. Breiter HC, Aharon I, Kahneman D, Dale A, Shizgal P. 2001. Functional imaging of neural responses to expectancy and experience of monetary gains and losses. *Neuron* 30: 619–639.

17. Burke KA, Franz TM, Miller DN, Schoenbaum G. 2008. The role of the orbitofrontal cortex in the pursuit of happiness and more specific rewards. *Nature* 454: 340–344.

18. Carmichael ST, Price JL. 1995. Sensory and premotor connections of the orbital and medial prefrontal cortex of macaque monkeys. *J Comp Neurol* 363: 642–664.

19. Cavada C, Company T, Tejedor J, Cruz-Rizzolo RJ, Reinoso-Suarez F. 2000. The anatomical connections of the macaque monkey orbitofrontal cortex: a review. *Cereb Cortex* 10: 220–242.

20. Christopoulos GI, Tobler PN, Bossaerts P, Dolan RJ, Schultz W. 2009. Neural correlates of value, risk, and risk aversion contributing to decision making under risk. *J Neurosci* 29: 12574–12583.

21. Coricelli G, Critchley HD, Joffily M, O'Doherty JP, Sirigu A, Dolan RJ. 2005. Regret and its avoidance: a neuroimaging study of choice behavior. *Nat Neurosci* 8: 1255–1262.

22. Cousins MS, Salamone JD. 1994. Nucleus accumbens dopamine depletions in rats affect relative response allocation in a novel cost/benefit procedure. *Pharmacol Biochem Behav* 49: 85–91.

23. Cromwell HC, Hassani OK, Schultz W. 2005. Relative reward processing in primate striatum. *Exp Brain Res* 162: 520–525.

24. Croxson PL, Johansen-Berg H, Behrens TE, Robson MD, Pinsk MA, Gross CG, Richter W, Richter MC, Kastner S, Rushworth MF. 2005. Quantitative investigation of connections of the prefrontal cortex in the human and macaque using probabilistic diffusion tractography. *J Neurosci* 25: 8854–8866.

25. Croxson PL, Walton ME, O'Reilly JX, Behrens TE, Rushworth MF. 2009. Effort-based cost-benefit valuation and the human brain. *J Neurosci* 29: 4531–4541.

26. de Araujo IE, Gutierrez R, Oliveira-Maia AJ, Pereira A, Jr, Nicolelis MA, Simon SA. 2006. Neural ensemble coding of satiety states. *Neuron* 51: 483–494.

27. De Araujo IE, Kringelbach ML, Rolls ET, McGlone F. 2003. Human cortical responses to water in the mouth, and the effects of thirst. *J Neurophysiol* 90: 1865–1876.

28. Denk F, Walton ME, Jennings KA, Sharp T, Rushworth MF, Bannerman DM. 2005. Differential involvement of serotonin and dopamine systems in cost-benefit decisions about delay or effort. *Psychopharmacology (Berl)* 179: 587–596.

29. Dum RP, Strick PL. 1993. Cingulate motor areas. In: Neurobiology of Cingulate Cortex and Limbic Thalamus: A Comprehensive Handbook (Vogt BA, Gabriel M, eds), pp 415–441. Cambridge, MA: Birkhaeuser.

30. Elliott R, Agnew Z, Deakin JF. 2008. Medial orbitofrontal cortex codes relative rather than absolute value of financial rewards in humans. *Eur J Neurosci* 27: 2213–2218.

31. Eslinger PJ, Damasio AR. 1985. Severe disturbance of higher cognition after bilateral frontal lobe ablation: patient EVR. *Neurology* 35: 1731–1741.

32. Fellows LK. 2006. Deciding how to decide: ventromedial frontal lobe damage affects information acquisition in multi-attribute decision making. *Brain* 129: 944–952.

33. Fellows LK, Farah MJ. 2005. Different underlying impairments in decision-making following ventromedial and dorsolateral frontal lobe damage in humans. *Cereb Cortex* 15: 58–63.

34. FitzGerald TH, Seymour B, Dolan RJ. 2009. The role of human orbitofrontal cortex in value comparison for incommensurable objects. *J Neurosci* 29: 8388–8395.

35. Floden D, Alexander MP, Kubu CS, Katz D, Stuss DT. 2008. Impulsivity and risk-taking behavior in focal frontal lobe lesions. *Neuropsychologia* 46: 213–223.

36. Fujiwara J, Tobler PN, Taira M, Iijima T, Tsutsui K. 2009. A parametric relief signal in human ventrolateral prefrontal cortex. *Neuroimage* 44: 1163–1170.

37. Fujiwara J, Tobler PN, Taira M, Iijima T, Tsutsui K. 2009. Segregated and integrated coding of reward and punishment in the cingulate cortex. *J Neurophysiol* 101: 3284–3293.

38. Gan JO, Walton ME, Phillips PE. 2010. Dissociable cost and benefit encoding of future rewards by mesolimbic dopamine. *Nat Neurosci* 13: 25–27.

39. Gershman SJ, Pesaran B, Daw ND. 2009. Human reinforcement learning subdivides structured action spaces by learning effector-specific values. *J Neurosci* 29: 13524–13531.

40. Glascher J, Hampton AN, O'Doherty JP. 2009. Determining a role for ventromedial prefrontal cortex in encoding action-based value signals during reward-related decision making. *Cereb Cortex* 19: 483–495.

41. Gottfried JA, O'Doherty J, Dolan RJ. 2003. Encoding predictive reward value in human amygdala and orbitofrontal cortex. *Science* 301: 1104–1107.

42. Grabenhorst F, Rolls ET. 2009. Different representations of relative and absolute subjective value in the human brain. *Neuroimage* 48: 258–268.

43. Haase L, Cerf-Ducastel B, Murphy C. 2009. Cortical activation in response to pure taste stimuli during the physiological states of hunger and satiety. *Neuroimage* 44: 1008–1021.

44. Hadland KA, Rushworth MF, Gaffan D, Passingham RE. 2003. The anterior cingulate and reward-guided selection of actions. *J Neurophysiol* 89: 1161–1164.

45. Hare TA, Camerer CF, Knoepfle DT, Rangel A. 2010. Value computations in ventral medial prefrontal cortex during charitable decision making incorporate input from regions involved in social cognition. *J Neurosci* 30: 583–590.

46. Hare TA, Camerer CF, Rangel A. 2009. Self-control in decision-making involves modulation of the vmPFC valuation system. *Science* 324: 646–648.

47. Hare TA, O'Doherty J, Camerer CF, Schultz W, Rangel A. 2008. Dissociating the role of the orbitofrontal cortex and the striatum in the computation of goal values and prediction errors. *J Neurosci* 28: 5623–5630.

48. Hayden BY, Pearson JM, Platt ML. 2009. Fictive reward signals in the anterior cingulate cortex. *Science* 324: 948–950.

49. Hayden BY, Platt ML. 2010. Neurons in anterior cingulate cortex multiplex information about reward and action. *J Neurosci* 30: 3339–3346.

50. Hikosaka K, Watanabe M. 2000. Delay activity of orbital and lateral prefrontal neurons of the monkey varying with different rewards. *Cereb Cortex* 10: 263–271.

51. Hillman KL, Bilkey DK. 2010. Neurons in the rat anterior cingulate cortex dynamically encode cost-benefit in a spatial decision-making task. *J Neurosci* 30: 7705–7713.

52. Holroyd CB, Coles MG. 2002. The neural basis of human error processing: reinforcement learning, dopamine, and the error-related negativity. *Psychol Rev* 109: 679–709.

53. Hsu M, Bhatt M, Adolphs R, Tranel D, Camerer CF. 2005. Neural systems responding to degrees of uncertainty in human decision-making. *Science* 310: 1680–1683.

54. Huettel SA, Stowe CJ, Gordon EM, Warner BT, Platt ML. 2006. Neural signatures of economic preferences for risk and ambiguity. *Neuron* 49: 765–775.

55. Izquierdo A, Suda RK, Murray EA. 2004. Bilateral orbital prefrontal cortex lesions in rhesus monkeys disrupt choices guided by both reward value and reward contingency. *J Neurosci* 24: 7540–7548.

56. Kable JW, Glimcher PW. 2007. The neural correlates of subjective value during intertemporal choice. *Nat Neurosci* 10: 1625–1633.

57. Kahneman D, Tversky A. 1979. Prospect theory: an analysis of decision under risk. *Econometrica* 47: 263–291.

58. Kennerley SW, Dahmubed AF, Lara AH, Wallis JD. 2009. Neurons in the frontal lobe encode the value of multiple decision variables. *J Cogn Neurosci* 21: 1162–1178.

59. Kennerley SW, Wallis JD. 2009. Encoding of reward and space during a working memory task in the orbitofrontal cortex and anterior cingulate sulcus. *J Neurophysiol* 102: 3352–3364.

60. Kennerley SW, Wallis JD. 2009. Evaluating choices by single neurons in the frontal lobe: outcome value encoded across multiple decision variables. *Eur J Neurosci* 29: 2061–2073.

61. Kennerley SW, Wallis JD. 2009. Reward-dependent modulation of working memory in lateral prefrontal cortex. *J Neurosci* 29: 3259–3270.

62. Kennerley SW, Walton ME, Behrens TE, Buckley MJ, Rushworth MF. 2006. Optimal decision making and the anterior cingulate cortex. *Nat Neurosci* 9: 940–947.

63. Kepecs A, Uchida N, Zariwala HA, Mainen ZF. 2008. Neural correlates, computation and behavioural impact of decision confidence. *Nature* 455: 227–231.

64. Kim S, Hwang J, Lee D. 2008. Prefrontal coding of temporally discounted values during intertemporal choice. *Neuron* 59: 161–172.

65. Knutson B, Taylor J, Kaufman M, Peterson R, Glover G. 2005. Distributed neural representation of expected value. *J Neurosci* 25: 4806–4812.

66. Kobayashi S, Nomoto K, Watanabe M, Hikosaka O, Schultz W, Sakagami M. 2006. Influences of rewarding and aversive outcomes on activity in macaque lateral prefrontal cortex. *Neuron* 51: 861–870.

67. Kobayashi S, Pinto de Carvalho O, Schultz W. 2010. Adaptation of reward sensitivity in orbitofrontal neurons. *J Neurosci* 30: 534–544.

68. Kurniawan IT, Seymour B, Talmi D, Yoshida W, Chater N, Dolan RJ. 2010. Choosing to make an effort: the role of striatum in signaling physical effort of a chosen action. *J Neurophysiol* 104: 313–321.

69. Labudda K, Woermann FG, Mertens M, Pohlmann-Eden B, Markowitsch HJ, Brand M. 2008. Neural correlates of decision making with explicit information about probabilities and incentives in elderly healthy subjects. *Exp Brain Res* 187: 641–650.

70. Lau B, Glimcher PW. 2008. Value representations in the primate striatum during matching behavior. *Neuron* 58: 451–463.

71. Litt A, Plassmann H, Shiv B, Rangel A. 2011. Dissociating valuation and saliency signals during decision-making. *Cereb Cortex* 21: 95–102.

72. Lohrenz T, McCabe K, Camerer CF, Montague PR. 2007. Neural signature of fictive learning signals in a sequential investment task. *Proc Natl Acad Sci USA* 104: 9493–9498.

73. Lohrenz T, McCabe K, Camerer CF, Montague PR. 2007. Neural signature of fictive learning signals in a sequential investment task. *Proc Natl Acad Sci USA* 104: 9493–9498.

74. Luk CH, Wallis JD. 2009. Dynamic encoding of responses and outcomes by neurons in medial prefrontal cortex. *J Neurosci* 29: 7526–7539.

75. Matsumoto K, Suzuki W, Tanaka K. 2003. Neuronal correlates of goal-based motor selection in the prefrontal cortex. *Science* 301: 229–232.

76. Matsumoto M, Matsumoto K, Abe H, Tanaka K. 2007. Medial prefrontal cell activity signaling prediction errors of action values. *Nat Neurosci* 10: 647–656.

77. Maunsell JH. 2004. Neuronal representations of cognitive state: Reward or attention? *Trends Cogn Sci* 8: 261–265.

78. McCoy AN, Crowley JC, Haghighian G, Dean HL, Platt ML. 2003. Saccade reward signals in posterior cingulate cortex. *Neuron* 40: 1031–1040.

79. Miller EK, Cohen JD. 2001. An integrative theory of prefrontal cortex function. *Annu Rev Neurosci* 24: 167–202.

80. Montague PR, Berns GS. 2002. Neural economics and the biological substrates of valuation. *Neuron* 36: 265–284.

81. Morrison SE, Salzman CD. 2009. The convergence of information about rewarding and aversive stimuli in single neurons. *J Neurosci* 29: 11471–11483.

82. Nakano Y, Oomura Y, Nishino H, Aou S, Yamamoto T, Nemoto S. 1984. Neuronal activity in the medial orbitofrontal cortex of the behaving monkey: modulation by glucose and satiety. *Brain Res Bull* 12: 381–385.

83. Nieuwenhuis S, Heslenfeld DJ, von Geusau NJ, Mars RB, Holroyd CB, Yeung N. 2005. Activity in human reward-sensitive brain areas is strongly context dependent. *Neuroimage* 25: 1302–1309.

84. Niv Y, Daw ND, Joel D, Dayan P. 2007. Tonic dopamine: opportunity costs and the control of response vigor. *Psychopharmacology (Berl)* 191: 507–520.

85. O'Neill M, Schultz W. 2010. Coding of reward risk by orbitofrontal neurons is mostly distinct from coding of reward value. *Neuron* 68: 789–800.

86. Ongur D, Price JL. 2000. The organization of networks within the orbital and medial prefrontal cortex of rats, monkeys and humans. *Cereb Cortex* 10: 206–219.

87. Ostlund SB, Balleine BW. 2007. The contribution of orbitofrontal cortex to action selection. *Ann NY Acad Sci* 1121: 174–192.

88. Owen AM. 1997. Cognitive planning in humans: neuropsychological, neuroanatomical and neuropharmacological perspectives. *Prog Neurobiol* 53: 431–450.

89. Padoa-Schioppa C. 2009. Range-adapting representation of economic value in the orbitofrontal cortex. *J Neurosci* 29: 14004–14014.

90. Padoa-Schioppa C, Assad JA. 2006. Neurons in the orbitofrontal cortex encode economic value. *Nature* 441: 223–226.

91. Padoa-Schioppa C, Assad JA. 2008. The representation of economic value in the orbitofrontal cortex is invariant for changes of menu. *Nat Neurosci* 11: 95–102.

92. Palminteri S, Boraud T, Lafargue G, Dubois B, Pessiglione M. 2009. Brain hemispheres selectively track the expected value of contralateral options. *J Neurosci* 29: 13465–13472.

93. Paton JJ, Belova MA, Morrison SE, Salzman CD. 2006. The primate amygdala represents the positive and negative value of visual stimuli during learning. *Nature* 439: 865–870.

94. Pears A, Parkinson JA, Hopewell L, Everitt BJ, Roberts AC. 2003. Lesions of the orbitofrontal but not medial prefrontal cortex disrupt conditioned reinforcement in primates. *J Neurosci* 23: 11189–11201.

95. Phillips PE, Walton ME, Jhou TC. 2007. Calculating utility: preclinical evidence for cost-benefit analysis by mesolimbic dopamine. *Psychopharmacology (Berl)* 191: 483–495.

96. Plassmann H, O'Doherty J, Rangel A. 2007. Orbitofrontal cortex encodes willingness to pay in everyday economic transactions. *J Neurosci* 27: 9984–9988.

97. Platt ML, Glimcher PW. 1999. Neural correlates of decision variables in parietal cortex. *Nature* 400: 233–238.

98. Preuschoff K, Bossaerts P, Quartz SR. 2006. Neural differentiation of expected reward and risk in human subcortical structures. *Neuron* 51: 381–390.

99. Quilodran R, Rothe M, Procyk E. 2008. Behavioral shifts and action valuation in the anterior cingulate cortex. *Neuron* 57: 314–325.

100. Rangel A, Camerer C, Montague PR. 2008. A framework for studying the neurobiology of value-based decision making. *Nat Rev Neurosci* 9: 545–556.

101. Rangel A, Hare T. 2010. Neural computations associated with goal-directed choice. *Curr Opin Neurobiol* 20: 262–270.

102. Rao SC, Rainer G, Miller EK. 1997. Integration of what and where in the primate prefrontal cortex. *Science* 276: 821–824.

103. Roesch MR, Olson CR. 2003. Impact of expected reward on neuronal activity in prefrontal cortex, frontal and supplementary eye fields and premotor cortex. *J Neurophysiol* 90: 1766–1789.

104. Roesch MR, Olson CR. 2004. Neuronal activity related to reward value and motivation in primate frontal cortex. *Science* 304: 307–310.

105. Roesch MR, Olson CR. 2005. Neuronal activity in primate orbitofrontal cortex reflects the value of time. *J Neurophysiol* 94: 2457–2471.

106. Roesch MR, Olson CR. 2007. Neuronal activity related to anticipated reward in frontal cortex: Does it represent value or reflect motivation? *Ann N Y Acad Sci* 1121: 431–446.

107. Roesch MR, Taylor AR, Schoenbaum G. 2006. Encoding of time-discounted rewards in orbitofrontal cortex is independent of value representation. *Neuron* 51: 509–520.

108. Rolls ET, Sienkiewicz ZJ, Yaxley S. 1989. Hunger modulates the responses to gustatory stimuli of single neurons in the caudolateral orbitofrontal cortex of the macaque monkey. *Eur J Neurosci* 1: 53–60.

109. Rudebeck PH, Behrens TE, Kennerley SW, Baxter MG, Buckley MJ, Walton ME, Rushworth MF. 2008. Frontal cortex subregions play distinct roles in choices between actions and stimuli. *J Neurosci* 28: 13775–13785.

110. Rudebeck PH, Buckley MJ, Walton ME, Rushworth MF. 2006. A role for the macaque anterior cingulate gyrus in social valuation. *Science* 313: 1310–1312.

111. Rudebeck PH, Walton ME, Smyth AN, Bannerman DM, Rushworth MF. 2006. Separate neural pathways process different decision costs. *Nat Neurosci* 9: 1161–1168.

112. Rushworth MF, Behrens TE. 2008. Choice, uncertainty and value in prefrontal and cingulate cortex. *Nat Neurosci* 11: 389–397.

113. Rushworth MF, Behrens TE, Rudebeck PH, Walton ME. 2007. Contrasting roles for cingulate and orbitofrontal cortex in decisions and social behaviour. *Trends Cogn Sci* 11: 168–176.

114. Salamone JD, Correa M, Farrar A, Mingote SM. 2007. Effort-related functions of nucleus accumbens dopamine and associated forebrain circuits. *Psychopharmacology (Berl)* 191: 461–482.

115. Salamone JD, Cousins MS, Bucher S. 1994. Anhedonia or anergia? Effects of haloperidol and nucleus accumbens dopamine depletion on instrumental response selection in a T-maze cost/benefit procedure. *Behav Brain Res* 65: 221–229.

116. Sallet J, Quilodran R, Rothe M, Vezoli J, Joseph JP, Procyk E. 2007. Expectations, gains, and losses in the anterior cingulate cortex. *Cogn Affect Behav Neurosci* 7: 327–336.

117. Samejima K, Ueda Y, Doya K, Kimura M. 2005. Representation of action-specific reward values in the striatum. *Science* 310: 1337–1340.

118. Scangos KW, Stuphorn V. 2010. Medial frontal cortex motivates but does not control movement initiation in the countermanding task. *J Neurosci* 30: 1968–1982.

119. Schoenbaum G, Roesch MR, Stalnaker TA, Takahashi YK. 2009. A new perspective on the role of the orbitofrontal cortex in adaptive behaviour. *Nat Rev Neurosci* 10: 885–892.

120. Schweimer J, Hauber W. 2006. Dopamine D1 receptors in the anterior cingulate cortex regulate effort-based decision making. *Learn Mem* 13: 777–782.

121. Schweimer J, Saft S, Hauber W. 2005. Involvement of catecholamine neurotransmission in the rat anterior cingulate in effort-related decision making. *Behav Neurosci* 119: 1687–1692.

122. Seo H, Lee D. 2007. Temporal filtering of reward signals in the dorsal anterior cingulate cortex during a mixed-strategy game. *J Neurosci* 27: 8366–8377.

123. Seo H, Lee D. 2009. Behavioral and neural changes after gains and losses of conditioned reinforcers. *J Neurosci* 29: 3627–3641.

124. Seymour B, McClure SM. 2008. Anchors, scales and the relative coding of value in the brain. *Curr Opin Neurobiol* 18: 173–178.

125. Shidara M, Richmond BJ. 2002. Anterior cingulate: single neuronal signals related to degree of reward expectancy. *Science* 296: 1709–1711.

126. Shima K, Tanji J. 1998. Role for cingulate motor area cells in voluntary movement selection based on reward. *Science* 282: 1335–1338.

127. Shizgal P. 1997. Neural basis of utility estimation. *Curr Opin Neurobiol* 7: 198–208.

128. Shuler MG, Bear MF. 2006. Reward timing in the primary visual cortex. *Science* 311: 1606–1609.

129. Small DM, Gregory MD, Mak YE, Gitelman D, Mesulam MM, Parrish T. 2003. Dissociation of neural representation of intensity and affective valuation in human gustation. *Neuron* 39: 701–711.

130. Smith DV, Hayden BY, Truong TK, Song AW, Platt ML, Huettel SA. 2010. Distinct value signals in anterior and posterior ventromedial prefrontal cortex. *J Neurosci* 30: 2490–2495.

131. Stephens DW, Krebs JR. 1986. Foraging Theory. Princeton, NJ: Princeton University Press.

132. Stevens JR, Rosati AG, Ross KR, Hauser MD. 2005. Will travel for food: spatial discounting in two new world monkeys. *Curr Biol* 15: 1855–1860.

133. Sul JH, Kim H, Huh N, Lee D, Jung MW. 2010. Distinct roles of rodent orbitofrontal and medial prefrontal cortex in decision making. *Neuron* 66: 449–460.

134. Takahashi YK, Roesch MR, Stalnaker TA, Haney RZ, Calu DJ, Taylor AR, Burke KA, Schoenbaum G. 2009. The orbitofrontal cortex and ventral tegmental area are necessary for learning from unexpected outcomes. *Neuron* 62: 269–280.

135. Talmi D, Seymour B, Dayan P, Dolan RJ. 2008. Human pavlovian-instrumental transfer. *J Neurosci* 28: 360–368.

136. Tobler PN, Christopoulos GI, O'Doherty JP, Dolan RJ, Schultz W. 2008. Neuronal distortions of reward probability without choice. *J Neurosci* 28: 11703–11711.

137. Tobler PN, Christopoulos GI, O'Doherty JP, Dolan RJ, Schultz W. 2009. Risk-dependent reward value signal in human prefrontal cortex. *Proc Natl Acad Sci USA* 106: 7185–7190.

138. Tobler PN, Dickinson A, Schultz W. 2003. Coding of predicted reward omission by dopamine neurons in a conditioned inhibition paradigm. *J Neurosci* 23: 10402–10410.

139. Tobler PN, Fiorillo CD, Schultz W. 2005. Adaptive coding of reward value by dopamine neurons. *Science* 307: 1642–1645.

140. Tobler PN, O'Doherty JP, Dolan RJ, Schultz W. 2007. Reward value coding distinct from risk attitude-related uncertainty coding in human reward systems. *J Neurophysiol* 97: 1621–1632.

141. Tom SM, Fox CR, Trepel C, Poldrack RA. 2007. The neural basis of loss aversion in decision-making under risk. *Science* 315: 515–518.

142. Tomlin D, Kayali MA, King-Casas B, Anen C, Camerer CF, Quartz SR, Montague PR. 2006. Agent-specific responses in the cingulate cortex during economic exchanges. *Science* 312: 1047–1050.

143. Tremblay L, Schultz W. 1999. Relative reward preference in primate orbitofrontal cortex. *Nature* 398: 704–708.

144. Tsujimoto S, Genovesio A, Wise SP. 2009. Monkey orbitofrontal cortex encodes response choices near feedback time. *J Neurosci* 29: 2569–2574.

145. Valentin VV, Dickinson A, O'Doherty JP. 2007. Determining the neural substrates of goal-directed learning in the human brain. *J Neurosci* 27: 4019–4026.

146. Wallis JD, Miller EK. 2003. Neuronal activity in primate dorsolateral and orbital prefrontal cortex during performance of a reward preference task. *Eur J Neurosci* 18: 2069–2081.

147. Walton ME, Bannerman DM, Rushworth MF. 2002. The role of rat medial frontal cortex in effort-based decision making. *J Neurosci* 22: 10996–11003.

148. Walton ME, Croxson PL, Rushworth MF, Bannerman DM. 2005. The mesocortical dopamine projection to anterior cingulate cortex plays no role in guiding effort-related decisions. *Behav Neurosci* 119: 323–328.

149. Walton ME, Groves J, Jennings KA, Croxson PL, Sharp T, Rushworth MF, Bannerman DM. 2009. Comparing the role of the anterior cingulate cortex and 6-hydroxydopamine nucleus accumbens lesions on operant effort-based decision making. *Eur J Neurosci* 29: 1678–1691.

150. Walton ME, Kennerley SW, Bannerman DM, Phillips PE, Rushworth MF. 2006. Weighing up the benefits of work: behavioral and neural analyses of effort-related decision making. *Neural Netw* 19: 1302–1314.

151. Wang XJ. 2008. Decision making in recurrent neuronal circuits. *Neuron* 60: 215–234.

152. Wang Y, Shima K, Isoda M, Sawamura H, Tanji J. 2002. Spatial distribution and density of prefrontal cortical cells projecting to three sectors of the premotor cortex. *Neuroreport* 13: 1341–1344.

153. Williams SM, Goldman-Rakic PS. 1993. Characterization of the dopaminergic innervation of the primate frontal cortex using a dopamine-specific antibody. *Cereb Cortex* 3: 199–222.

154. Williams ZM, Bush G, Rauch SL, Cosgrove GR, Eskandar EN. 2004. Human anterior cingulate neurons and the integration of monetary reward with motor responses. *Nat Neurosci* 7: 1370–1375.

155. Wunderlich K, Rangel A, O'Doherty JP. 2009. Neural computations underlying action-based decision making in the human brain. *Proc Natl Acad Sci USA* 106: 17199–17204.

6 A Comparative Perspective on Executive and Motivational Control by the Medial Prefrontal Cortex

Mark Laubach

The goal of this chapter is to describe recent efforts at understanding the functional significance of "prefrontal" areas in the cerebral cortex of rodents with regard to cognitive and motivational control. Previous discussions on the comparative anatomy of the prefrontal cortex have been framed around the question, "Do rats have prefrontal cortex?"[48,63] Researchers using rodents then tried to make the case that medial parts of the rodent frontal cortex are homologous to dorsolateral (granular) parts of frontal cortex that exist in primates. [63] Later, interest developed in medial regions of the prefrontal cortex and, though it was never resolved, the discussion about the precise nature of rodent prefrontal cortex seemed to go away. I would like to reexamine this issue, but from a different perspective. Rather than asking if rats have prefrontal cortex, I ask—to borrow a phrase from Jon Kaas[25]— "What, *if anything*, is rodent prefrontal cortex?" In this chapter, I try to answer this question based on studies of the anatomical connectivity between the medial prefrontal cortex (mPFC) and the hypothalamus, and on recent studies on mPFC during performance of simple reaction-time tasks. Together, these studies suggest that medial prefrontal regions have a privileged role in controlling the autonomic nervous system and thereby contribute at a most visceral level to cognitive and motivational control. A neural circuit model is proposed for the generation of persistent neural activity by medial prefrontal neurons based on competition between excitatory (reward expectation) and inhibitory (self-control) processing during the delay period of delayed response tasks. Finally, the evolutionary significance of cognitive and motivational control based on findings in the rodent mPFC is discussed.

What, *If Anything*, Is Rodent Prefrontal Cortex?

The prefrontal cortex in rodents and other "lower" mammals is located rostral to the genu of the corpus callosum and is comprised of three main regions: a dorsal area called anterior cingulate cortex, an intermediate area called the prelimbic cortex, and a ventral area called the infralimbic cortex. The relative locations of these areas are described in figure 6.1a, showing a saggital drawing of the rat brain.[60] A thick line denotes the location where our laboratory has worked to understand the functional properties of medial prefrontal neurons. A frontal section, illustrating the relative locations of the three main prefrontal regions, is shown in figure 6.1b. A notable feature of these cortical areas is that they are agranular, that is, they lack the thin layer of small, nonpyramidal neurons found in sensory regions of the cerebral cortex and also in granular regions of frontal cortex, such as the dorsolateral area 46.[48] The functional significance of this aspect of mPFC has remained a mystery as no study to date has compared neural activity patterns across layers in mPFC as has been done in other cortical regions, such as the somatosensory cortex.[31]

Studies in rodents, monkeys, and human beings have established that these cortical regions form a functionally connected network called the "medial" network.[44] A notable aspect of the medial network is its interconnectivity with the insular cortex and regions associated with the autonomic (or "visceral") nervous system (e.g., hypothalamus, nucleus of the solitary tract, parabrachial nucleus).[9,44] A clue to the functional significance of these connections may be the laminar patterns of corticocortical connections between the medial prefrontal and insular areas.[15] These connections are topographically organized such that the infralimbic region is most densely interconnected with oral and visceral sensory areas in the insular cortex,[23,66] the prelimbic area is densely interconnected with the dorsal agranular insular area, which contains neurons that are responsive to gustatory stimuli,[29] and the most dorsal cingulate region has relatively weak connectivity with insular areas. According to Gabbott,[15] insular-prefrontal connections are reciprocal and layer specific. Feedforward projections exist from the insular regions to the prelimbic and infralimbic cortices (i.e., neurons in layers II and III in the origin project to the same layers in the target[4]), and feedback connections exist between the medial prefrontal and insular cortices (i.e., neurons in layers II and III in the origin project to layers I and VI in the target[4]). As a result of these connections, specific subsets of medial and insular regions could become coactivated during behaviors that activate either brain network. However, as neurotransmitters such as dopamine have been shown to selectively enhance GABAergic processing in these cortical regions (e.g., ref. 61), it is also possible that medial and insular neurons could fire in reciprocal and sequential patterns when rewarding stimuli or other events lead to changes in dopamine release at a given location (or collection of locations) within the medial network. To date, no study has examined this issue by recording simultaneously in medial and insular regions in behaving animals.

In addition to differences in connectivity with the insular cortex, the three medial prefrontal areas can be distinguished on the basis of their efferent connectivity

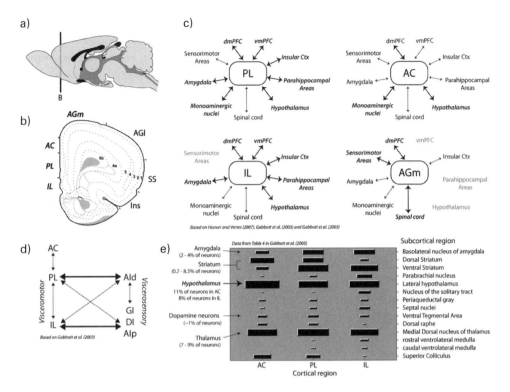

Figure 6.1

Anatomy of rodent medial prefrontal cortex. (a) Location of medial prefrontal cortex within the rat brain. A saggital view is shown for the rat brain (adapted from ref. 60). The thick line shows regions where reversible inactivation and neural recording studies have examined the role of medial prefrontal cortex in the top-down control of action. (b) Coronal section (adapted from ref. 60) at location denoted in (a). Primary cortical areas are given labels (IL, infralimbic; PL, prelimbic; AC, anterior cingulate; AGm, medial agranular; Agl, lateral agranular; SS, somatosensory; Ins, insula) and the four medial regions (IL, PL, AC, AGm) are highlighted in bold. Layers are shown as dashed lines. (c) Major anatomical connections of medial frontal areas. Ventromedial areas (IL and PL, termed vmPFC in the figure) are unique in having more connectivity with parahippocampal and amygdalar regions. Dorsomedial areas (AC and AGm, termed dmPFC in the figure) have more connectivity with sensorimotor areas, such the superior colliculus and spinal cord. The connections are based mostly on refs. 15, 16, 20, and 65. (d) Interconnections between medial and insular areas of frontal cortex, based on figure 5 in ref. 16. Connections between the prelimbic (PL) and dorsal agranular insular cortex (AId) and between the infralmbic (IL) and taste and visceral insular areas (granular, dysgranular, and posterior agranular insula) are more prominent than those between the immediately adjacent medial and insular areas. (e) Hinton diagram showing fractions of neurons projecting to various subcortical areas, based on table 4 in ref. 16. The main result from the analysis was that corticohypothalamic connections are the densest of all corticofugal connections from the three main parts of the medial prefrontal cortex.

(figure 6.1c, based primarily on refs. 16, 20, 56, 64, and 65; figure 6.1d, based on table 4 in ref. 16). The anterior cingulate area (AC) has extensive motor-related connectivity (including the motor cortex, superior colliculus, and spinal cord) that is similar to (although less than) its neighbor, the medial agranular area (AGm). The prelimbic area (PL) projects massively to the striatum (figure 6.1d), perhaps more than any other cortical area, and also to limbic system structures such as the basolateral amygdala and parahippocampal areas. The infralimbic area (IL) is most heavily connected with structures associated with the autonomic nervous system, such as the parabrachial nucleus, the nucleus of the solitary tract, and ventrolateral medulla, and it also projects to a unique subset of limbic areas (e.g., lateral septum, bed nucleus of stria terminalis[65]) that are not as heavily innervated by the more dorsal prefrontal areas. Importantly, projections from infralimbic cortex to brainstem autonomic centers may not be as extensive in primates.[14] Nevertheless, these overall patterns of connections suggest that the dorsomedial and ventromedial regions of prefrontal cortex differentially contribute to the control of skeletomotor and visceromotor functions, respectively.

To visualize the relative density of descending projections from medial prefrontal areas, I created a Hinton diagram (a graphical display developed for analyzing patterns of hidden units in neural networks) to understand the relative density of connections from medial prefrontal areas, as reported in table 4 in ref. 16 (see figure 6.1e). The plot revealed that all medial prefrontal regions project to the lateral hypothalamus and that these *projections are as dense as to any other brain area, including those to the mediodorsal thalamic nucleus (MD)*. This is of special note as projections to MD have traditionally been considered as the defining characteristic of rodent prefrontal cortex.[30] Unlike the connections from infralimbic cortex to brainstem autonomic centers, which may be weaker in primates,[14] projections to the hypothalamus are well developed in primates.[43] Far more neurons project to the hypothalamus than to other areas commonly featured in the literature, such as the amygdala, hippocampal formation, and midbrain dopamine neurons. Importantly, mPFC is also innervated directly by neurons in the hypothalamus.[53] Together with the connections from the insular cortex, these connections may serve as cortico-hypothalamic-cortical loops that encode persistent representations of visceral information.

In summary, medial prefrontal areas are distinct from other parts of the frontal cortex, especially with regard to their connections with "visceral" brain regions such as the hypothalamus. Rather than acting as a sort of "dorsolateral" PFC area in rodents,[63] medial prefrontal regions across species, especially those rostral to the genu of the corpus callosum,[65] have a special role in the integration of "limbic" and autonomic information.[9,44] By this view, the role of mPFC in cognitive and motivational control is likely to be *more like a coach than an executive*.

Top-Down Control over Action by Rodent Medial Prefrontal Cortex

Lesions in midline frontal areas of the human brain, including areas 24 and 32, result in slowed reactions to external stimuli,[59] and neuroimaging studies show that activations in mPFC can be correlated with reaction times[13,34] (but see ref. 36). These deficits may reflect a general role of medial parts of the prefrontal cortex in the executive control of behavior.[51] Executive control systems monitor ongoing actions and performance outcomes (success and failures) and enable adjustments of behavior. These processes are especially crucial as a behavioral procedure is learned for the first time.[18] Based on the anatomical data reviewed earlier, mPFC may serve to link recent actions to metabolically relevant outcomes during learning.

There are at least two potential interpretations of the change in reaction times following damage in mPFC. First, the effects could be due to impairments in assigning values to the action that must be made to the external stimulus, as expected based on lesions of mPFC impairing goal-directed aspects of instrumental learning.[10,28,45] Several recent neural recording studies in rats and monkeys support this interpretation, reporting neurons that fire selectively based on the outcome associated with a specific action.[2,3,11,27,33,38,39,49,50,57,62] For example, Matsumoto[33] found neurons in primate mPFC that responded to stimuli that indicated positive and negative outcomes, with changes in positive-outcome, but not negative-outcome, neurons occurring when monkeys learned new associations between actions and outcomes. Another study by Procyk[49] used a sequential motor task to study mPFC neural activity related to learning new action sequences. They found neurons in mPFC that responded when reward was delivered after the first correct performance of a movement sequence. Based on the anatomical data reviewed earlier, these signals could convey information about the animal's recent actions directly to the autonomic nervous system during learning.

A very different line of research suggests that mPFC has a role in inhibiting inappropriate actions in both rats[37,46,52] and humans.[6,12,17,24,47] For example, Passetti[46] found that lesions of rodent dorsal mPFC resulted in increased errors and loss of temporal control (e.g., increased premature responding) in a choice reaction-time task (similar to effects reported by our lab in the simple RT task[37]). By contrast, lesions within ventral mPFC led to increased perseverative responding, wherein rats persisted in responding at locations that were previously associated with reward. Similarly, Ishikawa[21,22] found that inactivation of the dorsal mPFC regions results in nonselective responding for sucrose rewards in a simple stimulus-response task and disrupts normal patterns of neural activity in the ventral striatum, especially for neurons that were activated when rats approached the reward port. These signals could control activity in the autonomic nervous system to minimize distracting influences of the animal's metabolic needs and emotions associated with making mistakes in performing a task.

My group has used simple reaction-time tasks (figure 6.2a[37]) to study the functional properties of mPFC in rodents. Our initial work using these tasks involved injecting fluorescent muscimol into the anterior cingulate and prelimbic areas and observing effects of reaction time performance as a function of the duration of the delay period. Fluorescent muscimol silences neural activity[1] and leads to profound increases in premature responding, that is, lever release before the end of the delay period (figure 6.2b). We find two other consistent results when using the muscimiol method. First, the distribution of response latencies (aka reaction times) is shifted to the left with muscimol in mPFC (figure 6.2c). This result suggests that rats with impaired medial prefrontal processing are unable to wait over the delay period to receive the stimulus. Second, response latencies are shorter than normal at short delay periods (figure 6.2d). This result suggests that mPFC is normally mediating an inhibitory control over response initiation.

To examine the neurophysiological basis for these effects of muscimol, we have implanted arrays of electrodes into mPFC and recorded neural activity during performance of the simple reaction-time task. Such recordings reveal that many neurons fire at elevated rates during the delay period.[39,41] These activity patterns are similar to those found in the monkey mPFC.[42] A striking finding was that most of the mPFC neurons showed slow modulations in firing rate around the start of the trial or around the scheduled time of the stimulus (figure 6.2c[41]). When we analyzed population activity using principal component analysis,[41] we found that more than 35% of the variance in the neural population could be explained by two simple functions (figure 6.2d). The first function (PC1) showed fluctuation around the start of the trial and then leveled off during the delay period. The second function (PC2) showed a persistent elevated signal during the delay period and until the scheduled time of the stimulus (and the reward). By taking the cumulative sum of the first principal component, we obtained a function that was highly similar to the second component (Pearson correlation coefficient: > 0.9). This result would be expected if the second component serves as an integral of the first component. We interpreted this finding as evidence for the medial prefrontal network serving as a type of neural integrator that tracks the time since the start of the trial or the confidence that the animal has pressed the lever. Inspired by earlier work,[32] we are currently examining how these signals change during the initial acquisition of the task.

We also examined functional dependencies between neural activity in the medial prefrontal and motor cortices. Following on our study of mPFC inactivation,[37] we combined inactivation of mPFC with neural ensemble recording in motor cortex, as in refs. 32 and 38, to examine how processing in mPFC controls activity in the motor system. Our initial hypothesis was that mPFC would control the level of

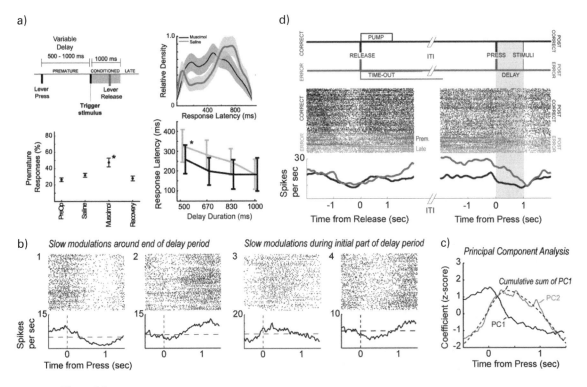

Figure 6.2
Neural activity in medial prefrontal cortex during a simple reaction-time task. (a) Design of the simple reaction-time task with variable delay periods.[37] Thirsty rats pressed down on a lever over a delay period of 0.5 to 1 sec until a tone was presented, and then promptly released the lever to obtain a drop of water. Errors occurred if the lever was released before the stimulus (premature response) or if the RT was > 1sec. Errors were punished by timeouts of 4 to 8 sec. Other panels show the effect of inactivating medial prefrontal cortex on premature responding.[37] Rats made more premature lever releases with muscimol in medial prefrontal cortex compared to control sessions. (b) Slow modulations of neural firing rates are integrated at the population level in medial prefrontal cortex. Rasters and perievent histograms are shown for four neurons from 0.5 sec before to 1.5 sec after lever press (from fig. 5 in ref. 41, used with permission). (c) Principal component analysis (PCA) was used to analyze population activity (fig. 8 in ref. 41, used with permission). The principal components (PC) accounted for temporal variations in neural firing rates. The leading PC was associated with slow modulations in firing rate, starting at lever press. The second PC was associated with a build-up pattern over the delay period. The cumulative sum of PC1 was highly similar to PC2 (Pearson correlation: > 0.9). The two leading components accounted for > 35% of variance over the neural population. (d) Persistent error activity in medial prefrontal cortex.[40] Task events are shown at the top of the panel. An example of persistent error-related firing is shown using raster plots (black: correct; dark gray: late; light gray: premature). This neuron lacked task-related modulation over all trials (left plots), but became persistently active when an error was made and maintained elevated firing rate throughout the intertrial interval until the next trial was performed correctly (right plots).

excitability in the motor cortex.[8] This hypothesis predicts that if mPFC is inactivated, neurons in motor cortex should show nonspecific increases in firing rates and other measures of neural activity, such as local field potentials (intracranial signals related to the electroencephalogram, or EEG). However, our recordings did not support the hypothesis. Instead, we found that delay-period firing in the motor cortex depended on the integrity of activity in mPFC. With mPFC inactivated, we observed many fewer neurons in the motor cortex that fired during the delay period (fig. 5 in ref. 39). A second major finding was that error-related firing was prominent in mPFC and motor cortex (fig. 3 in ref. 39) and that error-related firing in motor cortex was eliminated by inactivation of mPFC. This type of activity is interesting as it develops in the motor cortex during initial task acquisition[32] and is correlated over large groups of neurons.[38] Together, our results suggested that mPFC sends top-down control signals to the motor cortex to control the timing of action during the delay period in the simple reaction-time task.

Another finding from our recordings was what we now call "persistent error activity," that is, neurons that fire at elevated rates after rats make mistakes in the task. For example, if a rat makes a mistake in the reaction-time task by responding before the stimulus, these neurons maintain their delay-period firing rates throughout the intertrial interval until the next trial that is performed correctly. They show reduced activity only when the next reward is delivered.[40] Several other studies have reported such cross-trial encodings of behavioral outcomes in frontal cortex, striatum, and dopamine neurons.[2,3,5,19,35,49,55,62] If these signals track errors in task performance from one trial to the next, they could be used for improving performance during learning.[19] Based on the literature reviewed earlier in this chapter, a leading candidate for the generation of these signals is the reciprocal connectivity between mPFC and the insular cortex (where taste and tactile representations of fluid delivery are encoded[66]) and between these cortical areas and the hypothalamus. These connections may enable persistent representations of visceral information about recent behavioral outcomes that could be used to alter current and future task performance.

A Neural Circuit Model for Top-Down Control

As shown in figure 6.3a, we view the functions of mPFC more as a coach than as an executive. A coach is on the field with the players, takes part in daily practice sessions, and experiences the joys and pains of wins and losses. By contrast, an executive is usually distant from the workers, and knows little about their day-to-day activities. Based on the anatomical connectivity of mPFC, especially its connections to and from the hypothalamus, we believe the proper metaphor for describing mPFC function is as a coach and not as an executive. By this view, the

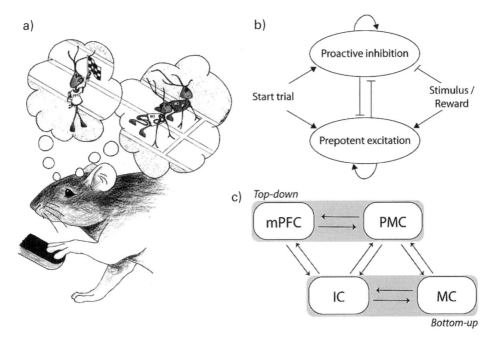

Figure 6.3
Computational model for top-down control of action by medial prefrontal cortex. (a) Cartoon depicting the role of medial prefrontal cortex in controlling action. This cortical region acts more like a coach than an executive. It suggests when to act and advises on future actions based on prior outcomes. (b) Neural circuit model for top-down control. Information about the start of the trial (e.g., limb position) is fed into two pools of mutually inhibitory neurons. One pool serves for "proactive inhibitory" control, and ensures that animals wait over the delay period before responding. This pool of neurons is thought to be in medial prefrontal cortex.[37] The other pool serves for "prepotent excitation" of the instrumental response (lever release), and ensures that rats respond for reward as quickly as possible. This pool of neurons is thought to be in the premotor cortex.[58] Presentation of the stimulus and/or the reward terminates the inhibitory pool and excites (or releases inhibition in) the excitatory pool, and leads to the release of the lever if the overall level of activity is above some threshold. Both pools of neurons serve to integrate information about the passage of time during the delay period. (c) Anatomical regions involved in top-down and bottom-up aspects of control. The medial prefrontal and premotor regions are suggested to function for top-down control, and to take part in the proactive inhibitory ("wait") and prepotent excitatory ("go") processes described in (b). Insular cortex contributes bottom-up information based on assessing the taste properties of fluids that are earned as rewards and the animal's homeostatic state. Sensorimotor cortex encodes bottom-up (proprioceptive) information about motor action in the task and controls activity in the corticospinal system that ultimately is responsible for lever release.

medial prefrontal coaching system takes part in guiding actions with regard to high-level goals, always with regard to the system's recent successes and failures and its current metabolic needs. The medial prefrontal coaching system understands the ability of the system to push itself harder than usual to overcome a bad streak in performance as well as to take it easy following a string of successes. We believe many dysfunctions of mPFC function are to be expected when viewed from this novel perspective.

To be more formal about the specific operations controlled by the medial prefrontal coaching system, Narayanan and Laubach[41] proposed a neural circuit model for the generation of persistent neural activity in mPFC during the performance of delayed-response tasks (figure 6.3b). The model is based on multielectrode recordings in rodent mPFC,[39–41] reviewed previously, and behavioral and EMG data collected in human subjects.[6,24] A key issue in the model is that variations in reaction-time performance are due to a dynamic competition between inhibitory (self-control) and excitatory (preparatory) processes during the delay period. These processes relate to the flag and whistle, respectively, in the cartoon in figure 6.3a. The model can explain effects of delay duration on response latency (delay-dependent speeding), accounts for lasting effects of errors on task-related activity,[40] and predicts that conflict-like signals (wait or go) should exist during the delay period of the simple reaction-time task.

The activity of neurons in this model could be interpreted in three ways. First, the signals could simply reflect that fact that the trial has been completed and it is no longer necessary for the animal to wait for reward. However, this interpretation does not explain the fact that *neurons fire differently in advance of errors* (fig. 3 in ref. 39). Second, the signals could reflect "reward expectation," that is, a signal in the animal that anticipates the forthcoming outcome of the trial. By this view, aberrant firing in advance of an error would reflect an overwhelming reward expectation in the animal. Such activity could be challenged by running sessions with variable outcomes given in blocks or by satiating the animals during the session. Bouret and Richmond[7] did exactly this second manipulation and found that neurons in the primate ventral mPFC were sensitive to the animal's overall level of thirst and that satiation altered neural activity for many neurons. A third interpretation, as suggested earlier, is that the signals reflect conflict between waiting for the stimulus and responding for reward. This issue is currently being addressed by our group, by analyzing RT distributions and examining spike and LFP data before and after the time of maximal conflict between waiting and going (i.e., the mode of the distribution of response durations). Based on our unpublished findings and the recent study by Bouret and Richmond,[7] it appears that neurons in ventral mPFC participate both in encoding information about the animal's current homeostatic state and in adjusting performance based on prior behavioral outcomes.

The anatomical literature predicts that these processes occur within a larger frontal control system (figure 6.3c). The medial prefrontal and premotor cortical areas serve as top-down controllers over the initiation of action, coaching the animal to adjust performance based on recent successes and failures and the current metabolic state of the organism. As such, the neurons normally serve to limit premature and inappropriate responses. After a mistake is made, the system could influence activity elsewhere in the control system to emphasize slower responding (i.e., post-error slowing). The premotor cortex serves to prepare the system for the forthcoming action. (We have recently reported evidence for exactly this behavioral process by a premotor area in the rat frontal cortex, located within the medial agranular cortex.[58]) These top-down areas receive bottom-up signals reflecting the state of the motor system (from the motor and somatosensory cortices) and the animal's homeostatic state and recent gustatory experience (from the insular cortices). Together, these systems enable a dynamic control over action so that the animal can adjust performance to achieve the best possible returns (rewards) over a long time scale.

Evolutionary Significance of Cognitive and Motivational Control

If the mPFC of rodents has a role in cognitive and motivational control, how does this bear on mPFC functions in "higher" animals, including human beings? From an evolutionary perspective, the mPFC is one of the most primordial parts of the cerebral cortex. It is found in all mammals.[26] As such, its functions should be fundamental to the survival of all mammalian species. Perhaps mPFC developed early due to its connections with the hypothalamus and the needs of animals to solve problems in foraging for food. Long-term success in foraging requires control over energy expenditures. Actions need to be taken at the right time and place. Self-control must be exerted to avoid being eaten by predators. As a result, the capacity for control over the autonomic nervous system and over the animal's other actions may have developed in parallel (coevolution) based on functional interactions within the corticohypothalamic system, as described in this chapter.

These evolutionary issues may be important for understanding neurological and psychiatric conditions that are associated with dysfunction in mPFC. Many symptoms of mPFC dysfunction involve problems with emotional control and the inability to inhibit inappropriate behaviors (e.g., vocal tics in Tourette syndrome, compulsive behaviors in OCD, excessive food consumption in morbid obesity). These symptoms are known to be exacerbated by stress, hunger and thirst, and thermal factors (e.g., increased tic frequency in some patients with Tourette syndrome with exposure to heat[54]), and may arise from dysfunction in the corticohypothalamic system.

Acknowledgments

I would like to thank the editors for allowing me to contribute this chapter despite my not being able to attend the Motivational and Cognitive Control Conference at Oxford in June 2010, due to a strike by British Air flight attendants. I would also like to thank Ivan de Araujo, Benjamine Liu, and the editors for helpful comments and discussions on this chapter. The research described in the chapter was supported by grants from the National Institute of Health, National Science Foundation, the American Federation for Aging Research, the Kavli Foundation, and the Tourette Syndrome Foundation.

Outstanding Questions

• Medial prefrontal areas have not acquired widely accepted functional titles like visual or motor cortex. Should they be considered as "hypothalamic" or visceral cortex? Three anatomical papers are suggested for further reading on this topic in the Further Reading list. The reader is encouraged to read related anatomical studies by Saper, Gabbott, Price, and Vertes.

• What specific aspects of rewarding stimuli, such as juice or liquid sucrose, influence neural activity in medial prefrontal cortex? How do the hedonic properties of the fluid (sweet taste), its nutrient content (calories), and the homeostatic state of the organisms (satiety) influence neural activity?

• What is the functional circuit for mediating lasting traces or preceding task events (such as prior trial outcomes) by persistent neural activity in the medial prefrontal cortex? What other brain areas (insular cortex, parahippocampal regions) and neurotransmitters (dopamine, norepinephrine, orexin) are crucial for this activity?

Further Reading

Gabbott PL, Warner TA, Jays PR, Bacon SJ. 2003. Areal and synaptic interconnectivity of prelimbic (area 32), infralimbic (area 25), and insular cortices in the rat. *Brain Res* 993: 59–71. This study carefully examined interconnections between medial and insular regions of the rat frontal cortex using anatomical tract-tracing methods. The authors found extensive and specific laminar patterns of connectivity between functionally related insular and medial subregions. The impact of these connections has yet to be examined using in vivo electrophysiological recordings or computational simulations.

Gabbott PJ, Warner TA, Jays PR, Salway P, Busby SJ. 2005. Prefrontal cortex in rat: projections to subcortical autonomic, motor, and limbic centers. *J Comp Neurol* 492: 145–177. The authors used advanced anatomical methods to examine the densities of neurons in various parts of the rat medial prefrontal cortex with regard to descending projections to subcortical regions. A key finding was that the densities of projections from medial prefrontal regions to the hypothalamus are as dense as those to the thalamus.

Hoover WB, Vertes RP. 2007. Anatomical analysis of afferent projections to the medial prefrontal cortex in the rat. *Brain Struct Funct* 212: 149–179. This is a comprehensive, and beautifully illustrated, examination of the afferent inputs to the medial prefrontal cortex in the rat. The study established that each subfield has a unique set of afferents, and suggests specialization for executive and motivational control as a function of depth. These cortical regions may no longer be considered as vaguely defined or to exist as a hodgepodge of neural connections.

References

1. Allen TA, Narayanan NS, Kholodar-Smith DB, Zhao Y, Laubach M, Brown TH. 2008. Imaging the spread of reversible brain inactivations using fluorescent muscimol. *J Neurosci Methods* 171: 30–38.

2. Amiez C, Joseph JP, Procyk E. 2005. Anterior cingulate error-related activity is modulated by predicted reward. *Eur J Neurosci* 21: 3447–3452.

3. Amiez C, Joseph JP, Procyk E. 2006. Reward encoding in the monkey anterior cingulate cortex. *Cereb Cortex* 16: 1040–1055.

4. Barbas H. 1995. Anatomic basis of cognitive-emotional interactions in the primate prefrontal cortex. *Neurosci Biobehav Rev* 19: 499–510.

5. Barraclough DJ, Conroy ML, Lee D. 2004. Prefrontal cortex and decision making in a mixed-strategy game. *Nat Neurosci* 7: 404–410.

6. Boulinguez P, Jaffard M, Granjon L, Benraiss A. 2008. Warning signals induce automatic EMG activations and proactive volitional inhibition: evidence from analysis of error distribution in simple RT. *J Neurophysiol* 99: 1572–1578.

7. Bouret S, Richmond BJ. 2010. Ventromedial and orbital prefrontal neurons differentially encode internally and externally driven motivational values in monkeys. *J Neurosci* 30: 8591–8601.

8. Brunia CH. 1999. Neural aspects of anticipatory behavior. *Acta Psychol (Amst)* 101: 213–242.

9. Cechetto D, Saper C. 1990. Role of the cerebral cortex in autonomic function. In: Central Regulation of Autonomic Functions (Loewy A, Spyer K, eds), pp 208–223. Oxford, UK: Oxford University Press.

10. Corbit LH, Balleine BW. 2003. The role of prelimbic cortex in instrumental conditioning. *Behav Brain Res* 146: 145–157.

11. Cowen SL, McNaughton BL. 2007. Selective delay activity in the medial prefrontal cortex of the rat: contribution of sensorimotor information and contingency. *J Neurophysiol* 98: 303–316.

12. Fassbender C, Hester R, Murphy K, Foxe JJ, Foxe DM, Garavan H. 2009. Prefrontal and midline interactions mediating behavioural control. *Eur J Neurosci* 29: 181–187.

13. Fellows LK, Farah MJ. 2005. Is anterior cingulate cortex necessary for cognitive control? *Brain* 128: 788–796.

14. Freedman LJ, Insel TR, Smith Y. 2000. Subcortical projections of area 25 (subgenual cortex) of the macaque monkey. *J Comp Neurol* 421: 172–188.

15. Gabbott PL, Warner TA, Jays PR, Bacon SJ. 2003. Areal and synaptic interconnectivity of prelimbic (area 32), infralimbic (area 25) and insular cortices in the rat. *Brain Res* 993: 59–71.

16. Gabbott PL, Warner TA, Jays PR, Salway P, Busby SJ. 2005. Prefrontal cortex in the rat: projections to subcortical autonomic, motor, and limbic centers. *J Comp Neurol* 492: 145–177.

17. Garavan H, Ross TJ, Murphy K, Roche RA, Stein EA. 2002. Dissociable executive functions in the dynamic control of behavior: inhibition, error detection, and correction. *Neuroimage* 17: 1820–1829.

18. Ghahremani DG, Monterosso J, Jentsch JD, Bilder RM, Poldrack RA. 2009. Neural components underlying behavioral flexibility in human reversal learning. *Cereb Cortex* 20: 1843–1852.

19. Histed MH, Pasupathy A, Miller EK. 2009. Learning substrates in the primate prefrontal cortex and striatum: sustained activity related to successful actions. *Neuron* 63: 244–253.

20. Hoover WB, Vertes RP. 2007. Anatomical analysis of afferent projections to the medial prefrontal cortex in the rat. *Brain Struct Funct* 212: 149–179.

21. Ishikawa A, Ambroggi F, Nicola SM, Fields HL. 2008. Contributions of the amygdala and medial prefrontal cortex to incentive cue responding. *Neuroscience* 155: 573–584.

22. Ishikawa A, Ambroggi F, Nicola SM, Fields HL. 2008. Dorsomedial prefrontal cortex contribution to behavioral and nucleus accumbens neuronal responses to incentive cues. *J Neurosci* 28: 5088–5098.

23. Ito S. 2002. Visceral region in the rat primary somatosensory cortex identified by vagal evoked potential. *J Comp Neurol* 444: 10–24.

24. Jaffard M, Longcamp M, Velay JL, Anton JL, Roth M, Nazarian B, Boulinguez P. 2008. Proactive inhibitory control of movement assessed by event-related fMRI. *Neuroimage* 42: 1196–1206.

25. Kaas JH. 1983. What, if anything, is SI? Organization of first somatosensory area of cortex. *Physiol Rev* 63: 206–231.

26. Kaas JH. 2006. Evolution of the neocortex. *Curr Biol* 16: R910–R914.

27. Kargo WJ, Szatmary B, Nitz DA. 2007. Adaptation of prefrontal cortical firing patterns and their fidelity to changes in action-reward contingencies. *J Neurosci* 27: 3548–3559.

28. Killcross S, Coutureau E. 2003. Coordination of actions and habits in the medial prefrontal cortex of rats. *Cereb Cortex* 13: 400–408.

29. Kosar E, Grill HJ, Norgren R. 1986. Gustatory cortex in the rat. I. Physiological properties and cytoarchitecture. *Brain Res* 379: 329–341.

30. Krettek JE, Price JL. 1977. The cortical projections of the mediodorsal nucleus and adjacent thalamic nuclei in the rat. *J Comp Neurol* 171: 157–191.

31. Krupa DJ, Wiest MC, Shuler MG, Laubach M, Nicolelis MA. 2004. Layer-specific somatosensory cortical activation during active tactile discrimination. *Science* 304: 1989–1992.

32. Laubach M, Wessberg J, Nicolelis MA. 2000. Cortical ensemble activity increasingly predicts behaviour outcomes during learning of a motor task. *Nature* 405: 567–571.

33. Matsumoto K, Suzuki W, Tanaka K. 2003. Neuronal correlates of goal-based motor selection in the prefrontal cortex. *Science* 301: 229–232.

34. Naito E, Kinomura S, Geyer S, Kawashima R, Roland PE, Zilles K. 2000. Fast reaction to different sensory modalities activates common fields in the motor areas, but the anterior cingulate cortex is involved in the speed of reaction. *J Neurophysiol* 83: 1701–1709.

35. Nakahara H, Itoh H, Kawagoe R, Takikawa Y, Hikosaka O. 2004. Dopamine neurons can represent context-dependent prediction error. *Neuron* 41: 269–280.

36. Nakamura K, Sakai K, Hikosaka O. 1999. Effects of local inactivation of monkey medial frontal cortex in learning of sequential procedures. *J Neurophysiol* 92: 1063–1068.

37. Narayanan NS, Horst NK, Laubach M. 2006. Reversible inactivations of rat medial prefrontal cortex impair the ability to wait for a stimulus. *Neuroscience* 139: 865–876.

38. Narayanan NS, Kimchi EY, Laubach M. 2005. Redundancy and synergy of neuronal ensembles in motor cortex. *J Neurosci* 25: 4207–4216.

39. Narayanan NS, Laubach M. 2006. Top-down control of motor cortex ensembles by dorsomedial prefrontal cortex. *Neuron* 52: 921–931.

40. Narayanan NS, Laubach M. 2008. Neuronal correlates of post-error slowing in the rat dorsomedial prefrontal cortex. *J Neurophysiol* 100: 520–525.

41. Narayanan NS, Laubach M. 2009. Delay activity in rodent frontal cortex during a simple reaction time task. *J Neurophysiol* 101: 2859–2871.

42. Niki H, Watanabe M. 1979. Prefrontal and cingulate unit activity during timing behavior in the monkey. *Brain Res* 171: 213–224.

43. Ongur D, An X, Price JL. 1998. Prefrontal cortical projections to the hypothalamus in macaque monkeys. *J Comp Neurol* 401: 480–505.

44. Ongur D, Price JL. 2000. The organization of networks within the orbital and medial prefrontal cortex of rats, monkeys and humans. *Cereb Cortex* 10: 206–219.

45. Ostlund SB, Balleine BW. 2005. Lesions of medial prefrontal cortex disrupt the acquisition but not the expression of goal-directed learning. *J Neurosci* 25: 7763–7770.

46. Passetti F, Chudasama Y, Robbins TW. 2002. The frontal cortex of the rat and visual attentional performance: dissociable functions of distinct medial prefrontal subregions. *Cereb Cortex* 12: 1254–1268.

47. Picton TW, Stuss DT, Alexander MP, Shallice T, Binns MA, Gillingham S. 2007. Effects of focal frontal lesions on response inhibition. *Cereb Cortex* 17: 826–838.

48. Preuss TM. 1995. Do rats have prefrontal cortex? The Rose-Woolsey-Akert program reconsidered. *J Cogn Neurosci* 7: 1–24.

49. Procyk E, Tanaka YL, Joseph JP. 2000. Anterior cingulate activity during routine and non-routine sequential behaviors in macaques. *Nat Neurosci* 3: 502–508.

50. Rich EL, Shapiro M. 2009. Rat prefrontal cortical neurons selectively code strategy switches. *J Neurosci* 29: 7208–7219.

51. Ridderinkhof KR, Ullsperger M, Crone EA, Nieuwenhuis S. 2004. The role of the medial frontal cortex in cognitive control. *Science* 306: 443–447.

52. Risterucci C, Terramorsi D, Nieoullon A, Amalric M. 2003. Excitotoxic lesions of the prelimbic-infralimbic areas of the rodent prefrontal cortex disrupt motor preparatory processes. *Eur J Neurosci* 17: 1498–1508.

53. Saper CB. 1985. Organization of cerebral cortical afferent systems in the rat. II. Hypothalamocortical projections. *J Comp Neurol* 237: 21–46.

54. Scahill L, Lombroso PJ, Mack G, Van Wattum PJ, Zhang H, Vitale A, Leckman JF. 2001. Thermal sensitivity in Tourette syndrome: preliminary report. *Percept Mot Skills* 92: 419–432.

55. Seo H, Barraclough DJ, Lee D. 2007. Dynamic signals related to choices and outcomes in the dorsolateral prefrontal cortex. *Cereb Cortex* 17(Suppl 1): i110–i117.

56. Sesack SR, Deutch AY, Roth RH, Bunney BS. 1989. Topographical organization of the efferent projections of the medial prefrontal cortex in the rat: an anterograde tract-tracing study with Phaseolus vulgaris leucoagglutinin. *J Comp Neurol* 290: 213–242.

57. Shidara M, Richmond BJ. 2002. Anterior cingulate: single neuronal signals related to degree of reward expectancy. *Science* 296: 1709–1711.

58. Smith NJ, Horst NK, Liu B, Caetano MS, Laubach M. 2010. Reversible inactivation of rat premotor cortex impairs temporal preparation, but not inhibitory control, during simple reaction-time performance. *Front Integr Neurosci* 4: 124.

59. Stuss DT, Alexander MP, Shallice T, Picton TW, Binns MA, Macdonald R, Borowiec A, Katz DI. 2005. Multiple frontal systems controlling response speed. *Neuropsychologia* 43: 396–417.

60. Swanson LW. 1999. Brain Maps: Structure of the Rat Brain: A Laboratory Guide with Printed and Electronic Templates for Data, Models, and Schematics. New York: Elsevier.

61. Tierney PL, Thierry AM, Glowinski J, Deniau JM, Gioanni Y. 2008. Dopamine modulates temporal dynamics of feedforward inhibition in rat prefrontal cortex in vivo. *Cereb Cortex* 18: 2251–2262.

62. Totah NK, Kim YB, Homayoun H, Moghaddam B. 2009. Anterior cingulate neurons represent errors and preparatory attention within the same behavioral sequence. *J Neurosci* 29: 6418–6426.

63. Uylings HB, Groenewegen HJ, Kolb B. 2003. Do rats have a prefrontal cortex? *Behav Brain Res* 146: 3–17.

64. Van Eden CG, Lamme VA, Uylings HB. 1992. Heterotopic cortical afferents to the medial prefrontal cortex in the rat. A combined retrograde and anterograde tracer study. *Eur J Neurosci* 4: 77–97.

65. Vertes RP. 2004. Differential projections of the infralimbic and prelimbic cortex in the rat. *Synapse* 51: 32–58.

66. Yamamoto T, Matsuo R, Kawamura Y. 1980. Localization of cortical gustatory area in rats and its role in taste discrimination. *J Neurophysiol* 44: 440–455.

7 Top-Down Control over the Motor Cortex

Rogier B. Mars, Franz-Xaver Neubert, and Matthew F. S. Rushworth

Goal-directed behavior requires the selection of task-relevant information and the suppression of task-irrelevant noise. A prominent element of most current models of cognitive control is that this is mediated by higher-level control signals that bias the state of lower-level neural processing.[14,15,31] The prefrontal cortex is commonly seen as the origin of these control signals.[31,43] In the context of action selection, top-down control is particularly needed during situations of response conflict, where a predominant response needs to be inhibited in favor of an alternative response or no response at all. In this chapter, we discuss recent advances in the study of top-down control over the motor cortex during action selection under conflict and action inhibition. We discuss the network of brain areas commonly indicated as having a role in the top-down control over the motor cortex and discuss the potential roles of some of these brain areas within the larger network.

Tasks evoking response conflict or response inhibition tend to consistently activate a large cortical and subcortical network. In one of the first imaging studies looking at action inhibition, Garavan and colleagues[21] reported that inhibition recruits a mostly right lateralized network of regions in addition to the normal action selection network. This network (figure 7.1) involves mostly frontal areas, including the presupplementary motor area (pre-SMA) and right inferior frontal gyrus (rIFG), but also subcortical structures, of which the subthalamic nucleus (STN) has recently received particular attention. In addition to this well-described network, parietal regions, particularly the right inferior parietal lobule, are also often found to be important in these tasks.[21,42] This network, or parts of it, is active in situations of response conflict,[45] action inhibition,[2] action reprogramming,[29] and task switching.[41] In the course of this chapter, we focus specifically on two nodes of this network that have been implicated in top-down control over the motor cortex, the pre-SMA and the right IFG.

This chapter is structured as follows. First, we present some evidence that such a thing as top-down control over the motor cortex indeed exists and that the pre-SMA

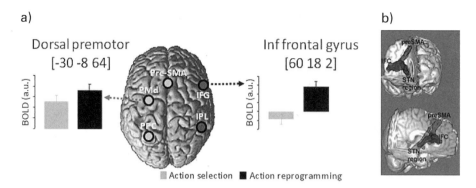

Figure 7.1
Areas commonly activated in conditions that require top-down control over the motor cortex. (a) Brain activity during action selection based on learned visual instructions and under conflict (action reprogramming[29]). Some areas in this network are activated exclusively during conflict trials, such as the right inferior parietal lobule (IPL) and the rIFG, whereas other areas are present during action selection both with and without conflict, such as left posterior parietal cortex (PPC) and left dorsal premotor cortex (PMd). During conflict, the regions active during normal action selection tend to be more active as well, as noticed most often for the pre-SMA. Based on data from Mars et al.[29] (b) Diffusion-weighted imaging shows that areas activated during response inhibition, such as pre-SMA, rIFG, and STN, are all connected with one another via direct white matter fibers. Adapted from Aron et al.[2] with permission.

and rIFG have some causal role in mediating this control. Then, we discuss how this control is exerted by looking at interactions between the frontal lobes and the motor cortex. We focus specifically on insights gained using recent advances in transcranial magnetic stimulation (TMS). Third, we look at the wider interactions within the frontal lobe and discuss how they influence top-down control. Finally, we discuss some caveats of the current approaches and open issues that remain to be investigated in the near future.

Evidence for Top-Down Control

In this section we review some of the evidence that there is indeed such a thing as top-down control from (pre)frontal cortex over the motor cortex. To establish this, we must first look at modulation of activity in the motor cortex to establish whether its activity shows patterns related to predominant responses during conflict tasks, indicating there is activity that needs to be controlled in the motor cortex at all rather than that all control is dealt with earlier in the processing stream, and whether the modulation of this activity during the course of a trial indicates this predominant action representation is modulated. Second, it has to be shown that this modulation is indeed the result of (pre)frontal activity.

Control in the Motor Cortex

The notion that multiple response alternatives can be simultaneously active in the motor cortex was already suggested in the 1980s,[13] and this notion is present in most current models of action selection.[5,10] Gratton and colleagues[22] provided early evidence that the presence of multiple, conflicting response alternatives influences activity all the way into the motor cortex. They used an event-related potential known as the lateralized readiness potential (LRP). The LRP is a measure reflecting the differential activation of the motor cortex in the two hemispheres. Participants were required to perform the Eriksen flanker task, in which participants have to respond with one of either hands in response to a stimulus array.[18] The array can contain both the target stimulus to which the participant needs to respond and distracters, which are designed to lure the participants into preparing the incorrect response (figure 7.2a). These "conflict trials" are generally associated with longer reactions times and more errors than trials without distracter information. Using the LRP, Gratton and colleagues were able to show that the motor cortex associated with the incorrect, distractor response was originally active as reflected by the "incorrect-dip" in the LRP (figure 7.2b). Later in the response period, presumably following increased processing of the stimulus, the preferential activity of the incorrect motor cortex was replaced by preferential activity of the correct motor cortex. These results provided early evidence that information associated with incorrect responses can be present in the motor cortex even when the trial ends in a correct response. Thus, under these conditions top-down control over the motor cortex is needed.

A problem with the LRP is that it is by definition a difference measure. Therefore, the disappearance of the incorrect-dip can be attributable to the inhibition of the incorrect response, the facilitation of the correct responses, or a mixture of both. This problem can be addressed by probing the excitability of the motor cortices with transcranial magnetic stimulation (TMS). A suprathreshold single pulse of TMS elicited over the representation in the motor cortex of the effector will elicit a motor-evoked potential (MEP) in the electromyogram (EMG) recorded from the effector muscle. The amplitude of the MEP is a measure of the excitability of the motor cortex and is modulated during the preparation and execution of a response.[46] A nice example of this approach is provided by a recent study of Verleger and colleagues,[49] who probed MEP amplitude during the time of the incorrect-dip in the LRP in the flanker task. They showed that on incongruent trials, the MEP associated with the incorrect response effector first increased and then decreased during the first 90 msec of the response period. Simultaneously with the decrease in the prematurely activated effector was an increase in MEP recorded from the correct response effector. These results thus detail the effects underlying the incorrect-dip

a)

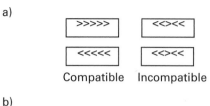

Compatible   Incompatible

b)

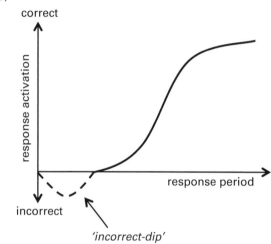

Figure 7.2
(a) Stimulus arrays typically employed in an arrow version of the Eriksen flanker task.[18] Participants are required to respond as quickly as possible with the response hand on the side indicated by the center arrow. (b) Schematic LRPs as expected during incompatible trials in this task show a preferential activation of the incorrect response hand due to the presence of the incompatible flankers in the stimulus array ("incorrect-dip") before preferential activation of the correct response hand. After Coles[12] and Gratton et al.[22]

in the LRP. There is indeed an incorrect activation of the effector associated with the incorrect response that is later inhibited, while the correct response effector is activated. Similar results have been obtained by Michelet and colleagues.[30]

Evidence for a Role of the Frontal Cortex

The most direct evidence for a necessary role of the frontal cortex in action inhibition comes from lesion studies. Early work by Aron and colleagues established the necessary role of the rIFG in inhibiting actions, but also in inhibiting task sets and during memory retrieval.[3] Lesion mapping showed that this was a unique contribution of rIFG along lateral frontal cortex regions. Similarly, applying repetitive transcranial magnetic stimulation (rTMS) over rIFG to create a so-called virtual lesion also impairs response inhibition, but not normal response execution.[8]

The involvement of pre-SMA in top-down control may be illustrated by a study by Isoda and Hikosaka in which they recorded activity from single neurons in the pre-SMA of monkeys during an action reprogramming task.[24] They report neurons that are active just before the initiation of successful reprogramming, early enough to cause the behavioral change. When the monkey fails to reprogram its action, however, the neurons are not active before the action, but show a delayed increase in activity. These results show that pre-SMA is a likely candidate for a role in top-down control over the motor cortex. As with rIFG, lesions in the pre-SMA offer evidence for a causal role. Although lesions in pre-SMA are rare, a recent study showed difficulty in action inhibition in a patient with just such a lesion,[34] dove-tailing with results showing increased activation of pre-SMA during inhibition in healthy participants performing the same task.[33]

Although lesion methods are quite informative and an improvement over correlative methods such as imaging and electrophysiology, they are not free of interpretational limitations. Lesions do not respect anatomical boundaries, and it is thus often difficult to establish which part of damaged tissue is responsible for the behavioral changes observed. Furthermore, the lesions act as a "global" influence that is always present, making it difficult to delineate the precise contribution of the neural structure in the number of processes involved in any task. Finally, the brain is remarkably adaptive and lesions in one brain area might lead to compensatory, or at least modulated, activity in other parts of the brain. Although the studies reviewed here were generally conducted quite carefully, often employing quite sophisticated lesion mapping techniques and carefully controlling for confounding effects of the lesions on behavior, more direct experimental evidence of the type of influence these regions exert in the normal brain would be beneficial.

More direct evidence for a top-down role of the pre-SMA was obtained by two studies using stimulation techniques to investigate brain function. First, Taylor and colleagues[44] combined rTMS with the LRP approach described previously. Using the Eriksen flanker paradigm, the researchers studied the incorrect-dip in the LRP. On some trials, rTMS was applied over the pre-SMA just before and during the presentation of the stimulus. Interfering with pre-SMA activity in this manner resulted in an increased incorrect-dip in the LRP, indicating that the top-down control influencing this resolution of this conflict is diminished. A second example is the study of Isoda and Hikosaka described earlier.[24] In a follow-up to the earlier experiments, instead of recording from the pre-SMA, the researchers artificially stimulated the same region on trial requiring action reprogramming. In 65% of the sessions, this stimulation increased the number of correct action reprogramming trials, at least for one response. Note that, although these studies show apparently opposite results, this comparison is not valid. rTMS globally affects an expanse of cortex, interfering with its normal function, whereas the microstimulations target very specific neuronal targets. The overall point of both studies, however, is that pre-SMA seems to have a causal influence on activity in the motor cortex and behavior.

How Control Is Exerted: Examples from Action Reprogramming

Paired-Pulse TMS Studies of Action Reprogramming

In the previous section we discussed evidence that there is indeed such a phenomenon as top-down control over the motor cortex. In this section we discuss some novel insights into the precise nature of the top-down control of both pre-SMA and rIFG on the primary motor cortex during action selection under conflict. We focus on the specific case of action reprogramming, that is, the inhibition of a prepared response in favor of an alternative in response to a change in the environment.[29] In a series of recent studies, we have explored top-down control of the pre-SMA and the rIFG over the motor cortex by means of the technique of paired-pulse transcranial magnetic stimulation (ppTMS). During ppTMS, two TMS coils are placed over an experimental subject's head. A "test" coil is placed over the primary motor cortex, over the representation of the response effector, in most cases the hand. As discussed previously, a single suprathreshold TMS pulse will elicit a motor-evoked potential (MEP) in the EMG recorded from the effector. A second, "conditioning" coil is placed over the region hypothesized to influence the motor cortex. PpTMS relies on the fact that the MEP elicited by the test coil can be modulated by a pulse through the conditioning coil a few milliseconds earlier (see chapter 11, figure 11.2). The ratio of the MEP elicited by the test pulse preceded by a pulse through the conditioning coil and the MEP elicited by a test coil pulse only indicate the influence of the area underneath the conditioning coil over the motor cortex. It is important to emphasize that ppTMS is thus a probing technique; the pulses are not applied continuously to achieve the "virtual lesion" as in rTMS. Paired-pulse TMS was first used within the motor cortex[27] and between the motor cortices of the different hemispheres,[19] before being applied outside the motor cortex, most notably in the dorsal premotor cortex.[26,32,40]

We applied this technique during an action reprogramming paradigm, modeled on the task developed by Isoda and Hikosaka.[24] In this task, participants are looking at a computer screen on which two colored boxes ("flankers") are presented, one to each side of fixation. After a short delay, a central fixation cue takes the color of one of the two flankers, instructing the participant to press a button using the index finger of the hand on the congruent side. The critical manipulation of the task was that the central fixation took the same color for three to seven consecutive trials, allowing participants to build up an expectation of the response required on each trial. Previous studies have shown that participants exploit these types of regularities in the trial sequence and prepare likely actions.[5] Following a number of trials that build up and confirm expectations (stay trials), the central fixation would take the opposite color (switch trials). On these switch trials, participants had to reprogram their response, by inhibiting the prepared response and selecting and executing the alternative. Behavioral data confirm the effectiveness of this experimental manipulation, with participants responding slower and making more errors on switch compared to stay trials. We then probed the influence of pre-SMA and rIFG during switch and stay trials just after the central fixation color change, signaling the participants to reprogram their action or simply execute the prepared action, respectively.

We first probed the pre-SMA/M1 interactions by applying pulses solely over M1 or over M1 preceded by a pre-SMA pulse 6 msec earlier.[28] Pulses were applied either 75, 125, or 175 msec after the central fixation color change. These time points were chosen based on the earlier monkey results[24] and the timing of conflict-related signals originating from the medial frontal cortex, such as the N2.[47] Pre-SMA had a strong facilitative influence over the motor cortex only on switch trials and only 125 msec following the reprogramming instruction. The effect of pre-SMA manifested itself by a facilitation of the MEP elicited by M1 stimulation. This effect was most prominent when participants were switching toward the stimulated M1. The effect was specific to reprogramming/switch trials. On stay trials, there was no significant effect of pre-SMA on M1. If anything, there was a trend toward an inhibitory effect. The effect of pre-SMA on M1 was thus specific to the action reprogramming condition and temporally specific in time.

To test whether this effect was also anatomically specific, we then repeated the experiment, but with the conditioning coil placed not over the pre-SMA, but over the rIFG.[38] Again, we probed the influence over the left M1, presenting either single pulses over M1 or pulses over M1 preceded by a pulse over rIFG 8 msec earlier. The effects were remarkably different from those of pre-SMA. Whereas pre-SMA had a facilitative effect on M1, rIFG stimulation resulted in an inhibition of the MEP elicited by M1 during stimulation on reprogramming trials. This influence was later than the pre-SMA influence, at 175 instead of 125 msec. Moreover, although the pre-SMA facilitation was most pronounced when participants switched toward the stimulated M1, the inhibitory effect of rIFG was more global, independent of whether the participant were switching toward or away from the stimulated M1. Thus, although pre-SMA and rIFG tend to often coactivate in fMRI studies of action inhibition or action reprogramming,[2,16] ppTMS shows that the effects are actually qualitatively and temporally distinct from one another.

White Matter Pathways Mediating Top-Down Control

Given this top-down control over the motor cortex, the question then is how the signal travels from the (pre)frontal cortex to the motor cortex. In the ppTMS studies described here, we are stimulating a precisely defined region and have a direct measurement of motor cortex activation, but we have no information over the route this signal is taking. In the action inhibition literature, there is a particular emphasis on a subcortical, hyperdirect pathway from the (pre)frontal cortex, via the subthalamic nucleus, globus palidus, and thalamus, to the motor cortex.[20,35]

One way to investigate which routes might be involved in transporting the information from the stimulated frontal region to M1 is to look at diffusion-weighted magnetic resonance imaging (DW-MRI).[25] DW-MRI allows one to obtain an estimate of the diffusion of water in the brain. In the brain's white matter, the water diffusion is directionally dependent. In a fiber bundle, the water diffusion is less constrained along the axis of the bundle, and hence more diffusion will be measured there. In contrast, water diffusion is more isotropic outside the white matter. This technique thus allows the quantification of white matter integrity on a voxel-by-voxel basis. One can then correlate individual differences in white matter in a given area with individual differences in the functional interactions measured by ppTMS. The rationale is that voxels in which individual differences in the structural white matter measure correlate with the functional ppTMS measure mediate the interaction between the area underneath the conditioning coil and M1. This technique was first used by Boorman et al. to study the pathways mediating premotor/M1 interactions during conditional action selection.[6]

We applied this technique to the data from the pre-SMA/M1 ppTMS study described earlier.[28] We found evidence for the involvement of direct cortical pathways between pre-SMA and M1, such as the white matter underlying the medial frontal cortex, the lateral premotor cortex, and M1. The same analysis was performed on the data obtained from a study investigating rIFG/M1 interactions during action reprogramming in a grasping task.[7] Again, there was evidence only for the involvement of direct cortical pathways between rIFG and M1.

At first glance, these results seem at odds with the results of imaging studies, which emphasize the importance of a subcortical route, the so-called hyperdirect route via the STN, in mediating action reprogramming.[2] However, it should be noted that the interval between the conditioning and test pulses in these experiments was 6 msec for the pre-SMA study and 8 msec for the rIFG. Although these interpulse intervals (IPIs) are normal in the ppTMS literature, any signal traveling through the hyperdirect pathway would be expected to take more time than this.[36] Therefore, the standard ppTMS setup would not be able to pick up signals traveling through this pathway.

To address this issue, we repeated the pre-SMA/M1 and rIFG/M1 interactions experiments using the Isoda and Hikosaka action reprogramming paradigm. Instead of using a constant short IPI, the IPI was varied between 3 and 18 msec.[38] The results are displayed in figure 7.3. During action reprogramming, we found a facilitatory effect of pre-SMA at an IPI of 6 msec, replicating our previous results,[28] but also at 9 and 12 msec. For the rIFG, we replicated the inhibitory effect at a short IPI, and

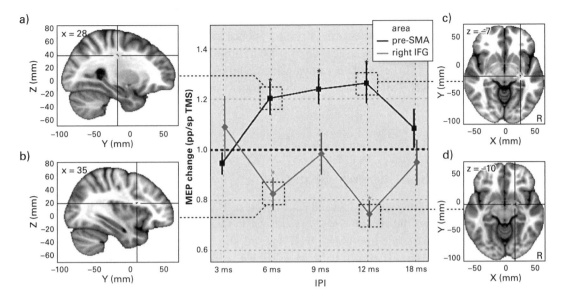

Figure 7.3
White matter pathways mediating rIFG/M1 and pre-SMA/M1 functional interactions. Middle panel shows the influence of a single pulse of TMS over pre-SMA (black) and rIFG (gray) on the motor-evoked potential elicited by a single TMS pulse over M1. X-axis indicates the interval between the pre-SMA or rIFG pulse and the M1 pulse. The effect sizes at 6-msec interpulse intervals correlate only with direct cortical pathways between the pre-SMA (a) and rIFG (b) and M1, while at 12-msec intervals there was also evidence for subcortical pathways (c, d). Adapted from Neubert et al.[38] with permission.

also found an inhibitory effect at a longer latency of 12 msec. Correlating the individual differences in effect sizes at different IPIs showed that, although short-IPI effect sizes are correlated with one another and long-IPI effect sizes are correlated with one another, the correlation between the effect sizes at short and long IPIs is much lower. This provides some preliminary indication that different systems might mediate the short- and long-IPI effects.

We then again correlated the effect sizes at short IPIs (6 msec) and long IPIs (12 msec) with white matter to investigate which pathways mediate these effects. At the short IPI, we found evidence only for the involvement of direct cortical pathways, replicating our previous results.[7,28] At the long IPI, however, we found additional white matter clusters in the vicinity of the STN correlating with effect size.[38] We then used the cluster found in the correlation analysis as the basis for probabilistic fiber tracking[4] to show which white matter pathways these clusters are part of. While at the short IPI there was evidence only for cortical pathways, at the long IPI there was evidence for additional subcortical pathways (figure 7.3). We then formally quantified this by counting the number of identified tracts passing through a region of interest around the STN. In both the pre-SMA and rIFG experiments there was strong evidence for involvement pathways around the STN at the long IPI, but not at the short IPI. These results show strong evidence favoring the view that separate pathways are mediating the influence of pre-SMA and rIFG over M1 during action reprogramming: a direct cortical pathway and an indirect, subcortical pathway, likely involving the STN. This second pathway is probed only in ppTMS experiments at longer IPIs.

Interactions within the Frontal Lobes

Interactions between Pre-SMA and rIFG

In the previous sections, we focused on the interactions between nodes within the frontal lobes and the motor cortex. However, it seems plausible that the frontal nodes interact with one another as well. Indeed, the regions involved in top-down control over the motor cortex have been shown to have direct white matter connections with one another[2] (figure 7.1b).

Duann and colleagues[16] used fMRI to study the interactions between the nodes of the action reprogramming network described in this chapter during action inhibition. They asked participants to perform a standard stop-signal task. They showed that during successful inhibition trials, rIFG activity correlated more with pre-SMA activity than during unsuccessful inhibition trials. Note that the functional connectivity measure used was purely correlative and as such cannot provide any information on whether rIFG was influencing pre-SMA, vice versa, or both.

Breaking the Network

An open question then is whether the interaction between pre-SMA and rIFG has some relevance to the top-down influence of either of these regions. This question can be investigated by probing the top-down control from one of these regions over the motor cortex while the influence of the other region is disrupted, either via lesions or by using repetitive TMS. We have done exactly that in a recent follow-up to our action reprogramming work described earlier.

Considering the timing of pre-SMA and rIFG effects found by Swann and colleagues and Neubert and colleagues, we chose to probe rIFG/M1 interactions following temporary interference with pre-SMA. Participants were asked to perform the same action reprogramming task as described previously while ppTMS was applied to rIFG and M1. Following an experimental session participants received 15 minutes of 1-Hz rTMS over the pre-SMA. Directly after this, they again performed the action reprogramming task. Administering 15 minutes of 1-Hz rTMS is a standard method to decrease the activity in a brain region, producing effects usually lasting up until 20 minutes. In the pre-TMS session, we replicated the earlier effect of an inhibitory influence of rIFG on M1 during action reprogramming. Following the rTMS over pre-SMA, however, this effect disappeared.[38] This breakdown of rIFG/M1 interactions was, however, not present following rTMS over a central parietal control area, indicating the specificity of pre-SMA rTMS.

Conclusions and Outlook

In this chapter, we have reviewed the evidence that a network of frontal regions, primarily pre-SMA and rIFG, exerts top-down control over the motor cortex during action selection under conflict. We found signals in the motor cortex that are modulated in a fashion consistent with the influence of top-down control. Furthermore, we have shown that when activity in frontal regions is disrupted, these M1 signals change in a different manner. We then looked at studies using paired-pulse TMS to study the nature of this top-down control in the situation of action reprogramming. Finally, we looked at some of the interactions within the frontal network itself and its role in shaping the top-down control signals. In this concluding section, we discuss some of the interpretational limitations of the reviewed results and present some questions that need to be addressed in the near future.

The Nature of Control

An important question is what the nature of the top-down control is. Although a number of studies focus on the role of rIFG on inhibition of irrelevant actions,[3] one prominent theory suggests that the prefrontal cortex exerts control through the amplification of task-relevant information, rather than via inhibition.[11] Support for this position was obtained by Egner and Hirsch, who investigated the nature of top-down control outside the motor cortex.[17] They asked participants to perform a variant of the Stroop task, in which the face and the name of a famous person were presented on top of each other and the participants had to choose whether the relevant stimulus dimension belonged to an "actor" or "politician" category. As an example, when a participant had to classify the face stimulus and was presented with the face of Robert de Niro and the name Mao Ze Dong, top-down control could either result in inhibition of activity in the visual word form area or amplify activity in the fusiform face area.[39] The results were consistent with the amplification model.

However, some of the TMS results reviewed here could be interpreted to argue the opposite. First, the MEP results obtained by Verleger and colleagues[49] showed that there was actual inhibition of the incorrect response tendency. However, one could argue that this is due not to top-down inhibition of the incorrect response tendency, but to lateral inhibition, which in turn is the result of amplification of activity related to the correct response. Second, the ppTMS results obtained by Neubert and Buch show a clear inhibitory effect of rIFG on the MEP elicited by

M1 stimulation during action reprogramming, consistent with the proposed role of this region in inhibition. However, although these results are certainly highly consistent with models assigning an inhibitory role of rIFG, it remains to be established whether the physiological inhibition measured with ppTMS is actually a reflected of cognitive inhibition.[1]

Apart from this uncertainty about the nature of inhibition, some recent studies have challenged the notion that rIFG is involved purely in inhibition, arguing instead for a more general role in either allocating attention to the stimulus or updating of the action representation. For instance, Hampshire and colleagues[23] found that rIFG was more active whenever important stimuli were detected, independent of whether that detection was followed by the inhibition of a motor response. One potential explanation for the divergence of results in the literature is an increasing appreciation that the region commonly referred to as the rIFG consists of subregions, each with different, albeit related, functions. For instance, Verbruggen and colleagues assign a role in updating the current action plan to the posterior ventral rIFG and a role in visual detection of changes in the environment to the more dorsal inferior frontal junction area.[48] A similar distinction has been suggested by Chikazoe and colleagues.[9]

Toward a Neurocomputational Framework

One drawback of most of the studies reviewed in this chapter is that they mostly distinguish only two conditions, those with and those without top-down control over M1. However, it is highly unlikely that the brain is organized along such a binary distinction. In a recent study, Vossel and colleagues[50] analyzed activity in the rIFG during attentional reorienting in a location cueing paradigm as a function of the number of preceding trials. They showed that activity in the rIFG increased on reorienting trials as a function of the number of preceding correct trials. Their results are interpreted in the context of Bayesian statistical theory, which—roughly—states that the brain continuously tries to predict the current state of the environment. Brain activity such as that described in rIFG in the study by Vossel and colleagues can then be described as a prediction error, implementing the need for adjustments and updating the brain's model of the environment. In this context, top-down control over the motor cortex is the implementation of control following a failure of the brain's predictive systems in adequately performing the task at hand. The advantages of such a model are that they provide a general framework for a large body of neural phenomena and they can be captured in formal computational models. The parameters of these computational models can be related to brain activity in parametric fashion, rather than the binary distinctions described previously, and can be used to dissociate some of the different processes described in the studies by Hampton, Chikazoe, and Verbruggen,[9,23,48] such as detection of the prediction violation, implementing of the behavioral adjustments, and updating of the brain's internal models[37] (see also chapter 23, this volume). In future, these formal computational models will hopefully be linked to these data on top-down control over the motor cortex described in this chapter.

Outstanding Questions

• What are the different contributions of subregions of the frontal lobes to top-down control and what are the functional properties of different routes mediating frontal/M1 interactions?

• What is the relationship between physiological inhibition and cognitive inhibition in top-down control?

• What is the relationship between top-down control over the motor cortex and other forms of top-down control?

• Can formal computation models be used to describe top-down control in a single framework?

Further Reading

Miller EK, Cohen JD. 2001. An integrative theory of prefrontal cortex function. *Annu Rev Neurosci* 24: 167–202. A comprehensive review that postulates a role for the prefrontal cortex in cognitive control via the biasing of information processing in posterior brain areas.

Aron AR. 2007. The neural basis of inhibition in cognitive control. *Neuroscientist* 13: 214–228. This review provides a wide-ranging discussion of the concept of inhibition, looking at inhibition in different domains and from a variety of perspectives.

References

1. Aron AR. 2007. The neural basis of inhibition in cognitive control. *Neuroscientist* 13: 214–228.

2. Aron AR, Behrens TE, Smith S, Frank MJ, Poldrack RA. 2007. Triangulating a cognitive control network using diffusion-weighted magnetic resonance imaging (MRI) and functional MRI. *J Neurosci* 27: 3743–3752.

3. Aron AR, Robbins TW, Poldrack RA. 2004. Inhibition and the right inferior frontal cortex. *Trends Cogn Sci* 8: 170–177.

4. Behrens TE, Johansen-Berg H, Jbabdi S, Rushworth MF, Woolrich MW. 2007. Probabilistic diffusion tractography with multiple fibre orientations: What can we gain? *Neuroimage* 34: 144–155.

5. Bestmann S, Harrison LM, Blankenburg F, Mars RB, Haggard P, Friston KJ, Rothwell JC. 2008. Influence of uncertainty and surprise on human corticospinal excitability during preparation for action. *Curr Biol* 18: 775–780.

6. Boorman ED, O'Shea J, Sebastian C, Rushworth MF, Johansen-Berg H. 2007. Individual differences in white-matter microstructure reflect variation in functional connectivity during choice. *Curr Biol* 17: 1426–1431.

7. Buch ER, Mars RB, Boorman ED, Rushworth MF. 2010. A network centered on ventral premotor cortex exerts both facilitatory and inhibitory control over primary motor cortex during action reprogramming. *J Neurosci* 30: 1395–1401.

8. Chambers CD, Bellgrove MA, Stokes MG, Henderson TR, Garavan H, Robertson IH, Morris AP, Mattingley JB. 2006. Executive "brake failure" following deactivation of human frontal lobe. *J Cogn Neurosci* 18: 444–455.

9. Chikazoe J, Jimura K, Asari T, Yamashita K, Morimoto H, Hirose S, Miyashita Y, Konishi S. 2009. Functional dissociation in right inferior frontal cortex during performance of go/no-go task. *Cereb Cortex* 19: 146–152.

10. Cisek P. 2007. Cortical mechanisms of action selection: the affordance competition hypothesis. *Philos Trans R Soc B Biol Sci* 362: 1585–1599.

11. Cohen JD, Servan-Schreiber D. 1992. Context, cortex, and dopamine: a connectionist approach to behaviour and biology in schizophrenia. *Psychol Rev* 99: 45–77.

12. Coles MGH. 1989. Modern mind-brain reading: psychophysiology, physiology, and cognition. *Psychophysiology* 26: 251–269.

13. Coles MGH, Gratton G, Bashore TR, Eriksen CW, Donchin E. 1985. A psychophysiological investigation of the continuous-flow model of human information-processing. *J Exp Psychol Human* 11: 529–533.

14. Corbetta M, Shulman GL. 2002. Control of goal-directed and stimulus-driven attention in the brain. *Nat Rev Neurosci* 3: 201–215.

15. Desimone R, Duncan J. 1995. Neural mechanisms of selective visual attention. *Annu Rev Neurosci* 18: 193–222.

16. Duann JR, Ide JS, Luo X, Li CS. 2009. Functional connectivity delineates distinct roles of the inferior frontal cortex and presupplementary motor area in stop signal inhibition. *J Neurosci* 29: 10171–10179.

17. Egner T, Hirsch J. 2005. Cognitive control mechanisms resolve conflict through cortical amplification of task-relevant information. *Nat Neurosci* 8: 1784–1790.

18. Eriksen BA, Eriksen CW. 1974. Effects of noise letters upon identification of a target letter in a nonsearch task. *Percept Psychophys* 16: 143–149.

19. Ferbert A, Priori A, Rothwell JC, Day BL, Colebatch JG, Marsden CD. 1992. Interhemispheric inhibition of the human motor cortex. *J Physiol* 453: 525–546.

20. Frank MJ. 2006. Hold your horses: a dynamic computational role for the subthalamic nucleus in decision making. *Neural Netw* 19: 1120–1136.

21. Garavan H, Ross TJ, Stein EA. 1999. Right hemispheric dominance of inhibitory control: an event-related functional MRI study. *Proc Natl Acad Sci USA* 96: 8301–8306.

22. Gratton G, Coles MGH, Sirevaag EJ, Eriksen CW, Donchin E. 1988. Prestimulus and poststimulus activation of response channels—a psychophysiological analysis. *J Exp Psychol Human* 14: 331–344.

23. Hampshire A, Chamberlain SR, Monti MM, Duncan J, Owen AM. 2010. The role of the right inferior frontal gyrus: inhibition and attentional control. *Neuroimage* 50: 1313–1319.

24. Isoda M, Hikosaka O. 2007. Switching from automatic to controlled action by monkey medial frontal cortex. *Nat Neurosci* 10: 240–248.

25. Johansen-Berg H, Rushworth MF. 2009. Using diffusion imaging to study human connectional anatomy. *Annu Rev Neurosci* 32: 75–94.

26. Koch G, Franca M, Del Olmo MF, Cheeran B, Milton R, Alvarez Sauco M, Rothwell JC. 2006. Time course of functional connectivity between dorsal premotor and contralateral motor cortex during movement selection. *J Neurosci* 26: 7452–7459.

27. Kujirai T, Caramia MD, Rothwell JC, Day BL, Thompson PD, Ferbert A, Wroe S, Asselman P, Marsden CD. 1993. Corticocortical inhibition in human motor cortex. *J Physiol* 471: 501–519.

28. Mars RB, Klein MC, Neubert FX, Olivier E, Buch ER, Boorman ED, Rushworth MF. 2009. Short-latency influence of medial frontal cortex on primary motor cortex during action selection under conflict. *J Neurosci* 29: 6926–6931.

29. Mars RB, Piekema C, Coles MG, Hulstijn W, Toni I. 2007. On the programming and reprogramming of actions. *Cereb Cortex* 17: 2972–2979.

30. Michelet T, Duncan GH, Cisek P. 2010. Response competition in the primary motor cortex: corticospinal excitability reflects response replacement during simple decisions. *J Neurophysiol* 104: 119–127.

31. Miller EK, Cohen JD. 2001. An integrative theory of prefrontal cortex function. *Annu Rev Neurosci* 24: 167–202.

32. Mochizuki H, Huang YZ, Rothwell JC. 2004. Interhemispheric interaction between human dorsal premotor and contralateral primary motor cortex. *J Physiol* 561: 331–338.

33. Nachev P, Rees G, Parton A, Kennard C, Husain M. 2005. Volition and conflict in human medial frontal cortex. *Curr Biol* 15: 122–128.

34. Nachev P, Wydell H, O'Neill K, Husain M, Kennard C. 2007. The role of the pre-supplementary motor area in the control of action. *Neuroimage* 36(Suppl 2): T155–T163.

35. Nambu A, Kaneda K, Tokuno H, Takada M. 2002. Organization of corticostriatal motor inputs in monkey putamen. *J Neurophysiol* 88: 1830–1842.

36. Nambu A, Tokuno H, Hamada I, Kita H, Imanishi M, Akazawa T, Ikeuchi Y, Hasegawa N. 2000. Excitatory cortical inputs to pallidal neurons via the subthalamic nucleus in the monkey. *J Neurophysiol* 84: 289–300.

37. Neubert FX, Klein MC. 2010. What is driving inhibition-related activity in the frontal lobe? *J Neurosci* 30: 4830–4832.

38. Neubert FX, Mars RB, Buch ER, Olivier E, Rushworth MFS. 2010. Cortical and subcortical interactions during action reprogramming and their related white matter pathways. *Proc Natl Acad Sci USA* 107: 13240–13245.

39. Nieuwenhuis S, Yeung N. 2005. Neural mechanisms of attention and control: losing our inhibitions? *Nat Neurosci* 8: 1631–1633.

40. O'Shea J, Sebastian C, Boorman ED, Johansen-Berg H, Rushworth MF. 2007. Functional specificity of human premotor-motor cortical interactions during action selection. *Eur J Neurosci* 26: 2085–2095.

41. Rushworth MFS, Hadland KA, Paus T, Sipila PK. 2002. Role of the human medial frontal cortex in task switching: a combined fMRI and TMS study. *J Neurophysiol* 87: 2577–2592.

42. Rushworth MFS, Taylor PCJ. 2006. TMS in the parietal cortex: updating representations for attention and action. *Neuropsychologia* 44: 2700–2716.

43. Sakai K, Passingham RE. 2003. Prefrontal interactions reflect future task operations. *Nat Neurosci* 6: 75–81.

44. Taylor PCJ, Nobre AC, Rushworth MFS. 2007. Subsecond changes in top-down control exerted by human medial frontal cortex during conflict and action selection: a combined transcranial magnetic stimulation electroencephalography study. *J Neurosci* 27: 11343–11353.

45. Ullsperger M, von Cramon DY. 2001. Subprocesses of performance monitoring: a dissociation of error processing and response competition revealed by event-related fMRI and ERPs. *Neuroimage* 14: 1387–1401.

46. Van den Hurk P, Mars RB, van Elswijk G, Hegeman J, Pasman JW, Bloem BR, Toni I. 2007. Online maintenance of sensory and motor representations: effects on corticospinal excitability. *J Neurophysiol* 97: 1642–1648.

47. Van Veen V, Carter CS. 2002. The timing of action-monitoring processes in the anterior cingulate cortex. *J Cogn Neurosci* 14: 593–602.

48. Verbruggen F, Aron AR, Stevens MA, Chambers CD. 2010. Theta burst stimulation dissociates attention and action updating in human inferior frontal cortex. *Proc Natl Acad Sci USA* 107: 13966–13971.

49. Verleger R, Kuniecki M, Moller F, Fritzmannova M, Siebner HR. 2009. On how the motor cortices resolve an inter-hemispheric response conflict: an event-related EEG potential-guided TMS study of the flankers task. *Eur J Neurosci* 30: 318–326.

50. Vossel S, Weidner R, Fink GR. 2011. Dynamic coding of events within the inferior frontal gyrus in a probabilistic selective attention task. *J Cogn Neurosci* 23: 414–424.

8 A Role for Posterior Cingulate Cortex in Policy Switching and Cognitive Control

John M. Pearson, Benjamin Y. Hayden, and Michael L. Platt

Despite the fact that early hypometabolism and neural degeneration in posterior cingulate cortex (CGp) predict cognitive decline in Alzheimer's disease, and CGp hyperactivity predicts cognitive dysfunction in schizophrenia as well as first-degree relatives, the function of this brain area remains unclear. The disparate evidence for CGp involvement in a variety of cognitive and behavioral processes has belied any simple functional description. Here we develop a new model that proposes that CGp integrates the recent history of rewards, errors, volatility, and context for the purpose of detecting changes in the environment and signaling the need for consequent changes in behavioral policy. In this model, suppressed CGp activity favors operation within the current behavioral policy and cognitive set, with few "open channels" for information to gain access to cognition and behavior. By contrast, increased CGp activity reflects a change in large-scale environmental contingencies or internal state and promotes flexibility, exploration, and renewed learning. In light of this new hypothesis, we review known electrophysiological responses of single neurons in CGp, and discuss the relationship of our model to the role of CGp in the so-called default mode of resting state activity.

The Basics: Anatomy and Physiology of CGp

Cingulate cortex, within the depths of the cingulate sulcus as well as along the medial wall of the cingulate gyrus, has long been recognized as an important site integrating sensory, motor, visceral, motivational, emotional, and mnemonic information.[44,60] Electrical microstimulation of various regions within cingulate cortex can evoke visceral or "emotional" responses, such as changes in heart rate or blood pressure, as well as vocalizations and movements of the limbs,[39,75,79,87] and can support self-stimulation behavior.[63] Neurophysiological studies in animals indicate that neurons in CGp respond to both sensory events[16,17,58] and the motivational and informational significance of those events.[20,34,47,62] Humans with posterior cingulate dysfunction may show emotional disturbances, such as schizophrenia and obsessive-compulsive disorder,[18] spatial impairments similar to the deficits of patients with parietal lesions, or memory deficits.[37,50,51]

In addition to its prominent reciprocal anatomical connections with areas involved in spatial attention—areas 7a, LIP, and 7, or PGm[1,2,6,9,53,59,83]—CGp is also strongly connected with brain areas known to be involved in learning and motivation, and to areas sensitive to reinforcement contingencies, including the anterior and lateral thalamic nuclei,[22] the caudate nucleus,[2,64,91] and orbitofrontal cortex.[2,54,59] In addition, CGp is strongly and reciprocally interconnected with anterior cingulate cortex (ACC), which contains neurons carrying nociceptive[73] and reward-related information,[35,57,72] and is capable of engaging reinforcement-related circuitry when artificially activated.[28,76]

CGp is also well-positioned to contribute to processes of memory and association formation. In particular, it forms strong, reciprocal connections with the medial temporal lobe, long known to be crucial for associative learning and episodic memory.[68,77] In the monkey, injections of horseradish peroxidase (HRP) have revealed substantial afferents from parahippocampal gyrus, including both entorhinal and perirhinal divisions.[84] CGp also sends projections to the medial temporal lobe, specifically back to parahippocampal areas TF and TH, as well as to entorhinal cortex.[93] Similarly, BOLD activity in parahippocampal gyrus and CGp is correlated with activity in the CGp in humans,[82] and modulations in CGp activity occur during both spatial and face-based working memory tasks.[5,11]

More recently, a number of studies in both humans and animals have suggested a role for CGp in encoding reward-related information. Many CGp neurons respond equivalently to the delivery of larger-than-average rewards and the omission of predicted rewards.[47] Further, information about reward outcomes is often maintained by relatively slow (multisecond), long-lasting changes in CGp firing rates across a variety of tasks.[34,47,48,62] In addition, a recent fMRI experiment offering individuals choices between small, immediate rewards and larger, delayed rewards found levels of CGp activation correlated strongly with subjective values inferred from the individuals' measured preference functions.[40,43,74]

Finally, numerous neuroimaging studies in humans have linked CGp to the so-called default network of cortical areas, including ventromedial prefrontal cortex and CGp, which show high metabolic and hemodynamic activity while at rest that is suppressed during active task engagement.[30,66,67] Activation in the default network is anticorrelated with activation of the dorsal frontoparietal network, a set of brain areas implicated in selective attention, and its concomitant benefits in accuracy and task performance.[10,19,38] Deactivation of the default network has been implicated in attention, arousal, and task engagement, and increases in hemodynamic response in these areas predict occasional lapses in attention,[89] failures to encode memories,[13] and failures to perceive near-threshold sensory stimuli.[7] Variations in the activity of the default network have been linked to self-directed cognition,[30,49] environmental monitoring,[45] and motivated behavior.[65] Monkeys show strikingly similar patterns of intrinsic metabolic activity within this network,[81] and tonic firing rates of single neurons in CGp predict variations in reaction times and error rates within a single task.[36] These data suggest that the default network in general, and CGp in particular, may track moment-to-moment variations in the balance of exteroceptive vigilance and interoceptive cognition needed to monitor the external environment and internal milieu.

Learning, Change Detection, and Policy Switching

Since the discovery that dopaminergic neurons of the substantia nigra pars compacta (SNc) and the ventral tegmental area (VTA) respond to rewarding events by signaling the difference in expected and received rewards—the so-called reward prediction error (RPE)—theories of reinforcement learning (RL) have come to dominate discussions of the neurobiology of learning and conditioning.[46,52,71,78,85] In fact, the sufficiency of these signals for simple conditioning has recently been demonstrated,[80] lending further credence to the hypothesis that dopaminergic signals impinging on the basal ganglia implement an RL-like learning algorithm.

Recent work suggests that other brain areas, in particular cortical areas lying along the midline, also contribute to conditioning and other types of associative learning. The orbitofrontal and anterior cingulate cortices (OFC and ACC) receive dopaminergic projections and maintain strong reciprocal connections with other structures in the basal ganglia.[31,32] Several hypotheses suggest that these areas are necessary for maintaining representations of and deciding among outcomes, actions, or cues,[41,69,70] as well as facilitating changes in action.[86] Areas such as the dorsolateral prefrontal cortex (DLPFC) are then thought to incorporate these representations into the process of strategic decision making and action planning.[3,42]

Missing from this picture, however, is the process by which organisms detect environmental change and begin the process of either switching between or learning entirely new behavioral strategies. Such a process should successfully handle changes in both the statistical parameters of the environment (alterations in volatility, outcome probability, and outliers) and its contingency structure (changes in the state space, its transition properties, and the introduction of new event types). In typical RL algorithms, agents begin with either a model of the world (model-based algorithms) or merely a set of outcomes observed in various states (model-free algorithms), and adjust the values assigned to states and actions by an amount proportional to the difference between their estimated and experienced values, the reward prediction error, or RPE.[78] In principle, such algorithms are capable of finding at least a local optimum for the decision policy under very generic assumptions.[78] Nevertheless, because the update process is incremental, naïve implementations may require many thousands of observations to converge on stable behavior.[88] Thus, in an environment rapidly alternating between several fixed, distinct reward structures, crude RL agents might find themselves forever playing catch-up, unable to do more than gradually adjust in response to abrupt transitions.

Clearly, this scenario fails to reflect the capability of many animals, including humans, to successfully implement a wide variety of behavioral strategies, each of which may be adjusted independently and deployed with minimal switching costs. Thus, though several classical theories of conditioning posit surprise (formalized as the absolute value of RPE) or similar violations of expectation as a means of dynamically adjusting reward rates and stimulating new learning,[61] such models are still based on the idea of a single policy subject to gradual updates. This is to be contrasted with the problem of change detection, in which expected variation in outcomes must be distinguished from a true shift in the underlying structure of the environment.[4,12,15,55,92] In such cases, rather than forever reshaping a single strategy in the face of constant change, agents may do better to learn an entire menu of behavioral strategies (or a meta-strategy with a small number of rapidly adjustable parameters), with the option of switching between them when a large enough shift in the environment is detected. Such a model accords well with the observed rapidity of behavioral adjustment in the face of sudden changes in the reward structure of the environment,[14,23] and operates similarly to more sophisticated theories of conditioning that invoke Bayesian mechanisms to dynamically adjust learning rates.[12,33] In this scenario, outcomes would be tracked not only for the purpose of adjusting the current strategy (and learning rate within that strategy), but for determining whether or not the environment has changed enough to warrant a completely different approach. Reinforcement learning would then operate as a subprocess within the change detection system, which would incorporate Bayesian inference and a suite of inborn or derived models of the world.[12,29,55]

Figure 8.1 depicts a schematic of the process by which such change detection might take place. Outcome data from single events are passed to the change detection system, which recombines these variables into strategy-specific measures of Bayesian evidence for environmental change. As in other models of information accumulation,[26,27] this signal, representing the log posterior odds of a given hypothesis (in this case, environmental change) increases until reaching a threshold, after which the agent switches strategy. However, in contrast with typical accumulation models of sensory evidence, these decision signals are maintained across multiple outcomes, and possess only a single threshold, as is appropriate for an all-or-none switching process that allows full Bayesian inference to be reduced to a simple update model.[55] Equally important, the decision variables accumulated by the

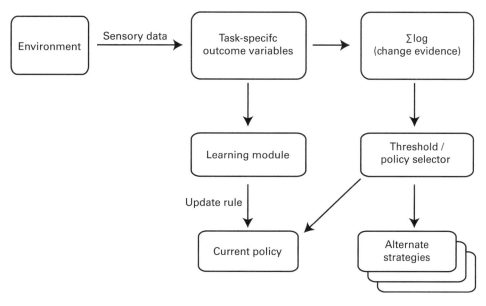

Figure 8.1
A simplified model of change detection and policy selection. Sensory feedback from reward outcomes is divided into task-specific variables and passed on to both a reinforcement learning module and a change detector. The learning module computes an update rule based on the difference between expectations and outcomes in the current model of the world, and updates the policy accordingly. The change detector calculates an integrated log probability that the environment has undergone a change to a new state. If this variable exceeds a threshold, the policy selection mechanism substitutes a new behavioral strategy, which will be updated according to subsequent reward outcomes.

change detector may vary between strategies, depending on the expected distribution of outcomes from the environment. That is, the correct statistical test for agents to perform in change detection depends not only on the environment, but also on current and alternative strategies. Thus, in an environment where the appropriate strategy may depend heavily on the relative frequency of outliers, the correct tracking statistic may be neither the mean nor the variance of outcomes, but a simple proportion of occurrence above a threshold.

Moreover, decision variables should not be sensitive to aspects of the current strategy adjustable through incremental learning, since such slow changes can be accommodated through gradual RL adjustment of current parameters, and change detection becomes superfluous. For example, in a foraging arena with randomly distributed returns (a fish pond or a spider's web), detecting a change in the environmental richness of the current location depends on the nature of the location itself (we shall assume that such changes may necessitate adopting an entirely separate strategy, like abandoning the site). If the site's mean and variance change slowly, reinforcement learning using a Kalman filter will yield reliable richness estimates.

If, on the other hand, the mean is subject to sudden jumps (with variance remaining stable), a simple average of recent returns will allow such shifts to be detected. However, if slow changes in variance also occur, the appropriate change detection statistic becomes the coefficient of variation (CV), since changes in the mean must be measured relative to the (evolving) variance. Put simply, decision makers must choose statistics that simultaneously track those environmental changes relevant to strategy switching (sudden jumps, contingency switches) while remaining insensitive to change acceptable within the current strategy (slow variation of parameters). Thus, we expect decision makers to encode and accumulate a wide variety of evidentiary variables in the process of change detection, perhaps arrived at through a type of principal component analysis applied to the complete range of available statistics. In such a framework, the best statistic is the one that maximizes the area under the receiver operating characteristic (ROC) curve for the strategy switching problem, balancing false positives against false negatives in accordance with the cost-benefit analysis that obtains in the current environment.

Posterior Cingulate Cortex as Change Detector

Here, we review several recent lines of evidence from single-unit electrophysiology implicating CGp as a key locus in the environmental change detection network. Though most of the experiments reviewed here examined short-term variations in firing rates within a single strategy rather than changes in firing rates across events that evoked changes in strategy, it is nonetheless possible, as in studies of learning, to search for traces of the underlying algorithm by studying perturbations about the stable state on a trial-to-trial basis. That is, just as learning-related circuits continue to track RPE even when learning has reached steady state,[46,52,71,78,85] so neurons involved in the process of change detection should continue to encode relevant variables even when the environment is stable. Thus, even in the absence of explicit policy switching, single-unit activity offers clues to the function of putative change detection areas.

The first such piece of evidence comes from single-unit recording studies in monkeys performing a simple rewarded saccade task.[47] That study found that neurons in CGp respond in graded fashion not only to varying amounts of liquid reward associated with a saccade, but to the unexpected omission of these same rewards.[47] Thus, CGp neurons track both a behaviorally relevant variable (for, say, updating the expected value of a saccade) and deviations from expectation within the current reward environment. Expanding on these results, a second line of evidence comes from a two-alternative forced choice task offering two options: a "safe" option with fixed associated liquid reward (J_s) and a "risky" option with a 50% probability of a very small reward (J_l) and a 50% probability of a larger reward (J_w

$> J_s > J_l$).[34,48] The magnitudes J_w and J_l varied across blocks, but always with the restriction that $\frac{1}{2}(J_l + J_w) = J_s$ so that each target had the same expected value (EV).

What is important to note about the structure of the task is not simply that environmental returns are stochastic, but that their variance also changes across blocks. As a result, change detection requires not only the encoding of individual reward outcomes, but also, as discussed earlier, some measure of variance. In fact, single neurons in CGp encoded not only reward size but also reward variance (specifically the CV in reward) in this task.[48]

Moreover, monkeys' choices were well characterized by a probabilistic version of the win-stay lose-shift (WSLS) heuristic. Specifically, monkeys showed high probabilities of repeating risky choices following the larger reward from the risky option and high probabilities of choosing the safe option following the low reward from the same option. Notably, firing rates of CGp neurons were highest following small and medium-sized rewards and lowest following large rewards, and these responses predicted the likelihood that the monkey would shift strategy. Importantly, single-trial injections of microcurrent into CGp changed the probability that the monkeys would shift strategy following large rewards delivered for choosing the variable option—as if they had erroneously detected a bad outcome.[34] Finally, tonic firing rates in CGp maintained information about previous reward outcomes reaching back multiple trials, implying that single neurons incorporated past environmental returns into firing rates predictive of future choices (figure 8.2).[34,48] Taken together, these data suggest that CGP neurons encode environmental outcomes—rewards, omissions, and variance—maintain this information online (in a leaky fashion), and contribute to adjusting subsequent behavior.

In a follow-up study, we asked whether the representation of this information generalized to strategic situations by recording from single neurons in monkeys performing a variant of the four-armed-bandit task.[62] In this task, reward amounts for four targets varied independently on each trial, slowly changed over time,[15] and thus provided a richer set of environmental returns and strategic behavioral options. As a result, monkeys' behavior could be characterized as a true change between strategies—explore and exploit—that depended crucially on their recent history of reward outcomes.[15,25,90] As expected, firing rates of CGp neurons not only signaled single-trial reward outcomes, but also predicted the probability of subsequent changes in strategy in graded fashion. These observations confirm the prediction that CGp participates in a circuit that monitors environmental outcomes for purposes of change detection and subsequent modifications in strategy (figure 8.2).[62] Equally important in such a task is that average reward rates in the bandit task depend crucially on integrating past information into current decisions. Once again, firing rates of CGp neurons in the pre- and postdecision epochs significantly

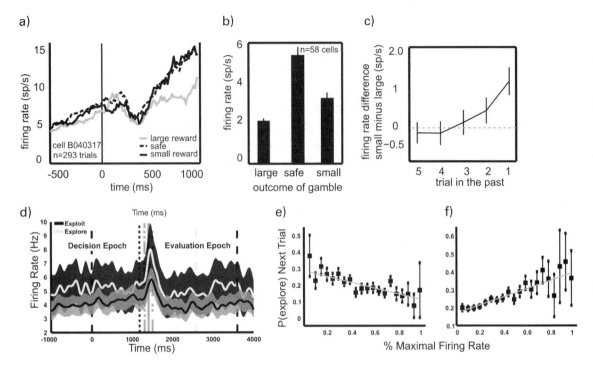

Figure 8.2
CGp encodes reward outcomes over multiple trials and predicts changes in strategy. (a) PSTH for example neuron following reward delivery when monkeys choose between variably rewarded outcomes and deterministically rewarded outcomes with the same mean reward rate. Firing rates were significantly greater following small or medium rewards than following large rewards. (b) Bar graph showing the average firing of all neurons in the population following delivery of large, medium, and small rewards. Firing rates are averaged over a 1-sec epoch beginning at the time of reward offset (t = 0). Tick marks indicate one standard error. (c) Average effect of reward outcome on neuronal activity up to five trials in the future. Bars indicate one standard error. (d) PSTH for example neuron in the 4-armed-bandit task, showing significant differences in firing for exploratory and exploitative strategies in both the decision and evaluation epochs. Exploit trials are in black, explore trials in white. The task begins at time 0. Onset of the "go" cue (dotted black line), reward delivery (solid gray line), and end of trial (rightmost dashed black line) are mean times. Dashed gray lines indicate ± 1 standard deviation in reward onset. Shaded areas represent SEM. (e, f) Neurons in CGp encode probability of exploring on the next trial. Points are probabilities of exploring next trial as a function of percent maximal firing rate in the decision epoch, averaged separately over negatively and positively tuned populations of neurons (e and f, respectively). Error bars: SEM. Adapted from refs. 34 and 62.

predicted upcoming choice, implicating this brain area in the integrative processes that inform decisions. Thus, even in a more mathematically complex environment, one in which changes in returns are gradual rather than sudden, the activity of CGp neurons both tracks and maintains strategically relevant information associated with the likelihood of policy switching.

Change Detection in the Default Mode Network

Given the prominent role of posterior cingulate cortex in the default mode network, it stands to reason that any purported role for CGp in the process of change detection may likewise have implications for the default network as a whole. In the case of CGp itself, we recently reported that firing rates of CGp neurons are elevated outside of task contexts and suppressed during task performance, and that spontaneous firing rates predict behavioral indices of task engagement on a trial-by-trial basis—with higher firing rates associated with poorer performance of simple orienting and memory tasks (figure 8.3).[74] Moreover, cued rest periods, in which monkeys were temporarily liberated from exteroceptive vigilance, evoked the highest firing rates of CGp neurons. Importantly, local field potentials (LFPs) in the gamma band, which has been closely linked to synaptic activity (and by extension, the fMRI BOLD signal), was also suppressed by active task performance.

Thus, firing rates of CGp neurons track levels of task engagement, consistent with the idea that monitoring functions in CGp are suppressed when agents are operating within a stable, well-learned environmental context. By contrast, periods of rest may be accompanied by more generalized exploratory behavior—that is, a state in which task-related attention is reduced and the current cognitive set is adjusted toward maximum flexibility. Along these lines, CGp may play a broader role in basic cognitive processes that are usually suppressed during the performance of well-learned tasks, including memory retrieval, internal monitoring, and the global balance of internal versus external information processing. As a result, modulations in the firing rates of CGp neurons are expected to be largest during the initial phases of learning, in response to sudden, drastic environmental changes, and in the midst of self-initiated switches between strategic modes of behavior.

Discussion

We have proposed, on the basis of several recent studies, that posterior cingulate cortex comprises a key node in the network responsible for environmental change detection and subsequent changes in decision policy and behavior. This proposed

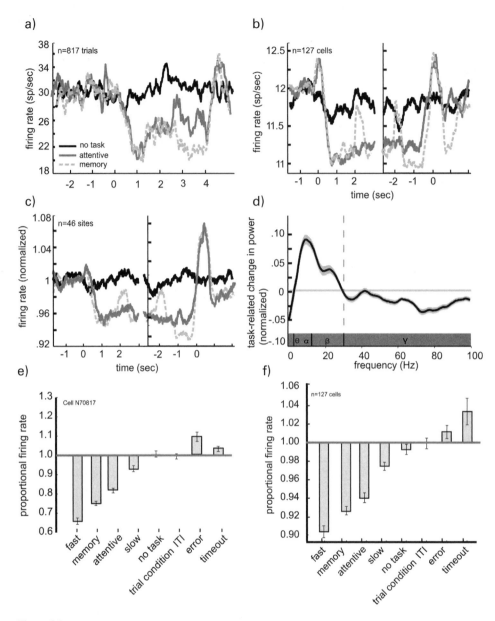

Figure 8.3

Exogenous task engagement suppresses activity of CGp neurons. (a) PSTHs plot average firing rates of a single CGp neuron during attentive task (solid gray line), working memory task (dashed gray line), and no-task condition (black line). Traces are aligned to cue fixation. Firing rates were suppressed during all tasks, although activity was phasically enhanced at the beginning and end of trials. (b) PSTHs showing average firing rates of all CGp neurons in the population (*n* = 127). Late portion of neural response is aligned to acquisition of target. Conventions as in (a). (c) PSTHs showing average multiunit activity at all CGp sites in the population (n = 43). Conventions as in (b). (d) Differential power spectra of LFPs for attentive task minus control condition. Vertical axis indicates proportional difference in power between the two tasks for all neurons (normalized). Power in the gamma band was suppressed relative to the intertrial interval, whereas power in lower-frequency bands was enhanced. (e, f) Neuronal activity in CGp as a function of exteroceptive vigilance. Bars show average normalized firing rate of a single example neuron (e) and the entire population (f) of CGp neurons in response to a variety of task conditions. Adapted from ref. 36.

network, which sits atop the reinforcement learning module in the cognitive hierarchy, would enable organisms to learn and implement a variety of behavioral policies in response to diverse environmental demands, refining each independently and employing them as changes in the pattern of environmental outcomes are detected. Evidence for this claim comes from simple binary decision tasks, in which firing rates of CGp neurons encode reward outcomes, reward omissions, and reward outcome variance, as well as more complex decision contexts such as the k-armed bandit, in which neuronal activity predicts policy switches in a graded fashion. Crucially, data from microstimulation studies demonstrate that the activity of these neurons has a causal effect on implementation of the current decision strategy by shifting it away from a previously stable state. Finally, evidence from studies of default-mode processing indicates that CGp activity is suppressed by engagement and attention within the context of a well-learned and static task environment, but that errors, task disengagement, and liberation from exteroceptive vigilance are all associated with overall higher firing rates in this area. These observations are consistent with a broader interpretation of change detection that encompasses an evaluation of not only task-related reward outcomes, but of balancing between endogenous and exogenous sources of information relevant for shifting between modes of behavior.

Several key predictions result from this model. First, CGp should encode task-specific variables for the purpose of change detection and subsequent changes in strategy, as suggested by single-unit studies involving changing CV[48] and strategy selection.[62] That such variables are not universal but task-specific implies that the same neuron may encode different variables in different decision contexts. The coefficient of variation in reward may be useful when returns are Gaussian, with abrupt jumps in means, but not when means and variances vary together, or when options are nonindependent. Furthermore, the choice of what information is encoded should depend on the set of available policies. In the case that agents can respond to slow environmental changes by (relatively) slow reinforcement learning, change detection is not necessary. Neither will it be necessary if agents are capable of devising only a single strategy. But when the environment may be modeled as a series of slow changes superimposed on sudden jumps, change detection becomes a necessary and readily applicable ingredient in optimal behavior.[4,12,23]

Likewise, CGp activity should show pronounced enhancement over time in scenarios that demand endogenously driven (as opposed to exogenously cued) changes in behavior. That is, when statistical inference becomes necessary to detect a change in task and alter behavior accordingly, CGp should exhibit a concomitant rise in firing rate as evidence mounts, followed by a gradual fall-off as behavior crystallizes into a single strategy. Naturally, this behavior requires that information be maintained and integrated across trials, and thus that firing rates in the present exhibit correlations with outcomes in the past, with an effective memory window dependent on the Bayesian prior estimate of the rate of environmental change.

In addition, the process of learning entirely new associations should result in increased CGp activity. That this should be true not only follows from the anatomical connections between CGp and parahippocampal gyrus, known to be necessary for long-term memory formation,[82,93] but from the results of classic conditioning experiments showing enhancement in CGp global activity during learning.[20–22] Here, however, we may be able to reveal the function of CGp by performing experiments in which new cues, while providing information, may pertain more or less directly to the problem of strategy switching. That is, changes in CGp activity should be larger following cues predicting environmental changes necessitating a strategy switch than to cues predicting strategically irrelevant changes. Likewise, self-detected or inferred changes in environment should elicit larger changes in CGp activity than cued change points, since no process of inference (and thus no evidence accumulation) is necessary in the latter.

Finally, the change detection hypothesis opens up new possibilities for investigating the default mode network function. If the canonical activations seen in fMRI studies merely represent, as is supposed, one end on a continuum of attentional allocation, the idea of changes in behavioral mode casts manipulations of this state in a new light. In this framework, default areas may be crucial for initiating the transition between basic behavioral modes, or even overriding them in cases where cognitive control is exercised. We might expect this to be particularly relevant in the case of schizophrenia, in which patients are highly prone to overdetecting behaviorally salient events in the environment, along with a diminished ability to "turn down" the internal milieu.[8,24] Likewise, the early degeneration of CGp in Alzheimer's disease may cripple a key node in the interface between cognitive set and memory networks, resulting in disorientation and impaired memory access.[56,94] Together, these data suggest a key role for CGp in organizing flexible behavior in response to an ever-changing environment, one that mediates learning, memory, control, and reward systems to promote adaptive behavior.

Acknowledgments

We want to thank Sarah Heilbronner and David Barack for stimulating discussions of the ideas in this paper. In addition, the authors were supported by NIH grants EY103496 (MLP) and EY019303 (JP), and by a career development award (DA027718) and a NIDA postdoctoral fellowship (DA023338) and a fellowship from the Tourette Syndrome Association (BYH), as well as by the Duke Institute for Brain Sciences.

Outstanding Questions

• How general is the proposed change detection mechanism in CGp? For example, does it extend to volatility in the social environment as well as the physical environment?

• What role do other default network regions such as vmPFC play in the process of altering behavioral policy in response to changing environmental contingencies?

• What is the link between change detection and other putative default mode functions such as mind-wandering, creativity, and prospection?

Further Reading

Courville AC, Daw ND, Touretzky DS. 2006. Bayesian theories of conditioning in a changing world. *Trends Cogn Sci* 10: 294–300. Summarizes several key models of Bayesian inference in the context of classical conditioning, extending them to the case of changing environmental contingencies. Demonstrates that altered learning rates observed in latent inhibition, blocking, and overshadowing have computational explanations in terms of change detection.

Behrens TE, Woolrich MW, Walton ME, Rushworth MF. 2007. Learning the value of information in an uncertain world. *Nat Neurosci* 10: 1214–1221. Presents evidence that a key variable for learning in changing environments, the current estimate of volatility, is correlated with BOLD signals in anterior cingulate cortex. As predicted by Bayesian considerations, subsequent learning rates are determined by this measure.

References

1. Andersen RA, Bracewell RM, Barash S, Gnadt JW, Fogassi L. 1990. Eye position effects on visual, memory, and saccade-related activity in areas LIP and 7a of macaque. *J Neurosci* 10: 1176–1196.

2. Baleydier C, Mauguiere F. 1980. The duality of the cingulate gyrus in monkey. Neuroanatomical study and functional hypothesis. *Brain* 103: 525–554.

3. Barraclough DJ, Conroy ML, Lee D. 2004. Prefrontal cortex and decision making in a mixed-strategy game. *Nat Neurosci* 7: 404–410.

4. Behrens TE, Woolrich MW, Walton ME, Rushworth MF. 2007. Learning the value of information in an uncertain world. *Nat Neurosci* 10: 1214–1221.

5. Belger A, Puce A, Krystal J, Gore J, Goldman-Rakic P, McCarthy G. 1998. Dissociation of mnemonic and perceptual processes during spatial and nonspatial working memory using fMRI. *Hum Brain Mapp* 6: 14–32.

6. Blatt GJ, Andersen RA, Stoner GR. 1990. Visual receptive field organization and cortico-cortical connections of the lateral intraparietal area (area LIP) in the macaque. *J Comp Neurol* 299: 421–445.

7. Boly M, Balteau E, Schnakers C, Degueldre C, Moonen G, Luxen A, Phillips C, Peigneux P, Maquet P, Laureys S. 2007. Baseline brain activity fluctuations predict somatosensory perception in humans. *Proc Natl Acad Sci USA* 104: 12187–12192.

8. Broyd SJ, Demanuele C, Debener S, Helps SK, James CJ, Sonuga-Barke EJS. 2009. Default-mode brain dysfunction in mental disorders: a systematic review. *Neurosci Biobehav Rev* 33: 279–296.

9. Cavada C, Goldman-Rakic PS. 1989. Posterior parietal cortex in rhesus monkey: I. Parcellation of areas based on distinctive limbic and sensory corticocortical connections. *J Comp Neurol* 287: 393–421.

10. Corbetta M, Kincade JM, Shulman GL. 2002. Neural systems for visual orienting and their relationships to spatial working memory. *J Cogn Neurosci* 14: 508–523.

11. Courtney SM, Ungerleider LG, Keil K, Haxby JV. 1996. Object and spatial visual working memory activate separate neural systems in human cortex. *Cereb Cortex* 6: 39–49.

12. Courville AC, Daw ND, Touretzky DS. 2006. Bayesian theories of conditioning in a changing world. *Trends Cogn Sci* 10: 294–300.

13. Daselaar SM, Prince SE, Cabeza R. 2004. When less means more: deactivations during encoding that predict subsequent memory. *Neuroimage* 23: 921–927.

14. Daw N, Courville A. 2007. The rat as particle filter. In: Advances in Neural Information Processing 20 (Platt JC, Koller D, Singer Y, Roweis S, eds), pp 369–376. Cambridge, MA: MIT Press.

15. Daw ND, O'Doherty JP, Dayan P, Seymour B, Dolan RJ. 2006. Cortical substrates for exploratory decisions in humans. *Nature* 441: 876–879.

16. Dean HL, Crowley JC, Platt ML. 2004. Visual and saccade-related activity in macaque posterior cingulate cortex. *J Neurophysiol* 92: 3056–3068.

17. Dean HL, Platt ML. 2006. Allocentric spatial referencing of neuronal activity in macaque posterior cingulate cortex. *J Neurosci* 26: 1117–1127.

18. Devinsky O, Luciano D. 1993. The contributions of cingulate cortex to human behavior. In: Neurobiology of Cingulate Cortex and Limbic Thalamus: A Comprehensive Handbook (Vogt BA, Gabriel M, eds), pp 527–556. Boston: Birkhäuser.

19. Fox MD, Snyder AZ, Vincent JL, Corbetta M, Van Essen DC, Raichle ME. 2005. The human brain is intrinsically organized into dynamic, anticorrelated functional networks. *Proc Natl Acad Sci USA* 102: 9673–9678.

20. Gabriel M, Foster K, Orona E. 1980. Interaction of laminae of the cingulate cortex with the anteroventral thalamus during behavioral learning. *Science* 208: 1050.

21. Gabriel M, Sparenborg SP, Stolar N. 1987. Hippocampal control of cingulate cortical and anterior thalamic information processing during learning in rabbits. *Exp Brain Res* 67: 131–152.

22. Gabriel M, Vogt B, Kubota Y, Poremba A, Kang E. 1991. Training-stage related neuronal plasticity in limbic thalamus and cingulate cortex during learning: a possible key to mnemonic retrieval. *Behav Brain Res* 46: 175–185.

23. Gallistel C, Mark T, King A, Latham P. 2001. The rat approximates an ideal detector of changes in rates of reward: implications for the law of effect. *J Exp Psychol Anim Behav Process* 27: 354–372.

24. Garrity AG, Pearlson GD, McKiernan K, Lloyd D, Kiehl KA, Calhoun VD. 2007. Aberrant "default mode" functional connectivity in schizophrenia. *Am J Psychiatry* 164: 450–457.

25. Gittins J. 1979. Bandit processes and dynamic allocation indices. *J R Stat Soc, B* 41: 148–177.

26. Gold JI, Shadlen MN. 2002. Banburismus and the brain: decoding the relationship between sensory stimuli, decisions, and reward. *Neuron* 36: 299–308.

27. Gold JI, Shadlen MN. 2007. The neural basis of decision making. *Annu Rev Neurosci* 30: 535–574.

28. Goodall E, Carey R. 1975. Effects of d-versus l-amphetamine, food deprivation, and current intensity on self-stimulation of the lateral hypothalamus, substantia nigra, & medial frontal cortex of the rat. *J Comp Physiol Psychol* 89: 1029–1045.

29. Green CS, Benson C, Kersten D, Schrater P. 2010. Alterations in choice behavior by manipulations of world model. *Proc Natl Acad Sci USA* 107: 16401–16406.

30. Gusnard DA, Akbudak E, Shulman GL, Raichle ME. 2001. Medial prefrontal cortex and self-referential mental activity: relation to a default mode of brain function. *Proc Natl Acad Sci USA* 98: 4259–4264.

31. Haber S. 2003. The primate basal ganglia: parallel and integrative networks. *J Chem Neuroanat* 26: 317–330.

32. Haber S, Fudge J, McFarland N. 2000. Striatonigrostriatal pathways in primates form an ascending spiral from the shell to the dorsolateral striatum. *J Neurosci* 20: 2369.

33. Hampton AN, Bossaerts P, O'Doherty JP. 2008. Neural correlates of mentalizing-related computations during strategic interactions in humans. *Proc Natl Acad Sci USA* 105: 6741–6746.

34. Hayden BY, Nair AC, McCoy AN, Platt ML. 2008. Posterior cingulate cortex mediates outcome-contingent allocation of behavior. *Neuron* 60: 19–25.

35. Hayden BY, Pearson JM, Platt ML. 2009. Fictive reward signals in the anterior cingulate cortex. *Science* 324: 948–950.

36. Hayden BY, Smith DV, Platt ML. 2009. Electrophysiological correlates of default-mode processing in macaque posterior cingulate cortex. *Proc Natl Acad Sci USA* 106: 5948–5953.

37. Hirono N, Mori E, Ishii K, Kitagaki H, Sasaki M, Ikejiri Y, Imamura T, Shimomura T, Ikeda M, Yamashita H. 1998. Alteration of regional cerebral glucose utilization with delusions in Alzheimer's disease. *J Neuropsychiatry Clin Neurosci* 10: 433–439.

38. Hopfinger JB, Buonocore MH, Mangun GR. 2000. The neural mechanisms of top-down attentional control. *Nat Neurosci* 3: 284–291.

39. Jürgens U, Ploog D. 1970. Cerebral representation of vocalization in the squirrel monkey. *Exp Brain Res* 10: 532–554.

40. Kable JW, Glimcher PW. 2007. The neural correlates of subjective value during intertemporal choice. *Nat Neurosci* 10: 1625–1633.

41. Lee D, Rushworth MF, Walton ME, Watanabe M, Sakagami M. 2007. Functional specialization of the primate frontal cortex during decision making. *J Neurosci* 27: 8170–8173.

42. Lee D, Seo H. 2007. Mechanisms of reinforcement learning and decision making in the primate dorsolateral prefrontal cortex. *Ann N Y Acad Sci* 1104: 108–122.

43. Levy I, Snell J, Nelson A, Rustichini A, Glimcher P. 2010. Neural representation of subjective value under risk and ambiguity. *J Neurophysiol* 103: 1036.

44. MacLean P. 1949. Psychosomatic disease and the "visceral brain": recent developments bearing on the Papez theory of emotion. *Psychosom Med* 11: 338.

45. Mason MF, Norton MI, Van Horn JD, Wegner DM, Grafton ST, Macrae CN. 2007. Wandering minds: the default network and stimulus-independent thought. *Science* 315: 393–395.

46. McClure SM, Berns GS, Montague PR. 2003. Temporal prediction errors in a passive learning task activate human striatum. *Neuron* 38: 339–346.

47. McCoy AN, Crowley JC, Haghighian G, Dean HL, Platt ML. 2003. Saccade reward signals in posterior cingulate cortex. *Neuron* 40: 1031–1040.

48. McCoy AN, Platt ML. 2005. Risk-sensitive neurons in macaque posterior cingulate cortex. *Nat Neurosci* 8: 1220–1227.

49. McKiernan KA, Kaufman JN, Kucera-Thompson J, Binder JR. 2003. A parametric manipulation of factors affecting task-induced deactivation in functional neuroimaging. *J Cogn Neurosci* 15: 394–408.

50. Mesulam MM. 1999. Spatial attention and neglect: parietal, frontal and cingulate contributions to the mental representation and attentional targeting of salient extrapersonal events. *Philos Trans R Soc Lond B Biol Sci* 354: 1325–1346.

51. Minoshima S, Giordani B, Berent S, Frey KA, Foster NL, Kuhl DE. 1997. Metabolic reduction in the posterior cingulate cortex in very early Alzheimer's disease. *Ann Neurol* 42: 85–94.

52. Montague PR, Berns GS. 2002. Neural economics and the biological substrates of valuation. *Neuron* 36: 265–284.

53. Morecraft RJ, Van Hoesen GW. 1993. Frontal granular cortex input to the cingulate (M3), supplementary (M2) and primary (M1) motor cortices in the rhesus monkey. *J Comp Neurol* 337: 669–689.

54. Müller-Preuss P, Jürgens U. 1976. Projections from the cingular vocalization area in the squirrel monkey. *Brain Res* 103: 29–43.

55. Nassar MR, Wilson RC, Heasly B, Gold JI. 2010. An approximately Bayesian delta-rule model explains the dynamics of belief updating in a changing environment. *J Neurosci* 30: 12366–12378.

56. Nestor PJ, Fryer TD, Ikeda M, Hodges JR. 2003. Retrosplenial cortex (BA 29/30) hypometabolism in mild cognitive impairment (prodromal Alzheimer's disease). *Eur J Neurosci* 18: 2663–2667.

57. Niki H, Watanabe M. 1979. Prefrontal and cingulate unit activity during timing behavior in the monkey. *Brain Res* 171: 213–224.

58. Olson CR, Musil SY, Goldberg ME. 1996. Single neurons in posterior cingulate cortex of behaving macaque: eye movement signals. *J Neurophysiol* 76: 3285–3300.

59. Pandya DN, Van Hoesen GW, Mesulam MM. 1981. Efferent connections of the cingulate gyrus in the rhesus monkey. *Exp Brain Res* 42: 319–330.

60. Papez J. 1937. A proposed mechanism of emotion. *Arch Neurol Psychiatry* 38: 725–743.

61. Pearce JM, Hall G. 1980. A model for Pavlovian learning: variations in the effectiveness of conditioned but not of unconditioned stimuli. *Psychol Rev* 87: 532–552.

62. Pearson JM, Hayden BY, Raghavachari S, Platt ML. 2009. Neurons in posterior cingulate cortex signal exploratory decisions in a dynamic multioption choice task. *Curr Biol* 19: 1532–1537.

63. Porrino L. 1993. Cortical mechanisms of reinforcement. In: Neurobiology of Cingulate Cortex and Limbic Thalamus: A Comprehensive Handbook (Vogt BA, Gabriel M, eds), pp 445–460. Boston: Birkhäuser.

64. Powell E. 1978. The cingulate bridge between allocortex, isocortex and thalamus. *Anat Rec* 190: 783–793.

65. Raichle ME, Gusnard DA. 2005. Intrinsic brain activity sets the stage for expression of motivated behavior. *J Comp Neurol* 493: 167–176.

66. Raichle ME, MacLeod AM, Snyder AZ, Powers WJ, Gusnard DA, Shulman GL. 2001. A default mode of brain function. *Proc Natl Acad Sci USA* 98: 676–682.

67. Raichle ME, Mintun MA. 2006. Brain work and brain imaging. *Annu Rev Neurosci* 29: 449–476.

68. Schacter D, Wagner A. 1999. Medial temporal lobe activations in fMRI and PET studies of episodic encoding and retrieval. *Hippocampus* 9: 7–24.

69. Schoenbaum G, Esber G. 2010. How do you (estimate you will) like them apples? Integration as a defining trait of orbitofrontal function. *Curr Opin Neurobiol* 20: 205–211.

70. Schoenbaum G, Roesch M, Stalnaker T, Takahashi Y. 2009. A new perspective on the role of the orbitofrontal cortex in adaptive behaviour. *Nat Rev Neurosci* 10: 885–892.

71. Schultz W, Dayan P, Montague P. 1997. A neural substrate of prediction and reward. *Science* 275: 1593.

72. Shidara M, Richmond BJ. 2002. Anterior cingulate: single neuronal signals related to degree of reward expectancy. *Science* 296: 1709–1711.

73. Sikes R, Vogt B. 1992. Nociceptive neurons in area 24 of rabbit cingulate cortex. *J Neurophysiol* 68: 1720.

74. Smith DV, Hayden BY, Truong TK, Song AW, Platt ML, Huettel SA. 2010. Distinct value signals in anterior and posterior ventromedial prefrontal cortex. *J Neurosci* 30: 2490–2495.

75. Smith WK. 1945. The functional significance of the rostral cingulate cortex as revealed by its responses to electrical excitation. *J Neurophysiol* 8: 241–255.

76. Spence S, Silverman J, Corbett D. 1985. Cortical and ventral tegmental systems exert opposing influences on self-stimulation from the prefrontal cortex. *Behav Brain Res* 17: 117–124.

77. Squire LR, Knowlton B, Musen G. 1993. The structure and organization of memory. *Annu Rev Psychol* 44: 453–495.

78. Sutton RS, Barto AG. 1998. Reinforcement Learning: An Introduction. Cambridge, MA: MIT Press.

79. Talairach J, Bancaud J, Geier S, Bordas-Ferrer M, Bonis A, Szikla G, Rusu M. 1973. The cingulate gyrus and human behaviour. *Electroencephalogr Clin Neurophysiol* 34: 45–52.

80. Tsai H, Zhang F, Adamantidis A, Stuber G, Bonci A, de Lecea L, Deisseroth K. 2009. Phasic firing in dopaminergic neurons is sufficient for behavioral conditioning. *Science* 324: 1080–1084.

81. Vincent JL, Patel GH, Fox MD, Snyder AZ, Baker JT, Van Essen DC, Zempel JM, Snyder LH, Corbetta M, Raichle ME. 2007. Intrinsic functional architecture in the anaesthetized monkey brain. *Nature* 447: 83–86.

82. Vincent JL, Snyder AZ, Fox MD, Shannon BJ, Andrews JR, Raichle ME, Buckner RL. 2006. Coherent spontaneous activity identifies a hippocampal-parietal memory network. *J Neurophysiol* 96: 3517–3531.

83. Vogt BA, Pandya DN, Rosene DL. 1987. Cingulate cortex of the rhesus monkey: I. Cytoarchitecture and thalamic afferents. *J Comp Neurol* 262: 256–270.

84. Vogt BA, Rosene DL, Pandya DN. 1979. Thalamic and cortical afferents differentiate anterior from posterior cingulate cortex in the monkey. *Science* 204: 205–207.

85. Waelti P, Dickinson A, Schultz W. 2001. Dopamine responses comply with basic assumptions of formal learning theory. *Nature* 412: 43–48.

86. Walton ME, Croxson PL, Behrens TE, Kennerley SW, Rushworth MF. 2007. Adaptive decision making and value in the anterior cingulate cortex. *Neuroimage* 36(Suppl 2): T142–T154.

87. Ward A, Jr. 1948. The anterior cingulate gyrus and personality. *Res Publ Assoc Res Nerv Ment Dis* 27: 438.

88. Watkins C, Dayan P. 1992. Q-learning. *Mach Learn* 8: 279–292.

89. Weissman DH, Roberts KC, Visscher KM, Woldorff MG. 2006. The neural bases of momentary lapses in attention. *Nat Neurosci* 9: 971–978.

90. Whittle P. 1988. Restless bandits: activity allocation in a changing world. *J Appl Probab* 25: 287–298.

91. Yeterian E, Van Hoesen G. 1978. Cortico-striate projections in the rhesus monkey: the organization of certain cortico-caudate connections. *Brain Res* 139: 43–63.

92. Yu AJ, Dayan P. 2005. Uncertainty, neuromodulation, and attention. *Neuron* 46: 681–692.

93. Yukie M, Shibata H. 2009. Temperocingulate interactions in the monkey. In: Cingulate Neurobiology and Disease (Vogt B, ed), pp 145–162. Oxford: Oxford University Press.

94. Zhou Y, Dougherty J, Jr, Hubner K, Bai B, Cannon R, Hutson R. 2008. Abnormal connectivity in the posterior cingulate and hippocampus in early Alzheimer's disease and mild cognitive impairment. *Alzheimers Dement* 4: 265–270.

III A SUBCORTICAL PERSPECTIVE ON THE FUNCTIONAL BASIS OF CONTROL

The four chapters in this section focus on interactions between cortical and subcortical systems. The first two chapters explore the neuroanatomical and neurochemical basis of motivational control. On the basis of results from different conditioning paradigms, Liljeholm and O'Doherty emphasize important functional divisions among motivational control mechanisms. For instance, the shell and core parts of the nucleus accumbens (NAcc) and the central and basolateral parts of the amygdala are suggested to play distinct roles in global versus specific Pavlovian-instrumental transfer. Walton and colleagues, in the second chapter, consider the role of dopamine (DA) in motivational control. DA's rise to prominence in the control literature is mostly due to the popular idea that DA neurons encode errors in reward prediction; that is, the difference between the expected and the obtained value of an outcome.[12] However, as discussed in the chapter by Walton and colleagues, the information conveyed by dopaminergic neurons is more complex than a simple scalar reward prediction error signal. Based on their DA recordings in the NAcc, they suggest that the phasic DA signal should be seen as a signal motivating explorative behavior.

The chapter by Greenhouse and colleagues focuses on the role of cortical-subcortical interactions in action inhibition, one of the hallmark functions of cognitive control. There are a number of models of the role of the basal ganglia in action selection and action inhibition. These models often dissociate two major projection systems through the basal ganglia: the direct pathway from cortex via striatum to the globus pallidus interna (GPi)/substantia nigra (SN), and the indirect pathway from cortex via striatum, globus pallidus externa (GPe), subthalamic nucleus (STN), and GPi/SN. These pathways are thought to interact to produce successful response selection.[10] Recently, particular emphasis has been placed on the so-called hyperdirect pathway, in which the STN forms the input to the basal ganglia, bypassing the striatum.[10] It has been suggested that these different pathways interact to ensure that appropriate actions can be selected, executed, and terminated with the required timing, whereas other motor programs are inhibited.[9,10] In particular, the hyperdirect pathway has been implicated in action inhibition.[1] In their chapter, Greenhouse and colleagues discuss the role of these different pathways and their interaction with frontal cortical structures such as the presupplementary motor area and the right inferior frontal cortex. These cortical-basal ganglia circuits are heavily influenced by dopamine function, as evidenced by their impairment in Parkinson's and Huntington's diseases. Furthermore, Greenhouse and colleagues highlight the role of these circuits not just in reactive stopping, but also in preparing to stop, that is, in adopting a more cautious response strategy.[3]

In the first section, Ullsperger already discussed the role of norepinephrine (NE) in cognitive control, focusing particularly on the locus coeruleus-norepinephrine (LC-NE) system with its widely distributed, ascending projections to the neocortex. Original proposals on the role of the LC-NE system suggested a role for NE in mediating arousal. Although intuitively appealing, this characterization lacks precise neural and computational mechanization. In recent years, a fundamental change has occurred in understanding of the LC-NE system, starting with the adaptive gain theory of Aston-Jones and colleagues.[2] This theory proposes that LC neurons exhibit phasic and tonic modes of activity, which facilitate exploitative or explorative behavior, respectively. Phasic LC activity is suggested to modulate the gain of target neurons to facilitate the execution of appropriate behavioral responses. The chapter by Nieuwenhuis takes the integration between work on the LC-NE and more traditional cognitive control work even further. Nieuwenhuis discusses his influential framework suggesting that the P300 component of the event-related brain potential is a reflection of precisely this type of phasic NE signal.[11] His earlier work focused on similarities in antecedent conditions of phasic NE responses and P300, and on the overlap in P300 sources and NE projections in the cortex. Here, Nieuwenhuis explores another important relationship between NE and the P300, namely, the roles of both in learning. In reviewing these similarities, he suggests possible homologs between recent computational theories of phasic LC function[5] and one of the most prominent theories of P300, the context-updating hypothesis.[7]

DA and NE are often considered as independent systems, but have been shown to interact with each other. Stimulation of ventral tegmental area (VTA) can induce discharges of LC cells,[6] and VTA cells receive projections from the locus coeruleus.[8] Integrative theories incorporating the roles of DA and NE are only now being contructed.[4]

References

1. Aron AR, Poldrack RA. 2006. Cortical and subcortical contributions to Stop signal response inhibition: role of the subthalamic nucleus. *J Neurosci* 26: 2424–2433.

2. Aston-Jones G, Cohen JD. 2005. An integrative theory of locus coeruleus-norepinephrine function: adaptive gain and optimal performance. *Annu Rev Neurosci* 28: 403–450.

3. Bogacz R, Wagenmakers EJ, Forstmann BU, Nieuwenhuis S. 2010. The neural basis of the speed-accuracy tradeoff. *Trends Neurosci* 33: 10–16.

4. Cohen JD, Aston-Jones G, Gilzenrat MS. 2004. A systems-level perspective on attention and cognitive control: guided activation, adaptive gating, conflict monitoring, and exploitation versus exploration. In: Cognitive Neuroscience of Attention (Posner MI, ed), pp 71–90. New York: Guilford Press.

5. Dayan P, Yu AJ. 2006. Phasic norepinephrine: a neural interrupt signal for unexpected events. *Network* 17: 335–350.

6. Deutch AY, Goldstein M, Roth RH. 1986. Activation of the locus coeruleus induced by selective stimulation of the ventral tegmental area. *Brain Res* 363: 307–314.

7. Donchin E, Coles MGH. 1988. Is the P300 component a manifestation of context updating? *Psychophysiology* 11: 357–374.

8. Fields HL, Hjelmstad GO, Margolis EB, Nicola SM. 2007. Ventral tegmental area neurons in learned appetitive behavior and positive reinforcement. *Annu Rev Neurosci* 30: 289–316.

9. Frank MJ. 2006. Hold your horses: a dynamic computational role for the subthalamic nucleus in decision making. *Neural Netw* 19: 1120–1136.

10. Nambu A, Tokuno H, Takada M. 2002. Functional significance of the cortico-subthalamo-pallidal 'hyperdirect' pathway. *Neurosci Res* 43: 111–117.

11. Nieuwenhuis S, Aston-Jones G, Cohen JD. 2005. Decision making, the P3, and the locus coeruleus-norepinephrine system. *Psychol Bull* 131: 510–532.

12. Schultz W. 1999. The reward signal of midbrain dopamine neurons. *News Physiol Sci* 14: 249–255.

9 Subcortical Contributions to the Motivational and Cognitive Control of Instrumental Performance by Pavlovian and Discriminative Stimuli

Mimi Liljeholm and John P. O'Doherty

Instrumental actions allow organisms to manipulate their environment for the purpose of achieving goals and avoiding punishment and, as such, provide the basis for a range of human behaviors, such as decision making, social interactions, tool use, and addiction. In a basic instrumental learning paradigm, initially arbitrary responses are acquired, and become operant, based on their ability to produce rewarding outcomes. However, a key finding from studies in both humans and rodents is that instrumental performance is often under the cognitive and motivational control of environmental cues. Indeed, as all instrumental actions occur in some kind of setting, their basis is often difficult to separate from processes tied to the stimuli that guide them.

While there is an extensive literature on the role of the prefrontal cortex in goal-directed control, more recent evidence has highlighted the contribution of subcortical structures, including the striatum and the amygdala, to instrumental performance. In this chapter, we consider subcortical mediation of the motivational and cognitive control exerted by environmental cues on instrumental performance. We begin with a discussion of some well-established motivational interactions between Pavlovian cues and instrumental responding. We then address more cognitive, nonmotivational, control of instrumental performance by environmental cues, specifically with respect to the eliciting properties of discriminative stimuli. Finally, we cover the distinction between stimuli that set the stage for a cognitive and motivational evaluation of a particular action, and those that compulsively trigger actions, thus serving as their sole determinants.

Motivational Control of Pavlovian Cues over Instrumental Performance

Pavlovian conditioning involves the pairing of a neutral (conditioned) stimulus (i.e., one that does not elicit any overt behavioral response) with a (unconditioned) stimulus that has biological relevance for the organism and that, consequently, triggers an apparent, unconditioned, response (UR). Given sufficient pairings of the conditioned stimulus (CS) with the unconditioned stimulus (US), the overt behavioral UR elicited by the US comes to be elicited by the CS. Unlike instrumental responses, which are initially arbitrary and acquired solely on the basis of their ability to produce rewards, conditioned responses are reflexive, intrinsic to the organism, and simply transferred from the US to CS through the process of conditioning.

While Pavlovian and instrumental conditioning are often studied, and conceived of, as separate learning processes, there is now ample evidence for the notion that Pavlovian cues provide motivational support for a modulation of the vigor, or rate, of instrumental performance. According to *Two-Process Theory*,[36] this is due to the fact that two types of associative structures support instrumental performance; an instrumental S-R association (established through the reinforcement contingent on performing a response in the presence of a particular stimulus) and a Pavlovian S-O association (based on the contiguity between stimuli and outcomes). Thus, this theory suggests that the two forms of associative learning interact, such that the S-O association activates an emotional state, which then motivates the instrumental behavior. These emotional states are general, except for their valence, which is either appetitive or aversive.

In this section, we begin by describing some of the behavioral evidence for the motivational control by Pavlovian cues over instrumental performance. We then discuss subcortical substrates that may be mediating such effects.

Behavioral Evidence for Motivational Control by Pavlovian Cues

The most frequently demonstrated support for a motivational role of Pavlovian cues in guiding instrumental performance comes from a paradigm called Pavlovian-instrumental transfer (PIT). Generally, PIT is studied by training subjects on two separate relationships: a Pavlovian relationship between a perceptual stimulus (CS+) and some rewarding outcome, and an instrumental relationship between an action and a contingently delivered reward. During test, the vigor or rate with which subjects perform the instrumental response in the presence of the CS+ is compared to instrumental performance in the presence of a control stimulus (CS−), which was also previously presented but has not been paired with any consequence. The effect is an apparent increase in instrumental responding during presentations of the CS+ over that observed during presentation of the CS−. Such increases in responding occur even when the rewarding outcome signaled by the CS+ is different from that earned by the instrumental response, indicating a general motivational process. The motivational basis of the PIT effect is further supported by evidence from rodent studies, showing that when animals are satiated (i.e., given free access to food prior to the test) the effect disappears.[12]

Although the transfer effect has been most frequently shown in rodents, a recent neuroimaging study with humans also provided evidence for an increase in the vigor of an instrumental response due to the presentation of a conditioned stimulus. Talmi et al.[38] trained participants to squeeze a hand-grip to obtain monetary reward. In a subsequent Pavlovian conditioning phase, two CSs, each consisting of a fractal image combined with a distinct sound, were presented; one of these CSs was paired with a monetary reward (CS+) while the other was not (CS−). Finally, in an extinction test, the two CSs were presented in a pseudo-random order, while participants were free to perform the hand-grip response at will. Consistent with Pavlovian-instrumental transfer results from the animal conditioning literature, the results showed that participants gripped more frequently in the presence of the CS+ than the CS−.

Another effect that speaks to the role of general motivational processes guiding instrumental performance is *instrumental reinstatement*. Generally, reinstatement is assessed by first training an instrumental response (e.g., lever-pressing) using standard instrumental conditioning procedures, and then extinguishing that response by eliminating the delivery of reward previously contingent on the response. Following extinction, noncontingent delivery of the reward reinstates the instrumental response.[35] As with Pavlovian-instrumental transfer, such reinstatement effects are sensitive to motivational shifts.[33] Although it is possible that the noncontingently delivered reward itself triggers motivational processes that result in an increase in responding, a series of experiments conducted by Baker et al.[2] demonstrated that it is most likely the *context* in which acquisition and performance of the response occurs that mediates this effect: Baker et al. showed that manipulations known to attenuate context conditioning (e.g., extinguishing the context, or assessing reinstatement in a different context from that in which noncontingent rewards were delivered) significantly reduced the reinstatement effect. Thus, it appears that the context, which is paired with the reward throughout acquisition and performance, and then again when rewards are noncontingently delivered, serves as a Pavlovian stimulus that influences instrumental responding in a manner akin to that observed in Pavlovian-instrumental transfer.

Subcortical Contributions to Motivational Control

At the neural level, evidence from rodent lesion studies suggest that the motivational aspect of the Pavlovian-instrumental transfer effect is mediated by the ventral tegmental area (VTA), the central nucleus of the amygdala (CeA), and the nucleus accumbens (NAcc): Inactivation of each of these areas attenuates, or completely abolishes, the transfer effect.

For example, using a very simple paradigm with rodents, involving a single instrumental response earning grain pellets, a CS+, also predicting grain pellets, and a

CS–, Murschall and Hauber[31] found that pretraining inactivation of the VTA (a dopaminergic midbrain structure) completely abolished the transfer effect. Interestingly, Corbit et al.[12] used a more complex experimental protocol, in which multiple instrumental responses were trained up, each earning a unique reward (see the final section) and found that inactivation of the VTA attenuated only the PIT effect. Thus, it is possible that complex training procedures, requiring more elaborate representations of responses, stimuli, and outcomes, recruit additional areas that also contribute to the PIT effect.

Another subcortical structure known to play a role in PIT is the CeA.[9,22,24] Together with the basolateral nucleus of the amygdala (BLA; discussed in more detail in the final section), the CeA is involved in several aspects of Pavlovian conditioning, including conditioned suppression[28] and orienting responses toward appetitive CSs.[20] Given its projections to the hypothalamus, reticular formation, and brainstem nuclei, the CeA has been argued to regulate both behavioral and autonomic responses,[6] consistent with its role in the invigoration of instrumental responding by Pavlovian cues.

A third subcortical structure found to be involved in PIT is the nucleus accumbens (NAcc), a collection of neurons in the ventral striatum. Specifically, Hall et al.[22] found that lesions to the core, but not the shell, of the NAcc abolished PIT while sparing conditioned and instrumental responding in general. Importantly, although the CeA does not directly project to the NAcc, it does affect this area indirectly through its projections to the dopaminergic cells in the VTA,[19] which in turn innervate the NAcc.[7] Interestingly, a neuroimaging study assessing PIT in humans has also identified the amygdala and NAcc. Talmi et al.[38] found that activity in the NAcc was positively correlated with instrumental response frequency during the CS+ and negatively correlated with response frequency during the CS–. In addition, activity in the NAcc and in the right amygdala was correlated with PIT such that the difference in activity in these areas across the CS+ and CS– was stronger in participants who exhibited a stronger PIT effect.

Finally, not surprisingly, the NAcc also appears to be involved in mediating instrumental reinstatement: Janak et al.[26] recorded extracellular single-unit neural activity using electrode arrays implanted into the NAcc of rats during initial acquisition, extinction, and reinstatement of an instrumental response for sucrose reward. They found that a large subset of NAcc neurons changed their response profiles across the sessions of the experiment. Specifically, during initial acquisition, while performance was rewarded, 54% of recorded neurons exhibited a change in activity around the time of the retrieval of the reward, including a subset whose altered responses were maintained from the time of the operant response until the delivery of reinforcement. During extinction, a large subset of neural responses were absent, but reappeared during reinstatement. Interestingly, 27% of neural responses observed during the reinstatement period were not present during initial training, suggesting that the representation was perhaps specific to reinstatement. More generally, the apparent role of the NAcc in both PIT and instrumental reinstatement suggests that these two behavioral effects may involve common underlying motivational processes.

Cognitive Control of Pavlovian Cues over Instrumental Performance

Though it is clear that general motivational processes can guide instrumental performance, two-process theory is challenged by the finding that both transfer and reinstatement effects often exhibit a selectivity suggesting the involvement of cognitive representations of the outcomes of instrumental actions. In addition to this being beyond the scope of general motivational accounts, such outcome-selective effects are also unaffected by shifts in motivational state, providing further support for the notion that they are independent of incentive processes.

There is, however, an alternative *expectancy* version of two-process theory that accounts for outcome-selective effects. Unlike motivational two-process theory, this theory postulates that the sensory-specific features of outcomes constitute discriminative stimuli that trigger actions based on S-R associations.[40] Specifically, on this account, Pavlovian cues, and noncontingent reward deliveries, elicit not motivational, but cognitive representations of rewarding outcomes. These cognitive, or sensory, representations of reward are then allowed to enter into S-R associations just like any other discriminative stimulus. Notably, while this version of two-process theory accounts for outcome-selective effects, it does not cover the motivational effects discussed in the previous section. Thus, a full theoretical account of the influence of Pavlovian cues on instrumental performance has not yet been worked out.

In this section, we first briefly discuss the behavioral evidence for an outcome-selective influence of Pavlovian cues on instrumental performance, and then review data from neuroscientific studies, suggesting that the subcortical structures that mediate these effects are dissociable from those involved in motivational control.

Behavioral Evidence for Cognitive Control

The studies that have provided evidence for outcome-selective transfer and reinstatement use procedures similar to those discussed in the previous section, except that subjects are trained on multiple actions, each generating a unique outcome. For example, Corbit and Balleine[8] trained rats to press one lever for a sucrose solution and another lever for grain pellets (in separate sessions). In a subsequent phase of the experiment, the rats received Pavlovian conditioning training, in which one conditioned stimulus signaled the availability of sucrose and another signaled the availability of grain pellets. During an extinction test phase, the two CSs were presented in random order while one or the other of the two levers was present. Interestingly, each stimulus only elevated lever pressing, relative to the prestimulus period, on the lever that had earned the *same* outcome as the stimulus, suggesting that the sensory-specific (i.e., cognitive) features of the signaled outcome played a critical role in mediating instrumental performance. Importantly, a subsequent study[12] demonstrated that a shift from a hungry to a relatively satiated state (i.e., motivational shift) did not affect this outcome-selective transfer effect.

More recently, Bray et al.[5] conducted a similar experiment with humans in which simple geometric figures were initially paired with rewarding liquid outcomes (i.e., chocolate milk, cola, and orange juice). In a subsequent instrumental conditioning phase, these outcomes were contingent on distinct instrumental responses. Finally, in a third session, Pavlovian and instrumental trials were randomly intermixed. During the transfer test, one of the Pavlovian cues was presented simultaneously with the availability of two alternative instrumental responses. As with rodents, human participants showed a clear bias toward the instrumental response that produced the same outcome as that signaled by the presented Pavlovian cue.

Reinstatement effects (i.e., an increase in the performance of an extinguished instrumental response due the noncontingent presentation of the outcome associated with that response) exhibit an outcome selectivity akin to that demonstrated with Pavlovian-instrumental transfer. For example, Ostlund and Balleine[33] trained rats on two alternative instrumental actions (i.e., right and left lever press) each of which earned a unique outcome (sucrose solution or grain pellet). During a reinstatement test, both levers were available but, for the first 15 minutes, neither yielded any reward. After this 15-minute extinction period, one of the two outcomes was delivered noncontingently (i.e., 5 sec after neither response had been performed). The results of this test showed that the outcome delivery selectively reinstated performance of the response that had earned the reinstating outcome, relative to the other response. Importantly, a subsequent experiment showed that the noncontingently delivered outcome's ability to reinstate responding was unaffected by a reduction in its motivational value, suggesting a purely cognitive basis for its modulation of performance[33] consistent with the *expectancy* version of two-process theory.

Subcortical Contributions Cognitive Control

The apparent behavioral differences between outcome-selective and general Pavlovian-instrumental interactions, with respect to the influence of motivational shifts, raise the question of whether dissociable neural substrates support these different effects. Although very little work has been done assessing dissociable neural substrates for general and selective instrumental reinstatement (although see ref. 32), a substantial body of research indicates that this does indeed appear to be the case for PIT effects.

For example, Corbit et al.[13] found that lesions to the NAcc shell but not the core abolished outcome-selective PIT. Although these results may appear to contradict those of Hall et al.,[22] who found that lesions to the core but not the shell eliminated PIT, the important difference is that Hall et al. were assessing general PIT. Taken together, these results suggest a dissociation within the NAcc, such that the shell of this structure is needed for outcome-selective PIT, whereas the core mediates the motivational processes supporting general PIT. Additional evidence for the role of the NAcc shell in selective PIT comes from Wyvell and Berridge,[44] who found that amphetamine microinjection into the NAcc shell enhanced PIT; importantly, though they only used a single rewarding outcome, their experiment included a control lever that did not yield any reward; no increases due to the presentation of the CS+ was seen on this lever, consistent with outcome-selective PIT.

A dissociation between selective and general PIT has also been observed with respect to the BLA and CeA. Corbit and Balleine[9] (experiment 3) found that BLA lesions abolished the outcome-selective PIT effect, but spared general PIT whereas, in contrast, CeN lesions abolished the general excitatory influence of Pavlovian cues on instrumental responding, but spared the outcome-selective effect. Interestingly, unlike the dissociations between general and selective PIT found for the shell and core of the NAcc, and for the BLA and CeA, the VTA appears to be needed for both forms of transfer. Corbit et al.[12] found that, although motivational shifts had a clearly differential effect on general and selective transfer, attenuating the former but not affecting the latter, inactivation of the VTA during the transfer test eliminated both the general and selective effects. Indeed, VTA inactivation produced a general reduction in responding, significant even for the baseline period, during which no Pavlovian cues were presented; it is possible, therefore, that this structure plays a more general role in response initiation.[12]

As described previously, outcome-selective PIT has recently been demonstrated in human subjects: Bray et al.[5] scanned human subjects with functional magnetic resonance imaging while they were choosing between instrumental responses that produced liquid rewards in the presence of Pavlovian cues that had previously been paired with those same rewards. In addition to finding clear behavioral evidence for outcome-selective PIT (such that participants tended to choose the response that had produced the same outcome as the currently presented Pavlovian cue), Bray et al. found that activity in the ventrolateral putamen was greater when subjects chose the response compatible with the Pavlovian cue than when they chose the incompatible response. Notably, control conditions revealed that, rather than an increase in activity in this area during compatible choices, this effect was due to a decrease in activity during incompatible choices, suggesting, perhaps, that the withholding of the compatible, not the incompatible, choice required inhibitory processes.

Goal-Directed and Habitual Instrumental Performance

A major finding in the animal operant conditioning literature is an apparent shift from voluntary to compulsive action selection. Specifically, during early stages of training, instrumental performance is goal directed, reflecting changes in the causal efficacy with which actions produce rewards, and in the subjective value, or utility, of those rewards. However, with extensive training, action selection becomes *habitual*; largely stimulus driven and insensitive to both contingency and utility manipulations. Both associative and computational models suggest that, rather than the habit system replacing goal-directed action selection, the two sources of behavioral control develop together, and flexibly compete or cooperate.

In this section we begin by describing some behavioral evidence, from both rodents and humans, for goal-directed and habitual performance. We then give a brief account of associative and computational models of the two behavioral control systems and, finally, discuss dissociable subcortical substrates.

Behavioral Evidence for Habitual and Goal-Directed Processes

Under normal training conditions, rats that have learned to perform an instrumental response for some natural reward will decrease their rate of responding if that reward has been *devalued* by pairing it with an aversive event, or by feeding the animal on it to satiety.[1] This decrease in responding indicates that behavior is sensitive to the subjective value of the anticipated outcome, and thus that performance is goal directed. Likewise, the goal-directedness of instrumental performance is frequently demonstrated by the finding that rats will suppress their performance of an instrumental response if the causal relationship, or contingency, between that response and its outcome is degraded by delivering the outcome irrespective of lever-press performance.[3] Importantly, given extensive training, instrumental actions exhibit an insensitivity to both devaluation and contingency degradation,[15,16] suggesting that they are no longer based on any consideration of their consequences (i.e., that they have become habitual).

As with demonstrations of Pavlovian-instrumental interactions, the majority of behavioral and neuroscientific studies on goal-directed and habitual action selection have been conducted with rodents. However, there now exists a fair amount of evidence for similar processes, and homologous neural substrates, in humans. For example, sensitivity to both devaluation[43] and contingency degradation[30] has been demonstrated in human subjects, as has insensitivity to such manipulations.[37,41] Nonetheless, obtaining clear demonstrations of habitual performance in human subjects, using appropriate behavioral assays, has proven remarkably challenging, perhaps in part because humans, by virtue of a highly developed goal-directed system, often remain goal directed, or rapidly switch from habitual control to goal-directed control when they notice changes in the environment or detect that their behavior is being evaluated

Theoretical Accounts of Habitual and Goal-Directed Learning

As described in the previous sections, traditional theories of instrumental learning postulate a compulsory elicitation of actions by discriminative stimuli, through stimulus-response (S-R) associations, as well as motivational modulation by stimulus-outcome (S-O) associations and underlying incentive processes. In addition, contemporary associative theories attempt to provide a description of the processes supporting voluntary, or goal-directed, instrumental performance, and do so in terms of associations between instrumental actions and their outcomes. For example, according to the associative-cybernetic model,[4] action selection is largely controlled by the retrieval of a response by the sensory-specific features of a present, or associatively retrieved, outcome (i.e., through O-R associations). This action selection then initiates a process of action evaluation through the R-O association, such that the estimated value of an action is based on the efficacy with which the action produces an outcome, and on the subjective value of that outcome. Actual performance of an action occurs when its representation is sufficiently activated by the response selection and evaluation processes. In addition to updating the strength of the R-O association and allowing estimation of outcome value, the delivery of response-contingent, appetitive outcomes give rise to a reinforcement signal that strengthens contiguously active S-R associations, including those between the sensory-specific features of the outcome and the response (i.e., O-R).

On a computational level of analysis, goal-directed and habitual action selection has been proposed to depend on two distinct classes of reinforcement learning.[14] According to this theory, the first, so-called model-based class is suggested to support goal-directed performance by constructing a model of the environment and deriving optimal decisions using estimates of the probabilities and utilities of outcomes, as well as of the probabilities of transitioning from one state to another given a particular action. In contrast, the model-free, habitual, system learns based on trial-and-error, such that the stored, or *cached*, value of an action depends strictly on the previously experienced long-run average reward contingent on that action: Thus, just as with S-R learning, rewards are not explicitly represented, but rather serve to increase the probability of performing an action in a particular state. The model-free system is computationally more efficient than the model-based one, since the former does not have to search a complex tree of states and outcomes to arrive at decisions. However, it is also much less flexible; since cached values are divorced from the actual outcomes of actions, they are slow to reflect changes in the probabilities and utilities of rewards.

It is worth noting that neither of these RL models, nor a Pavlovian version of model-free RL (the actor-critic model), can account for the Pavlovian-instrumental interactions discussed in the two previous sections. Specifically, in order to do so, these models would have to include a dynamic representation of incentive value (to account for general PIT and reinstatement; see ref. 46 for a possible solution) as well as representations that reflect the discriminative stimulus properties of mediating outcomes (to account for outcome-selective effects).

Subcortical Contributions to Habitual and Goal-Directed Processes

Evidence from rodent lesion studies suggests that, whereas the acquisition of action-outcome associations depends on the prelimbic region of prefrontal cortex, and the medial area of dorsal striatum to which this region of cortex projects, the formation and expression of S-R associations is mediated by the dorsolateral striatum (DLS). Interestingly, lesions of the DLS have also been shown to disrupt outcome-selective PIT,[10] further supporting the notion that such effects involve the elicitation of actions based on the discriminative properties of outcomes signaled by Pavlovian cues. With respect to the DMS and its role in goal-directed performance, Yin et al.[45] found that whereas inactivation of the posterior DMS abolished sensitivity to contingency degradation (i.e., to the delivery of noncontingent rewards), inactivation of the anterior DMS had no effect, suggesting a dissociation along the anterior-posterior axis of this structure. Likewise, Corbit and Janak[11] found that the posterior DMS was critical for the acquisition of both response-outcome and stimulus-outcome relationships, while the anterior DMS appeared to be needed only for response-outcome encoding.

Similarly, in humans, neuroimaging studies have shown that the anterior caudate plays a critical role in encoding the action-outcome relationship. For example, Tanaka et al.[39] found that activity in the anterior caudate increased with an increase in the contingency between pressing a button and receiving monetary reward, whereas Tricomi et al.[42] found robust activity in the caudate only when subjects believed that their actions determined the valence of a contingent outcome (i.e., gain or loss of money). Perhaps most pertinently, Liljehom et al.[30] found that, whereas activity in the anterior caudate correlated with the probability of receiving reward given that an instrumental action was performed, activity in the posterior caudate correlated with the probability of noncontingent rewards.

As mentioned, with respect to habitual performance in humans, very little is known about both behavioral and neural processes. Indeed, to our knowledge, only a single study has shown neural correlates of the behavioral development of habits in human subjects.[41] In that study, extensive training was used to induce habits in one group, compared to a moderately trained group. In both groups, after initial training in which two distinct instrumental responses were paired with pictures of unique food outcomes, one of the outcomes was devalued through selective satiation (i.e., participants were asked to eat one of the food outcomes until it was no longer desirable to them). In the subsequent test phase, participants in the moderately trained group suppressed their responding for the devalued outcome. In contrast, participants in the overtrained group continued to respond for the devalued outcome, suggesting that their behavior had become insensitive to outcome value, consistent with a habitual mode of performance. Tricomi et al.[41] found a significant increase in the posterior lateral putamen, across sessions and across days of training, for the overtrained group, suggesting that activity in this structure correlates with the behavioral development of habits in humans.

Summary and Conclusions

In this chapter, we have identified several instances where environmental stimuli take complete or partial control over instrumental performance, with respect to both cognitive and motivational constraints. In particular, we addressed the role of incentive processes in the interactions between Pavlovian stimuli and instrumental responding, as well as the influence exerted over instrumental performance by sensory-specific, cognitive aspects of Pavlovian predictions. Finally, we covered the distinction between stimuli that prompt an evaluation of the consequences of performing a particular action and those that lead directly to action execution.

However, two major issues remain: First, although the focus in this chapter has been on the role of subcortical structures, such areas interact with cortical structures in distinct yet partially anatomically overlapping corticostriatal loops.[21] For example, in the section on subcortical contributions to goal-directed and habitual performance, we emphasized the roles of dorsomedial and dorsolateral striatum, respectively. It is well known that these striatal areas are subcomponents of distinct corticostriatal loops. Specifically, with respect to goal-directed action selection in rodents, lesion studies have identified the prelimbic cortex, an area that projects heavily to the dorsomedial striatum.[3,8] Analogously, in humans, the medial, ventromedial, and orbitofrontal cortex have been implicated, together with the anterior caudate, in goal-directed instrumental performance.[30,39,43] In contrast, evidence from skill-learning studies suggests that automatic, or habitual, performance in humans depends on interactions between the posterior putamen and motor cortices, such as the supplementary and premotor areas.[27,34]

Another factor that is integral to each of the topics addressed here, but that we have not dealt with explicitly, is the role of dopamine in the functions of the relevant neural substrates. Indeed, dopamine has been implicated in several of the behaviors discussed in this chapter. For example, recall that microinjections of amphetamine (a dopamine agonist) into the NAcc shell enhance PIT.[44] In addition, dopamine antagonists have been shown to attenuate both PIT[17] and reinstatement.[25] Finally, dopamine appears to play a critical role in habit formation; Faure et al.[18] found that rats that had been subjected to dopamine depletion in the lateral striatum remained sensitive to outcome devaluation relative to non-depleted, control animals, suggesting that dopamine in this area may be necessary for the development of habits. Another recent rodent study found that infusion of a dopamine antagonist into the posterior DMS reduced sensitivity to contingency degradation while leaving sensitivity to outcome devaluation intact.[29] Notably, while this study[29] found sensitivity to both contingency degradation and outcome devaluation intact when the same antagonist was infused into the PL, others have shown that dopamine depletion in this area does indeed reduce sensitivity to outcome value[23]; further research is needed to establish the role of PL dopamine in goal-directed performance. What is clear is that a comprehensive account of the motivational and cognitive bases of instrumental performance requires careful consideration of subcortical-cortical interactions, as well as related dopamine systems.

Outstanding Questions

• How can computational RL be modified so as to account for general and selective PIT and reinstatement effects?

• Are the neural bases of general and selective reinstatement dissociable in the same manner as those mediating general and selective PIT?

• Are there neural systems (separate from those discussed here) that mediate flexible transitions between goal-directed and habitual action selection?

Further Reading

Balleine BW, Daw ND, O'Doherty JD. 2008. Multiple forms of value learning and the function of dopamine. In: Neuroeconomics: Decision Making and the Brain (Glimcher PW, Camerer DF, Fehr E, Poldrack RA, eds), pp 367–387. Amsterdam: Academic Press. An overview of different types of reinforcement learning and their neural basis, including a discussion of the role of dopamine.

Balleine BW, Liljeholm M, Ostlund SB. 2009. The integrative function of the basal ganglia in instrumental conditioning. *Behav Brain Res* 199: 43–52. Discussion of the role of the basal ganglia in instrumental conditioning and, through this, a number of higher-order executive functions.

Daw ND, Niv Y, Dayan P. 2005. Uncertainty-based competition between prefrontal and dorsolateral striatal systems for behavioral control. *Nat Neurosci* 8: 1704–1711. This paper describes a computational theory for goal-directed and habitual learning based on two variants of reinforcement learning algorithms: a "model-based" version that uses a forward-model to compute optimal choices, and a model-free version, that selects actions based on previous reinforcement history.

References

1. Adams CD, Dickinson A. 1981. Instrumental responding following reinforcer devaluation. *Q J Exp Psychol* 33B: 109–122.

2. Baker AG, Steinwald H, Bouton ME. 1991. Contextual conditioning and reinstatement of extinguished instrumental responding. *Q J Exp Psychol* 43B: 199–218.

3. Balleine BW, Dickinson A. 1998. Goal-directed instrumental action: contingency and incentive learning and their cortical substrates. *Neuropharmacology* 37: 407–419.

4. Balleine BW, Ostlund SB. 2007. Still at the choice point: action selection and initiation in instrumental conditioning. *Ann N Y Acad Sci* 1104: 147–171.

5. Bray S, Rangel A, Shimojo S, Balleine BW, O'Doherty JP. 2008. The neural mechanisms underlying the influence of pavlovian cues on human decision making. *J Neurosci* 28: 5861–5866.

6. Cardinal RN, Parkinson JA, Hall J, Everitt BJ. 2002. Emotion and motivation: the role of the amygdala, ventral striatum, and prefrontal cortex. *Neurosci Biobehav Rev* 26: 321–352.

7. Carr DB, Sesack SR. 2000. Projections from the rat prefrontal cortex to the ventral tegmental area: target specificity in the synaptic associations with mesoaccumbens and mesocortical neurons. *J Neurosci* 20: 3864–3873.

8. Corbit LH, Balleine BW. 2003. The role of the prelimbic cortex in instrumental conditioning. *Behav Brain Res* 146: 145–157.

9. Corbit LH, Balleine BW. 2005. Double dissociation of basolateral and central amygdala lesions on the general and outcome-specific forms of Pavlovian-instrumental transfer. *J Neurosci* 25: 962–970.

10. Corbit LH, Janak PH. 2007. Inactivation of the lateral but not medial dorsal striatum eliminates the excitatory impact of Pavlovian stimuli on instrumental responding. *J Neurosci* 27: 13977–13981.

11. Corbit LH, Janak PH. 2010. Posterior dorsomedial striatum is critical for both selective instrumental and Pavlovian reward learning. *Eur J Neurosci* 31: 1312–1321.

12. Corbit LH, Janak PH, Balleine BW. 2007. General and outcome-specific forms of Pavlovian-instrumental transfer: the effect of shifts in motivational state and inactivation of the ventral tegmental area. *Eur J Neurosci* 26: 3141–3149.

13. Corbit LH, Muir JL, Balleine BW. 2001. The role of the nucleus accumbens in instrumental conditioning: evidence for a functional dissociation between accumbens core and shell. *J Neurosci* 21: 3251–3260.

14. Daw N, Niv Y, Dayan P. 2005. Uncertainty-based competition between prefrontal and dorsolateral striatal systems for behavioral control. *Nat Neurosci* 8: 1701–1711.

15. Dickinson A. 1985. Actions and habits: the development of behavioral autonomy. *Philos Trans R Soc Lond B Biol Sci* 308: 67–78.

16. Dickinson A. 1998. Omission learning after instrumental pretraining. *Q J Exp Psychol* 51: 271–286.

17. Dickinson A, Smith J, Mirenowicz J. 2000. Dissociation of Pavlovian and instrumental incentive learning under dopamine antagonists. *Behav Neurosci* 114: 468–483.

18. Faure A, Haberland U, Conde F, Massioui NE. 2005. Lesion to the nigrostriatal dopamine system disrupts stimulus-response habit formation. *J Neurosci* 25: 2771–2780.

19. Fudge JL, Haber SN. 2000. The central nucleus of the amgdala projection to dopamine subpopulations in primates. *Neuroscience* 97: 479–494.

20. Gallagher M, Graham PW, Holland PC. 1990. The amygdala central nucleus and appetitive Pavlovian conditioning: lesions impair one class of conditioned behavior. *J Neurosci* 10: 1906–1911.

21. Haber SN. 2003. The primate basal ganglia: parallel and integrative networks. *J Chem Neuroanat* 26: 317–330.

22. Hall J, Parkinson JA, Connor TM, Dickinson A, Everitt BJ. 2001. Involvement of the central nucleus of the amygdala and nucleus accumbens core in mediating Pavlovian influences on instrumental behavior. *Eur J Neurosci* 13: 1984–1992.

23. Hitchcott PK, Quinn J, Taylor JR. 2007. Bidirectional modulation of goal-directed actions by prefrontal cortical dopamine. *Cereb Cortex* 17: 1680–1694.

24. Holland PC, Gallagher M. 2003. Double dissociation of the effects of lesions of basolateral and central amygdala in conditioned stimulus-potentiated feeding and Pavlovian-instrumental transfer. *Eur J Neurosci* 17: 1680–1694.

25. Horvitz JC, Ettenberg A. 1988. Haloperidol blocks the response-reinstating effects of food reward: a methodology for separating neuroleptic effects on reinforcement and motor processes. *Pharmacol Biochem Behav* 31: 861–865.

26. Janak PH, Chen MT, Caulder T. 2004. Dynamics of neural coding in the accumbens during extinction and reinstatement of rewarded behavior. *Behav Brain Res* 154: 125–135.

27. Jenkins IH, Brooks DJ, Nixon PD, Frackowiak RSJ, Passingham RE. 1994. Motor sequence learning——a study with positron emission tomography. *J Neurosci* 14: 3775–3790.

28. Killcross S, Robbins TW, Everitt BJ. 1997. Different types of fear-conditioned behavior mediated by separate nuclei within amygdala. *Nature* 388: 377–380.

29. Lex B, Hauber W. 2010. The role of dopamine in the prelimbic cortex and the dorsomedial striatum in instrumental conditioning. *Cereb Cortex* 40: 873–883.

30. Liljeholm M, Tricomi E, O'Doherty JP, Balleine BW. 2011. Neural correlates of instrumental learning: dissociable effects of action-outcome conjuctions and disjunctions. *J Neurosci* 31: 2474–2480.

31. Murschall A, Hauber W. 2006. Inactivation of the ventral tegmental area abolished the general excitatory influence of Pavlovian cues on instrumental performance. *Learn Mem* 13: 123–126.

32. Ostlund SB, Balleine BW. 2005. Lesions of medial prefrontal cortex disrupt the acquisition but not the expression of goal-directed learning. *J Neurosci* 25: 7763–7770.

33. Ostlund SB, Balleine BW. 2007. Selective reinstatement of instrumental performance depends on the discriminative stimulus properties of the mediating outcome. *Learn Behav* 35: 43–52.

34. Poldrack RA, Sabb FW, Foerde K, Tom SM, Asarnow RF, Bookheimer SY, Knowlton BJ. 2005. The neural correlates of motor skill automaticity. *J Neurosci* 25: 5356–5364.

35. Rescorla RA, Skucy JC. 1969. The effect of response-independent reinforcers during extinction. *J Comp Physiol Psychol* 67: 381–389.

36. Rescorla RA, Solomon RL. 1967. Two-process learning theory: relationships between Pavlovian conditioning and instrumental learning. *Psychol Rev* 74: 151–182.

37. Schwabe L, Wolf OT. 2009. Stress prompts habit behavior in humans. *J Neurosci* 29: 7191–7198.

38. Talmi D, Seymour B, Dayan P, Dolan RJ. 2008. Human pavlovian-instrumental transfer. *J Neurosci* 28: 360–368.

39. Tanaka SC, Balleine BW, O'Doherty JP. 2008. Calculating consequences: brain systems that encode the causal effects of actions. *J Neurosci* 28: 6750–6755.

40. Trapold MA, Overmier JB. 1972. The second learning process in instrumental learning. In: Classical Conditioning II: Current Research and Theory (Black AH, Prokasy WF, eds). New York: Appleton-Century-Crofts.

41. Tricomi E, Balleine BW, O'Doherty JP. 2009. A specific role for posterior dorsolateral striatum in human habit learning. *Eur J Neurosci* 29: 2225–2232.

42. Tricomi E, Delgado MR, Fiez JA. 2004. Modulation of caudate activity by action contingency. *Neuron* 41: 281–292.

43. Valentin VV, Dickinson A, O'Doherty JP. 2007. Determining the neural substrates of goal-directed learning in the human brain. *J Neurosci* 27: 4019–4026.

44. Wyvell CL, Berridge KC. 2000. Intra-accumbens amphetamine increases the conditioned incentive salience of sucrose reward: enhancement of reward "wanting" without enhanced "liking" or response reinforcement. *J Neurosci* 20: 8122–8130.

45. Yin HH, Ostlund SB, Knowlton BJ, Balleine BW. 2005. The role of the dorsomedial striatum in instrumental conditioning. *Eur J Neurosci* 22: 513–523.

46. Zhang J, Berridge KC, Tindell AJ, Smith KS, Aldridge JW. 2009. A neural computational model of incentive salience. *PLOS Comput Biol* 5: e1000437.

10 The Influence of Dopamine in Generating Action from Motivation

Mark E. Walton, Jerylin O. Gan, and Paul E. M. Phillips

There is cognitive separation between evaluating what one finds desirable or rewarding and working out how and whether to obtain such goals. Traditionally, the study of central nervous system function divided neatly between these two faculties: one approach looking at how an organism maintains the equilibrium in its internal milieu, and another focusing on the regulation of movements in the external environment.[67] Many contemporary studies of cognitive control have also tended to treat these processes as separate, and have generally concentrated on the latter faculty. Classic paradigms such as the Stroop task or Erikson flanker task provide response selection problems through the combination of distracting stimuli and deterministic task rules, and might seem to have little particular regard to how this might be influenced by the internal motivation of the participants, though see "emotional" Stroop tasks for examples of how even this task can be tacitly adapted to tap into unconscious motivations.[114]

Working from the premise that a primary function of the control of action stems from a requirement to place the organism in a position to satisfy its needs and ultimately to ensure its survival, however, this separation of systems into either "motivation" or "action" might be argued to be artificial and potentially limiting. Instead, an important question arises as to which neural systems bridge the divide between motivation and action and how they allow us to translate often competing desires into a coherent action plan. It is not difficult to imagine that such a basic and necessary behavior as deciding whether to perform an action for reward would require coordinated action across multiple brain regions. While there have been several recent candidate regions, particularly in the frontal and parietal lobes,[45,77,80] the focus of this chapter is on parts of the striatum and the dopamine projections to this region, with special emphasis on the nucleus accumbens (NAc), which was arguably the first structure proposed to act as a "limbic-motor interface."[64]

The dopamine projection to the NAc arises from a midbrain nucleus called the ventral tegmental area (VTA) and is referred to as the "mesolimbic" dopamine system, to differentiate it nominally from the fibers originating in the dorsal substantia nigra known as the "nigrostriatal" dopamine system. This division has also been, respectively, associated with a reward versus motor functional dichotomy.[119] Although there is little doubt that mesolimbic dopamine is important for modulating behavioral control, its exact role has remained controversial. One potential reason for this is limited appreciation of the types of incentives that might drive an organism to engage in or desist with a particular course of action. Much work has looked at how the anticipation of reinforcers and rewards might guide response selection, but there has been less appreciation of other factors that may modulate choices, such as the costs of a course of action, the novelty of exploring options, or current motivational state.

In the present chapter, we address the question of what role or roles the mesolimbic dopamine projection might play in helping translate motivation into action and in allowing one course of action to be selected in the face of competing, beneficial alternatives. We first investigate how mesolimbic dopamine came to be implicated in signaling reward and motivating an animal to action. We then discuss how dopamine transmission may promote responding to environmental cues and how this may be important for promoting control of action in some situations and disinhibition in others. Finally, we consider the limitations of the dopamine signal, focusing particularly on its role in guiding decisions when the utility of an outcome depends on the expected costs to be overcome as well as, or instead of, the anticipated benefits to be obtained.

Anatomy and Physiology of Mesolimbic Dopamine

The importance of dopamine as a chemical neurotransmitter in its own right and its function in motivation and reinforcement were realized only in the second half of the 20th century.[18,116] Dopamine is a modulatory neurotransmitter, classically thought to modulate coincident glutamatergic input in neighboring terminals. Whereas glutamatergic neurons make asymmetric synapses on the heads of dendritic spines, dopaminergic neurons synapse symmetrically on dendritic shafts and the necks of spines. In fact, the dopamine innervation of the striatum is so dense, it is thought that every structure in the striatum will be within range of a concentration of dopamine sufficient to stimulate both low- and high-affinity receptors following activation of dopamine neurons.[66]

Dopamine acts on a family of G-protein–coupled receptors classified as either D1-like (D1 and D5) or D2-like (D2, D3, D4). These receptors regulate intracellular signaling cascades in a cyclic adenosine monophosphate (cAMP)–dependent manner, where D1-like receptors increase and D2-like receptors decrease cAMP production.[69] D2-like receptors are expressed both pre- and postsynaptially, whereas

D1-like-receptor expression is limited to postsynaptic locations. In addition to their action on cAMP production, D2-like receptors regulate ion-channel conductance through the G-protein βγ complex, generally reducing cell excitability; and, as was shown recently, they participate in β-arrestin-2-dependent cell signaling using the protein-kinase-B/glycogen-synthase-kinase-3 pathway.[9] Thus, while D1-like receptors are generally considered to be excitatory and D2-like receptors inhibitory, these inferences are clearly oversimplifications. DA neurons exhibit multiple firing patterns: quiescence, tonic, slow-oscillatory/pacemaker (2–10 Hz), and phasic (bursting, 15–30 Hz) firing.[42–44,58,97,113] The pacemaker-like pattern results in a "tonic" extracellular concentration of dopamine (5–20 nM) assessable on a minute-by-minute time scale with microdialysis.[113] "Phasic" firing arises from short-latency (70–100 msec), short duration (100–200 msec) bursts of dopaminergic neuron firing that result in transient elevations of extracellular dopamine up to 1 μM.[113] It is believed that the temporally distinct patterns of dopaminergic firing convey information that subserves distinct but related behaviors, although the precise roles of tonic and phasic signals and their interaction remain to be fully elucidated.[94,113]

The majority of dopamine neurons arise from ventroanterior midbrain nuclei, which include the substantia nigra pars compacta (SNc: areas A8 and A9) and VTA (area A10) (fig. 10.1). Afferent inputs into the VTA include glutamatergic input from many parts of the brain,[41] including prefrontal cortex, amygdala, lateral hypothalamus, superior colliculus, along with the adjacent pedunculopontine tegmental nucleus (PPTg) and laterodorsal tegmental nucleus (LDT).[34] The PPTg and LDT also send cholinergic and GABAergic projections to the VTA.[96] Other GABAergic projections to the VTA originate from the ventral pallidum, the NAc, and the rostromedial tegmentum, as well as from local-circuit connections within the VTA. Additionally, the VTA receives serotonergic input from the dorsal raphe and noradrenergic input from the locus coeruleus.[34] Unlike the VTA, the major inputs to the SNc are inhibitory, consisting of GABAergic innervation from the striatum, globus pallidus, ventral pallidum, and the substantia nigra pars reticulata (SNr).[63] Excitatory inputs, though in the minority, arise from the subthalamic nucleus, amygdale, and PPTg.[63,72]

Dopaminergic projections from these nuclei comprise three main projection pathways: the nigrostriatal, the mesolimbic and the mesocortical pathway (figure 10.1). The nigrostriatal and mesolimbic dopaminergic pathways heavily but differentially innervate the striatum. SNc A8 dopaminergic neurons of the nigrostriatal pathway mainly innervate the dorsolateral striatum, while mesolimbic VTA neurons mainly innervate the ventral striatum, including NAc. Other neurons of the nigrostriatal pathway originating from A9 innervate a broad, intermediate area primarily in the dorsolateral striatum but reaching areas considered in the ventromedial striatum.[51,109] This anatomical gradient from the dorsolateral to ventromedial striatum

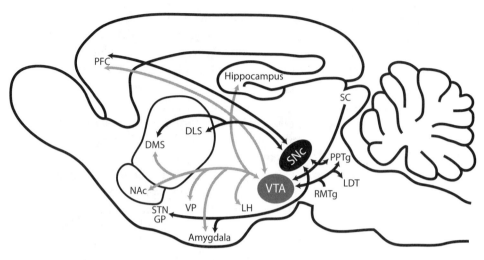

Figure 10.1
Schematic of the primary afferents and efferents of the midbrain dopaminergic nuclei depicted on a
rodent brain. Although the correspondence between the midbrain dopamine pathways in rodents and
primates is large, there are some important differences in both the putative definitions of the VTA and
SNc and the density of projections to regions such as mediodorsal nucleus of the thalamus and non-
prefrontal cortex; for example, see ref. 30 for a more detailed discussion of these differences. As the focus
of this chapter is on rodent studies, the anatomy and physiology where described will be consistent with
the rodent dopamine system.

mirrors a functional differentiation demonstrated by both recording and interference studies across mammalian species: while dorsolateral striatum is implicated in
a range of sensorimotor functions, ventromedial striatum has a more direct connection with rewards and motivated behavior. For the purposes of this chapter, we
largely concentrate on control of behavior by phasic changes in dopamine in mesolimbic pathways, although a number of the principles may well be common to
both systems.

Dopamine, Drives, and Reward

One of the earliest sets of experiments to investigate how motivations might
be translated into actions in the brain came from the accidental discovery that
electrical stimulation delivered to parts of the limbic forebrain when an animal
made a particular response would cause an animal to repeat that action.[74] These
responses might be as simple as pressing a lever or positioning in a box or may
involve navigating correctly in a complex maze. In some situations, the intracranial
self-stimulation (ICSS) would act as such a potent positive reinforcer that animals
would overcome electric shocks or even forgo food when starving to achieve the

stimulation.[73] More recently, it has been argued that stimulation parameters can be titrated so that animals will trade off stimulation for other positive reinforcers such as sucrose or saline dependent on their internal state, suggesting that ICSS might be acting as a "payoff" signal in a computation of the overall subjective utility of the available options.[99] ICSS sites included parts of the cortex, hippocampus, lateral hypothalamus, NAc, and "as far back as the tegmentum."[74]

Although the relationship between ICSS and natural rewards and the anatomical basis for ICSS is not fully resolved, the coincidence between some of the potent sites for electrical stimulation and the location of either the cell bodies, axons, or major terminal regions of mesolimbic dopamine neurons suggested a possible connection between dopamine and control of motivated behavior. However, it should be noted that characterization of threshold and optimal electrical-stimulation parameters favors the primary activation of small myelinated fibers, rather than dopamine axons, which are large and unmyelinated.[98] Nonetheless, support for an important role of dopamine transmission in ICSS-mediated reinforcement comes from pharmacological and lesion studies that showed injections of dopamine antagonists into the median forebrain bundle, which carries mesolimbic dopamine fibers, or large dopaminergic lesions could attenuate ICSS with electrodes placed around the VTA, whereas amphetamine, an indirect dopaminergic agonist, caused a reduction in the stimulation threshold required to sustain responding.[33] Microdialysis studies in the NAc have reported persistent raised dopamine tone during repeated VTA-centered ICSS, and there is also separate evidence that animals would acquire ICSS only if electrical stimulation resulted in this phasic elevation of extracellular dopamine concentrations as detected by fast-scan cyclic voltammetry.[40] At a cellular level, it has been shown that the rate of learning of ICSS correlates with the dopamine-dependent potentiation of corticostriatal synapses.[84] Although it is likely that ICSS can occur in certain circumstances without direct activation of dopaminergic neurons or phasic increases in dopamine concentration,[40,61] the persistent impression nonetheless remains of a role for subcortical dopamine in providing a component of a reward signal that can motivate or even entirely control current behavior.

A second line of evidence implicating dopamine in the translation of drives into actions comes from research into a situation paradigmatic of the loss of control, namely, addiction. Addiction is defined as a loss of control over some aspect of behavior accompanied by a compulsive drive to continue with such behavior in spite of negative consequences.[32] As mentioned earlier, psychostimulants such as amphetamine are known to enhance ICSS, suggesting a link between the drugs, reward, and dopamine.[33] Many drugs of abuse increase dopamine levels in NAc and in other parts of the striatum,[28,78,107] and the direct effects of these drugs on motor function can be attenuated by low levels of dopamine antagonists.[26] More recently, several lines of evidence have implicated striatal dopamine release and dopamine receptor availability in NAc in aspects of vulnerability to addiction, which in turn seems connected with aspects of impulse control.[23,27,68] It is not just drugs of abuse that are associated changes in dopamine function. Other compulsive behaviors such as pathological levels of gambling, shopping, or binge eating have been observed in patients taking dopamine agonists.[21,108] Although the complex functional and neurobiological facets of addiction and compulsion are beyond the scope of this chapter, and certainly extend beyond NAc dopamine, the preceding findings nonetheless again underline an indelible link between subcortical dopamine and aspects of behavioral control.

A third indication of the role subcortical dopamine might play in aiding the translation from motivation to action comes from studies of Parkinson's disease. Although Parkinson's disease primarily causes the progressive loss of dopamine neurons in SNc, there is also some depletion of dopamine within mesolimbic pathways, particularly at later stages of the disease.[52] Though this disorder is usually associated with a variety of motor disturbances such as akinesia, rigidity, and tremor, another extremely common symptom is apathy, believed to occur in as many as 70% of patients.[56] The degree of apathy has been correlated with catecholamine levels in the ventral striatum,[83] and levodopa can help increase levels of motivation in at least a proportion of patients with Parkinson's disease.[20] More recently, it has been suggested that some symptoms classified as problems with general motor function, such as bradykinesia, might be partly based on changes in motivation to act.[60] In a speed-accuracy trade-off task, patients with Parkinson's disease were found to be just as able as controls to make the appropriate movements accurately within the required speed range. However, these patients were shown to make significantly more slow movements when the task was made more difficult, as if they had become more sensitive to the energetic demands of the movement. Therefore, a deficit that had been previously classified as a pure motor impairment was instead shown to be a problem with correctly integrating the costs and benefits of a response, implying that dopamine may be critical not just for making movements, but also for motivating a desire to act.[70]

Dopamine, Cue Control, and Prediction

The preceding lines of evidence strongly implicate mesolimbic dopamine as playing a critical role in motivating actions and the control of behavior. Nonetheless, taking evidence from ICSS, addiction, and Parkinson's disease in isolation—each of which provides a heterogenous model of behavior and is underpinned by a complex underlying neurobiology—does not easily allow us to specify what that role might be. This is partly because dopamine transmission and the effects of dopamine disruption vary substantially in different parts of the striatum (and cortex) based on both ascending and descending anatomical projections,[2,5,91,103] even though many electrophysiological studies have tended to report largely similar responses across their sampled putative dopamine neurons during behavior, whether recording from the VTA or SNc.[93]

Up until now, we have treated both the terms "motivation" and "action" as unitary concepts. However, it has been long appreciated that the former can be divided behaviorally and neurobiologically into a preparatory, anticipation phase prior to the receipt of a reward and a consummatory phase once reward has been obtained.[47,85] This partially overlaps with the psychological idea that an animal might be motivated by incentive properties to "want" to gain a particular reward separate from the degree to which the reward may cause any pleasure or "liking" when received.[11] Equally, appetitive actions can be guided by associations with stimuli or with particular instrumental responses, each of which may either evoke a rich representation of the predicted contingent outcome (i.e., when behavior is "goal-directed"), or may instead control either automatic responses that are largely impervious to changes in current motivational state ("habit"-like behavior).[4,25]

Therefore, to try to understand how dopamine might modulate the control of behavior, it is necessary to probe further the types of situation where dopamine transmission is elicited and necessary for appropriate responses to be selected. Although it has been shown that feeding or the presentation of appetitive rewards, as well as a variety of other positive reinforcers such as companionship or drugs of abuse, can cause increased dopamine cell firing and release in various areas of the striatum,[5,78,87,90,95,115] mesolimbic dopamine does not appear to be required for feeding behavior. Lesions to the mesolimbic dopamine pathways to NAc do not cause deficits, whereas lesions to the pathways going to dorsal striatum do.[118] Indeed, feeding remains impaired in genetically targeted dopamine-deficient mice following restored dopamine production only in NAc,[102] but is rescued by selective restoration of dopamine function in the nigrostriatal pathway. Moreover, if facial expressions are taken as an indicator of the hedonic pleasure associated with food, neither dopamine agonists nor antagonists appear to alter the degree to which animals like or dislike the taste of foods,[11,104] a finding supported by more direct measures of subjective pleasantness in patients with Parkinson's disease.[100] Dopamine-deficient mice can also develop preferences for one reward type over another (e.g., sucrose versus water) to a degree similar to wild-type littermates.[16]

Instead, several lines of evidence suggest that the mesolimbic dopamine pathways are involved with signaling the potential availability of positive reinforcers, particularly when this is predicted by some external cue. Dopamine lesions or antagonism of NAc attenuate the usual increases in locomotor activity in the presence of food and profoundly reduce levels of operant responding for reward guided by predictive cues.[54,120] Stimuli associated with primary rewards reliably cause rapid increases in activity in dopamine neurons and in dopamine transmission in NAc.[6,19,57] Though such changes in dopamine activity in response to the presentation of cues known to predict reward can occur before any movement takes place,[57,62] there is also evidence that NAc dopamine transmission is permissive, and arguably causally related, to allowing motivated responses to be directed by these cues. In well-trained animals, Roitman and colleagues found that a rewarded lever-press response tended to occur at the peak of the phasic rise in dopamine transmission in NAc, even on trials where animals failed to respond for some time after cue onset.[90] More directly, Phillips and colleagues not only showed increases in dopamine concentration in this region just as an animal chooses to approach a lever to obtain infusions of cocaine in the presence of a cue indicating the drug's availability, but also demonstrated that briefly electrically evoking dopamine release by stimulating the VTA significantly increased the likelihood of drug-seeking response being initiated.[78]

It is notable that in both of the preceding studies, presentation of cues that had explicitly not previously been paired with reward and/or where there was no possibility to respond failed to elicit any detectable increase in NAc dopamine concentration. It has been clearly established that the timing of putative midbrain dopamine cell activity is adaptive, as exemplified during acquisition of an auditory reaction-time task where initial phasic increases in activity of dopamine neurons to the presentation of liquid reward progressively diminish as the task is learned while the activity at the time of an earlier predictive auditory cue simultaneously develops.[62] Comparably, in a Pavlovian conditioning experiment, increased phasic changes in dopamine transmission in NAc has been shown within a single animal across several sessions to move from being triggered by the presentation of a reward to being elicited by a predictive cue,[19] and NAc dopamine depletion or antagonism receptor activation disrupts the expression and later consolidation of new appetitive learning.[22,24,29]

Such findings have led to suggestions that dopamine might be crucial to facilitating associations between a conditioned stimulus (CS) and reward or an unconditioned stimulus (UCS)[5,117] or to enhance the CS-UCS relationship in order to form habits.[31] An influential, formal computational theory has proposed that dopamine activity and release relays reward prediction errors—the difference between the predicted future reward in the current state and the actual experience reward—that are important in learning.[95] In trained animals, if the amount of reward is in compliance with the CS-predicted value, there is no phasic dopaminergic activity at the UCS. However, in situations where greater-than-predicted reward is delivered, the UCS causes a phasic increase in firing in dopamine neuron activity, whereas situations where less-than-predicted reward is delivered are marked with a brief cessation of dopaminergic cell firing at the time of the UCS.

These findings suggest that a primary role of mesolimbic dopamine transmission in control of behavior is simply to use discrepancies in these reward predictions to improve performance. However, it is important to note that animals in which mesolimbic dopamine transmission is disrupted either pharmacologically or genetically can still display evidence of learning. Dopamine-deficit mice, if activated by caffeine (acting via extra-dopaminergic mechanisms), are able to learn a T-maze spatial discrimination.[88] Moreover, NAc-dopamine lesioned animals can acquire Pavlovian conditioned approach responses, although at a retarded rate compared to controls, and it has recently been shown that mice lacking NMDA receptors on midbrain dopamine neurons, which attenuate phasic dopamine transmission in NAc, also learn certain cue-reward associations at a similar rate to normal animals.[19,76] There are likely multiple ways to learn associations between stimuli and outcomes,[25,110] and therefore likely multiple influences even on the performance of a simple action in response to a cue. The preceding evidence indicates that dopamine in NAc may be particularly important early in training for learning about and representing predictions of future reward states based on cues at times when the structure of the task environment is not fully known.

Dopamine and the Representation of the Benefits of a Goal

The majority of studies investigating the role of dopamine in motivated appetitive behavior have examined situations where there is only a single appropriate, externally rewarded response to learn about. However, in more natural settings, animals are faced with multiple possible options, each of which may be associated with different likelihoods of success and different potential outcomes, and the appropriate choice may depend on the animal's current motivational state as well as on any externally determined task rules. Parameters such as reward size, quality, and hunger have measurable effects on motivation and the choices that animals make.[17,46]

Internal states, such as hunger, thirst, sexual arousal, or stress, have been shown to affect dopamine activation. Tonic changes in NAc dopamine levels, as measured by microdialysis, are modulated by levels of food deprivation and also by the sensory properties of consumed food such that, after an initial meal of one foodstuff, a second meal of the same palatable food would hardly be eaten and there would be little increase in dopamine levels, whereas animals given a different type of food that was readily consumed did cause significant dopamine efflux.[1,115] Several peptides that regulate food intake are known to affect dopamine signaling. Leptin, a satiety signal released by nondepleted adipose cells, inhibits feeding-evoked dopamine release in NAc,[55] while ghrelin and orexin, which promote feeding, enhance dopamine signaling.[12,50] To date, few studies have investigated how such changes in state affect dopamine firing rates or fast release properties, which will be important for addressing the degree to which current motivation is related to modulations in phasic dopaminergic signaling and, if so, how rapidly any changes in motivation are transmitted to the mesolimbic dopamine system.

However, several studies have demonstrated that the firing rates of putative mid-brain dopamine neurons in response to sensory stimuli correlate with fundamental economic parameters relating to future rewards such as reward magnitude and probability.[36,65,89,105] To test whether this would be translated into terms of NAc dopamine release, Gan and colleagues used fast-scan cyclic voltammetry during a two-option decision-making task where animals were trained to select between a "reference" option, which gained them a single food pellet after a certain number of responses, and an alternative where the same response requirement would result in a greater reward in one condition or a lesser reward in another.[39] Blocks of trials were divided into "forced" trials, where only one option was available, and "choice" trials, where both options were presented (figure 10.2a). In keeping with the elec-trophysiological findings, once the reward contingencies were learned and animals were consistently choosing the high reward option, the size of phasic dopamine release in NAc on forced trials scaled with anticipated reward magnitude in response to predictive cues (figure 10.2b and c). Such reporting of reward size remained after extended experience with the reward contingencies (figure 10.2c).

Some data also that suggest dopamine neurons change their activity as a function of the timing of future rewards, with cues indicating sooner reward delivery having slightly higher or more persistent increases in firing rates.[35,53,89] However, it is not yet clear to what degree this modulation of activity represents a temporally dis-counted reward value signal or the increased uncertainty about future reward timing and contingency between the cue and the reward as delays increase.

To have a controlling effect on behavior, dopamine would be expected to play an important role in guiding trial-by-trial decisions between different rewarding options. To date, the evidence speaking to this issue is sparse and somewhat con-tradictory. In a two-option decision-making task where visual stimuli were associ-ated with different probabilities of reward delivery, the firing rate of putative SNc

Figure 10.2
Dopaminergic signaling to the NAc in a two-option reward-based decision-making task.[39] (a) Schematic of a set of eight trials comprising the behavioral task. Animals were presented with either "forced trials" (white background) or "choice trials" (gray background). Forced and choice trials occurred in blocks of four trials (two forced trials for each lever in the forced blocks, pseudorandomly presented). (b) Repre-sentative dopaminergic recordings from two forced trials, one where a cue predicts four food pellets (top left-hand panel) and the other where the alternative cue predicts one food pellet (top right-hand panel). Color plots represent cyclic voltammograms across time with the oxidation potential of dopamine indi-cated by a red arrow. Bottom panels represent extracted dopamine traces for those trials. (c) Postbehav-ioral criterion choices (upper panels) and average peak dopaminergic transmission to cues (lower panels) in animals that had either ≤ 9 or > 9 sessions experience with the four-pellet versus one-pellet condition. Data redrawn from Gan et al.,[39] with permission.

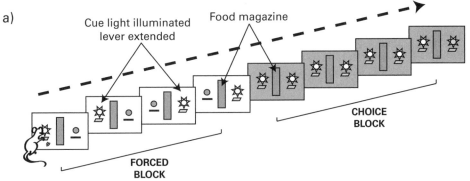

a)

Cue light illuminated
lever extended

Food magazine

FORCED
BLOCK

CHOICE
BLOCK

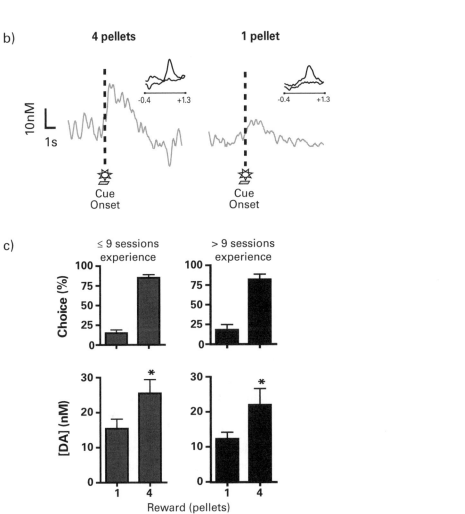

b)

4 pellets

1 pellet

10nM

1s

-0.4   +1.3

-0.4   +1.3

Cue
Onset

Cue
Onset

c)

≤ 9 sessions
experience

> 9 sessions
experience

Choice (%)

[DA] (nM)

*

*

1   4

1   4

Reward (pellets)

dopamine neurons in monkeys correlated with the average reward associated with the subsequently chosen option, even if the animal chose the lower value of the two available options.[65] By contrast, in another two-option decision-making study in rats where a particular odor was associated with a choice between options that differed either in the delay to reward (short versus long delay) or in reward magnitude (large versus small reward), the activity of putative dopamine neurons in VTA instead encoded the value of the best of the two options, regardless of which was subsequently chosen.[89]

Whether these differences are indicative of functional separation within the VTA and SNc or are caused by the different paradigms (one in which firing rates are correlated to the appearance of two cues, the other where a separate cue is associated with both options being available) remains to be seen. Using a task where choice trials were indicated by presentation of both response options, Gan and colleagues showed that NAc dopamine release on trials when the animal subsequently chose the high-value option was comparable to release on forced trials when only the high-value option was available,[39] and preliminary evidence suggests that signals prior to low reward choices are similar to those on low-reward forced trials (Walton, Gan, and Phillips, unpublished observations). In all these tasks to date, however, the questions as to why animals might choose a lower-value option and whether the factors that might promote such behavior—such as exploration bonuses or, in changeable paradigms, representations of previous task contingencies—are influencing dopamine firing patterns and release remain. Ideally, these questions should be investigated using a task where more than one factor could influence a choice and where these factors might have differing weightings on the mesolimbic dopamine system.

Although behavioral preferences are strongly influenced by rewards and reward-predictive cues and, in at least some situations, the firing rates of dopamine neurons and dopamine release seem to reflect the choices being made, this does not necessarily imply that mesolimbic dopamine has a primary role in setting behavioral policy. In the study by Gan et al., the assignment of the high- and low-utility options reversed in each session, meaning animals were required to relearn the cost-benefit contingencies. As can be observed in figure 10.3a, cue-evoked NAc dopamine release on forced trials developed rapidly within a testing session to reflect the magnitude of future reward delivery as the animals learned the reward contingencies associated with each option.[39] If these data are time-locked to the point in the session when animals reached a behavioral criterion of making more than 75% of high-value option choices, it becomes evident that dopamine often scales with pending reward size several blocks of trials before they have learned to display a consistent preference for the high-reward option (figure 10.3b). Even when an animal failed to reach the behavioral criterion during a single session, it was nonetheless apparent that the differential reward magnitudes were being reflected by dopamine release (figure 10.3c).

These data are comparable to those in a saccade timing task where monkeys had to use trial-and-error feedback to determine when to make an eye movement.[8] Even though the firing rate of dopamine neurons accurately relayed errors in reward prediction, these signals only weakly correlated with subsequent changes in reaction time following receipt of some magnitude of reward, suggesting that decisions about when to move were being mainly controlled via a different mechanism. Therefore, although mesolimbic dopamine might rapidly adapt to represent current predictions of future outcomes, this may be providing only one motivating influence on the actions that are taken at any particular moment.

Dopamine, Utility, and the Intersection of Reward and Action

Given the large literature implicating dopamine as critical to enabling a large number of rewarded behaviors, this disconnection between NAc dopamine release and decision making raises the question of what role it does play in the control of behavior, particularly in instrumental settings. Up until here, the discussion of how motivation is translated to action has concentrated on how rewards help guide response selection, with little regard for how the reward is obtained. However, in order to make appropriate decisions, it is important to evaluate not only the potential benefits of a course of action, but also the costs, such as the anticipated amount of work that will be required to obtain such payoffs. All other factors being equal, animals will usually prefer to pursue goals that require less effort to achieve,[101] and several lines of evidence demonstrate that animals' choices are weighted by both the costs and benefits of the available options, with animals tolerating increasing costs for higher-value rewards.[7,38,111] Moreover, such decisions are influenced by the current motivational state of the animal, with food-deprived animals being more willing to put in work to achieve reward than those who have recently been given access to a meal.[37]

Importantly, lesion and pharmacology studies have implicated dopamine specifically in the NAc as being important to enabling cues to energize behavior and, in particular circumstances, to allowing animals to overcome effort constraints to obtain larger or more palatable reward.[91] This is particularly prominent in tasks where the less beneficial outcome is a readily available primary reward (for instance, laboratory chow freely available in an operant box) whereas the availability of the larger reward at greater response cost is signaled by a conditioned stimulus (e.g., the presence of the lever in the operant box).

To address how response costs are represented by phasic NAc dopamine release, Gan and colleagues tested animals on the two-option decision-making task described

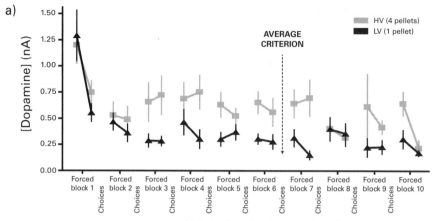

a)

Forced blocks from beginning of session

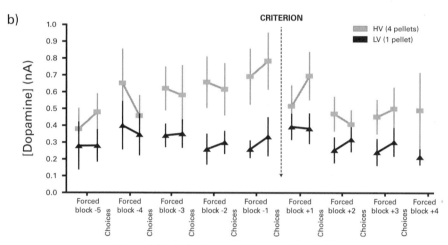

b)

Forced Blocks before and after reaching behavioral criterion

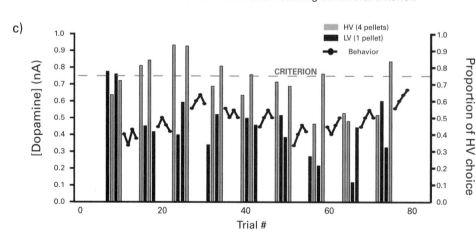

c)

earlier (figure 10.2a), except that now the reward magnitude associated with each option was the same and value was instead manipulated by altering the number of lever presses required to obtain the reward.[39] The cost parameters were set such that they had comparable motivating effects on choice behavior as the reward manipulation had, with animals rapidly learning to prefer the low-cost option. Nonetheless, in spite of this preference, in most cases, dopamine did not encode an effort-discounted value signal (figure 10.4). One exception was in situations where the response cost was unexpectedly lower than the reference cost, where dopamine release preferentially encoded the low-cost option; however, after repeated experience of these contingencies, even this scaling with net value disappeared. This lack of encoding of upcoming response costs by NAc phasic dopamine was also recently observed in a more dynamic, progressive ratio paradigm where responses costs escalate as a function of the animals' past choices.[112]

These findings may initially seem surprising given that disruption of dopamine affects allocation of effortful actions. However, they can be reconciled by considering such cost-benefit trade-offs in terms of utility curves depicting the amount of effort expenditure an animal would put in to obtain an expected future payoff given its current motivational state.[79] In such a framework, mesolimbic dopamine might participate in encoding the availability of particular sizes of future payoffs with reference to the work required to reach these goals such that appropriate cost expenditures can be set. Somewhat paradoxically, to provide useful input to such a computation, the phasic dopamine signal elicited by a predictive cue would itself have to be impartial to movement-related response costs. Moreover, this would allow for separate updating of predictions about the costs and benefits of a course of action when discrepancies are detected, something that would not be possible if dopamine signaled the overall net utility of a course of action.

Dopamine, Salience, and a Motivation to Learn?

Under this model, the mesolimbic dopamine system plays an important but limited role in translating motivation into action. Specifically, phasic dopamine release

Figure 10.3
Dopamine, learning, and choices. (a) Average dopamine release in forced trials from the beginning of the session (signals on choice trials are not depicted). On average, animals reached the ≥75% high-reward choices between forced blocks 6 and 7. (b) Average dopamine release in forced trials centered on the point at which each animal reached the behavioral criterion in each session. As signals were, on average, 1.5 to 2 times as large on the first of the forced trials as on any other trial in a session, data from these first high- and low-reward forced trials have been removed. (c) Behavioral choice and dopamine release for an example animal that never reached the behavioral criterion in one particular session. Smoothed choice performance is depicted by the black dots, peak forced trial dopamine by the red and blue bars.

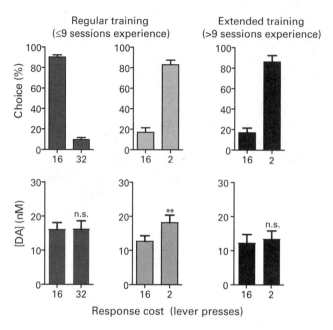

Figure 10.4
Post-behavioral criterion choices (upper panels) and average dopamine release (lower panels) to cues predicting different effort requirements (lever presses) to gain the reward in the two-option decision-making task of Gan et al.,[39] redrawn with permission. Animals were tested after having either ≤ 9 (left-hand and center panels) or > 9 sessions experience (right-hand panel) of the effort contingencies prior to recording session.

enables environmental stimuli to promote, but not control, responses as a function of their anticipated benefits in allowing animals to seek potentially costly rewards. This naturally raises the question of what in a natural environment might be considered "beneficial" to an animal? Moreover, how does this fit in with the abundant evidence suggesting an important role for dopamine in learning?

It has been known for some time that novel, salient stimuli cause rapid increases in the firing rates of putative dopamine neurons, sometimes even in the absence of appetitive consequences.[15,49,57] Redgrave and colleagues have pointed out that the latency of firing of dopamine neurons to the presentation of a simple visual stimulus is sufficiently fast to normally occur prior to any orienting response to that stimulus,[82] suggesting that dopamine serves as a marker for unpredictable events rather than as an indicator of upcoming reward value.[81]

Even in situations where the task rules are known, there is still evidence that the initial presentation of cues can cause increased levels of phasic dopamine activity, if the task contingencies (for example, the reward sizes or response costs) are not known. Analyzing NAc dopamine release from interleaved sessions of discrete trial fixed and progressive ratio tasks, Wanat and colleagues found that phasic signals to the first cue signaling the opportunity to response evoked on average about 50 to 100% more dopamine than that in all other trials.[112] As there was only one available response option, such increased release could be caused either by the unpredictable timing of the start of the session or by a prediction error for the incentive properties of the entire session.

However, neither of these explanations easily accounts for the patterns of release observed early in a session during the two-option decision-making task of Gan and colleagues.[39] In each session, the first four trials of each session were forced (two presentations of either the left or right option in pseudorandom order). As can be observed in figure 10.3a, phasic changes in dopamine transmission elicited by the first presentation of cues to be associated with high reward or low reward was substantially larger than anything else in the session. This was not dependent on the cost-benefit contingencies in the previous session or the order of presentation of the forced trials, demonstrating that it does not simply reflect previous associations or anticipation of all the rewards to be obtained in the coming session. Moreover, when the same option was presented on both of the first two forced trials of a session, the dopamine signal on the next trial to the alternative cue was significantly larger than release to the second presentation on the previous trial of the other cue (Walton, Gan, and Phillips, unpublished observations).

While the general setup did not change from session to session in this paradigm, the assignment cost-benefit contingencies consistently reversed between sessions, meaning that animals were required to learn new cue-outcome associations to guide appropriate behavior. In a separate study, dopamine neuron activity was modulated by the requirement to learn about an outcome in a multistep-decision task where animals had to learn using positive and negative reinforcement a three-target sequence and then repeat it twice.[92] Firing rates were lower on the first repeat trial than on the second or third search trial despite the expected value of the repeat trial (i.e., the reward probability) being higher than either of the search trials. Moreover, here, as in the earlier studies of Pavlovian conditioning, dopamine also seemed permissive of responding, with responses to cues of identical value being larger when reaction times were shorter. The size of cue-evoked responses also correlated positively with activity at the time of reward delivery, suggesting that moment-by-moment fluctuations in drive to learn about cues might have influenced the effectiveness of reinforcers update predictions. In a separate study, the responses of dopamine neurons correlated with a strong bias that monkeys exhibited to seek advanced information about future rewards.[13]

In the wild, the future benefits of a course of action are frequently not fully known. Yet in spite of this uncertainty, which should logically reduce the expected value of an outcome, all foraging species are believed to have a drive to explore unknown elements of their surroundings.[75] It is known that, as well as the connection between dopamine and novelty, NAc dopamine lesions can disrupt the long-lasting potentiation of so-called adjunctive motivated behaviors such as drinking, gnawing, or wheel running evoked by cues following receipt of a food reward.[86] The preceding evidence suggests that one function of phasic mesolimbic dopamine may be to provide an opportunistic drive in response to environmental stimuli to motivate animals to seek out potential future rewards to satisfy their current needs. Simultaneously, dopamine release might in turn facilitate learning about predictors of the structure of their environment by changing synaptic plasticity and modulating the excitability of output neurons within the targets of the mesolimbic dopamine system. This might explain why phasic dopamine release in the study by Gan and colleagues did represent the net utility of effort when the cost contingency was unexpectedly low compared to the standard response cost, yet after extended training reflected only the pending reward magnitude of the benefit and not the associated costs. Collectively, such a system would provide what Horwitz and colleagues have called a "good parent,"[48] promoting appropriate behaviors to help reduce uncertainty and gain benefits even when costs have to be overcome. Future experiments comparing changeable versus static environments will be important to further elucidate these functions.

Caveats and Conclusions

It is worth noting that several important issues concerning the role of dopamine in translating motivation to action have largely been sidestepped in this chapter. First, what role does dopamine release at different time scales play in these functions? We have concentrated here on phasic changes in dopamine-mediated activity and release. However, modulations in background tonic dopamine levels can be detected across minutes. Even within the phasic range, alterations in the firing rate of midbrain dopamine cells can happen as rapidly as 70 to 100 msec following the presentation of a salient visual stimulus, yet can also occur across several seconds during states such as uncertainty.[94] Moreover, it has recently been suggested that the dynamics of firing rates within hundreds of seconds may convey different types of information, including salience, timing, and value.[13,71] It will be important to determine how these different modes of transmission affect control of behavior.

Second, all the studies discussed have investigated how dopamine modulates animals' responses to positive reinforcers. However, it is evident that aversive events may also be strongly motivating. While it had been thought for a long time that dopamine neurons mainly coded positive prediction errors and were uniformly inhibited by negative prediction errors or aversive events,[94,106] new evidence indicates that this may have been a simplification, as dopamine cells, particularly those more dorsolateral within SNc, have been found to be excited by stimuli associated with aversive consequences as well as the aversive air puff itself.[59]

This also relates to a third important area requiring consideration, namely, how the modulatory role ascribed to the mesolimbic dopamine system relates to the functions of the nigrostriatal dopamine projection to dorsal parts of the striatum and to the mesocortical projection to thalamus and cortex. Do the same computational principles apply to each set of pathways, with the specific function of each being determined by the connectivity and local circuits of the terminal regions, or is the information conveyed by each system markedly distinct? Does this separation relate in any way to the nature of the representations, in terms of stimulus versus action values and goal-directed versus habitual response selection? Though the answers to these questions are far from clear, it is apparent that the different dopamine systems interact during learning and choice behavior to promote appropriate adaptive behavior.[3,10]

Manipulations of the mesolimbic dopamine pathways affect the motivation of humans and animals to act and the decisions they ultimately take. The firing patterns of midbrain dopamine neurons and dopamine release in the NAc reflect predictions of future benefits evoked by environmental stimuli. This appears to be important for prompting animals to seek rewards to satisfy their internal needs, particularly in situations where the structure of the environment remains unknown. Nonetheless, phasic dopamine release appears to be only indirectly related to the choices made by an animal in instrumental situations. Instead, by signaling the benefits of pending payoffs separate to response costs, dopamine may provide a positive component to computations of the overall utility of a course of action in enabling animals to overcome response costs. This may be crucial in uncertain environments to allowing animals to explore novel options and motivating animals to learn. However, in situations where the dopamine system fails to be appropriately regulated, such as certain neuropsychiatric disorders or through the effects of pharmacological agents, this may cause loss of control over behavior and an increase in impulsive choices.[14,23]

Acknowledgments

The preparation of this manuscript was supported by a Wellcome Trust Research Career Development Fellowship to MEW. The work depicted in figures 10.2 through 10.4 was funded by the National Institutes of Health (R01-MH079292, R21-AG030775, P.E.M.P.). The authors have no competing interests.

Outstanding Questions

• What role does dopamine release in different striatal (and cortical) regions play in the control of behavior? Are the dynamics of phasic dopamine release different in these regions? If so, what factors control when, where, and how much dopamine is released within restricted regions?

• There are multiple influences on behavior and multiple representations of value in the brain. Theoretically, phasic dopamine cell firing and release seem to correlate better with predictions of a "habitlike" system. However, little work has been done to date probe how dopamine might represent richer "goal" values. The presence of anatomical connections allowing midbrain dopamine cells to receive information and to influence hypothalamic motivational state signals makes this a pressing question.

• Dopamine is clearly involved in learning and representing the predicted state of the world. But what factors are included in such a representation: simply the mean expected benefits in a particular context, or a complex set of factors such as the mean and known variance of reward, uncertainty in these estimates, and learning rates?

Further Reading

Special issue of the journal *Psychopharmacology* (2007, 191; 3). Many detailed and differing perspectives on dopamine can be found within this special issue, including a paper by two of this chapter's authors that sets out the theoretical framework behind many of the ideas contained here.

Kehagia AA, Murray GK, Robbins TW. 2010. Learning and cognitive flexibility: frontostriatal function and monoaminergic modulation. *Curr Opin Neurobiol* 20: 199–204. An interesting recent review looking at dopamine, cognitive control, and behavioral flexibility, and also broadening out the question to include other monoamines and frontostriatal circuits.

References

1. Ahn S, Phillips AG. 1999. Dopaminergic correlates of sensory-specific satiety in the medial prefrontal cortex and nucleus accumbens of the rat. *J Neurosci* 19(RC29): 21–26.

2. Aragona BJ, Day JJ, Roitman MF, Cleaveland NA, Wightman RM, Carelli RM. 2009. Regional specificity in the real-time development of phasic dopamine transmission patterns during acquisition of a cue-cocaine association in rats. *Eur J Neurosci* 30: 1889–1899.

3. Ashby FG, Turner BO, Horvitz JC. 2010. Cortical and basal ganglia contributions to habit learning and automaticity. *Trends Cogn Sci* 14: 208–215.

4. Balleine BW, Dickinson A. 1998. Goal-directed instrumental action: contingency and incentive learning and their cortical substrates. *Neuropharmacology* 37: 407–419.

5. Bassareo V, De Luca MA, Di Chiara G. 2002. Differential expression of motivational stimulus properties by dopamine in nucleus accumbens shell versus core and prefrontal cortex. *J Neurosci* 22: 4709–4719.

6. Bassareo V, Di Chiara G. 1999. Modulation of feeding-induced activation of mesolimbic dopamine transmission by appetitive stimuli and its relation to motivational state. *Eur J Neurosci* 11: 4389–4397.

7. Bautista LM, Tinbergen J, Kacelnik A. 2001. To walk or to fly? How birds choose among foraging modes. *Proc Natl Acad Sci USA* 98: 1089–1094.

8. Bayer HM, Glimcher PW. 2005. Midbrain dopamine neurons encode a quantitative reward prediction error signal. *Neuron* 47: 129–141.

9. Beaulieu JM, Gainetdinov RR, Caron MG. 2007. The Akt-GSK-3 signaling cascade in the actions of dopamine. *Trends Pharmacol Sci* 28: 166–172.

10. Belin D, Jonkman S, Dickinson A, Robbins TW, Everitt BJ. 2009. Parallel and interactive learning processes within the basal ganglia: relevance for the understanding of addiction. *Behav Brain Res* 199: 89–102.

11. Berridge KC, Robinson TE. 1998. What is the role of dopamine in reward: hedonic impact, reward learning, or incentive salience? *Behav Brain Res Rev* 28: 309–369.

12. Borgland SL, Taha SA, Sarti F, Fields HL, Bonci A. 2006. Orexin A in the VTA is critical for the induction of synaptic plasticity and behavioral sensitization to cocaine. *Neuron* 49: 589–601.

13. Bromberg-Martin ES, Hikosaka O. 2009. Midbrain dopamine neurons signal preference for advance information about upcoming rewards. *Neuron* 63: 119–126.

14. Buckholtz JW, Treadway MT, Cowan RL, Woodward ND, Li R, Ansari MS, Baldwin RM, et al. 2010. Dopaminergic network differences in human impulsivity. *Science* 329: 532.

15. Bunzeck N, Duzel E. 2006. Absolute coding of stimulus novelty in the human substantia nigra/VTA. *Neuron* 51: 369–379.

16. Cannon CM, Palmiter RD. 2003. Reward without dopamine. *J Neurosci* 23: 10827–10831.

17. Caraco T, Martindale S, Whittam T-S. 1980. An empirical demonstration of risk-sensitive foraging preferences. *Anim Behav* 28: 820–830.

18. Carlsson A, Lindqvist M, Magnusson T. 1957. 3,4-Dihydroxyphenylalanine and 5-hydroxytryptophan as reserpine antagonists. *Nature* 180: 1200.

19. Clark JJ, Sandberg SG, Wanat MJ, Gan JO, Horne EA, Hart AS, Akers CA, et al. 2010. Chronic microsensors for longitudinal, subsecond dopamine detection in behaving animals. *Nat Methods* 7: 126–129.

20. Czernecki V, Pillon B, Houeto JL, Pochon JB, Levy R, Dubois B. 2002. Motivation, reward, and Parkinson's disease: influence of dopatherapy. *Neuropsychologia* 40: 2257–2267.

21. Dagher A, Robbins TW. 2009. Personality, addiction, dopamine: insights from Parkinson's disease. *Neuron* 61: 502–510.

22. Dalley JW, Chudasama Y, Theobald DE, Pettifer CL, Fletcher CM, Robbins TW. 2002. Nucleus accumbens dopamine and discriminated approach learning: interactive effects of 6-hydroxydopamine lesions and systemic apomorphine administration. *Psychopharmacology (Berl)* 161: 425–433.

23. Dalley JW, Fryer TD, Brichard L, Robinson ES, Theobald DE, Laane K, Pena Y, et al. 2007. Nucleus accumbens D2/3 receptors predict trait impulsivity and cocaine reinforcement. *Science* 315: 1267–1270.

24. Dalley JW, Laane K, Theobald DE, Armstrong HC, Corlett PR, Chudasama Y, Robbins TW. 2005. Time-limited modulation of appetitive Pavlovian memory by D1 and NMDA receptors in the nucleus accumbens. *Proc Natl Acad Sci USA* 102: 6189–6194.

25. Dayan P, Balleine BW. 2002. Reward, motivation, and reinforcement learning. *Neuron* 36: 285–298.

26. De Wit H, Wise RA. 1977. Blockade of cocaine reinforcement in rats with the dopamine receptor blocker pimozide, but not with the noradrenergic blockers phentolamine or phenoxybenzamine. *Can J Psychol* 31: 195–203.

27. Deminiere JM, Piazza PV, Le Moal M, Simon H. 1989. Experimental approach to individual vulnerability to psychostimulant addiction. *Neurosci Biobehav Rev* 13: 141–147.

28. Di Chiara G, Imperato A. 1988. Drugs abused by humans preferentially increase synaptic dopamine concentrations in the mesolimbic system of freely moving rats. *Proc Natl Acad Sci USA* 85: 5274–5278.

29. Di Ciano P, Cardinal RN, Cowell RA, Little SJ, Everitt BJ. 2001. Differential involvement of NMDA, AMPA/kainate, and dopamine receptors in the nucleus accumbens core in the acquisition and performance of pavlovian approach behavior. *J Neurosci* 21: 9471–9477.

30. Duzel E, Bunzeck N, Guitart-Masip M, Wittmann B, Schott BH, Tobler PN. 2009. Functional imaging of the human dopaminergic midbrain. *Trends Neurosci* 32: 321–328.

31. Everitt BJ, Dickinson A, Robbins TW. 2001. The neuropsychological basis of addictive behaviour. *Brain Res Brain Res Rev* 36: 129–138.

32. Everitt BJ, Robbins TW. 2005. Neural systems of reinforcement for drug addiction: from actions to habits to compulsion. *Nat Neurosci* 8: 1481–1489.

33. Fibiger HC, LePiane FG, Jakubovic A, Phillips AG. 1987. The role of dopamine in intracranial self-stimulation of the ventral tegmental area. *J Neurosci* 7: 3888–3896.

34. Fields HL, Hjelmstad GO, Margolis EB, Nicola SM. 2007. Ventral tegmental area neurons in learned appetitive behavior and positive reinforcement. *Annu Rev Neurosci* 30: 289–316.

35. Fiorillo CD, Newsome WT, Schultz W. 2008. The temporal precision of reward prediction in dopamine neurons. *Nat Neurosci* 11: 966–973.

36. Fiorillo CD, Tobler PN, Schultz W. 2003. Discrete coding of reward probability and uncertainty by dopamine neurons. *Science* 299: 1898–1902.

37. Floresco SB, Ghods-Sharifi S. 2007. Amygdala-prefrontal cortical circuitry regulates effort-based decision making. *Cereb Cortex* 17: 251–260.

38. Floresco SB, Onge JR, Ghods-Sharifi S, Winstanley CA. 2008. Cortico-limbic-striatal circuits subserving different forms of cost-benefit decision making. *Cogn Affect Behav Neurosci* 8: 375–389.

39. Gan JO, Walton ME, Phillips PE. 2010. Dissociable cost and benefit encoding of future rewards by mesolimbic dopamine. *Nat Neurosci* 13: 25–27.

40. Garris PA, Kilpatrick M, Bunin MA, Michael D, Walker QD, Wightman RM. 1999. Dissociation of dopamine release in the nucleus accumbens from intracranial self-stimulation. *Nature* 398: 67–69.

41. Geisler S, Derst C, Veh RW, Zahm DS. 2007. Glutamatergic afferents of the ventral tegmental area in the rat. *J Neurosci* 27: 5730–5743.

42. Grace AA, Bunney BS. 1983. Intracellular and extracellular electrophysiology of nigral dopaminergic neurons—2. Action potential generating mechanisms and morphological correlates. *Neuroscience* 10: 317–331.

43. Grace AA, Bunney BS. 1984. The control of firing pattern in nigral dopamine neurons: burst firing. *J Neurosci* 4: 2877–2890.

44. Grace AA, Bunney BS. 1984. The control of firing pattern in nigral dopamine neurons: single spike firing. *J Neurosci* 4: 2866–2876.

45. Hare TA, Camerer CF, Rangel A. 2009. Self-control in decision-making involves modulation of the vmPFC valuation system. *Science (New York, NY)* 324: 646–648.

46. Hodos W. 1961. Progressive ratio as a measure of reward strength. *Science* 134: 943–944.

47. Holland PC, Rescorla RA. 1975. Second-order conditioning with food unconditioned stimulus. *J Comp Physiol Psychol* 88: 459–467.

48. Horvitz JC, Choi WY, Morvan C, Eyny Y, Balsam PD. 2007. A "good parent" function of dopamine: transient modulation of learning and performance during early stages of training. *Ann N Y Acad Sci* 1104: 270–288.

49. Horvitz JC, Stewart T, Jacobs BL. 1997. Burst activity of ventral tegmental dopamine neurons is elicited by sensory stimuli in the awake cat. *Brain Res* 759: 251–258.

50. Jiang H, Betancourt L, Smith RG. 2006. Ghrelin amplifies dopamine signaling by cross talk involving formation of growth hormone secretagogue receptor/dopamine receptor subtype 1 heterodimers. *Mol Endocrinol* 20: 1772–1785.

51. Joel D, Weiner I. 2000. The connections of the dopaminergic system with the striatum in rats and primates: an analysis with respect to the functional and compartmental organization of the striatum. *Neuroscience* 96: 451–474.

52. Kish SJ, Shannak K, Hornykiewicz O. 1988. Uneven pattern of dopamine loss in the striatum of patients with idiopathic Parkinson's disease. Pathophysiologic and clinical implications. *N Engl J Med* 318: 876–880.

53. Kobayashi S, Schultz W. 2008. Influence of reward delays on responses of dopamine neurons. *J Neurosci* 28: 7837–7846.

54. Koob GF, Riley SJ, Smith SC, Robbins TW. 1978. Effects of 6-hydroxydopamine lesions of the nucleus accumbens septi and olfactory tubercle on feeding, locomotor activity, and amphetamine anorexia in the rat. *J Comp Physiol Psychol* 92: 917–927.

55. Krugel U, Schraft T, Kittner H, Kiess W, Illes P. 2003. Basal and feeding-evoked dopamine release in the rat nucleus accumbens is depressed by leptin. *Eur J Pharmacol* 482: 185–187.

56. Leentjens AF, Dujardin K, Marsh L, Martinez-Martin P, Richard IH, Starkstein SE, Weintraub D, et al. 2008. Apathy and anhedonia rating scales in Parkinson's disease: critique and recommendations. *Mov Disord* 23: 2004–2014.

57. Ljungberg T, Apicella P, Schultz W. 1992. Responses of monkey dopamine neurons during learning of behavioral reactions. *J Neurophysiol* 67: 145–163.

58. Martinelli M, Rudick CN, Hu XT, White FJ. 2006. Excitability of dopamine neurons: modulation and physiological consequences. *CNS Neurol Disord Drug Targets* 5: 79–97.

59. Matsumoto M, Hikosaka O. 2009. Two types of dopamine neuron distinctly convey positive and negative motivational signals. *Nature* 459: 837–841.

60. Mazzoni P, Hristova A, Krakauer JW. 2007. Why don't we move faster? Parkinson's disease, movement vigor, and implicit motivation. *J Neurosci* 27: 7105–7116.

61. Miliaressis E, Emond C, Merali Z. 1991. Re-evaluation of the role of dopamine in intracranial self-stimulation using in vivo microdialysis. *Behav Brain Res* 46: 43–48.

62. Mirenowicz J, Schultz W. 1994. Importance of unpredictability for reward responses in primate dopamine neurons. *J Neurophysiol* 72: 1024–1027.

63. Misgeld U. 2004. Innervation of the substantia nigra. *Cell Tissue Res* 318: 107–114.

64. Mogenson GJ, Jones DL, Yim CY. 1980. From motivation to action: functional interface between the limbic system and the motor system. *Prog Neurobiol* 14: 69–97.

65. Morris G, Nevet A, Arkadir D, Vaadia E, Bergman H. 2006. Midbrain dopamine neurons encode decisions for future action. *Nat Neurosci* 9: 1057–1063.

66. Moss J, Bolam JP. 2010. The relationship between dopaminergic axons and glutamatergic synapses in the striatum: Structual considerations. In: Dopamine Handbook (Iversen LL, Iversen SD, Dunnett SB, Bjorklund A, eds), pp 49–59. New York: Oxford University Press.

67. Mountcastle VB. 1974. Medical Physiology, 13th Ed. St Louis: Mosby & Co.

68. Nader MA, Czoty PW, Gould RW, Riddick NV. 2008. Positron emission tomography imaging studies of dopamine receptors in primate models of addiction. *Philos Trans R Soc Lond B Biol Sci* 363: 3223–3232.

69. Neve KA, Seamans JK, Trantham-Davidson H. 2004. Dopamine receptor signaling. *J Recept Signal Transduct Res* 24: 165–205.

70. Niv Y, Rivlin-Etzion M. 2007. Parkinson's disease: fighting the will? *J Neurosci* 27: 11777–11779.

71. Nomoto K, Schultz W, Watanabe T, Sakagami M. 2010. Temporally extended dopamine responses to perceptually demanding reward-predictive stimuli. *J Neurosci* 30: 10692–10702.

72. Oakman SA, Faris PL, Kerr PE, Cozzari C, Hartman BK. 1995. Distribution of pontomesencephalic cholinergic neurons projecting to substantia nigra differs significantly from those projecting to ventral tegmental area. *J Neurosci* 15: 5859–5869.

73. Olds J. 1969. The central nervous system and the reinforcement of behavior. *Am Psychol* 24: 114–132.

74. Olds J, Milner P. 1954. Positive reinforcement produced by electrical stimulation of septal area and other regions of rat brain. *J Comp Physiol Psychol* 47: 419–427.

75. Panksepp J. 1998. Affective Neuroscience. New York: Oxford University Press.

76. Parkinson JA, Dalley JW, Cardinal RN, Bamford A, Fehnert B, Lachenal G, Rudarakanchana N, Halkerston KM, Robbins TW, Everitt BJ. 2002. Nucleus accumbens dopamine depletion impairs both acquisition and performance of appetitive Pavlovian approach behaviour: implications for mesoaccumbens dopamine function. *Behav Brain Res* 137: 149–163.

77. Paus T. 2001. Primate anterior cingulate cortex: where motor control, drive and cognition interface. *Nat Rev Neurosci* 2: 417–424.

78. Phillips PE, Stuber GD, Heien ML, Wightman RM, Carelli RM. 2003. Subsecond dopamine release promotes cocaine seeking. *Nature* 422: 614–618.

79. Phillips PE, Walton ME, Jhou TC. 2007. Calculating utility: preclinical evidence for cost-benefit analysis by mesolimbic dopamine. *Psychopharmacology (Berl)* 191: 483–495.

80. Platt ML, Glimcher PW. 1999. Neural correlates of decision variables in parietal cortex. *Nature* 400: 233–238.

81. Redgrave P, Gurney K. 2006. The short-latency dopamine signal: a role in discovering novel actions? *Nat Rev Neurosci* 7: 967–975.

82. Redgrave P, Prescott TJ, Gurney K. 1999. Is the short-latency dopamine response too short to signal reward error? *Trends Neurosci* 22: 146–151.

83. Remy P, Doder M, Lees A, Turjanski N, Brooks D. 2005. Depression in Parkinson's disease: loss of dopamine and noradrenaline innervation in the limbic system. *Brain* 128: 1314–1322.

84. Reynolds JN, Hyland BI, Wickens JR. 2001. A cellular mechanism of reward-related learning. *Nature* 413: 67–70.

85. Robbins TW, Everitt BJ. 1992. Functions of dopamine in the dorsal and ventral striatum. *Semin Neurosci* 4: 119–127.

86. Robbins TW, Koob GF. 1980. Selective disruption of displacement behaviour by lesions of the mesolimbic dopamine system. *Nature* 285: 409–412.

87. Robinson DL, Heien ML, Wightman RM. 2002. Frequency of dopamine concentration transients increases in dorsal and ventral striatum of male rats during introduction of conspecifics. *J Neurosci* 22: 10477–10486.

88. Robinson S, Sandstrom SM, Denenberg VH, Palmiter RD. 2005. Distinguishing whether dopamine regulates liking, wanting, and/or learning about rewards. *Behav Neurosci* 119: 5–15.

89. Roesch MR, Calu DJ, Schoenbaum G. 2007. Dopamine neurons encode the better option in rats deciding between differently delayed or sized rewards. *Nat Neurosci* 10: 1615–1624.

90. Roitman MF, Stuber GD, Phillips PE, Wightman RM, Carelli RM. 2004. Dopamine operates as a subsecond modulator of food seeking. *J Neurosci* 24: 1265–1271.

91. Salamone JD, Correa M, Farrar A, Mingote SM. 2007. Effort-related functions of nucleus accumbens dopamine and associated forebrain circuits. *Psychopharmacology (Berl)* 191: 461–482.

92. Satoh T, Nakai S, Sato T, Kimura M. 2003. Correlated coding of motivation and outcome of decision by dopamine neurons. *J Neurosci* 23: 9913–9923.

93. Schultz W. 1998. Predictive reward signal of dopamine neurons. *J Neurophysiol* 80: 1–27.

94. Schultz W. 2007. Multiple dopamine functions at different time courses. *Annu Rev Neurosci* 30: 259–288.

95. Schultz W, Dayan P, Montague P. 1997. A neural substrate of prediction and reward. *Science* 275: 1593.

96. Semba K, Fibiger HC. 1992. Afferent connections of the laterodorsal and the pedunculopontine tegmental nuclei in the rat: a retro- and antero-grade transport and immunohistochemical study. *J Comp Neurol* 323: 387–410.

97. Shi WX. 2005. Slow oscillatory firing: a major firing pattern of dopamine neurons in the ventral tegmental area. *J Neurophysiol* 94: 3516–3522.

98. Shizgal P. 1989. Toward a cellular analysis of intracranial self-stimulation: contributions of collision studies. *Neurosci Biobehav Rev* 13: 81–90.

99. Shizgal P. 1997. Neural basis of utility estimation. *Curr Opin Neurobiol* 7: 198–208.

100. Sienkiewicz-Jarosz H, Scinska A, Kuran W, Ryglewicz D, Rogowski A, Wrobel E, Korkosz A, Kukwa A, Kostowski W, Bienkowski P. 2005. Taste responses in patients with Parkinson's disease. *J Neurol Neurosurg Psychiatry* 76: 40–46.

101. Solomon RL. 1948. The influence of work on behavior. *Psychol Bull* 45: 1–40.

102. Szczypka MS, Kwok K, Brot MD, Marck BT, Matsumoto AM, Donahue BA, Palmiter RD. 2001. Dopamine production in the caudate putamen restores feeding in dopamine-deficient mice. *Neuron* 30: 819–828.

103. Takada M, Tokuno H, Hamada I, Inase M, Ito Y, Imanishi M, Hasegawa N, Akazawa T, Hatanaka N, Nambu A. 2001. Organization of inputs from cingulate motor areas to basal ganglia in macaque monkey. *Eur J Neurosci* 14: 1633–1650.

104. Tindell AJ, Berridge KC, Zhang J, Pecina S, Aldridge JW. 2005. Ventral pallidal neurons code incentive motivation: amplification by mesolimbic sensitization and amphetamine. *Eur J Neurosci* 22: 2617–2634.

105. Tobler PN, Fiorillo CD, Schultz W. 2005. Adaptive coding of reward value by dopamine neurons. *Science* 307: 1642–1645.

106. Ungless MA, Magill PJ, Bolam JP. 2004. Uniform inhibition of dopamine neurons in the ventral tegmental area by aversive stimuli. *Science* 303: 2040–2042.

107. Volkow ND, Wang GJ, Telang F, Fowler JS, Logan J, Childress AR, Jayne M, Ma Y, Wong C. 2006. Cocaine cues and dopamine in dorsal striatum: mechanism of craving in cocaine addiction. *J Neurosci* 26: 6583–6588.

108. Voon V, Fernagut PO, Wickens J, Baunez C, Rodriguez M, Pavon N, Juncos JL, Obeso JA, Bezard E. 2009. Chronic dopaminergic stimulation in Parkinson's disease: from dyskinesias to impulse control disorders. *Lancet Neurol* 8: 1140–1149.

109. Voorn P, Vanderschuren LJ, Groenewegen HJ, Robbins TW, Pennartz CM. 2004. Putting a spin on the dorsal-ventral divide of the striatum. *Trends Neurosci* 27: 468–474.

110. Walton ME, Behrens TE, Buckley MJ, Rudebeck PH, Rushworth MF. 2010. Separable learning systems in the macaque brain and the role of orbitofrontal cortex in contingent learning. *Neuron* 65: 927–939.

111. Walton ME, Kennerley SW, Bannerman DM, Phillips PE, Rushworth MF. 2006. Weighing up the benefits of work: behavioral and neural analyses of effort-related decision making. *Neural Netw* 19: 1302–1314.

112. Wanat MJ, Kuhnen CM, Phillips PE. 2010. Delays conferred by escalating costs modulate dopamine release to rewards but not their predictors. *J Neurosci* 30: 12020–12027.

113. Wanat MJ, Willuhn I, Clark JJ, Phillips PE. 2009. Phasic dopamine release in appetitive behaviors and drug addiction. *Curr Drug Abuse Rev* 2: 195–213.

114. Whalen PJ, Bush G, Shin LM, Rauch SL. 2006. The emotional counting Stroop: a task for assessing emotional interference during brain imaging. *Nat Protoc* 1: 293–296.

115. Wilson C, Nomikos GG, Collu M, Fibiger HC. 1995. Dopaminergic correlates of motivated behavior: importance of drive. *J Neurosci* 15: 5169–5178.

116. Wise RA. 1978. Catecholamine theories of reward: a critical review. *Brain Res* 152: 215–247.

117. Wise RA. 2004. Dopamine, learning and motivation. *Nat Rev Neurosci* 5: 483–494.

118. Wise RA. 2006. Role of brain dopamine in food reward and reinforcement. *Philos Trans R Soc Lond B Biol Sci* 361: 1149–1158.

119. Wise RA. 2009. Roles for nigrostriatal—not just mesocorticolimbic—dopamine in reward and addiction. *Trends Neurosci* 32: 517–524.

120. Yun IA, Wakabayashi KT, Fields HL, Nicola SM. 2004. The ventral tegmental area is required for the behavioral and nucleus accumbens neuronal firing responses to incentive cues. *J Neurosci* 24: 2923–2933.

11 Fronto-Basal-Ganglia Circuits for Stopping Action

Ian Greenhouse, Nicole C. Swann, and Adam R. Aron

Imagine you are sitting on your bicycle at an intersection waiting for the traffic light to turn green. When the light changes, you are about to press down on the pedal when suddenly a motorist runs a light. You must quickly stop the incipient action. This example highlights an important kind of control that we refer to as "reactive stopping." The tendency to move is stopped outright (i.e., completely) and in response to an external signal. Many neuroscience studies now suggest that a relatively specific fronto-basal-ganglia circuit is important for this kind of control. The first section of this chapter reviews this evidence. However, reactive stopping is not the only kind of stopping. Consider a different example. You are a trying-to-abstain nicotine addict who is on your way to a party where you know cigarettes will be available. When offered a cigarette at the party, you are able to resist because you have your abstinence goal in mind, and you use this goal to target your urge. This is a different kind of control that we refer to as "proactive stopping"—the stopping system is prepared in advance. This kind of stopping may be more prevalent in everyday life than reactive stopping. Yet, its neural basis is only now being investigated. The second section of this chapter summarizes preliminary evidence for a neural mechanism underlying proactive stopping.

Reactive Stopping

Behavioral Tasks

Many experimental paradigms exist for studying how people—and, in some cases, experimental animals—control their response tendencies. These include stop signal, go/no-go, response switching, antisaccade, flanker, Stroop, Simon, Wisconsin Card Sort, continuous performance, reversal learning, and many others. These all require control over a prepotent response tendency. Here, we consider the first three in brief detail.

The stop signal task requires people to stop an already initiated response[44] (see figure 11.1A). On each trial, the subject is presented with a Go signal (e.g., a leftward pointing arrow requiring a left-button response or a rightward pointing arrow requiring a right-button response). On a minority of trials, a stop signal is presented after the Go signal. The subject is instructed to respond as fast as possible on Go trials, and to do his or her best to stop the response when the stop signal occurs. If the delay between Go and stop signals is short, the subject is more likely to stop, whereas if the delay is long, the subject is less likely to stop. The various metrics from this task can be used to calculate the internal speed of stopping, that is, stop signal reaction time (SSRT).[67]

In a typical Go/No-Go paradigm the subject is presented with a stream of letter stimuli, and is required to quickly respond to all letters except the letter "X." The key dependent variable is how many times the subject fails to withhold the response on the No-Go trials—referred to as "commission errors." While there are variants of this task (see figure 11.1D), they typically create a prepotent response tendency by having more Go than No-Go trials. An important difference between Go/No-Go and the stop signal paradigm is that in the latter the stop signal is presented after the Go cue.

Another paradigm that also requires stopping a response that is already underway is the response-switching task, typified by Isoda and Hikosaka[35] (see figure 11.2A). Each trial begins with two differently colored cues presented to the left and right of center screen. In the target period, a cue in one of the flanker colors is presented at center screen. This indicates which of the two responses is to be executed. Importantly, the color of the target stays the same for several consecutive trials (i.e., stay trials). When the target color switches, the "preactivated" tendency toward the incorrect response must be stopped.

While the Go/No-Go and response-switching paradigms do not measure exactly the same behavior or the same psychological processes as the stop signal task, they also require rapid stopping in response to an external signal, and many lines of

Figure 11.1
(A) The stop signal task. This requires responding with a button press to a Go stimulus (arrow). On a minority of trials, the arrow is followed by a stop signal presented at a variable delay. (B) A representative rIFC electrode for an electrocorticography study. The precentral sulcus and inferior frontal sulcus are also shown. (C) Electrocorticography results from rIFC. Successful stopping is associated with an increased response in the beta band (~16 Hz) compared to failed stopping. Stop signal occurs at 0 msec. (A–C reproduced with permission from Swann et al.[63]). (D) The Go/No-Go task used by Kühn and colleagues.[41] A cue indicated which response would need to be made, followed by a 2.5-sec delay and then either a Go signal (80% of trials) or a No-Go signal (20% of trials). (E) A representative anatomical scan showing STN electrode placement. (F) Local field potential results from the STN. Beta power (averaged across subjects) is plotted over time for No-Go compared to go. Data represent cumulative percent increase above a baseline period. The Go/No-Go cue is at 0 msec (D–F reproduced with permission from Kühn et al.[41]).

A. Stop Signal Task

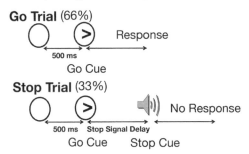

Go Trial (66%)
500 ms
Go Cue
Response

Stop Trial (33%)
500 ms   Stop Signal Delay
Go Cue   Stop Cue
No Response

D. Go/NoGo Task

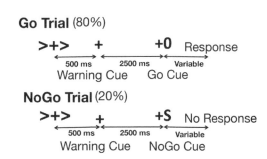

Go Trial (80%)
>+>   +   +0   Response
500 ms   2500 ms   Variable
Warning Cue   Go Cue

NoGo Trial (20%)
>+>   +   +S   No Response
500 ms   2500 ms   Variable
Warning Cue   NoGo Cue

B. RIFC Electrode

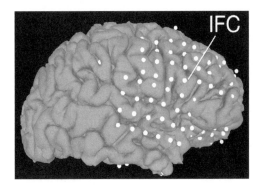

IFC

E. STN Electrode

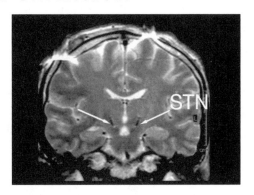

STN

C. RIFC Stop. Response

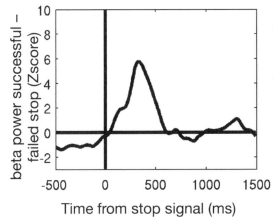

Time from stop signal (ms)

F. STN NoGo Response

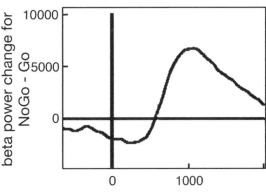

Time from Go/NoGo (ms)

evidence suggest that they engage common neural circuits. Thus, evidence from these paradigms will also be considered when motivating a model of the neural circuitry underlying reactive stopping.

Key Fronto-Basal-Ganglia Regions

A brief overview of the neural circuit for reactive stopping is as follows: Sensory information about the stop signal is quickly relayed to the prefrontal cortex, where the stopping command is presumably generated. Two broad regions of the prefrontal cortex are apparently critical for stopping behavior—the right inferior frontal cortex (rIFC) and the dorsomedial frontal cortex (especially the presupplementary motor area, pre-SMA). These two regions appear to work together to send a stop command to intercept the Go process, via the basal ganglia (figure 11.3). The consequence could be suppression of basal ganglia output with downstream inhibitory effects on the primary motor cortex (M1). Here, we consider each of these key regions in turn: the rIFC, the pre-SMA, the basal ganglia, and M1.

The region referred to here as the rIFC corresponds to areas of lateral prefrontal cortex that are anterior to the precentral sulcus and inferior to the inferior frontal sulcus (see figure 11.1B). The critical importance of the rIFC for stopping in humans has been established by lesion studies. A key study used the stop signal task to compare a large sample of patients with either right or left lateral frontal damage and controls.[2] It was found that right frontal damage affected stopping (made SSRT longer), while left frontal damage did not (also see ref. 55). It was also found that a specific region of importance was the rIFC. This has been confirmed by three studies with transcranial magnetic stimulation (TMS) using the "virtual lesion" approach (i.e., disruptive stimulation followed by behavioral testing).[14,15,66]

While these loss-of-function methodologies show that the rIFC is causally important for stopping, they do not speak to its precise functional role. It might be critical for inhibitory control itself—for example, by projecting directly, or indirectly, to the basal ganglia to block the incipient response[3,63]; and/or it may be critical for attentional monitoring/detection of the stop signal.[22,30,60] A recent study used TMS to directly test the inhibitory versus attention accounts.[66] TMS was applied over two rIFC regions. In one session, this was the posterior inferior frontal gyrus and, in a different session, a more dorsal IFC region known as the inferior frontal junction. Although disruption of both regions affected the speed of stopping (SSRT), it did so by affecting different processes. The results suggest that the right inferior frontal junction implements attentional detection whereas the more ventral sector of rIFC (the posterior inferior frontal gyrus) implements inhibitory control (also see ref. 17). Thus, different sectors of rIFC could implement both attentional monitoring/detection and inhibitory control functions. This makes sense from the view that a subject needs to detect a signal in the environment to stop motor output, and that, in the brain, these functions might be tightly coupled.

Other recent evidence supports an inhibitory control function for the rIFC. Electrocorticography recordings from the surface of the brain revealed activity increases in the inferior frontal gyrus at around 150 to 300 msec following the stop signal, especially in the beta frequency band (13 to 30 Hz)[63] (see figure 11.1A–C). The timing of the response is consistent with an inhibitory control function that occurs within the time scale of the behavioral stopping process (SSRT). The observation of increased activity in the beta band is consistent with the possibility of long-range functional coupling with the basal ganglia to implement the stop (discussed in the following).

Some recent studies have used paired-pulse TMS to probe the functional role of the rIFC (figure 11.2B). In this technique, one coil is held over the rIFC and another over the hand area of M1. On each trial, there is either an M1 pulse alone (with the motor-evoked potential recorded from the hand muscles with electromyography) or an M1 pulse preceded by a rIFC pulse (with a very short delay, e.g., 8 msec). If the rIFC has an inhibitory effect on M1, then the size of the motor evoked potential recorded from the hand should be smaller when rIFC stimulation precedes M1 stimulation than when there is M1 stimulation alone. This is what was found in two studies in which subjects needed to cancel an initiated action in favor of making another.[12,51] These results strongly suggest that the rIFC has an inhibitory effect on the motor system.

In monkeys, lesions, microstimulation, and neurophysiological recordings during performance of the Go/No-Go task all point to the importance of a possibly homologous region (the inferior frontal convexity) for stopping motor responses.[31,37,57,58]

Taken together, these studies show that the rIFC's role in behavioral stopping includes an inhibitory control function (for the right inferior frontal gyrus region), as well as an attentional monitoring/detection function (for the dorsal inferior frontal junction region). Another cortical region that is important for stopping is the pre-SMA. This is a region of dorsomedial frontal cortex. It is in the medial wall of the superior frontal gyrus, dorsal to the anterior cingulate, and anterior to the supplementary motor area proper (see figure 11.2B). The importance of the pre-SMA for stop signal, Go/No-Go, response switching and other related behavioral paradigms is suggested by many studies in humans (lesion, TMS, and fMRI) and monkeys (recording and stimulation).[16,47,49]

Yet the precise functional role of pre-SMA and its relation to rIFC in these forms of behavioral control are still unclear. There have been numerous conceptual accounts for the functional role of the pre-SMA including "selecting superordinate sets of action-selection rules,"[56] action reprogramming,[45] motivation,[59] conflict resolution/monitoring,[35,54] and modulating the tradeoff between speed and accuracy.[8]

These accounts might predict that pre-SMA generates a control signal and rIFC implements the stopping. In the following section, we consider evidence for communication between the pre-SMA and rIFC. Here, we consider how the stop command intercepts the Go process at the level of the basal ganglia.

One basal ganglia region that is well-positioned for stopping action is the subthalamic nucleus (STN). The STN is a basal ganglia input region located bilaterally beneath the thalamus (figure 11.1E). Its role in stopping is supported by anatomical and functional evidence. The STN broadly excites the globus pallidus pars interna (GPi), which increases the neural inhibition on thalamocortical output to the motor system (figure 11.3A). In this way, the massively connected STN may lead to widespread pulses that could inhibit basal ganglia output and the motor system generally.[28] The STN also receives direct input (no intervening synapses) from the cortical foci reviewed above, namely, pre-SMA and rIFC.[3,34] Thus, these cortical regions could quickly activate the STN via a so-called hyperdirect pathway[50] with cortical-STN effects occurring in less than 10 msec.

Functional/behavioral studies also point to the importance of the STN for stopping. A single-unit recording study found neurons in the monkey STN that increased their response on both switch and No-Go trials.[36] In rodents, lesions to the STN produced a generalized stopping impairment for the stop signal task.[23] A high-resolution fMRI study in humans demonstrated activation of the STN region on successful stop trials[4] (also see ref. 43). Modulation of the STN with deep brain stimulation in patients with Parkinson's disease affects SSRT and No-Go commission error rates, although not always in consistent directions.[7,32,52,65]

Other, indirect evidence for the importance of the STN in stopping comes from the observation that when reactive stopping occurs it has global effects on the motor system. For example, when subjects stopped a thumb movement, there was significant, below-baseline suppression of corticomotor excitability of the tibia muscles of the leg.[6] As the leg was not relevant for task performance, this implies there is a brain mechanism for stopping that has global effects on the motor system (such as the STN with its massive output to the GPi). Similarly, behavioral studies have shown that stopping one effector leads to long delays when continuing with another,[5,20] also consistent with a global stop command.

An alternative way of implementing reactive stopping is via inputs to the striatum. This is a frontostriatal system for control rather than a frontosubthalamic one (figure 11.3B). Yet the evidence implicating the striatum in reactive stopping is mixed. Functional MRI studies of the stop signal task do show striatal activation (e.g., refs. 3 and 4). However, this could reflect a variety of processes including the slower speed of the Go process on stop than on Go trials,[4] feedback concerning a successful outcome, or preparation for stopping. Additionally, two stop signal studies of patients with manifest Huntington's disease revealed no deficit in stopping,[2] though up to 50% of the striatum had been lost at that stage of the disease. Other studies have observed that patients with basal ganglia damage are slow to stop their responses,[55] but that could relate to generalized damage (including to the STN). Similarly, patients with Parkinson's disease are slow to stop,[27] but that is also likely to reflect alterations in general basal ganglia function. Lesions to the medial striatum in rodents did lead to overall longer SSRT, but the results were complex, with better stopping at earlier delays, increased Go RT, and increased omission errors.[24] Overall, therefore, while the striatum is implicated in tasks that require reactive stopping, its precise role is still is unclear. Notably, an fMRI study that examined activation on Go trials in a stop signal task found a parametric increase of striatal activation the more stopping was anticipated.[69,70] This points to the possible importance of the striatum for proactive rather than reactive stopping, and is further discussed later.

The primary motor cortex is the last cortical site before movement commands descend the corticospinal tract. The pyramidal cells that generate the corticospinal volleys are embedded in a network of local connections, including many GABAergic inhibitory interneurons. Generating a movement requires driving the pyramidal cells as well as removing the GABAergic inhibition.[53] Reactive stopping has measurable effects in human M1. TMS studies show that stopping an initiated response leads to reductions of corticomotor excitability as well as increased GABAergic inhibition reviewed by Stinear et al.[62] Consistent with this, electrocorticography recordings over M1 in humans show a characteristic pattern of oscillatory change in the alpha/beta range on stop trials that may also relate to GABAergic effects.[63] In standard stop paradigms, it appears as if reactive stopping leads to a "global" effect on the motor system. As we saw previously, a TMS study with the stop signal paradigm showed that stopping a finger movement was associated with suppression of the task-irrelevant leg.[6] This could be the "TMS signature" of a stopping command generated by inputs to the STN with global downstream effects on M1.

Communication between Key Regions in Fronto-Basal-Ganglia Circuits

The rIFC, the pre-SMA, and the STN appear to make up a structurally connected network. Connectivity studies using tract tracing in the monkey and diffusion tensor imaging in humans show that the pre-SMA is connected with the rIFC[40] and also with the basal ganglia input nuclei—the striatum and subthalamic nucleus.[3,34,40] Recent studies have begun to investigate the functional connectivity within this network. This could help to validate the importance of these regions, the relative timing of their recruitment, and their true functional roles. As we saw earlier, there are several possible ways to account for the functional roles of the pre-SMA and rIFC. The pre-SMA may be important for "selecting superordinate sets of action-selection rules,"[56] action reprogramming,[45] motivation,[59] conflict resolution/

monitoring,[35,54] and modulating the tradeoff between speed and accuracy.[8] The rIFC appears to have subregions for action control (including inhibitory control) and attentional orienting.[66] Taken together, these accounts might suggest that the pre-SMA has higher-level representations about the task-to-be-performed, whereas the rIFC may implement stopping. Thus, when control is needed, the pre-SMA may signal to the rIFC to implement the stopping.

Some evidence for this theory was provided by a recent TMS study.[51] Paired-pulse TMS was delivered either over pre-SMA and M1 or over the rIFC and M1 during the performance of a switching task (figure 11.2). This task requires the subject to overcome a prepotent tendency to make one response, and instead to quickly make another. The dependent measure was the motor-evoked potential recorded from the responding hand on switch trials. This method can address whether there is a functional influence of pre-SMA over M1 or of rIFC over M1, and also the timing of any effects. Thus, it can be used to determine if the pre-SMA has its effect before or after rIFC when switching is required. It was found that TMS delivered over the pre-SMA modulated the motor evoked potentials 125 msec after presentation of a switch stimulus, whereas pulsing over rIFC, then M1, modulated the amplitude of motor evoked potentials 175 msec after the switch stimulus (figure 11.2C). This shows that the pre-SMA is involved in control before the rIFC. However, a study using Granger Causal analysis of fMRI data for a stop signal task came to the reverse conclusion—that is, that rIFC precedes the pre-SMA.[22] Yet there are concerns about the use of such causality methods with fMRI data, related to varying hemodynamic responses in different regions.[21]

Other recent studies suggest that the message to stop might be communicated across the network within a particular oscillatory frequency band. This can be measured with extracellular recordings of electrical activity from populations of neurons, for example, using local field potentials or electrocorticography at the surface of the brain. Local field potential recordings within the STN in human patients showed increases in the beta frequency band for No-Go compared to Go trials[41] (see figure 11.1E,F). This is especially interesting insofar as enhancement of beta band power was also observed in the right IFC for stop trials[63] (see above and figure 11.1A–C). Taking these results together, it appears to be possible that inhibitory control is mediated via a right hemisphere pre-SMA–IFC–STN structurally connected functional circuit operating in the beta band (~16 Hz). A better understanding of this system in health and disease is important. It has been suggested, for example, that oversynchronization in the beta band may explain the symptoms in Parkinson's disease.[11]

Summary

Reactive stopping depends on a fronto-basal-ganglia network in the right hemisphere. The network includes the pre-SMA, the rIFC, the basal ganglia, and M1.

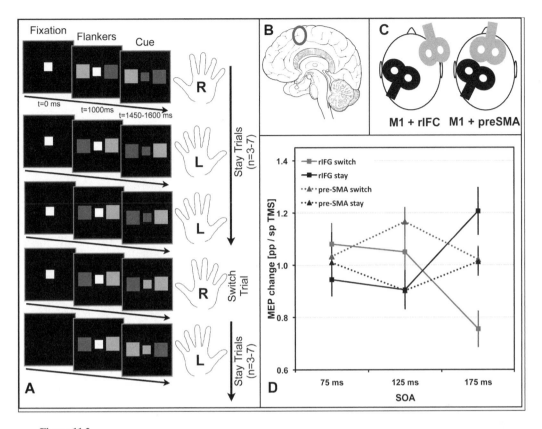

Figure 11.2
(A) The response switching task. This consists of two colored spatial cues that correspond with two possible response outcomes. A target matches one or the other colored cue to indicate an appropriate response. The target color remains the same for a string of three to seven consecutive trials and then switches to the other color. (B) The presupplementary motor area (pre-SMA) is highlighted. (C) Transcranial magnetic stimulation (TMS) coil configurations. TMS was applied over the right inferior frontal cortex (rIFC), then M1 or pre-SMA, then M1. (D) TMS over the rIFC and pre-SMA had differential effects on the amplitudes of motor-evoked potentials recorded from the responding hand on switch trials (solid line) relative to stay trials (dashed line). Pre-SMA exerted its influence at 125 msec, whereas rIFC exerted its influence at 175 msec following the target. (Reproduced with permission from Mars et al.[45] and Neubert et al.[51])

Within the rIFC, two regions seem important—the inferior frontal junction and the posterior inferior frontal gyrus. When a stop signal occurs, the inferior frontal junction may implement attentional detection, while the posterior inferior frontal gyrus may implement inhibitory control. This latter region may implement inhibitory control via inputs to the basal ganglia, perhaps specifically via the STN, using a hyperdirect pathway (figure 11.3A). This is consistent with the observation that reactive stopping has global effects on the motor system.

The relative functional roles of the pre-SMA versus rIFC in reactive stopping are not yet clear. Some evidence suggests the pre-SMA is recruited before the rIFC; so it may be involved in setting up and/or triggering the rIFC. The relative functional roles of the STN versus striatum are not entirely clear either. The frontosubthalamic route may be favored when stopping is an emergency, whereas the frontostriatal route may be used when stopping can be prepared, and perhaps when stopping needs to be selective, as we will see in the following section.

Proactive Stopping

We saw earlier that reactive stopping may be important in everyday life. One example is preventing yourself from stepping on your bike pedal when you detect oncoming traffic. Another is in sports requiring fast action control, such as stopping and switching movements in response to changing environmental signals. Yet, the number of scenarios requiring fast stopping, and especially stopping that has global effects on the motor system, is probably limited. Some examples from psychiatry might make this clearer. It seems doubtful that a child with a premonitory urge to tic is using a brain mechanism that reactively stops responses in a global fashion. Tic suppression, if it involves top-down control at all, is likely to be extended over time, and also selectively targeted at a particular urge. The same goes for the control of urges in the context of substance abuse, such as cigarette smoking. A brain mechanism for rapid, stimulus-driven, reactive stopping of response tendencies, with global effects, seems unsuitable for these cases. Instead, such control appears to require both preparation to stop, and selectivity (i.e., control that is targeted at particular response tendencies). The remainder of this chapter focuses on paradigms of stopping that address these criteria.

Preparing to Stop in Standard Stop Signal and Go/No-Go Tasks

Whereas standard stop signal or Go/No-Go tasks require a minimal working memory load and rapid stopping at the time of the signal, other behavioral paradigms require the subject to prepare to stop an upcoming response. This can occur trial-by-trial in response to control cues (e.g., on this very trial you may have to stop),[18] or at the level of blocks of trials (e.g., when performing a mixed Go and No-Go block of trials,)[68] or in a strategic sense when instructions specify the importance of accuracy over speed.[8]

The behavioral manifestation of proactive stopping is that response times are slower. To examine the neural basis of this behavioral slowing, we consider studies with stop signal and Go/No-Go tasks. However, we note that the neural basis of proactive control has been investigated with several other paradigms (e.g., refs. 10, 26, and 38).

One study addressed proactive stopping using a conditional stop paradigm.[39] Subjects were given a rule that if they initiated (for example) a right-button response and a stop signal occurred, then they would have to stop (critical direction), but if they initiated a left-button response and a stop signal occurred they could ignore it (noncritical direction). Thus, as soon as the Go signal occurs, and it is the critical direction, subjects can proactively prepare to stop. It was found that RT was longer for critical than noncritical Go trials, and those subjects who slowed more were able to stop more quickly. Using fMRI it was found that the network for "reactive stopping" (i.e., rIFC, pre-SMA, and the STN region) was more activated the greater the degree of slowing on Go critical trials. These results suggest that the brain network for reactive stopping could be prepared in advance, that is, control is proactive. Similar findings of proactive activation of the stopping network—including some or all of the pre-SMA, rIFC, and the STN region—have been reported for variants of the stop signal task[18,69,70,72] and the Go/No-Go task.[36] Notably, in some of these studies, there was also dorsolateral prefrontal cortex (DLPFC) and striatal activation. This could reflect the increased working memory demands when preparation is needed. The striatal activation could also reflect use of an indirect fronto-basal-ganglia pathway when the subject is preparing to stop a particular response tendency rather than using a global stop. This will be considered later.

Other evidence for the neural systems underlying proactive control comes from a study examining STN stimulation in humans.[7] The key behavioral index was the difference in RT for mixed blocks of Go and No-Go versus pure blocks of Go trials. When the patients were on stimulation, this slowing (or braking) effect was found to be smaller and rIFC activation was less than when patients were off stimulation. Thus, STN stimulation may have altered the "stopping network," leading to a poorer ability to apply proactive inhibitory control.

Considered together, these studies suggest that regions important for reactive stopping, including the pre-SMA, the rIFC, and the STN, are also activated in situations in which No-Go or stop signals are anticipated. Since recruitment of this stopping network is also often accompanied by slowing of response emission,[18,39,69,70,72] the possibility exists that the stopping network can act as a brake on motor output (without stopping it completely). Further, if the stopping network is preactivated by preparing to stop, then stopping should be quicker when it is needed. Two studies have shown that this is in fact the case.[18,39]

Preparing to Stop a Specific Response Tendency

We saw that the STN is involved in both stop signal and Go/No-Go paradigms. We also saw that the STN may lead to widespread pulses that could inhibit basal ganglia output generally. Behavioral studies and TMS studies with the stop signal paradigm are consistent with the idea that such global suppression has functional consequences in the motor system. Other evidence, reviewed earlier, points to a role for the STN in proactive inhibitory control. Yet, a widespread pulse from the STN appears unsuitable for situations in which the subject is required to stop selectively.

One study attempted to dissociate mechanistically global and selective stopping using a selective stop signal paradigm.[5] On each trial, participants initiated a coupled response with fingers of both hands, and when a stop signal occurred, they tried to stop one response while continuing with the other one. This task provides a measurement of the selectivity of stopping in terms of the degree of interference that is produced in the alternative (unstopped) response—referred to as the "stopping interference effect." When a stopping goal was provided in advance (i.e., "Maybe stop left" or "Maybe stop right"), the stopping interference effect was reduced (i.e., stopping was more selective) whereas SSRT was increased (i.e., stopping was slower).

Mechanistically selective stopping may be slower because selective stopping could be implemented by the indirect pathway of the basal ganglia. One form of this is a projection from the striatum to the globus pallidus pars externa (GPe) and then to the globus pallidus pars interna (GPi),[9] as depicted in figure 11.3B (dotted arrows). The projection of striatal neurons onto the GPe, and the projection from GPe to GPi has a very focused effect on GPi (unlike, for example, the effect of the STN on the GPi, which is very diffuse). Thus, the striatum–GPe–GPi pathway offers a means to selectively control a particular response tendency. A puzzle, however, is that the other (more standard) form of the indirect pathway is a projection from the striatum to the GPe to the STN, and only then to the GPi—and, notably, this standard form itself includes the STN (figure 11.3B, solid arrows). If the STN sends a widespread pulse to the GPi, this would appear to be ill-suited to selective stopping. It is possible that the standard pathway is not used in the circumstance when selective stopping is required, or that it corresponds to a more specific set of STN neurons with more specific effects on GPi than does the cortico-STN-GPi pathway (for review of these complex issues about the indirect pathway of the basal ganglia, see ref. 61). Regardless of the precise way in which selective stopping may be implemented in the basal ganglia, circuitry considerations motivate the indirect pathway via the striatum as a more selective control mechanism than the cortico-STN hyperdirect pathway.

Several studies point to a role for the striatum in preparing to stop, and perhaps especially in preparing to stop selectively. Three fMRI studies found increases of striatal activation when stopping was anticipated.[39,69,70] Other evidence for striatal involvement in selective stopping comes from the antisaccade task. On each trial of this task, a cue indicates whether a saccadic eye movement should be made toward an upcoming spatial target (prosaccade) or away from it (antisaccade). When the

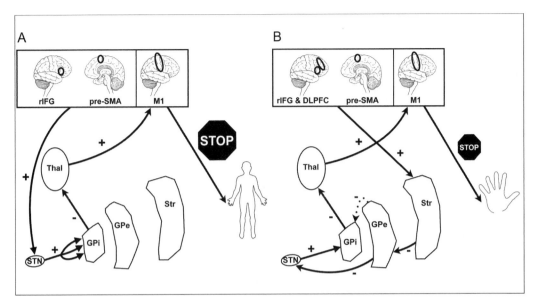

Figure 11.3
(A) A fronto-basal-ganglia system for reactive stopping. The network comprises the pre-SMA and rIFC, which send signals to the STN. The STN sends diffuse output to the globus pallidus pars interna (GPi), which inhibits thalamic output to the primary motor cortex (M1). This stopping mechanism is believed to have global inhibitory effects on the motor system due to the diffuse STN-GPi projections. (B) A fronto-basal-ganglia system for proactive/selective stopping. The network comprises a frontostriatal pathway that could allow for more selective motor control. The standard indirect pathway is depicted with solid arrows, and alternative projections that may allow for more focused selective stopping are depicted with dotted arrows. The dorsolateral prefrontal cortex (DLPFC) represents stopping goals in working memory.

target occurs, a reflexive eye movement is generated; thus correct performance on antisaccade trials requires inhibiting the reflexive tendency while generating a new saccade. In one such study, neurophysiological recordings were made from the striatum of monkeys performing the antisaccade task.[25] This showed that some neurons specifically increased their activity for antisaccades, but not for prosaccades. It was postulated that the suppression of the eye movement on antisaccade trials was due to activation of the indirect pathway of the basal ganglia, with suppressive effects on the superior colliculus. For a similar result using microstimulation in the striatum, see ref. 71.

Preparing to stop selectively may thus be implemented via a frontostriatal rather than a frontosubthalamic pathway. An additional region of importance in the frontal cortex may be the dorsolateral PFC (DLPFC). This spans the middle frontal gyrus in humans. The DLPFC is key for working memory.[13,29,48] Furthermore, stopping goals are a form of working memory—and consistent with this, DLPFC is activated in stop signal or Go/No-Go paradigms with increased working memory load.[18,39,46] The DLPFC is also known to be connected with the striatum via a so-called associative frontostriatal-pallidal-thalamic loop.[1,42] Thus, the subject's goal of what to stop may be implemented in a signal from the DLPFC to the striatum, which inhibits the GPe, which in turn removes inhibition from the GPi, thus targeting particular representations in M1. This circuit may be used to set up a stopping system that can target a particular response tendency. At the time that stopping is needed, this network could be triggered by the pre-SMA or rIFC. This is a speculative model that needs to be tested with further research.

Summary

The candidate brain network for reactive stopping—the pre-SMA, rIFC, and STN—may also be used to prepare to stop. The behavioral consequence of proactive stopping is that subjects slow down, and if stopping is required, they may stop more quickly.

If selective stopping is required by the behavioral paradigm, then subjects may be able to use a selective mechanism to stop. This selective mechanism could engage the indirect pathway of the basal ganglia, rather than the hyperdirect pathway that may be used in reactive stopping. Selective stopping could also be prepared in advance—perhaps via an influence of DLPFC over the striatum.

Conclusion

Converging evidence from the study of reactive stopping using behavioral paradigms such as the stop signal, go/no-go, and switching tasks validates the existence of a functional stopping network comprised of the pre-SMA, rIFC, and STN. This network is believed to send a fast inhibitory signal to the motor system that is widespread or global and might be engaged when stopping is an emergency (e.g., urgently stopping yourself from pushing down on your bike pedal). The identification of this network is leading to efforts that characterize its subcomponents. For example: What are the relative roles of different nodes in the network such as the pre-SMA versus the rIFC,[51] and what is the relative role of the STN versus the striatum?[8] How do attention and inhibitory control functions map to the network?[60,66]

Yet reactive stopping has limitations as a model for control in both everyday life and psychiatric disorders. First, there are scenarios in which a rapid, punctate, stopping process appears ill-suited, for example, when someone has to tonically control an urge to tic. Second, whereas reactive stopping appears to have global effects on the motor system, many scenarios require selective stopping. Third, in everyday life, control is specified according to one's goals, which are monitored over seconds, minutes, or longer, and periodically retrieved from long-term memory in particular contexts. Thus, the control must be set up in advance, extended across time, and it must be targeted internally rather than externally at particular tendencies as these emerge.

It appears that some forms of proactivity, such as preparing to stop in stop signal or Go/No-Go paradigms, or favoring accuracy over speed, engage the same brain network that is used for reactive stopping—but in a partial mode (leading to response slowing).[8,18,39] Further studies are needed to verify these findings and to understand the relative roles of the STN versus the striatum.

Other research suggests that mechanistically selective stopping is possible. When subjects are given a stopping goal, and they use this to prepare to stop a particular response tendency, they can stop one response and continue making another with very little interference.[5,19] Further research is required to examine the neural basis of selective stopping. It is predicted that it will engage the striatum and the indirect pathway, and that it is made possible by a top-down influence from DLPFC.

The research summarized here has focused on motor response control. However, there are fronto-basal-ganglia circuits with a highly similar organization for motivational and emotional control.[64] Further research is needed to develop behavioral paradigms that can measure such limbic control, and to examine whether the fronto-basal-ganglia circuits that are important for stopping action are also important in these domains.

Outstanding Questions

• What are the relative functional roles of the pre-SMA versus the rIFC in stopping?

• Are global and selective stopping dissociable in terms of hyperdirect versus indirect fronto-basal-ganglia circuits?

• Do the fronto-basal-ganglia circuits for stopping action have their counterpart in fronto-basal-ganglia circuits for motivational and emotional control?

Further Reading

Chambers CD, Garavan H, Bellgrove MA. 2009. Insights into the neural basis of response inhibition from cognitive and clinical neuroscience. *Neurosci Biobehav Rev* 33:631–646. A thorough review that looks at the contributions of clinical neuroscience to the understanding of response inhibition. Focuses on, among others, ADHD and obsessive-compulsive disorder, but also on the effects of drug addiction.

Verbruggen F, Logan GD. 2008. Response inhibition in the stop-signal paradigm. *Trends Cogn Sci* 12:418–424. A recent review of one of the most popular paradigms in cognitive psychology and cognitive neuroscience to study action inhibition.

Chikazoe J. 2010. Localizing performance of go/no-go tasks to prefrontal cortical subregions. *Curr Opin Psychiatry* 23: 267–272. A recent review on the neural basis of inhibition. Apart from implicating pre-SMA and rIFC, it focuses on the contributions of different subregions of the IFC to response inhibition.

References

1. Alexander GE, Crutcher MD. 1990. Functional architecture of basal ganglia circuits: neural substrates of parallel processing. *Trends Neurosci* 13: 266–271.

2. Aron AR. 2003. The neural basis of inhibitory mechanisms in executive function. PhD thesis: Cambridge University.

3. Aron AR, Behrens TE, Smith S, Frank MJ, Poldrack RA. 2007. Triangulating a cognitive control network using diffusion-weighted magnetic resonance imaging (MRI) and functional MRI. *J Neurosci* 27: 3743–3752.

4. Aron AR, Poldrack RA. 2006. Cortical and subcortical contributions to Stop signal response inhibition: role of the subthalamic nucleus. *J Neurosci* 26: 2424–2433.

5. Aron AR, Verbruggen F. 2008. Stop the presses: dissociating a selective from a global mechanism for stopping. *Psychol Sci* 19: 1146–1153.

6. Badry R, Mima T, Aso T, Nakatsuka M, Abe M, Fathi D, Foly N, Nagiub H, Nagamine T, Fukuyama H. 2009. Suppression of human cortico-motoneuronal excitability during the Stop-signal task. *Clin Neurophysiol* 120: 1717–1723.

7. Ballanger B, Van Eimeren T, Moro E, Lozano AM, Hamani C, Boulinguez P, Pellecchia G, Houle S, Poon YY, Lang AE, Strafella AP. 2009. Stimulation of the subthalamic nucleus and impulsivity: release your horses. *Ann Neurol* 66: 817–824.

8. Bogacz R, Wagenmakers EJ, Forstmann BU, Nieuwenhuis S. 2010. The neural basis of the speed-accuracy tradeoff. *Trends Neurosci* 33: 10–16.

9. Bolam JP, Smith Y. 1992. The striatum and the globus pallidus send convergent synaptic inputs onto single cells in the entopeduncular nucleus of the rat: a double anterograde labelling study combined with postembedding immunocytochemistry for GABA. *J Comp Neurol* 321: 456–476.

10. Boulinguez P, Ballanger B, Granjon L, Benraiss A. 2009. The paradoxical effect of warning on reaction time: demonstrating proactive response inhibition with event-related potentials. *Clin Neurophysiol* 120: 730–737.

11. Brown P. 2007. Abnormal oscillatory synchronisation in the motor system leads to impaired movement. *Curr Opin Neurobiol* 17: 656–664.

12. Buch ER, Mars RB, Boorman ED, Rushworth MF. 2010. A network centered on ventral premotor cortex exerts both facilitatory and inhibitory control over primary motor cortex during action reprogramming. *J Neurosci* 30: 1395–1401.

13. Bunge SA, Ochsner KN, Desmond JE, Glover GH, Gabrieli JD. 2001. Prefrontal regions involved in keeping information in and out of mind. *Brain* 124: 2074–2086.

14. Chambers CD, Bellgrove MA, Gould IC, English T, Garavan H, McNaught E, Kamke M, Mattingly JB. 2007. Dissociable mechanisms of cognitive control in prefrontal and premotor cortex. *J Neurophysiol* 98: 3638–3647.

15. Chambers CD, Bellgrove MA, Stokes MG, Henderson TR, Garavan H, Robertson IH, Morris AP, Mattingley JB. 2006. Executive "brake failure" following deactivation of human frontal lobe. *J Cogn Neurosci* 18: 444–455.

16. Chambers CD, Garavan H, Bellgrove MA. 2009. Insights into the neural basis of response inhibition from cognitive and clinical neuroscience. *Neurosci Biobehav Rev* 33: 631–646.

17. Chikazoe J, Jimura K, Asari T, Yamashita K, Morimoto H, Hirose S, Miyashita Y, Konishi S. 2009. Functional dissociation in right inferior frontal cortex during performance of go/no-go task. *Cereb Cortex* 19: 146–152.

18. Chikazoe J, Jimura K, Hirose S, Yamashita K, Miyashita Y, Konishi S. 2009. Preparation to inhibit a response complements response inhibition during performance of a stop-signal task. *J Neurosci* 29: 15870–15877.

19. Claffey MP, Sheldon S, Stinear CM, Verbruggen F, Aron AR 2009. Having a goal to stop action is associated with advance control of specific motor representations. *Neuropsychologia*.

20. Coxon JP, Stinear CM, Byblow WD. 2007. Selective inhibition of movement. *J Neurophysiol* 97: 2480–2489.

21. David O, Guillemain I, Saillet S, Reyt S, Deransart C, Segebarth C, Depaulis A. 2008. Identifying neural drivers with functional MRI: an electrophysiological validation. *PLoS Biol* 6: 2683–2697.

22. Duann JR, Ide JS, Luo X, Li CS. 2009. Functional connectivity delineates distinct roles of the inferior frontal cortex and presupplementary motor area in stop signal inhibition. *J Neurosci* 29: 10171–10179.

23. Eagle DM, Baunez C, Hutcheson DM, Lehmann O, Shah AP, Robbins TW. 2008. Stop-signal reaction-time task performance: role of prefrontal cortex and subthalamic nucleus. *Cereb Cortex* 18: 178–188.

24. Eagle DM, Robbins TW. 2003. Inhibitory control in rats performing a stop-signal reaction-time task: effects of lesions of the medial striatum and d-amphetamine. *Behav Neurosci* 117: 1302–1317.

25. Ford KA, Everling S. 2004. Neural activity in primate caudate nucleus associated with pro- and antisaccades. *J Neurophysiol* 102: 2334–2341.

26. Forstmann BU, Dutilh G, Brown S, Neumann J, von Cramon DY, Ridderinkhof KR, Wagenmakers EJ. 2008. Striatum and pre-SMA facilitate decision-making under time pressure. *Proc Natl Acad Sci USA* 105: 17538–17542.

27. Gauggel S, Rieger M, Feghoff TA. 2004. Inhibition of ongoing responses in patients with Parkinson's disease. *J Neurol Neurosurg Psychiatry* 75: 539–544.

28. Gillies AJ, Willshaw DJ. 2009. A massively connected subthalamic nucleus leads to the generation of widespread pulses. *Proc Biol Sci* 265: 2101–2109.

29. Goldman-Rakic PS. 1990. Cellular and circuit basis of working memory in prefrontal cortex of non-human primates. *Prog Brain Res* 85: 325–335.

30. Hampshire A, Chamberlain SR, Monti MM, Duncan J, Owen AM. 2010. The role of the right inferior frontal gyrus: inhibition and attentional control. *Neuroimage* 50: 1313–1319.

31. Hasegawa RP, Peterson BW, Goldberg ME. 2004. Prefrontal neurons coding suppression of specific saccades. *Neuron* 43: 415–425.

32. Hershey T, Revilla FJ, Wernle A, Gibson PS, Dowling JL, Perlmutter JS. 2004. Stimulation of STN impairs aspects of cognitive control in PD. *Neurology* 62: 1110–1114.

33. Hester RL, Murphy F, Foxe JJ, Foxe DM, Javitt DC, Garavan H. 2004. Predicting success: patterns of cortical activation and deactivation prior to response inhibition. *J Cogn Neurosci* 16: 776–785.

34. Inase M, Tokuno H, Nambu A, Akazawa T, Takada M. 1999. Corticostriatal and corticosubthalamic input zones from the presupplementary motor area in the macaque monkey: comparison with the input zones from the supplementary motor area. *Brain Res* 833: 191–201.

35. Isoda M, Hikosaka O. 2007. Switching from automatic to controlled action by monkey medial frontal cortex. *Nat Neurosci* 10: 240–248.

36. Isoda M, Hikosaka O. 2008. Role for subthalamic nucleus neurons in switching from automatic to controlled eye movement. *J Neurosci* 28: 7209–7218.

37. Iversen SD, Mishkin M. 1970. Perseverative interference in monkeys following selective lesions of the inferior prefrontal convexity. *Exp Brain Res* 11: 376–386.

38. Jaffard M, Longcamp M, Velay JL, Anton JL, Roth M, Nazarian B, Boulinguez P. 2008. Proactive inhibitory control of movement assessed by event-related fMRI. *Neuroimage* 42: 1196–1206.

39. Jahfari S, Stinear CM, Claffey M, Verbruggen F, Aron AR. 2009. Responding with restraint: What are the neurocognitive mechanisms? *J Cogn Neurosci* 22: 1479–1492.

40. Johansen-Berg H, Behrens TE, Robson MD, Drobnjak I, Rushworth MF, Brady JM, Smith SM, Higham DJ, Matthews PM. 2004. Changes in connectivity profiles define functionally distinct regions in human medial frontal cortex. *Proc Natl Acad Sci USA* 101: 13335–13340.

41. Kühn AA, Williams D, Kupsch A, Limousin P, Hariz M, Schneider GH, Yarrow K, Brown P. 2004. Event-related beta desynchronization in human subthalamic nucleus correlates with motor performance. *Brain* 127: 735–746.

42. Lehéricy S, Ducros M, Van de Moortele PF, Francois C, Thivard L, Poupon C, Swindale N, Ugurbil K, Kim DS. 2004. Diffusion tensor fiber tracking shows distinct corticostriatal circuits in humans. *Ann Neurol* 55: 522–529.

43. Li CS, Yan P, Sinha R, Lee TW. 2008. Subcortical processes of motor response inhibition during a stop signal task. *Neuroimage* 41: 1352–1363.

44. Logan GD, Cowan WB, Davis KA. 1984. On the ability to inhibit simple and choice reaction time responses: a model and a method. *J Exp Psychol Hum Percept Perform* 10: 276–291.

45. Mars RB, Klein MC, Neubert FX, Olivier E, Buch ER, Boorman ED, Rushworth MF. 2009. Short-latency influence of medial frontal cortex on primary motor cortex during action selection under conflict. *J Neurosci* 29: 6926–6931.

46. Mostofsky SH, Schafer JG, Abrams MT, Goldberg MC, Flower AA, Boyce A, Courtney SM, Calhoun VD, Kraut MA, Denckla MB, Pekar JJ. 2003. fMRI evidence that the neural basis of response inhibition is task-dependent. *Brain Res Cogn Brain Res* 17: 419–430.

47. Mostofsky SH, Simmonds DJ. 2008. Response inhibition and response selection: two sides of the same coin. *J Cogn Neurosci* 20: 751–761.

48. Müller NG, Knight RT. 2006. The functional neuroanatomy of working memory: contributions of human brain lesion studies. *Neuroscience* 139: 51–58.

49. Nachev P, Kennard C, Husain M. 2008. Functional role of the supplementary and pre-supplementary motor areas. *Nat Rev Neurosci* 9: 856–869.

50. Nambu A, Tokuno H, Takada M. 2002. Functional significance of the cortico-subthalamo-pallidal 'hyperdirect' pathway. *Neurosci Res* 43: 111–117.

51. Neubert FX, Mars RB, Buch ER, Olivier E, Rushworth MFS. 2010. Cortical and subcortical interactions during action reprogramming and their related white matter pathways. *Proc Natl Acad Sci USA* 107: 13240–13245.

52. Ray NJ, Jenkinson N, Brittain J, Holland P, Joint C, Nandi D, Bain PG, Yousif N, Green A, Stein JS, Aziz TZ. 2009. The role of the subthalamic nucleus in response inhibition: evidence from deep brain stimulation for Parkinson's disease. *Neuropsychologia* 47: 2828–2834.

53. Reynolds C, Ashby P. 1999. Inhibition in the human motor cortex is reduced just before a voluntary contraction. *Neurology* 53: 730–735.

54. Ridderinkhof KR, Ullsperger M, Crone EA, Nieuwenhuis S. 2004. The role of the medial frontal cortex in cognitive control. *Science* 306: 443–447.

55. Rieger M, Gauggel S, Burmeister K. 2003. Inhibition of ongoing responses following frontal, non-frontal, and basal ganglia lesions. *Neuropsychology* 17: 272–282.

56. Rushworth MF, Walton ME, Kennerley SW, Bannerman DM. 2004. Action sets and decisions in the medial frontal cortex. *Trends Cogn Sci* 8: 410–417.

57. Sakagami M, Tsutsui K, Lauwereyns J, Koizumi M, Kobayashi S, Hikosaka O. 2001. A code for behavioral inhibition on the basis of color, but not motion, in ventrolateral prefrontal cortex of macaque monkey. *J Neurosci* 21: 4801–4808.

58. Sasaki K, Gemba H, Tsujimoto T. 1989. Suppression of visually initiated hand movement by stimulation of the prefrontal cortex in the monkey. *Brain Res* 495: 100–107.

59. Scangos KW, Stuphorn V. 2010. Medial frontal cortex motivates but does not control movement initiation in the countermanding task. *J Neurosci* 30: 1968–1982.

60. Sharp DJ, Bonnelle V, De Boissezon X, Beckmann CF, James SG, Patel MC, Mehta MA. 2010. Distinct frontal systems for response inhibition, attentional capture, and error processing. *Proc Natl Acad Sci USA* 107: 6106–6111.

61. Smith Y, Bevan MD, Shink E, Bolam JP. 1998. Microcircuitry of the direct and indirect pathways of the basal ganglia. *Neuroscience* 86: 353–387.

62. Stinear CM, Coxon JP, Byblow WD. 2009. Primary motor cortex and movement prevention: where Stop meets Go. *Neurosci Biobehav Rev* 33: 662–673.

63. Swann N, Tandon N, Canolty R, Ellmore TM, McEvoy LK, Dreyer S, DiSano M, Aron AR. 2009. Intracranial EEG reveals a time- and frequency-specific role for the right inferior frontal gyrus and primary motor cortex in stopping initiated responses. *J Neurosci* 29: 12675–12685.

64. Temel Y, Blokland A, Steinbusch HW, Visser-Vandewalle V. 2005. The functional role of the subthalamic nucleus in cognitive and limbic circuits. *Prog Neurobiol* 76: 393–413.

65. Van den Wildenberg WPM, Van Boxtel GJ, Van der Molen MW, Bosch DA, Speelman JD, Brunia CH. 2006. Stimulation of the subthalamic region facilitates the selection and inhibition of motor responses in Parkinson's disease. *J Cogn Neurosci* 18: 626–636.

66. Verbruggen F, Aron AR, Stevens MA, Chambers CD. 2010. Theta burst stimulation dissociates attention and action updating in human inferior frontal cortex. *Proc Natl Acad Sci USA* 107: 13966–13971.

67. Verbruggen F, Logan GD. 2008. Response inhibition in the stop-signal paradigm. *Trends Cogn Sci* 12: 418–424.

68. Verbruggen F, Logan GD. 2009. Proactive adjustments of response strategies in the stop-signal paradigm. *J Exp Psychol Hum Percept Perform* 35: 835–854.

69. Vink M, Kahn RS, Raemaekers M, van den Heuvel M, Boersma M, Ramsey NF. 2005. Function of striatum beyond inhibition and execution of motor responses. *Hum Brain Mapp* 25: 336–344.

70. Vink M, Ramsey NF, Raemaekers M, Kahn RS. 2006. Striatal dysfunction in schizophrenia and unaffected relatives. *Biol Psychiatry* 60: 32–39.

71. Watanabe M, Munoz DP. 2010. Saccade suppression by electrical microstimulation in monkey caudate nucleus. *J Neurosci* 30: 336–344.

72. Zandbelt B, Van Buuren M, Gladwin TE, Hoogendam R, Kahn S, Vink M. 2008. Brain regions involved in response inhibition are also activated during anticipation of inhibition. Presented at the Annual Meeting of the Society for Neuroscience 2008.

12 Learning, the P3, and the Locus Coeruleus-Norepinephrine System

Sander Nieuwenhuis

Recent research has suggested that the neuromodulatory brainstem nucleus locus coeruleus (LC) is critical for the regulation of cognitive performance.[2,29,39,57] The LC exhibits a strong phasic increase in activity during the processing of motivationally relevant stimuli, leading to the release of the neuromodulatory neurotransmitter norepinephrine (NE) in the hippocampus, neocortex, and many other projection areas. This LC-mediated noradrenergic innervation increases the responsivity (or gain) of efferent target neurons.[6] It has been shown that, when applied in a temporally strategic manner (e.g., when driven by the identification and evaluation of motivationally relevant stimuli), increases in gain produce an increase in the signal-to-noise ratio of subsequent processing and a concomitant improvement in the efficiency and reliability of behavioral responses.[48] Accordingly, it has been found that LC phasic activation reliably precedes and is temporally linked to behavioral responses to attended stimuli.[8,11] The idea that the LC may serve as a temporal filter—facilitating responses to task-relevant information at the moment that such information is being actively represented—is a key component of the adaptive gain theory,[2] which posits an important role for the LC-NE system in optimizing task performance.

In recent work, I and others have proposed that the neuromodulatory effect of phasic NE release in the neocortex can be measured noninvasively in human subjects by recording the P3(00) component of the scalp-recorded event-related potential (ERP).[37] The P3 is a prominent positive large-amplitude ERP component with a broad, midline scalp distribution, and a typical peak latency between 300 and 400 msec following presentation of stimuli in any sensory modality (for a review, see ref. 43). First reported in 1965,[51] the P3 has undoubtedly been the single most studied ERP component. Yet, until recently, psychologists and neuroscientists had failed to come up with a precise, mechanistic account that elucidates the functional role in information processing of the process underlying the P3, as well as its neural basis. The LC-P3 theory was the first account of the P3 that was both mechanistically explicit and based on firm neuroscientific knowledge. The theory claims that the P3 reflects the response of the LC-NE system to the outcome of internal decision-making processes and the consequent effects of noradrenergic potentiation of information processing.

The goal of this chapter is twofold: First we review similarities between the P3 and phasic LC-NE responses in terms of their relationship with learning. The original discussion of the LC-P3 theory focused on the relationship between the P3, LC activity, and performance in two-choice reaction-time tasks, and emphasized the importance of the LC-P3 response in facilitating rapid action—a key tenet of adaptive gain theory. In contrast, there was little discussion of the empirical evidence suggesting a close relationship between the LC-P3 response and learning. One goal of this chapter is to fill this hiatus. The second goal is to briefly review recent accounts of the role of the LC-NE system in learning, and to show that one of these accounts[14] is strikingly similar to the context-updating hypothesis,[15] the most influential account of the functional significance of the P3. This analysis is meant to elucidate the relationship between the LC-P3 theory and the context-updating hypothesis, showing that the two are more closely related than previously thought.

The LC-P3 Theory

The hypothesis that the P3 reflects the LC-mediated phasic enhancement of neural responsivity in the cortex is supported by a wealth of data from intracranial recordings, lesion studies, psychopharmacology, functional imaging, and other methods, as summarized in this chapter (for an extensive review, see ref. 37). First, the antecedent conditions for the P3 are similar to those reported for the LC phasic response. In general, P3 amplitude is more closely related to the overall motivational significance and/or arousing nature of a given stimulus than to the affective valence of the stimulus. Important factors affecting the amplitude of the P3 are the subjective probability of the eliciting stimulus, its task relevance, and its salience (e.g., intensity, novelty). Like the LC phasic response, the P3 is also enlarged for stimuli with intrinsic significance such as emotionally valent stimuli, whether experienced as positive or negative.

Second, the distribution and timing of intracranial and scalp-recorded P3 activity are consistent with the anatomical and physiological properties of the noradrenergic system. For example, functional imaging studies, intracranial recordings, and lesion studies have indicated that brain areas showing or contributing to P3 activity are scattered across the brain,[49] consistent with the widespread projections from the LC to cortical and subcortical areas. In addition, the pattern of P3 generators shows a spatial specificity that mirrors the projection density of the LC. Furthermore, P3 onset latency in simple two-alternative forced-choice tasks is consistent with the latency of LC phasic activity (~150–200 msec), if one takes into account the relatively slow conduction velocity of LC fibers. Additionally, the relatively early timing of P3 activity in frontal and subcortical areas (e.g., thalamus) is consistent with the trajectory of LC fibers, which first reach these areas and only then veer backward to innervate posterior cortical areas.

Third, several studies have reported direct evidence for an LC generator of the P3. These include psychopharmacological studies, which have shown that P3 amplitude is modulated in a systematic fashion by noradrenergic agents such as clonidine, and entirely abolished following drug-induced NE depletion.[52] Also, a recent study found that individual differences in the noradrenergic gene that affects the activity of the alpha-2a receptor are a key determinant of P3 amplitude.[33] In addition, lesion studies have demonstrated a selective effect on P3 amplitude of LC lesions.[42]

Finally, larger and faster P3s are associated with more accurate and faster behavioral responses and stronger stimulus-related sympathetic nervous system responses.[38] This pattern mirrors the relation between LC phasic activity, task performance, and sympathetic nervous system activity, and is consistent with the functional role ascribed to the noradrenergic system by the adaptive gain theory: to afford rapid action in response to motivationally significant stimuli. The LC-P3 theory does not claim that the P3 process is necessary for responding; of course, subjects can decide to respond before their perceptual system has fully analyzed the stimulus. The theory claims that *if* the P3 occurs before the response, then the response will be facilitated and more efficient.

The Role of the LC-NE System in Learning: Neurophysiological Data

Because it built on the framework of adaptive gain theory, the LC-P3 theory focused primarily on the role of the LC-NE system in optimizing the speed and accuracy of responding in choice reaction-time tasks. However, neurophysiological data also suggest an important role for the LC-NE system in learning.

Kety[30] was the first to propose that phasic NE release might serve as a learning signal, by producing persistent facilitation of synaptic inputs occurring in conjunction with the NE release: "The aroused state induced by novel stimuli, or by stimuli genetically recognized as significant, is pervasive and affects synapses throughout the central nervous system, suppressing most, but permitting or even accentuating activity in those that are transmitting the novel or significant stimuli." Thus, the phasic NE release associated with motivationally significant stimuli selectively acts on synapses that are actively involved at the time of learning, thus strengthening the corresponding memory trace. Such strengthening of synaptic connections is the predominant neuroscientific model of learning in the nervous system.

Various basic properties of the LC-NE system support its role in learning. Phasic LC responses occur following both positive and negative reinforcers, and following novel, unexpected, and other stimuli requiring animals to update their representation of the environment. The LC's widespread projection system is consistent with the distribution of representations of the elements that constitute a memory across multiple sensory processing areas according to their content. The timing of LC activity at several time scales is also consistent with a role in learning. LC neurons increase their activity during learning of new stimulus associations, habituate rapidly, and respond again when the stimulus changes its predictive value, well before learning is visible at the behavioral level. The timing of LC-NE phasic activity within a trial is also sufficiently rapid to afford modulation of the neural trace of the stimulus that triggered the phasic response.

NE also has several postsynaptic effects that support Kety's original hypothesis.[25,47] First, NE can enhance or even permit cellular responses to synaptic input, and thus promote the impact of stimuli in LC projection areas. For example, iontophoretically applied NE can reduce spontaneous neuronal activity in various brain areas while at the same time preserving or enhancing neuronal responses to potent and specific synaptic input. Second, considerable evidence indicates that NE is able to modulate long-term potentiation (LTP) in the hippocampus, the prevalent cellular model of memory.[6] LTP is a long-lasting enhancement in synaptic strength between two neurons that results when the synapse is rapidly stimulated for a brief period. NE promotes LTP through actions at beta-adrenergic receptors.[23] A critical precondition is the close temporal proximity of the NE release and evoked synaptic activity.[44] Finally, there is evidence that NE suppresses intracortical and feedback synaptic transmission, while sparing, or even boosting, thalamocortical processing.[31] For example, NE can change the mode of activity of thalamic neurons from burst to spike mode, necessary for the accurate transfer of incoming information to the neocortex[35]; and LC activation enhances the processing of concomitant sensory input by reducing feedforward inhibitory interneuron activity, and reduces "binding" oscillations hypothesized to stabilize existing memories.[10] These actions promote learning by favoring bottom-up, sensory signals at the expense of top-down, expectation-driven signals (cf. ref. 57).

The Relationship Between the P3 and Learning

The neurophysiological evidence for an important effect of phasic LC-NE responses on learning is mirrored by similar evidence for a close relationship between the P3 and learning.

Numerous ERP studies have reported a "Dm effect," a broad positive ERP deflection during encoding of stimuli that are later remembered compared to stimuli that are later forgotten (reviewed in ref. 56). Although some studies have reported Dm effects that do not appear to be restricted to the P3, Fabiani and Donchin reported that a P3 amplitude difference generally makes up an important part of the effect.[18] The Dm effect has been found when trials are sorted on the basis of both recall performance and recognition performance,[41] and is larger for stimuli that are both recalled and recognized than for stimuli that are neither recalled nor recognized; stimuli that are recognized but not recalled elicit an intermediate positive deflection.[18] Fabiani and Donchin have also replicated the Dm effect using the reverse procedure: sorting and binning trials on the basis of single-trial P3 amplitudes, and then comparing recall and recognition performance between these bins.

In incidental encoding tasks (i.e., when subjects do not know their memory for the stimuli will be tested), the Dm effect is larger for stimuli that are processed more deeply (e.g., semantically) during encoding, but it is also observed in shallow encoding tasks.[22] Additionally, the Dm effect has been examined using tasks in which a small proportion of the stimuli are physically or semantically different from the majority of the stimuli.[20,28] These "isolated" stimuli are remembered significantly more often than "nonisolated" stimuli and elicit a larger P3 during encoding. However, the correlation between P3 amplitude and later memory is also found within stimulus categories; for example, nonisolated stimuli are associated with a larger P3 amplitude if they are later remembered. Interestingly, there is some evidence that the Dm effect is absent during the encoding of abstract visual stimuli.[53] This suggests that the presence of a Dm effect may, at least in some situations, depend on whether stimuli can access or be integrated with preexisting semantic or other knowledge.[56]

In intentional encoding tasks (i.e., subjects know their memory for the stimuli will be tested), researchers have also found typical Dm effects on P3 amplitude, but only in subjects who engaged in "rote" rehearsal (e.g., silent repetition of the to-be-encoded stimuli), either by choice or by instruction.[19,21,28] Subjects who used elaborate encoding strategies (e.g., forming images or sentences based on the to-be-encoded stimuli) performed better in the test phase and showed a normal centroparietal P3 during the study phase, but this P3 did not correlate with subsequent memory performance. Instead, these subjects showed another neural correlate of subsequent learning: a later positive component that was largest at frontal scalp electrodes. These findings suggest that the P3 process is most strongly related to later memory when subjects engage in relatively simple rehearsal strategies. If subjects engage in further processing of the stimuli, then other processes (perhaps supported by the prefrontal cortex) influence the accuracy of memory and the relative contribution of the P3 process is reduced.

These P3 findings are consistent with the notion that phasic NE signals influence learning in a bottom-up way. That is, subsequent memory effects on P3 amplitude may reflect sources of variability in the strength of the LC-NE responses associated with the to-be-encoded stimuli: systematic variability due to experimental manipulations (e.g., manipulations that make an item "stand out" in a physical or semantic sense) and uncontrolled variability due to (subject-specific) differences in the motivational significance of the encoded stimuli (e.g., some words are more meaningful to a subject than other words). The contribution of these NE signals to learning may be reduced to the extent that subjects engage in top-down strategies for learning. The effect of these (e.g., prefrontal) strategies tends to de-correlate the relationship between P3 amplitude and learning.

The Role of the LC-NE System in Learning: Recent Theories

Since the publication of the LC-P3 theory,[37] researchers have advanced several new accounts that build on the role of phasic LC responses in learning.[9,14,55] These accounts may enhance our understanding of the P3 literature.

The work of Verguts and Notebaert[55] builds on the effect of LC activity on strengthening synaptic connections (see section on the role of the LC-NE system in learning: above), and was inspired by recent findings of item-specific conflict adaptation effects. A hallmark finding in cognitive control experiments is that congruency effects (e.g., in the Stroop task) are smaller on trials immediately following an incongruent trial. Botvinick and colleagues have explained such conflict-adaptation effects by assuming that high conflict signals in anterior cingulate cortex (ACC) on trial n-1 are used to strengthen task representations (e.g., a color-naming representation) in prefrontal cortex on trial n, thus increasing cognitive control and reducing congruency effects. This conflict-control loop model has successfully accounted for a wide range of phenomena in the cognitive control literature.[7] However, the task-level representations in this model cannot account for recent findings that conflict-adaptation effects are stronger for some stimulus-stimulus and stimulus-response associations within a given task than for others. For example, if in a Stroop task some color words are presented mostly congruently, and other color words mostly incongruently, the congruency effect is larger for the former type of stimuli. These item-specific conflict-adaptation effects have led Verguts and Notebaert[54,55] to propose a new model of conflict adaptation.

According to this model, ACC conflict signals are not (directly) relayed to the prefrontal cortex, but instead trigger a phasic response of the LC. The consequent phasic release of the NE enhances ongoing (LTP-mediated) Hebbian learning as discussed earlier, and thus strengthens associations between active (i.e., usually task-relevant) representations. Item-specific conflict-adaptation effects occur because the NE-dependent modification of synaptic weights is proportional to the degree of conflict associated with particular stimulus-stimulus or stimulus-response associations. For example, conflict is larger for incongruent red color words if the color red is usually paired with the congruent word "red." More formally, in the Hebbian learning rule, weight changes between two connected cells are proportional to the product of presynaptic and postsynaptic activity:

$$\Delta w_{ij} = \lambda \times x_i \times x_j \qquad \qquad (12.1)$$

where x_i and x_j are the activation of the sending cell i and receiving cell j, respectively. According to Verguts and Notebaert, the learning-rate parameter λ is modulated by trial-to-trial changes in conflict-dependent phasic NE release. This model is consistent with the hypothesized ACC-LC interactions in adaptive gain theory[2] and with recent findings that ACC activity and pupil diameter (a correlate of LC activity[24]) correlate with trial-to-trial changes in learning rate in volatile environments.[4,36] In recent work, Notebaert and colleagues have started investigating the relationship between the P3 and conflict-related adaptations in cognitive control parameters.[40]

Dayan and Yu's[14] account of phasic LC-NE function and learning builds on the role of NE in promoting bottom-up as opposed to top-down processing, and hence learning about the external environment (see preceding section on the role of the LC-NE system in learning; see also ref. 57). According to this account, phasic NE signals encode unexpected uncertainty about the current state within a task, and serve to interrupt the ongoing processing associated with the default task state. Dayan and Yu implemented their ideas in a Bayesian model of the oddball task, the most commonly used task for studying the P3:

For the [oddball] task modeled here, the specific effect of the NE-mediated interrupt is to arouse the animal from default inaction to release a continuously pressed bar in response to an unexpected target stimulus. More general roles for such an interrupt include organizing more general aspects of behavioral responding as well as ensuring that top-down influences on sensory processing associated with the default, current state are immediately nullified once their statistical foundations have been undermined. . . . NE's fast responses and diffuse projections make it particularly suitable for signaling the detection of such unexpected state changes. The actual maintenance of the contextual model, and the computation of the posterior probabilities, are likely to be subserved by the prefrontal cortex . . . and also the anterior cingulate cortex. . . . Both these neural structures exert a powerful influence over the locus coeruleus, as indeed do subcortical structures, which could occasion interrupts based on more primitively assessed unexpected events. (pp. 342–343)

Dayan and Yu showed that their model captures some key aspects of monkey LC activity observed in the oddball task.

This account is consonant with Bouret and Sara's[9] view of NE as a neural interrupt signal that promotes learning (see also refs. 8 and 13): "these [LC] neurons are activated within behavioral contexts that require a cognitive shift—that is, interruption of ongoing behavior and adaptation. This LC activation occurs whenever there is a change in environmental imperative, such as the appearance of a novel, unexpected event, or a change in stimulus-reinforcement contingencies within a formal learning situation."

The ideas reviewed here are also broadly consistent with the adaptive gain theory.[2] Although primarily a theory of the role of the LC-NE system in the regulation of attention and performance, the adaptive gain theory implicitly suggests a role for this system in modulating learning rate and long-term memory. Specifically, higher levels of NE and, through an increased gain, greater neural activity at the time of the stimulus (i.e., increased x_i and x_j in equation 12.1; cf. ref. 55 may promote larger adjustments in current probabilistic beliefs, speeding learning and enhancing memory.

The Context-Updating Hypothesis of the P3

Dayan and Yu's[14] account of phasic LC function shows a striking correspondence with the prevalent account of the functional significance of the P3, the context-updating hypothesis.[15-17]

Donchin and colleagues hypothesized that the function of the P3 process is to update the mental model (or schema) that we maintain of the environment. For example, Donchin[15] proposed that

[T]he process manifested by the P300 is not elicited for the purpose of tactically responding to a given stimulus in a given trial, but rather to what I call strategic information processing. This is the information processing that will affect the manner in which we respond to *future* stimuli. . . . *These are activities that affect our schema rather than our actions.* . . . The schema may be conceptualized as a large and complex map representing all available data about the environment. . . . When there is a need, the model is revised by building novel representations through the incorporation of incoming data into schema[ta] based on long-term memory data. It is likely that it is this updating process that we see manifested by the P300. . . . It is the degree to which the event requires a revision of the model, not its inherent attributes, that is the crucial determinant of P300 [amplitude]. (pp. 507–508)

In later work, Donchin and Coles[16] described the mental model as representing the probabilistic structure of the environment. Furthermore, to explain why task-relevant stimuli elicit larger P3s, they assumed that "Only those segments of the context that are central to the tasks performed by the subject are likely to bring about the changes in the model of the environment" (p. 369).

The context-updating hypothesis led Donchin and colleagues to investigate the possible effect of the P3 process on subsequent performance through the restructuring of the subject's model of the environment. In this context they asked to what extent P3 amplitude predicts the probability that items will be remembered. As discussed in the section on the relationship between the P3 and learning, Donchin's group and, subsequently, other researchers found strong evidence for a close relationship between these variables. The finding that the target probability effect on

P3 amplitude in the oddball task diminishes with increasing interstimulus intervals (with changes on the order of seconds[17]) provides further evidence that the P3 reflects a decaying memory representation of the task structure. The context-updating hypothesis also offers a possible account of why the Dm effect is not observed during encoding of abstract visual stimuli[53]: Subjects do not have an existing mental model of these stimuli, and therefore stimuli differ little in terms of the evoked mismatch with already present knowledge.

The similarities between the context-updating hypothesis and Dayan and Yu's[14] account are clear: Both hold that the subject has an (implicit or explicit) internal model of the external environment, for example, a model that reflects the current task's statistical structure. If the corresponding expectations are violated by sensory observations (e.g., an infrequent target in the oddball task), the system produces an LC phasic response (Dayan and Yu) or P3 (Donchin). A result of that process is that the internal model is updated and the subject is learning.

Unexpected Uncertainty, Surprise, the LC-NE System, and the P3

According to Dayan and Yu,[14] phasic NE encodes a decision variable that is important for learning: unexpected uncertainty, or surprise, about the current state within a task. More specifically, they proposed that in tasks such as the oddball task, phasic NE reports on the ratio between the posterior probability of a target being present (given the sensory data) and its prior probability. Thus, infrequent targets elicit a phasic LC response because of their low prior probability. Furthermore, increasing the prior probability of a target (i.e., the denominator of the equation) should reduce the magnitude of the phasic NE signal associated with a target. This prediction is consistent with the finding that increasing target frequency reduces the magnitude of phasic LC responses.[1] As noted earlier, Dayan and Yu believe that prior probability is represented and posterior probability is computed by brain structures projecting to the LC, not by the LC itself. Indeed, if Dayan and Yu's hypothesis is right, this does not imply that surprise is the only variable encoded by the LC: The LC may receive and encode various other signals, for example, about the task relevance or intrinsic motivational significance of a stimulus.

The hypothesis that phasic NE reports on the ratio between posterior probability and prior probability of a task state is consistent with the well-known sensitivity of the P3 to (subjective) prior probability (e.g., refs. 12 and 50, see also ref. 3). For example, P3 amplitude is highly sensitive to expectations elicited by the recent stimulus-sequence history in an oddball task: The P3 to an oddball target stimulus is larger when the target stimulus is preceded by a series of nontarget stimuli than when it is preceded by a series of other targets[50] (but see ref. 26). Presumably, increasing the number of preceding nontarget stimuli decreases the subjective prior probability of a target. Other evidence suggests that the P3 also closely tracks unexpected uncertainty in the oddball task when there are frequent reversals of the probabilities of the target and nontarget stimuli (i.e., a volatile environment[27]). Donchin[15] argued that "on the basis of data like these we can assert that *surprising* events elicit a large P300 component" (p. 498, italics added).

Other evidence indicates that in addition to prior probability, P3 amplitude is sensitive to posterior probability, the numerator in Dayan and Yu's[14] surprise equation.[45,46] This variable reflects the subject's uncertainty about having correctly perceived the stimulus: the smaller the posterior probability associated with a task state (e.g., "a target is presented on the screen"), the lower the amplitude of the corresponding P3. For example, P3 amplitudes become smaller if stimuli are degraded and cannot be easily classified, and when there is uncertainty about the anticipated time of stimulus onset.

Some researchers have related the P3 to alternative but similar definitions of surprise. Kopp[32] has proposed that P3 amplitude varies as a function of the difference (not ratio) between prior probability and posterior probability, that is, as a function of the magnitude of the evidence-based probability revision. Mars and colleagues have shown that single-trial amplitudes of the P3 can be well explained by an information-theoretic definition of surprise—a monotonically decreasing function of the subjective prior probability of a given stimulus on a particular trial.[34] They showed that this model could account for the data better than a model based on blockwise (objective) stimulus probabilities and some alternative models based on information theory. Regardless of which specific definition of surprise does best describe P3 amplitudes, the sensitivity to violations of expectations provides yet another similarity between the P3 and LC-NE activity.

Conclusion

In 1981, Emanuel Donchin already noticed the similarities between the P3 and the LC-NE system in terms of their relationship with learning: "The model I propose assumes that the P300 is intimately involved with the process of memory modification or, if you will, learning. . . . Things appear to be learned if, and only if, they are surprising. In the neurophysiological literature, we find increasing emphasis on the role of the norepinephrine system in the incorporation of memories. . . . Things are apparently learned if, and only if, they activate this system" (p. 508).[15]

In this chapter, I discussed the intimate relationship between phasic LC activity, the P3, and learning, and suggested how these phenomena may be related: Phasic NE release, for example, following a surprising stimulus, promotes learning about the eliciting stimulus. Stimuli that elicit a larger LC-NE response are more likely to be remembered. Assuming that phasic NE release is reflected in the P3, this explains why stimuli that elicit a larger P3 are more likely to be remembered. I also tried to highlight the marked similarities between recent theories of phasic LC-NE function[9,14] and the context-updating hypothesis of the P3.[15,16] These accounts suggest that phasic NE and the P3 reflect unexpected uncertainty or surprise, and that these signals promote updating of the internal model of the environment. Altogether, this analysis provides strong additional support for the LC-P3 theory. It also suggests that the LC-P3 theory and context-updating hypothesis are not competing accounts of the P3: Context updating in response to surprising and motivationally significant stimuli and facilitating behavioral responses to such stimuli are each consistent with the broad temporal filtering function of phasic LC-NE activity.[2] Therefore, the LC-P3 theory explains both the close relationship between the P3 and learning (as proposed by Donchin and reviewed here) and the link betiween the P3 and the speed and accuracy of responding in reaction-time tasks (as reviewed in ref. 37).

Of course, the LC-P3 theory remains a theory. The relationship between LC activity and the P3 may be much more indirect than proposed. Also, there is some evidence that subcomponents of the P3 are influenced by other neuromodulators, such as dopamine.[43] But critical tests of the LC-P3 theory are underway: Various labs are currently using newly developed optogenetic manipulation methods[5] to test the LC-P3 theory in monkeys. In these monkeys, LC neurons will be genetically modified so that they become highly sensitive to a particular light frequency. Careful light stimulation at this frequency then allows the experimenters to selectively activate or suppress these LC neurons with extremely high temporal precision (in the millisecond range) while the monkeys are performing a task. The critical questions that can then be addressed are: What happens if a target stimulus is presented while the LC is suppressed? Is the LC response necessary for observing a P3 at the scalp? And what happens if we present no stimulus but briefly activate the LC under optical control? Is such an LC response sufficient for observing a P3 at the scalp? Or is it necessary that the monkey is doing a task, so that there is sufficient cortical activity that can be modulated by NE? Eventually, these methods will also be an extremely powerful means for directly testing the role of LC-NE activity in learning.

Acknowledgments

The author thanks Christopher Warren and Jonathan Cohen for fruitful discussions about LC function and learning. This research was supported by a VIDI grant from the Netherlands Organization for Scientific Research.

Outstanding Questions

• Is the P3 to a stimulus that produces response conflict predictive of the degree of item-specific conflict adaptation associated with that stimulus?[55]

• What is the formal relationship between information-theoretic and Bayesian models of surprise and the phasic P3-norepinephrine signal?

• Is the P3 elicited during the decision process, as evidence about the current stimulus accumulates?[14] Or is it elicited when the decision process crosses the decision threshold and terminates?[2]

Further Reading

Dayan P, Yu AJ. 2006. Phasic norepinephrine: a neural interrupt signal for unexpected events. *Network* 17:335–350. Dayan and Yu propose that phasic norepinephrine responses encode unexpected uncertainty about the current state within a task, and serve to interrupt ongoing processing associated with the default task state. A Bayesian model that formalizes this account in the context of a visual discrimination task captures some key aspects of monkey LC activity observed in this task.

Aston-Jones G, Cohen JD. 2005. An integrative theory of locus coeruleus-norepinephrine function: adaptive gain and optimal performance. *Annu Rev Neurosci* 28:403–450. The authors review animal studies of locus coeruleus activity in two-alternative forced-choice tasks. On the basis of this review, they propose a novel theory about the role of the central noradrenergic system in optimizing task performance. Phasic locus coeruleus activation driven by the outcome of stimulus-related decision processes is proposed to facilitate ensuing responses to the stimulus.

Nieuwenhuis S, Aston-Jones G, Cohen JD. 2005. Decision making, the P3, and the locus coeruleus-norepinephrine system. *Psychol Bull* 131:510–532. Nieuwenhuis and colleagues propose that the P3 reflects the response of the central noradrenergic system to the outcome of internal decision-making processes and the consequent effects of noradrenergic potentiation of information processing. This theory is supported by a review of data from intracranial recordings in animals and humans, functional brain imaging, lesion studies, and psychopharmacology.

References

1. Alexinsky T, Aston-Jones G, Rajkowski J, Revay RS. 1990. Physiological correlates of adaptive behavior in a visual discrimination task in monkeys. *Soc Neurosci Abstracts* 16: 164.

2. Aston-Jones G, Cohen JD. 2005. An integrative theory of locus coeruleus-norepinephrine function: adaptive gain and optimal performance. *Annu Rev Neurosci* 28: 403–450.

3. Barceló F, Periáñez JA, Knight RT. 2002. Think differently: a brain orienting response to task novelty. *Neuroreport* 13: 1887–1892.

4. Behrens TE, Woolrich MW, Walton ME, Rushworth MF. 2007. Learning the value of information in an uncertain world. *Nat Neurosci* 10: 1214–1221.

5. Berdyyeva TK, Reynolds JH. 2009. The dawning of primate optogenetics. *Neuron* 62: 159–160.

6. Berridge CW, Waterhouse BD. 2003. The locus coeruleus-noradrenergic system: modulation of behavioral state and state-dependent cognitive processes. *Brain Res Brain Res Rev* 42: 33–84.

7. Botvinick MM, Cohen JD, Carter CS. 2004. Conflict monitoring and anterior cingulate cortex: an update. *Trends Cogn Sci* 8: 539–546.

8. Bouret S, Sara SJ. 2004. Reward expectation, orientation of attention and locus coeruleus–medial frontal cortex interplay during learning. *Eur J Neurosci* 20: 791–802.

9. Bouret S, Sara SJ. 2005. Network reset: a simplified overarching theory of locus coeruleus noradrenaline function. *Trends Neurosci* 28: 574–582.

10. Brown RA, Walling SG, Milway JS, Harley CW. 2005. Locus ceruleus activation suppresses feedforward interneurons and reduces beta-gamma electroencephalogram frequencies while it enhances theta frequencies in rat dentate gyrus. *J Neurosci* 25: 1985–1991.

11. Clayton EC, Rajkowski J, Cohen JD, Aston-Jones G. 2004. Phasic activation of monkey locus ceruleus neurons by simple decisions in a forced-choice task. *J Neurosci* 24: 9914–9920.

12. Daffner KR, Scinto LF, Calvo V, Faust R, Mesulam MM, West WC, Holcomb PJ. 2000. The influence of stimulus deviance on electrophysiologic and behavioral responses to novel events. *J Cogn Neurosci* 12: 393–406.

13. David-Johnson J. 2003. Neuroadrenergic control of cognition: global attenuation and an interrupt function. *Med Hypoth* 60: 689–692.

14. Dayan P, Yu AJ. 2006. Phasic norepinephrine: a neural interrupt signal for unexpected events. *Network* 17: 335–350.

15. Donchin E. 1981. Surprise! . . . Surprise? *Psychophysiology* 18: 493–513.

16. Donchin E, Coles MGH. 1988. Is the P300 component a manifestation of context updating? *Behav Brain Sci* 11: 357–374.

17. Donchin E, Karis D, Bashore TR, Coles MGH, Gratton G. 1986. Cognitive psychophysiology: systems, processes, and applications. In: Psychophysiology: Systems, Processes, and Applications (Coles MGH, Donchin E, Proges S, eds), pp 244–267. New York: Guilford Press.

18. Fabiani M, Donchin E. 1995. Encoding processes and memory organization: a model of the von Restorff effect. *J Exp Psychol Learn Mem Cogn* 21: 224–240.

19. Fabiani M, Karis D, Donchin E. 1985. Effects of strategy manipulation on P300 amplitude in a von Restorff paradigm. *Psychophysiology* 22: 588–589.

20. Fabiani M, Karis D, Donchin E. 1986. P300 and recall in an incidental memory paradigm. *Psychophysiology* 23: 298–308.

21. Fabiani M, Karis D, Donchin E. 1990. Effects of mnemonic strategy manipulation in a von Restorff paradigm. *Electroencephalogr Clin Neurophysiol* 75: 22–35.

22. Friedman D, Ritter W, Snodgrass JG. 1996. ERPs during study as a function of subsequent direct and indirect memory testing in young and old adults. *Brain Res Cogn Brain Res* 4: 1–13.

23. Gibbs ME, Summers RJ. 2002. Role of adrenoceptor subtypes in memory consolidation. *Prog Neurobiol* 67: 345–391.

24. Gilzenrat MS, Nieuwenhuis S, Jepma M, Cohen JD. 2010. Pupil diameter tracks changes in control state predicted by the adaptive gain theory of locus coeruleus function. *Cogn Affect Behav Neurosci* 10: 252–269.

25. Harley CW. 2004. Norepinephrine and dopamine as learning signals. *Neural Plast* 11: 191–204.

26. Holm A, Ranta-aho PO, Sallinen M, Karjalainen PA, Müller K. 2006. Relationship of P300 single-trial responses with reaction time and preceding stimulus sequence. *Int J Psychophysiol* 61: 244–252.

27. Johnson R, Donchin E. 1982. Sequential expectancies and decision making in a changing environment: an electrophysiological approach. *Psychophysiology* 9: 183–200.

28. Karis D, Fabiani M, Donchin E. 1984. "P300" and memory: individual differences in the von Restorff effect. *Cognit Psychol* 16: 117–216.

29. Kehagia AA, Murray GK, Robbins TW. 2010. Learning and cognitive flexibility: frontostriatal function and monoaminergic modulation. *Curr Opin Neurobiol* 20: 199–204.

30. Kety S. 1970. The biogenic amines in the central nervous system: their possible roles in arousal, emotion and learning. In: The Neurosciences: Second Study Program (Schmitt FO, ed), pp 324–335. New York: Rockefeller Press.

31. Kobayashi M. 2000. Selective suppression of horizontal propagation in rat visual cortex by norepinephrine. *Eur J Neurosci* 12: 264–272.

32. Kopp B. 2006. The P300 component of the event-related brain potential and Bayes' theorem. *Cogn Sci* 2: 113–125.

33. Liu J, Kiehl KA, Pearlson G, Perrone-Bizzozero NI, Eichele T, Calhoun VD. 2009. Genetic determinants of target and novelty-related event-related potentials in the auditory oddball response. *Neuroimage* 46: 809–816.

34. Mars RB, Debener S, Gladwin TE, Harrison LM, Haggard P, Rothwell JC, Bestmann S. 2008. Trial-by-trial fluctuations in the event-related electroencephalogram reflect dynamic changes in the degree of surprise. *J Neurosci* 28: 12539–12545.

35. McCormick DA. 1992. Neurotransmitter actions in the thalamus and cerebral cortex and their role in neuromodulation of thalamocortical activity. *Prog Neurobiol* 39: 337–388.

36. Nassar M, Wilson RC, Kalwani R, Heasly B, Gold JI 2010. Pupillometric evidence for a role of locus coeruleus in dynamic belief updating. Proc Comput Syst Neurosci 2010.

37. Nieuwenhuis S, Aston-Jones G, Cohen JD. 2005. Decision making, the P3, and the locus coeruleus-norepinephrine system. *Psychol Bull* 131: 510–532.

38. Nieuwenhuis S, De Geus EJ, Aston-Jones G. in press. The anatomical and functional relationship between the P3 and autonomic components of the orienting response. *Psychophysiology*.

39. Nieuwenhuis S, Jepma M. in press. Investigating the role of the noradrenergic system in human cognition. In: Attention & Performance XXIII: Decision Making, Affect, and Learning (Delgado MR, Phelps EA, Robbins TW, eds). Oxford: Oxford University Press.

40. Núñez Castellar E, Kühn M, Mayes AR. 1987. Outcome expectancy and not accuracy determines post-error slowing: ERP support. *Cogn Affect Behav Neurosci* 10: 270–278.

41. Paller KA, Kutas M, Mayes AR. 1987. Neural correlates of encoding in an incidental learning paradigm. *Electroencephalogr Clin Neurophysiol* 67: 360–371.

42. Pineda JA, Foote SL, Neville HJ. 1989. Effects of locus coeruleus lesions on auditory, long-latency event-related potentials in monkey. *J Neurosci* 9: 81–93.

43. Polich J. 2007. Updating P300: an integrative theory of P3a and P3b. *Clin Neurophysiol* 118: 2128–2148.

44. Reid AT, Harley CW. 2010. An associativity requirement for locus coeruleus-induced long-term potentiation in the dentate gyrus of the urethane-anesthetized rat. *Exp Brain Res* 200: 151–159.

45. Ruchkin DS, Sutton S. 1978. Emitted P300 potentials and temporal uncertainty. *Electroencephalogr Clin Neurophysiol* 45: 268–277.

46. Ruchkin DS, Sutton S. 1978. Equivocation and P300 amplitude. In: Multidisciplinary Perspectives in Event-Eelated Brain Potential Research (Otto D, ed), pp 175–177. Washington, DC: U.S. Government Printing Office.

47. Sara SJ, Vankov A, Herve A. 1994. Locus coeruleus-evoked responses in behaving rats: a clue to the role of noradrenaline in memory. *Brain Res Bull* 35: 457–465.

48. Servan-Schreiber D, Printz H, Cohen JD. 1990. A network model of catecholamine effects: gain, signal-to-noise ratio, and behavior. *Science* 249: 892–895.

49. Soltani M, Knight RT. 2000. Neural origins of the P300. *Crit Rev Neurobiol* 14: 199–224.

50. Squires KC, Wickens C, Squires NK, Donchin E. 1976. The effect of stimulus sequence on the waveform of the cortical event-related potential. *Science* 193: 1142–1146.

51. Sutton S, Braren M, Aubin J, John ER. 1965. Evoked-potential correlates of stimulus uncertainty. *Science* 150: 1187–1188.

52. Swick D, Pineda JA, Foote SL. 1994. Effects of systemic clonidine on auditory event-related potentials in squirrel monkeys. *Brain Res Bull* 33: 79–86.

53. Van Petten C, Senkfor AJ. 1996. Memory for words and novel visual patterns: repetition, recognition, and encoding effects in the event-related brain potential. *Psychophysiology* 33: 491–506.

54. Verguts T, Notebaert W. 2008. Hebbian learning of cognitive control: dealing with specific and non-specific adaptation. *Psychol Rev* 115: 518–525.

55. Verguts T, Notebaert W. 2009. Adaptation by binding: a learning account of cognitive control. *Trends Cogn Sci* 13: 252–257.

56. Wagner AD, Koutstaal W, Schacter DL. 1999. When encoding yields remembering: insights from event-related neuroimaging. *Philos Trans R Soc Lond B Biol Sci* 354: 1307–1324.

57. Yu AJ, Dayan P. 2005. Uncertainty, neuromodulation, and attention. *Neuron* 46: 681–692.

IV INDIVIDUAL VARIATIONS IN CONTROL

The chapters in this section review three types of individual differences in control: those observed during development in ontogenesis, particularly during adolescence; those related to neurological and psychiatric syndromes; and those seen in natural variability within the healthy adult population.

With the availability of more sophisticated analysis techniques, variability within the normal population can now be studied at multiple levels of description, from the gene, via the structure of the nervous system, to brain activity and behavior. Individual differences in control have been studied at each of these levels. At the genetic level, a number of studies have focused on carriers of different alleles of genes associated with dopamine function. For instance, Klein and colleagues[7] have shown that the dopamine D2 receptor gene polymorphism DRD2-TAQ-IA, which is associated with different D2 receptor densities, correlates with differential ability to learn to avoid actions with negative consequences. These behavioral differences were accompanied at the neural level by reductions in activity in medial frontal cortex following negative feedback, and by reduced interactions between medial frontal cortex and the hippocampus. Frank and colleagues have similarly shown, in a number of studies, that genes associated with different aspects of dopamine function have dissociable effects on reward and avoidance learning in humans[5,6] (see also chapter 17, this volume).

The structural basis of individual differences has traditionally been assessed primarily postmortem or in patients with brain lesions. For instance, deficits in action inhibition in patients with lesions of the right inferior frontal gyrus and patients suffering from Parkinson's disease gave some indication of the frontal-basal ganglia network involved in this function. However, with the availability of better structural imaging methods such as voxel-based morphometry[1] and tract-based spatial statistics,[10] it has become possible to investigate the structural basis of the functional differences in the healthy brain. As discussed in their chapter, Ridderinkhof and colleagues relate individual differences in core aspects of control to differences in gray matter volume and white matter integrity. For instance, individual differences in action inhibition correlate with differences in white matter density of the frontal-occipital fascicle near the inferior frontal gyrus.[4] Similarly, gray matter density in the pre-SMA predicts people's ability to select correct actions voluntarily during response conflict.[11] Individual difference correlations with brain structure and function can also be derived from computational models' fit to dynamic variations in behavior. For instance, Behrens and colleagues have shown that activity in the medial frontal cortex can be predicted by individuals' estimates of environmental stability during a reward-based learning task.[2]

At more extreme ends of the distribution, one can look at patients who are particularly impaired in a certain function, as reviewed by De Bruijn and Ullsperger. A number of neurological and psychiatric disorders are associated with impairments in specific aspects cognitive control. For instance, as De Bruijn and Ullsperger discuss, obsessive-compulsive disorder is associated with hyperactivity of the anterior cingulate cortex whereas patients suffering from schizophrenia typically have a hypoactive ACC. These traits are already apparent in the subclinical population and also distinguish differences within the population of patients suffering from depression. Conversely, one can also focus on people who excel at a certain function. A common example of this approach is the study by Maguire and colleagues, who showed that hippocampal volume in London taxi drivers correlated with the amount of time spent driving taxis.[8] In the field of performance monitoring, Danielmeier and colleagues have shown that adjustments participants make following errors are correlated with white matter underneath the pre-SMA.[3] This finding could be extended by looking at groups of participants who excel at certain aspects of cognitive control and decision making, such as air traffic controllers[12] and footballers taking penalties.[9]

The relationship between these differences in brain structure and function and individuals' behavior are perhaps most apparent during the course of development. As discussed in the chapter by Van den Bos and Crone, changes in brain structure and brain function can be related to behavioral changes that manifest in the period of adolescence and into adulthood. Showing how far-ranging this approach can be, they focus on the development of particularly complex behavior, namely, social interactions and judgment of others. In turn, these results provide tremendous insight in the dissociability of different social decision-making processes.

The chapters in this section illustrate not only the effects of individual differences in brain structure and function on cognitive control, but also how these individual differences can in turn be used to understand the underlying processes of control. With increasing integration of research on individual differences at different levels of description, it seems likely that the study of individual differences is set to become increasingly important in the coming years.

References

1. Ashburner J, Friston KJ. 2000. Voxel-based morphometry—the methods. *Neuroimage* 11: 805–821.

2. Behrens TE, Woolrich MW, Walton ME, Rushworth MF. 2007. Learning the value of information in an uncertain world. *Nat Neurosci* 10: 1214–1221.

3. Danielmeier C, Eichele T, Forstmann BU, Tittgemeyer M, Ullsperger M. 2009. Top-down modulation of task-relevant perceptual brain areas after errors. *Neuroimage* 47: S177.

4. Forstmann BU, Jahfari S, Scholte HS, Wolfensteller U, van den Wildenberg WP, Ridderinkhof KR. 2008. Function and structure of the right inferior frontal cortex predict individual differences in response inhibition: a model-based approach. *J Neurosci* 28: 9790–9796.

5. Frank MJ, Doll BB, Oas-Terpstra J, Moreno F. 2009. Prefrontal and striatal dopaminergic genes predict individual differences in exploration and exploitation. *Nat Neurosci* 12: 1062–1068.

6. Frank MJ, Moustafa AA, Haughey HM, Curran T, Hutchison KE. 2007. Genetic triple dissociation reveals multiple roles for dopamine in reinforcement learning. *Proc Natl Acad Sci USA* 104: 16311–16316.

7. Klein TA, Endrass T, Kathmann N, Neumann J, von Cramon DY, Ullsperger M. 2007. Neural correlates of error awareness. *Neuroimage* 34: 1774–1781.

8. Maguire EA, Gadian DG, Johnsrude IS, Good CD, Ashburner J, Frackowiak RSJ, Frith CD. 2000. Navigation-related structural change in the hippocampi of taxi drivers. *Proc Natl Acad Sci USA* 97: 4398–4403.

9. Palacios-Huerta I. 2003. Professionals play minimax. *Rev Econ Stud* 70: 395–415.

10. Smith SM, Johansen-Berg H, Jenkinson M, Rueckert D, Nichols TE, Miller KL, Robson MD, Jones DK, Klein JC, Bartsch AJ, Behrens TE. 2007. Acquisition and voxelwise analysis of multi-subject diffusion data with tract-based spatial statistics. *Nat Protoc* 2: 499–503.

11. Van Gaal S, Scholte S, Lamme VAF, Fahrenfort JJ, Ridderinkhof KR. 2010. Pre-SMA gray-matter density predicts individual differences in action selection in the face of conscious and unconscious response conflict. *J Cogn Neurosci* 23: 382–390.

12. Vortac OU, Edwards MB, Fuller DK, Manning CA. 1993. Automation and cognition in air traffic control: an empirical investigation. *Appl Cogn Psychol* 7: 631–651.

13 The Neurocognitive Development of Social Decision Making

Wouter van den Bos and Eveline A. Crone

Humans grow up and live in highly complex social environments, and most of the decisions they make are in the context of social interactions. Already in infancy a large proportion of time is spent interacting with caretakers, and over the course of development, social interactions become more prevalent and particularly more complex.[40] One of the most salient developmental challenges is therefore to develop the ability to monitor and regulate thoughts and actions for adaptive behavior in social interactions. Adolescent-specific changes in brain and behavior have been examined in the framework of *social reorientation*.[50] During adolescence, defined as the period between approximately 10 and 22 years of age, there is a significant increase in peer interactions and interest; more time is spent with peers than in any other period in life.[36] Furthermore, adolescents become more self-conscious[67] and more sensitive to the opinion of their peers, which is reflected in a hypersensitivity to acceptance and rejection by peers[29] and increased sensitivity to peer influence.[71] The increased focus on others also contributes positively to adolescent development. For example, it is well known that early in adolescence, individuals are more inclined toward self-oriented thought and actions, whereas later in adolescence individuals become more inclined toward thinking about others, taking social responsibility, and engaging in more pro-social behavior.[17] Although these changes in social behavior have been extensively studied, the underlying neural mechanisms contributing to these changes are less well understood.

In this chapter we review evidence for the hypothesis that the development of social decision making is related to changes in different, but interacting, brain networks. The chapter focuses on the developmental period between late childhood and young adulthood, because this transitional period involves a process of major social reorientation.[6,50] We describe how these changes in social behavior are paralleled by a specific set of physical, cognitive, affective, and neurological changes.[18,69,70]

Social decision making is a complex process that involves the consideration of consequences for self versus others in combination with the ability to make future-oriented decisions. For example, one can consider taking the car to work or go with public transport; either decision will affect oneself but will obviously also affect others, and each decision has short-term and long-term consequences. Thus, where most decisions can often be described as the consideration of alternatives and choosing the optimal one on the basis of a subjective value,[57] social decisions also depend on the actions and mental states of others.[60] The combination of these different processes most likely drives our social decision making in a complex environment.

Researchers have begun to investigate the psychological and neural correlates of social decision making using game theoretical paradigms derived from experimental economics and social psychology.[7,63] In these experiments, participants interact with other people in simple bargaining or exchange games, often with real monetary consequences for both players. The advantage of these paradigms is their structural simplicity, which yields precise characterizations of complex social behavior, and can inform and constrain neuroscientific models of social decision making. One particular insight from these interdisciplinary studies is that social decision making is best understood as the product of multiple interacting systems.[2,22,63]

Whereas some neural accounts of social behavior have emphasized the importance of a specific "social brain" network involved in understanding others' beliefs and intentions,[31,34,83] others have identified the importance of brain regions with a more general role in learning from past experience[16,42] and cognitive control.[44,80] These systems, which can be further divided in several subcomponents, are associated with different brain networks. In the following sections, we describe the postulated social brain network in adults, followed by the scientific evidence from game paradigms. The hypothesis that this network is sensitive to developmental change is supported by studies that have examined changes in structural development. These changes are briefly summarized, followed by a summary of behavioral and developmental functional magnetic resonance imaging (fMRI) studies examining this relation in more detail. Finally, we show that computational modeling may be a fruitful approach to understanding the subprocesses that underlie development of social decision making in a dynamic environment.

Social Decision Making and the Brain

Social Decision Making and Game Theory

The contribution of different brain networks involved in social decision making has been demonstrated using the Trust Game and the Ultimatum Game. In these games, two players are asked to exchange or share a certain amount of money. In the Trust Game,[4] the first player can choose to divide the money equally between herself and the second player, or to give it all to the second player with the advantage that the

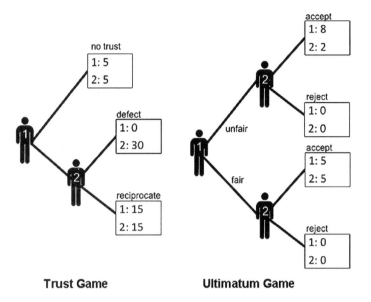

Figure 13.1
Schematic representation of the structure of two common games often used to study social decision making.

amount then increases in value (see figure 13.1). The second player has the choice to reciprocate and share the increased amount of money with the first player, or to defect and exploit the given trust by keeping the money for herself. The Ultimatum Game[33] is a bargaining game in which the first player (proposer) is given a sum of money to share with the second player (responder). If the responder accepts the amount offered by the proposer, the money is split between the two as proposed. However, if the responder considers the proposed split unfair and rejects the offer, neither player receives any money (see figure 13.1). Studies with the Ultimatum Game typically focus on the behavior of the responder in order to capture the tendency of individuals to reject unfairness. On average, responders start rejecting offers of less than 40% of the stake, suggesting that their decisions are not driven by material interests only but are also based on self-other comparisons, or "fairness considerations."[73] Furthermore, studies using a binary choice version of the Ultimatum Game, the mini-Ultimatum Game, have shown that responder behavior is intentionality dependent; responders are more likely to reject an unfair offer when the alternative for the proposer was a fair split, whereas they are more willing to accept an unfair offer when the alternative for the proposer was also unfair (i.e., the proposer had no other choice).[20,75] Both paradigms have previously been shown to rely, at least partly, on a social brain network.

Social Brain Networks

The social brain network,[25,87] thought to be involved in thinking about other people's believes and intentions, consists of the anterior medial prefrontal cortex (aMPFC), temporal poles (TP), posterior superior temporal sulcus (pSTS), and the temporal parietal junction (TPJ, see figure 13.2). Prior neuroimaging studies have considered the aMPFC together with the temporal-parietal-junction (TPJ) to be involved in taking the perspective of another person. For example, neuroimaging studies have demonstrated that aMPFC and TPJ are active during theory-of-mind tasks, such as tasks that require participants to infer mental states of characters in stories[21] and cartoons[26] or while watching animations.[8] Additionally, the aMPFC and the TPJ are thought to be involved in consideration of outcomes for self versus others in context of social interaction paradigms.[6,34,65] First, aMPFC activity has been reported when first players trust another individual, with the expectation of increasing their own payoff.[48] Furthermore, when the second player decides to exploit the given trust in order to increase personal gain, aMPFC activity has also been reported.[83] In contrast, TPJ is activated when the second player receives trust from the first player in the Trust Game, particularly when individuals are inclined to take the perspective of the other player into account. Consistent with these results, a neuroimaging study with the mini-Ultimatum Game showed that the TPJ played a role in intention consideration[31] when judging unfair proposals. Together, these results suggest that

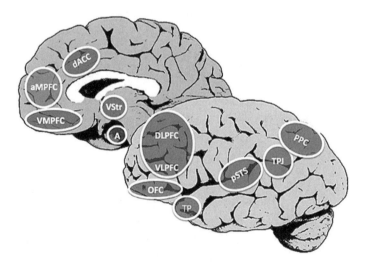

Figure 13.2
Schematic representation of the networks of brain areas involved in social decision making: aMPFC, anterior medial prefrontal cortex; TPJ, temporal parietal junction; pSTS, posterior superior temporal sulcus; TP, temporal poles; Vstr, ventral striatum; A, amygdala; VMPFC, ventromedial prefrontal cortex; OFC, orbitofrontal cortex; dACC, dorsal anterior cingulate cortex; DLPFC, dorsolateral prefrontal cortrex; VLPFC, ventrolateral prefrontal cortrex; PPC, posterior parietal cortex.

the aMPFC activity is important for the evaluation of own outcomes, whereas TPJ may indicate a focus on others in social decision making.

The second network, which is also referred to as the affective network because it is associated with approach and avoidance behavior in social context, consists of the striatum, amygdala, anterior insula, orbitofrontal cortex (OFC), and the ventral medial prefrontal cortex (VMPFC). Neuroimaging studies showed that unfair proposals in the Ultimatum Game are associated with increased activation in the insula,[49,64,78] and this region is also engaged during unreciprocated trust.[59] In contrast, striatum and VMPFC activity correlates positively with cooperation choices in the Trust Game.[61] Importantly, this network has been shown to be involved in tracking and predicting the behavior of other players in multiround Trust Games.[2,16,42,45] Thus, the ventral striatum and the insula seem to be involved in signaling *and* learning the pleasant and unpleasant aspects of social interactions, which may explain how lower-level affective processes can result in encouragement or discouragement of social behavior.[63]

These affective areas of the brain typically work together with areas that signal the control of impulses. This cognitive regulatory network, which includes the lateral prefrontal cortex (VLPFC and DLPFC), dorsal anterior cingulate cortex (dACC), and the posterior parietal cortex (PPC), is important for the control of self-oriented impulses and the selection of responses that represent a conflict between social norms and personal interest,[80] such as the rejection of unfair offers.[31] It has been suggested that, in those cases when there is competition between different motivational drives, the higher-level regulatory processes have a role in modulating the interactions of these lower-level motivational processes.[24]

Development of the Social Brain

Current developmental models hypothesize that structural changes in the developing brain during adolescence are associated with functional changes in brain networks, and that these changes contribute to the development of adolescent social behavior.[18,50,70] In general, studies on structural and functional brain development have been separate strands of research, although some studies have shown relations between brain maturation and behavioral development. The next section summarizes relevant findings of adolescent structural brain development and its relation to social behavior.

Structural Brain Development

Early studies of postmortem brain tissue revealed that particularly the prefrontal cortex (PFC) of the human brain still shows great changes in synaptic development well into the adolescent period.[39] Gray matter as measured with MRI is proposed to represent the cell bodies, synapses, unmyelinated axons, and neuropil. The developmental pattern of gray matter is thought to reflect, at least in part, the processes of synaptogenesis followed by synaptic elimination.[39] Several studies have reported a nonlinear "inverted-U" shaped pattern of gray matter development.[27,28,68] The general pattern of gray matter development increases across the cortex prior to puberty, followed by a postpuberty decline. The decline in gray matter follows nonlinear patterns and varies by region. The first to mature are the sensorimotor regions, followed by other parts of the cortex in a posterior to anterior direction, with the PFC being one of the last areas to develop.[28] Furthermore, the developmental trajectories of GM vary also within the prefrontal cortex,[28] which could account for differences in rate of development of different control functions associated with these areas.[13] Correlational studies have shown that differences in gray matter volume are associated with individual differences in (anti-)social behavior.[72] These data suggest that local quantities of gray matter density can be related to the regulation of social behavior.

In contrast to gray matter, white matter development follows a more linear trajectory, increasing in volume and density during the first two decades of life.[54] Increases in white matter volume have been associated with the myelination of axons (but see also ref. 53). Studies that have focused on structural connectivity by use of diffusion tensor imaging (DTI) demonstrated that there are still large changes in the fiber tracts that link different brain regions, particularly a rewiring of subcortical-cortical regions and a strengthening of corticocortical connectivity,[66,74] which have been related to individual differences in adolescent risk taking,[5] impulsivity,[51] and resistance to peer influence.[55] Thus, there is robust evidence of changes in cortical gray matter and connectivity that may also be related to individual differences in traits or behaviors. It should be noted that subcortical brain regions[79] also change during development; these studies indicate that subcortical structures have heterogeneity in developmental trajectories, where some structures show linear increases in gray matter (e.g., caudate, putamen, and cerebellum) and others show a nonlinear pattern (e.g., amygdala and hippocampus).

Coordinating Perspectives—Development of the Social Brain

Developmental studies using social interaction paradigms have shown that the increased capacity of perspective taking is related to changes in pro-social behavior during adolescence.[30,85] These studies show that, while most basic theory of mind tasks are passed around age 4,[23] the ability to take the perspective of the other still develops into late adolescence.[6] In the next section, we review recent behavioral and neuroimaging studies that have investigated the development of the social decision making in adolescence, with a focus on the networks involved in perspective taking.

Development of Trust and Reciprocity

Developmental studies using the TG have demonstrated an increase in both trust and reciprocity with increasing age.[76] Besides an increase in general levels of trust and reciprocity, we demonstrated that developmental differences in trust and reciprocity depend on the extent to which the other person's perspective is taken into account. The first study was conducted with four age groups (9, 12, 16, and 25 years), and we dissociated between different intentions for trust and reciprocity. Specifically, the task was adapted in such a way that the levels of risk for the trustor by trusting and the benefit for the trustee by being trusted were varied.[47] The goal of these manipulations was to examine how the decision to trust or to reciprocate trust depended on intentions of the other players. As anticipated, the results demonstrated that during development there was a general increase of pro-social behavior, but more significant, perspective taking was a more important factor in social decision making with increasing age.

To test the neural correlates of reciprocating behavior during adolescence, we performed a neuroimaging study that included adolescents and adults between ages 12 and 22 years.[84] In this study, we had participants of three different age groups (12–14 years, 15–17 years, and 18–22 years) play the role of the trustee in the scanner. Using a similar design as in the behavioral study, we could investigate the role of perspective taking in reciprocal behavior. The results of this study revealed that, with age, adolescents were increasingly sensitive to the perspective of the other player, as indicated by their reciprocal behavior. Furthermore, these advanced forms of social perspective taking were associated with increased involvement of the left TPJ (see figure 13.3). In contrast, the aMPFC showed more activity for the youngest participants. Additionally, there was an age-related increase in DLPFC activity that was also related to advanced forms of perspective taking, suggesting involvement in improved regulation of social behavior with increasing age. These results are consistent with recent developmental studies indicating that adolescents and adults activate the same social brain network during theory-of-mind tasks (e.g., reading stories, thinking about others), but there is an age-related shift in relative contribution of the aMPFC and the TPJ.[6,56,88] It is hypothesized that this shift is related to a decrease in self-referential thought and an increased focus of attention on the other.

Development of Fairness

Prior behavioral studies have demonstrated that children already have a strong sense of fairness at a very young age, but important developmental changes still occur until late adolescence.[30,75] With age, there is an increasingly important role for taking into consideration the intentions of the other person. For example, in one study using the mini-Ultimatum Game, the youngest participants (9 years old) were

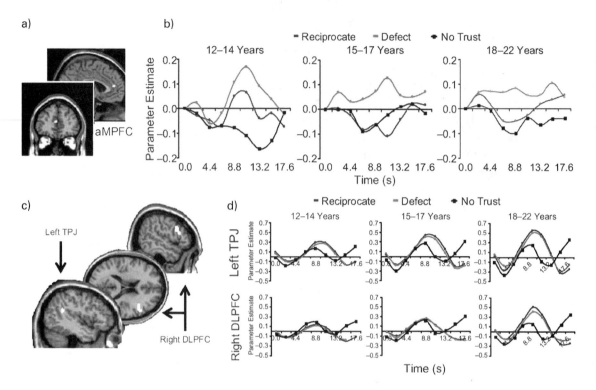

Figure 13.3
(a) Activation maps with the clusters that show an early increase in the difference in defect versus reciprocate activation. (b) The time course of activation in the aMPFC related to defect, reciprocate, and no trust. (c) Activation maps with the clusters that show linear and nonlinear increases in trust-related activation with age. (d) The time course of activation in the lTPJ and the rDLPFC related to defect, reciprocate, and no trust. Adapted from Van den Bos et al.,[84] reprinted with permission.

more likely to reject than to accept unfair offers, even when the proposer could not have chosen otherwise, whereas older participants (18 years) were more likely to accept unfair offers in that situation.[30]

We have performed a developmental neuroimaging study using the mini-Ultimatum Game to investigate the neural correlates of age differences in fairness considerations in participants between ages 10 and 20 years.[32] Replicating previous findings in adults, participants of all ages showed activation in the bilateral insula related to detecting norm violations. However, rejection of unintentional unfair offers involved increasing activation with age in the TPJ and the DLPFC. Consistent with the findings of the Trust Game, these findings provide evidence for an early developing affective network involved in detecting norm violations and gradually increasing involvement of temporal and prefrontal brain regions related to intentionality considerations in social reasoning.

Taken together, these two studies of the neural correlates of developmental changes in trust, reciprocity, and fairness confirm the involvement of the different control networks in reciprocal exchange and support the hypothesis that the asynchronous development of the different control systems underlies specific changes in social behavior across adolescence.

Monitoring Social Interactions—Development of Adaptive Learning

Prior research has demonstrated that, in social context, affective areas such as the striatum attach an affective tag to social partners, which ultimately results in the encouragement or discouragement of social behavior[63] (see also chapter 22, this volume). This is important for tracking and predicting the behavior of others as well as for learning which types of behavior are socially acceptable based on feedback from the environment.

This affective network is not specifically sensitive to social stimuli, and comprises brain regions that involve the computation of reward and punishment in general.[2] Theories in decision neuroscience describe specific systems that are involved in the updating and representation of expected outcomes,[11] which includes the striatum, amygdala, anterior insula, OFC, and the VMPFC. The VMPFC is thought to play a central role in representing the (expected) value for future outcome,[10] whereas the phasic activity of the mesolimbic dopamine system is thought to code signals that reflect the difference between the expected and experienced outcomes, also referred to as prediction errors.[58] Neuroimaging studies have shown that these prediction error signals correlate with activation in areas that receive input from the dopamine system, including the ventral striatum[52] and the medial prefrontal cortex[43] (mPFC). These learning signals are subsequently used to adapt future expectations and, if necessary, to adjust future behavior in order to optimize future outcomes.

Several studies suggest that the dorsal part of the mPFC (the dACC), plays an important role in using the learning signal to guide future behavior, because of its connections with the premotor cortex, motor cortex, and the DLPFC.[62] Results from several imaging studies have supported this role of the dACC, by showing that its response to errors predicts subsequent activation in DLFPC, which suggests the dACC sends signals to other areas to increase cognitive control following an unexpectedly negative outcome or mistake.[37,41] As such, the affective and control networks may work together to contribute to adaptive behavior.

Until now the development of these networks has not been studied specifically in the context of social interactions. However, age-related changes have been observed in other types of adaptive learning tasks, such as the Iowa Gambling Task[1] (IGT). In these studies, children and young adolescents apply a strategy that is advantageous in the short term but disadvantageous in the long run. Several studies have suggested that this developmental pattern is the result of unbalanced activity between frontal and subcortical systems involved in decision making (for review, see ref. 69).

Other studies that have focused on the development of processing negative reinforcers and performance errors identified age-related changes in the dACC and DLPFC. First, age-related increases in the error-related negativity (ERN), a scalp potential thought to reflect dACC activity, are consistently reported across studies,[15,46] and are suggested to reflect an age-related increase in the ability to use these signals to adapt subsequent behavior. Consistent with these results, recent neuroimaging studies from our lab have shown age-related changes in dACC, DLPFC, and posterior parietal cortex (PPC) in processing of negative reinforcers until late adolescence.[14,82,86] In the first study,[14] participants were instructed to infer rules based on positive and negative feedback that could change without warning. As anticipated, adults engaged dACC and the DLPFC when processing negative feedback, indicating a rule shift. A similar pattern was observed in 14- to 15-year-old adolescents, but 8- to 11-year-old children engaged these regions less following negative feedback compared with positive feedback. In the second study,[86] participants were instructed to guess which of two rules was correct. Again, adults engaged dACC, DLPFC, and PPC following negative feedback, but in this study 8-year-old children engaged DLPFC and PPC more following positive feedback than negative feedback. The developmental trajectory of the dACC followed a different pattern, as it slowly emerged in response to negative feedback at the age of 12, but it was not more active following negative than positive feedback at a younger age. Finally, a study in which children (8–11 years), adolescents (13–16 years), and adults (18–22 years) had to learn probabilistic rules revealed that DLPFC and dACC were more active in younger children following positive feedback and in adults following negative feedback, but only when exploring alternative rules. These findings suggest that developmental differences in the dACC and DLPFC are not related to valence per se, but that there is an age-related change in processing informative value. Finally, in a follow-up study we modeled the behavioral data using a reinforcement learning model[77] and investigated the developmental changes in network connectivity during this task.[81] Model-based analyses of imaging data revealed that age-related differences in feedback adjustment were associated with increased ventral striatum connectivity with the VMPFC. These findings indicate that developmental changes in adaptive behavior are not due to differences in the computation of the learning signal, but rather are related to changes in how the learning signal is subsequently used in action selection.

Together, these studies show that brain areas involved in learning from experience develop until late adolescence and are related to changes in adaptive behavior. Given the role of these areas in social behavior, we hypothesize that the reported developmental changes in brain activation contribute to the ability to use past experience to optimize social behavior. For example, prior research has shown that brain areas involved in reward processing are also involved in tracking and predicting the trustworthiness of other players in multiround Trust Games.[2,16,42] Given that areas such as the ventral striatum and the insula are involved in signaling *and* learning the pleasant and unpleasant aspects of social interactions, this may explain how lower-level affective processes can result in encouragement or discouragement of social behavior,[63] in this example trusting another person.

Conclusions and Future Directions

In this chapter we have demonstrated that different brain networks underlie social decision making, and develop at different rates. To improve our understanding of the development of cognitive and motivational control, it would be beneficial to develop integrative models that include the social brain network. The challenge for these models is not just recognizing the involvement of multiple processes, but also understanding how they interact. Promising recent developments for understanding these interactions are network analysis[19] and computational models.[22] These approaches have the following advantages and challenges for developmental research.

First, functional connectivity between the social brain network (TPJ) and the VMPFC has been associated with the amount of money participants are willing to give to charity,[35] supporting the hypothesis that not just the activity within but also the interaction between these separate networks contributes to social decision making. Furthermore, connectivity of the dACC with DLPFC increases from childhood through adolescence,[19] suggesting that improved dACC networking with the DLPFC may further contribute to the developmental changes in adaptive behavior. Based on research demonstrating developmental changes in structural connectivity until young adulthood,[66] it can be hypothesized that multimodal analyses of structural and functional connectivity provide a better framework for understanding how networks interact to give rise to behavior and how the network architecture shapes and constrains the development of social and control functions.

Second, current experimental designs allow only a limited view of the computational processes that underlie these changes[12,38] (see also chapter 23, this volume). Over the past decade, computational models of reward-based decision making in combination with neuroimaging techniques have proven successful in identifying computational subprocesses and their neural implementations (for review, see ref. 62). Several studies have successfully extended these models to include processes involved in social interactions.[3,9,34] Using these models, the experimenters were able to correlate activity in brain regions with different model parameters, demonstrating dissociations between social and nonsocial functional processing. Future developmental studies could use this model-based approach to gain more detailed insight into the computational processes that underlie changes in social behavior.

Finally, future studies on the neurocognitive development of social decision making may focus on more ecologically valid game theoretical paradigms that involve multiple interactions with the same partner. Currently, adult neuroimaging studies with these types of games have already produced promising results,[42,45] showing that the general networks involved in learning from past experience are involved in tracking and predicting the behavior of others.[24] Investigating the neural correlates of social behavior in multiple interactions of developmental populations will give us further insight into the role of the developing control networks in social development, particularly those involved in adaptive learning.

Outstanding Questions

• How do the different neural control networks interact in the process of making social decisions?

• What are the genetic and environmental influences on developmental trajectories of social decision making?

• How is the development of neural control networks related to neuroanatomical maturation, and how is this reflected to functional brain activity?

Further Reading

Blakemore SJ. 2008. The social brain in adolescence. *Nat Rev Neurosci* 9: 267–277. Review of changes that occur in the social brain during adolescence, particularly in the medial prefrontal cortex and the superior temporal sulcus. Integrates these recent findings of neurocognitive research with findings from developmental social psychology.

Sommerville LH, Casey BJ. 2010. Developmental neurobiology of cognitive control and motivational systems. *Curr Opin Neurobiol* 20: 236–241. This article provides a comprehensive overview of the most recent work on neurobiological changes supporting motivational and cognitive development, and a theoretical perspective that moves away from discussing singular functional regions toward considering functional circuitry.

Frank MJ, Cohen MX, Sanfey AG. 2009. Multiple systems in decision making: a neurocomputational perspective. *Curr Dir Psychol Sci* 8: 73–77. This paper argues for moving beyond dual-systems models of decision making and gives an elegant example of how a neurocomputational approach can contribute to more advanced models of behavior.

References

1. Bechara A, Damasio AR, Damasio H, Anderson SW. 1994. Insensitivity to future consequences following damage to the human prefrontal cortex. *Cognition* 50: 7–15.

2. Behrens TE, Hunt LT, Rushworth MF. 2009. The computation of social behavior. *Science* 324: 1160–1164.

3. Behrens TE, Hunt LT, Woolrich MW, Rushworth MF. 2008. Associative learning of social value. *Nature* 456: 245–249.

4. Berg J, Dickhaut J, McCabe K. 1995. Trust, reciprocity, and social history. *Games Econ Behav* 10: 122–142.

5. Berns GS, Moore S, Capra CM. 2009. Adolescent engagement in dangerous behaviors is associated with increased white matter maturity of frontal cortex. *PLoS ONE* 4: e6773.

6. Blakemore SJ. 2008. The social brain in adolescence. *Nat Rev Neurosci* 9: 267–277.

7. Camerer CF. 2003. Behavioral Game Theory: Experiments in Strategic Interaction. Princeton: Princeton University Press.

8. Castelli F, Happe F, Frith U, Frith C. 2000. Movement and mind: a functional imaging study of perception and interpretation of complex intentional movement patterns. *Neuroimage* 12: 314–325.

9. Chang LJ, Doll BB, van 't Wout M, Frank MJ, Sanfey AG. 2010. Seeing is believing: trustworthiness as a dynamic belief. *Cognit Psychol* 61: 87–105.

10. Chib VS, Rangel A, Shimojo S, O'Doherty JP. 2009. Evidence for a common representation of decision values for dissimilar goods in human ventromedial prefrontal cortex. *J Neurosci* 29: 12315–12320.

11. Cohen MX. 2008. Neurocomputational mechanisms of reinforcement-guided learning in humans: a review. *Cogn Affect Behav Neurosci* 8: 113–125.

12. Corrado G, Doya K. 2007. Understanding neural coding through the model-based analysis of decision making. *J Neurosci* 27: 8178–8180.

13. Crone EA, Wendelken C, Donohue S, van Leijenhorst L, Bunge SA. 2006. Neurocognitive development of the ability to manipulate information in working memory. *Proc Natl Acad Sci USA* 103: 9315–9320.

14. Crone EA, Zanolie K, Van Leijenhorst L, Westenberg PM, Rombouts SA. 2008. Neural mechanisms supporting flexible performance adjustment during development. *Cogn Affect Behav Neurosci* 8: 165–177.

15. Davies PL, Segalowitz SJ, Gavin WJ. 2004. Development of error-monitoring event-related potentials in adolescents. *Ann N Y Acad Sci* 1021: 324–328.

16. Delgado MR, Frank RH, Phelps EA. 2005. Perceptions of moral character modulate the neural systems of reward during the trust game. *Nat Neurosci* 8: 1611–1618.

17. Eisenberg N, Carlo G, Murphy BC, Van Court P. 1995. Prosocial development in late adolescence: a longitudinal study. *Child Dev* 66: 1179–1197.

18. Ernst M, Romeo R, Andersen S. 2008. Neurobiology of the development of motivated behaviors in adolescence window into a neural systems model. *Pharmacol Biochem Behav* 93: 199–211.

19. Fair DA, Cohen AL, Dosenbach NU, Church JA, Miezin FM, Barch DM, Raichle ME, Petersen SE, Schlaggar BL. 2008. The maturing architecture of the brain's default network. *Proc Natl Acad Sci USA* 105: 4028–4032.

20. Falk A, Fehr E, Fischbacher U. 2008. Testing theories of fairness—intentions matter. *Games Econ Behav* 62: 287–303.

21. Fletcher PC, Happe F, Frith U, Baker SC, Dolan RJ, Frackowiak RS, Frith CD. 1995. Other minds in the brain: a functional imaging study of "theory of mind" in story comprehension. *Cognition* 57: 109–128.

22. Frank MJ, Cohen MX, Sanfey AG. 2009. Multiple systems in decision making: a neurocomputational perspective. *Curr Dir Psychol Sci* 18: 73–77.

23. Frith CD, Frith U. 2007. Social cognition in humans. *Curr Biol* 17: R724–R732.

24. Frith CD, Singer T. 2008. The role of social cognition in decision making. *Philos Trans R Soc Lond B Biol Sci* 363: 3875–3886.

25. Frith U, Frith CD. 2003. Development and neurophysiology of mentalizing. *Philos Trans R Soc Lond B Biol Sci* 358: 459–473.

26. Gallagher HL, Jack AI, Roepstorff A, Frith CD. 2002. Imaging the intentional stance in a competitive game. *Neuroimage* 16: 814–821.

27. Giedd JN, Blumenthal J, Jeffries NO, Castellanos FX, Liu H, Zijdenbos A, Paus T, Evans AC, Rapoport JL. 1999. Brain development during childhood and adolescence: a longitudinal MRI study. *Nat Neurosci* 2: 861–863.

28. Gogtay N, Thompson PM. 2010. Mapping gray matter development: implications for typical development and vulnerability to psychopathology. *Brain Cogn* 72: 6–15.

29. Gunther Moor B, Crone EA, Van der Molen MW. 2010. The heart-brake of social rejection: a heart rate deceleration in response to unexpected peer rejection. *Psych Sci* 21: 1326–1333.

30. Güroğlu B, Van den Bos W, Crone EA. 2009. Fairness considerations: increasing understanding of intentionality during adolescence. *J Exp Child Psychol* 104: 398–409.

31. Güroğlu B, Van den Bos W, Rombouts SA, Crone EA. Unfair? It depends: neural correlates of fairness in social context. *Soc Cogn Affect Neurosci.* In press.

32. Güroğlu B, van den Bos W, Rombouts SARB, Crone EA. in preparation. Dissociable brain networks involved in development of fairness considerations.

33. Guth W, Schmittberger R, Schwarze B. 1982. An experimental analysis of ultimatum bargaining. *J Econ Behav Organ* 3: 367–388.

34. Hampton AN, Bossaerts P, O'Doherty JP. 2008. Neural correlates of mentalizing-related computations during strategic interactions in humans. *Proc Natl Acad Sci USA* 105: 6741–6746.

35. Hare TA, Camerer CF, Knoepfle DT, O'Doherty JP, Rangel A. 2010. Value computations in ventral medial prefrontal cortex during charitable decision making incorporate input from regions involved in social cognition. *J Neurosci* 30: 583–590.

36. Hartup WW, Stevens N. 1997. Friendships and adaptation in the life course. *Psychol Bull* 121: 355–370.

37. Hester R, Madeley J, Murphy K, Mattingley JB. 2009. Learning from errors: error-related neural activity predicts improvements in future inhibitory control performance. *J Neurosci* 29: 7158–7165.

38. Huizinga M, Dolan CV, van der Molen MW. 2006. Age-related change in executive function: developmental trends and a latent variable analysis. *Neuropsychologia* 44: 2017–2036.

39. Huttenlocher PR. 1979. Synaptic density in human frontal cortex—developmental changes and effects of aging. *Brain Res* 163: 195–205.

40. Johnson M, Grossmann T, Kadosh K. 2009. Mapping functional brain development: building a social brain through interactive specialization. *Dev Psychol* 45: 151–159.

41. Kerns JG. 2006. Anterior cingulate and prefrontal cortex activity in an fMRI study of trial-to-trial adjustments on the Simon task. *Neuroimage* 33: 399–405.

42. King-Casas B, Tomlin D, Anen C, Camerer CF, Quartz SR, Montague PR. 2005. Getting to know you: reputation and trust in a two-person economic exchange. *Science* 308: 78–83.

43. Klein TA, Neumann J, Reuter M, Hennig J, von Cramon DY, Ullsperger M. 2007. Genetically determined differences in learning from errors. *Science* 318: 1642–1645.

44. Knoch D, Nitsche MA, Fischbacher U, Eisenegger C, Pascual-Leone A, Fehr E. 2008. Studying the neurobiology of social interaction with transcranial direct current stimulation—the example of punishing unfairness. *Cereb Cortex* 18: 1987–1990.

45. Krueger F, McCabe K, Moll J, Kriegeskorte N, Zahn R, Strenziok M, Heinecke A, Grafman J. 2007. Neural correlates of trust. *Proc Natl Acad Sci USA* 104: 20084–20089.

46. Ladouceur CD, Dahl RE, Carter CS. 2004. ERP correlates of action monitoring in adolescence. *Ann N Y Acad Sci* 1021: 329–336.

47. Malhotra D. 2004. Trust and reciprocity decisions: the differing perspectives of trustors and trusted parties. *Organ Behav Hum Decis Process* 94: 61–73.

48. McCabe K, Houser D, Ryan L, Smith V, Trouard T. 2001. A functional imaging study of cooperation in two-person reciprocal exchange. *Proc Natl Acad Sci USA* 98: 11832–11835.

49. Montague PR, Lohrenz T. 2007. To detect and correct: norm violations and their enforcement. *Neuron* 56: 14–18.

50. Nelson EE, Leibenluft E, McClure EB, Pine DS. 2005. The social re-orientation of adolescence: a neuroscience perspective on the process and its relation to psychopathology. *Psychol Med* 35: 163–174.

51. Olson LA, Oberndorfer TA, Yang TT, Frank GK. 2008. Reactive aggressive youth brain activation is increased in response to emotional faces, but reduced during an impulsivity task. *Biol Psychol* 63: 47.

52. Pagnoni G, Zink CF, Montague PR, Berns GS. 2002. Activity in human ventral striatum locked to errors of reward prediction. *Nat Neurosci* 5: 97–98.

53. Paus T. 2010. Growth of white matter in the adolescent brain: myelin or axon? *Brain Cogn* 72: 26–35.

54. Paus T, Collins DL, Evans AC, Leonard G, Pike B. 2001. Maturation of white matter in the human brain: a review of magnetic resonance studies. *Brain Res Bull* 54: 255–266.

55. Paus T, Toro R, Leonard G, Lerner JV, Lerner RM, Perron M, Pike GB, Richer L, Steinberg L. 2008. Morphological properties of the action-observation cortical network in adolescents with low and high resistance to peer influence. *Soc Neurosci* 3: 303–316.

56. Pfeifer JH, Lieberman MD, Dapretto M. 2007. "I know you are but what am I?!": Neural bases of self- and social knowledge retrieval in children and adults. *J Cogn Neurosci* 19: 1323–1337.

57. Rangel A, Camerer C, Montague P. 2008. A framework for studying the neurobiology of value-based decision making. *Nat Rev Neurosci* 9: 545–556.

58. Rescorla RA, Wagner AR. 1972. A theory of Pavlovian conditioning: variations in the effectiveness of reinforcement and nonreinforcement. In: Classical Conditioning II (Black AH, Prokasy WF, eds), pp 64–99. New York: Appleton-Century-Crofts.

59. Rilling J, Goldsmith D, Glenn A, Jairam M, Elfenbein H, Dagenais J, Murdock C, Pagnoni G. 2008. The neural correlates of the affective response to unreciprocated cooperation. *Neuropsychologia* 46: 1256–1266.

60. Rilling J, King-Casas B, Sanfey AG. 2008. The neurobiology of social decision-making. *Curr Opin Neurobiol* 18: 159–165.

61. Rilling JK, Sanfey AG, Aronson JA, Nystrom LE, Cohen JD. 2004. The neural correlates of theory of mind within interpersonal interactions. *Neuroimage* 22: 1694–1703.

62. Rushworth MFS, Behrens TEJ. 2008. Choice, uncertainty and value in prefrontal and cingulate cortex. *Nat Neurosci* 11: 389–397.

63. Sanfey AG. 2007. Social decision-making: insights from game theory and neuroscience. *Science* 318: 598–602.

64. Sanfey AG, Rilling JK, Aronson JA, Nystrom LE, Cohen JD. 2003. The neural basis of economic decision-making in the Ultimatum Game. *Science* 300: 1755–1758.

65. Saxe R, Carey S, Kanwisher N. 2004. Understanding other minds: linking developmental psychology and functional neuroimaging. *Annu Rev Psychol* 55: 87–124.

66. Schmithorst VJ, Yuan WH. 2010. White matter development during adolescence as shown by diffusion MRI. *Brain Cogn* 72: 16–25.

67. Sebastian C, Burnett S, Blakemore SJ. 2008. Development of the self-concept during adolescence. *Trends Cogn Sci* 12: 441–446.

68. Shaw P, Kabani NJ, Lerch JP, Eckstrand K, Lenroot R, Gogtay N, Greenstein D, et al. 2008. Neurodevelopmental trajectories of the human cerebral cortex. *J Neurosci* 28: 3586–3594.

69. Somerville LH, Casey BJ. 2010. Developmental neurobiology of cognitive control and motivational systems. *Curr Opin Neurobiol* 20: 236–241.

70. Steinberg L. 2005. Cognitive and affective development in adolescence. *Trends Cogn Sci* 9: 69–74.

71. Steinberg L, Monahan KC. 2007. Age differences in resistance to peer influence. *Dev Psychol* 43: 1531–1543.

72. Sterzer P, Stadler C, Poustka F, Kleinschmidt A. 2007. A structural neural deficit in adolescents with conduct disorder and its association with lack of empathy. *Neuroimage* 37: 335–342.

73. Straub PG, Murnighan JK. 1995. An experimental investigation of ultimatum games—information, fairness, expectations and lowest acceptable offers. *J Econ Behav Organ* 27: 345–364.

74. Supekar K, Musen M, Menon V. 2009. Development of large-scale functional brain networks in children. *PLoS Biol* 7: e1000157.

75. Sutter M. 2007. Outcomes versus intentions: on the nature of fair behavior and its development with age. *J Econ Psychol* 28: 69–78.

76. Sutter M, Kocher MG. 2007. Trust and trustworthiness across different age groups. *Games Econ Behav* 59: 364.

77. Sutton RS, Barto AG. (1998) Reinforcement Learning: An Introduction. Cambridge, MA: MIT Press.

78. Tabibnia G, Satpute AB, Lieberman MD. 2008. The sunny side of fairness: preference for fairness activates reward circuitry (and disregarding unfairness activates self-control circuitry). *Psychol Sci* 19: 339–347.

79. Toga AW, Thompson PM, Sowell ER. 2006. Mapping brain maturation. *Trends Neurosci* 29: 148–159.

80. Van 't Wout M, Kahn RS, Sanfey AG, Aleman A. 2005. Repetitive transcranial magnetic stimulation over the right dorsolateral prefrontal cortex affects strategic decision-making. *Neuroreport* 16: 1849–1852.

81. Van den Bos W, Cohen MX, Kahnt T, Crone EA. 2010. Neurocognitive development of reinforcement learning. Paper presented at Annual Meeting of the Organization for Human Brain Mapping.

82. Van den Bos W, Guroglu B, van den Bulk BG, Rombouts S, Crone EA. 2009. Better than expected or as bad as you thought? The neurocognitive development of probabilistic feedback processing. *Front Hum Neurosci* 3: 52.

83. Van den Bos W, van Dijk E, Westenberg M, Rombouts S, Crone EA. 2009. What motivates repayment? Neural correlates of reciprocity in the Trust Game. *Soc Cogn Affect Neurosci* 4: 294–304.

84. Van den Bos W, Van Dijk E, Westenberg PM, Rombouts SARB, Crone EA. 2011. Changing brains, changing perspectives: the neurocognitive development of reciprocity. *Psychol Sci.* 22: 60–70.

85. Van den Bos W, Westenberg M, van Dijk E, Crone EA. 2010. Development of trust and reciprocity in adolescence. *Cogn Dev* 25: 90–102.

86. Van Duijvenvoorde AC, Zanolie K, Rombouts SA, Raijmakers ME, Crone EA. 2008. Evaluating the negative or valuing the positive? Neural mechanisms supporting feedback-based learning across development. *J Neurosci* 28: 9495–9503.

87. Van Overwalle F. 2009. Social cognition and the brain: a meta-analysis. *Hum Brain Mapp* 30: 829–858.

88. Wang AT, Lee SS, Sigman M, Dapretto M. 2006. Neural basis of irony comprehension in children with autism: the role of prosody and context. *Brain* 129: 932–943.

14 Motivational Modulation of Action Control: How Interindividual Variability May Shed Light on the Motivation-Control Interface and Its Neurocognitive Mechanisms

K. Richard Ridderinkhof, Michael X Cohen, and Birte U. Forstmann

Despite their importance in a wide variety of situations, the concepts of motivation and cognitive control have long remained intractable, due perhaps to their descriptive rather than mechanistic conceptualizations. Motivation refers to (internal or external) incentives that energize goal-oriented behavior. Cognitive control refers to the capacity to orchestrate, coordinate, and direct basic cognitive processes and their temporal structure, in accordance with internal goals and/or external demands, so as to optimize behavioral outcomes. Action control refers more specifically to a subset of adaptive cognitive control processes involved in the requirement to coordinate one's instantaneous urges vis-à-vis actions that concord with our intentions or instructions. Action control involves active preparation for upcoming decisions and actions, and the flexible switching between action plans or task sets.

Obviously, the anticipatory goal-oriented regulation aspect of action control requires effort. Because of this energetic component, action control is highly susceptible to modulation by motivational incentives. This observation may seem almost trivial, but today the neurocognitive mechanisms through which motivation influences action control remain surprisingly elusive. Here, we approach this interface from an individual-differences perspective (some individuals are more proficient in the control of goal-oriented actions than others, and individual differences also apply to the extent to which motivational modulations of action control are successful). Such a perspective sheds light on the neurobiological mechanisms that support motivation and action control, and suggests that capturing these individual differences in theories and models may be crucial to better understanding cognitive control processes.

Here's what the reader can expect. In the first section, we briefly outline the three central concepts of this chapter: motivation (why and how motivation is important for shaping action), action control (what is action control for, and what are its main constituents), and individual differences (how can we capitalize on interindividual variability to advance our understanding of neurocognitive mechanisms). In the next section, we elaborate on the processes and neural bases of online action control, and illustrate the additional advantages of an individual-differences approach by reviewing a few recent covariance-based functional magnetic resonance imaging (fMRI) studies. In the third section, we survey the neurocognitive processes involved in anticipatory regulation of action control. Specifically, as two prominent points in case, we discuss anticipatory processes involved in speed-accuracy balance setting and in action-rule switching, and highlight how our understanding of the mechanisms involved in these processes benefits from individual-differences studies. Finally, in the last section, we address the key issue: how action control is modulated by motivational incentives. Despite an increasing interest in this motivation-control interface, the neurocognitive mechanisms through which motivational factors impact action control processes remain surprisingly elusive. We discuss the current state of affairs, and suggest that a thorough appreciation of this interface function (and its neurocognitive bases) may, once more, benefit from an individual-differences approach. A few encouraging examples may convince the reader of the promise this approach holds.

Motivation, Action Control, and Individual Differences

Motivation

Already in the early days of experimental psychology, theorists recognized that motivational incentives influence behavior.[20,34] Motivational states are widely believed to regulate and prioritize action goals.[58] Today, the neural mechanisms through which motivational factors modulate action control remain surprisingly elusive,[71] but the motivational factors that shape human behavior appear to be closely tied to the anticipation of reward.

Hence, we concentrate on reward anticipation as one specific guise of external motivational incentive. By no means do we intend to argue that anticipation of reward is more central to motivation than other types of incentive (internal or external); we focus on reward anticipation simply because the neurocognitive architecture of this aspect of motivation has been studied more (in both animal and human work) than most other aspects.

Action Control

When interacting with the outside world, one is confronted with situations that present action affordances (alluring and potentiating opportunities for action in a particular situation, some more potent than others[35]). Our sensitivity to these affordances is shaped and guided by our current motivation, concerns, intentions, and prior experiences, such that we can prioritize our responsiveness to the different affordances. Some action affordances may present more potent solicitations than others, but it may not always be appropriate to give in to immediate captivation by the strongest action urge.

It is important to distinguish online action control from the anticipatory processes that regulate them.[10,77] Anticipatory and online control processes can be dissociated in terms of underlying neural networks, temporal dynamics, and sensitivity to experimental manipulations as well as individual differences.

Online action control is exerted to suppress and overcome incorrect, inappropriate, or undesirable actions in favor of intention-driven action selection.[6] Proficient traffic navigation, for instance, requires one to arrest conversation with a passenger when approaching a complex roundabout, and to overrule the habit of driving on the right side of the road when navigating traffic in England.

Anticipatory action regulation refers to those modulatory processes that either strengthen online action control proactively, or preempt the need for such online action control.[73,77] If a traffic accident (e.g., resulting from an experienced tendency to drive the right side of an English road) was barely avoided, anticipatory action regulation might lead one to tighten online action control to preempt further error. Anticipatory action regulation can be instigated by several kinds of processes that monitor for external and internal signals indicating the need to adjust behavior.[78] Online action control operates transiently, whereas anticipatory regulation operates in a more sustained fashion.

Individual Differences

Individual differences in the behavioral variables of interest usually end up sitting in the error variance. In recent years, however, it has been recognized that these individual differences can and should be turned from a weakness into a strength in terms of understanding neurocognitive processes.[56] Numerous examples illustrate how cardinal individual differences in the susceptibility to factor effects are concealed and overlooked in group averages.[17,76,109] Much information is lost by ignoring interindividual variability, sometimes resulting in misleading interpretations of results when, for example, effects are in opposite directions for different subjects or subgroups.

More important, however, we can potentially gain a deeper understanding of the importance of neural circuits in cognitive functions by examining which brain areas covary in their activation with individual differences in relevant behavioral parameters.[4,32,33,48,54] Beyond mere correlation analyses, individual differences in relevant behavioral parameters can be entered as covariates into the regression model for the BOLD signal in so-called covariance-based fMRI analysis. Covariance-based fMRI capitalizes on individual differences in parameters that quantify the efficiency of specific cognitive processes. Such parameters can be estimated for each individual on the basis of formal (mathematical) models,[17] theoretical (descriptive) models,[29] or personality variables.[63]

As an example, Haruno and Kawato[42] employed the Q-learning model of reinforcement learning[94] to quantify the effect of outcome processing and reward anticipation processes. More specifically, Haruno and Kawato[42] used the Q-learning algorithm to estimate outcome and reward anticipation processes on a trial-by-trial basis for each participant. These estimates were convolved with a hemodynamic response function to model the blood oxygen level–dependent (BOLD) signal representing outcome and reward anticipation processes, respectively. The results revealed that individual differences in these estimates correlated with BOLD activation in putamen and caudate nucleus, respectively.

In later sections, we briefly review individual differences in action control, focusing in particular on covariance-based fMRI analyses of these processes. We then evaluate initial individual-differences studies of motivational modulation of action control, hoping to show that this approach allows us to make headway in understanding the interface between motivation and action control.

Online Action Control

Online action control can involve a number of component processes.[77] Most important, the activation of appropriate actions is prompted based on *intention-driven action selection* in almost any action selection situation. In many situations, however, this process is impeded by the presence of competing action options, often in the form of alluring affordances implicitly presented by external stimuli. Thus, online action control often involves resisting the activation of inappropriate actions based on extraneous stimulus-action associations that are strong enough to incur *response capture*, and in some conditions also the suppression of this activation of inappropriate actions through *active response inhibition*. The magnitude of the mean interference effect on reaction time in conflict tasks (such as the Simon task) is considered to reflect the additional time needed to resolve the response conflict when selecting between two competing action alternatives, and to inhibit early response capture by the irrelevant stimulus dimension before the correct response is emitted.[90]

As one theoretical framework, the activation-suppression model[76] describes the effects of processing conflicting information on behavior. Importantly, this model generates specific individual parameters that represent the temporal aspects of the susceptibility to make fast impulsive reactions, and the proficiency of selective inhibitory control over unwanted actions to facilitate the selection of the appropriate response. Reaction-time distribution analysis techniques were developed to incorporate the temporal dynamics underlying the expression of impulsive errors followed by a gradual build-up of selective suppression as an act of cognitive control.

Based on these temporal dynamics, the model predicts that faster reactions on conflict trials should be more vulnerable to impulsive actions because selective suppression has not been fully engaged. Thus, plotting accuracy rates for noncorresponding trials as a function of reaction time (RT; i.e., conditional accuracy function or CAF; see figure 14.1) provides a means for studying the strength of automatic response capture in conflicting situations, with stronger capture associated with a higher frequency of fast errors,[102] as less time is available for the build-up of suppression to counter this incorrect activation.[55]

In contrast to the rapid engagement of the response capture mechanism, top-down suppression takes time to build up and, therefore, is most evident for responses that are relatively slow. For instance, the faster one responds, the less likely it is that suppression will have accrued to a level sufficient to counteract response capture. With slower responses, the selective inhibition process has had time to develop, and thus, the activation of the incorrect response along the direct capture route will be reduced. Consequently, correct slow responses to congruent stimuli will be less facilitated by position-driven response capture, whereas correct slow responses to conflict stimuli will be less delayed. Thus, plotting the Simon effect as a function of response speed (the so-called *delta plot*; see figure 14.1) should reveal a pattern of reduced interference in slower segments of the RT distribution as the suppression mechanism becomes more fully engaged. The slope of the reduction of interference at the slowest segment of the RT distribution serves as a sensitive metric of the proficiency of selective response inhibition.[102]

Online action control is thought to be supported largely through frontostriatal circuits in the brain, with the presupplementary motor area (pre-SMA) as a key node for action selection.[44,67] The pre-SMA may act as an action-selection director, modulating the action-selection gate through which the available action affordances are translated into actual actions. The inferior frontal cortex (IFC) is often recruited to aid in implementing selective response inhibition. Direct connections between the pre-SMA and IFC on the one hand and basal ganglia structures (most prominently the anterior dorsal striatum and the subthalamic nucleus, STN) on the other serve to keep basal ganglia output in check until intention-driven action selection has completed the final green signal received from upstream. Extraneous, impulsive action affordances may capture the action system nondeliberately. When multiple stimulus-action association alternatives compete for activation, the demands on action control are highest, and selecting the appropriate action engages stronger activation of the pre-SMA compared to when response capture is absent. Monitoring of action selection during conflict tasks, and of action outcomes in general, is believed to play a crucial role in task performance and has been associated with functioning of the dorsal and posterior portions of the mediofrontal cortex (MFC).[78]

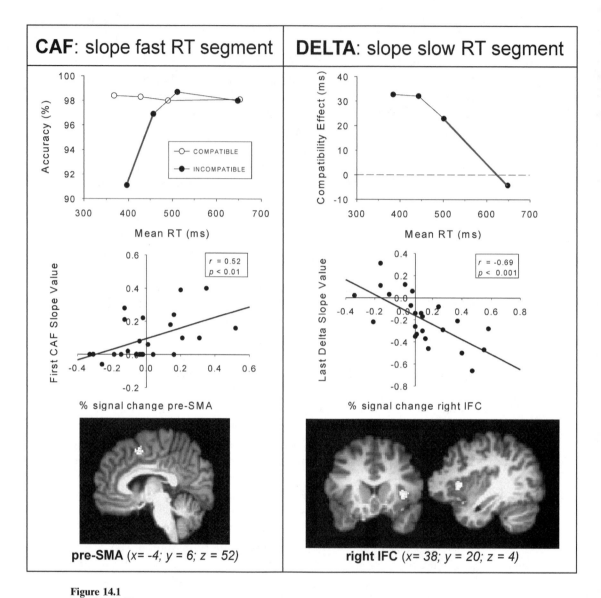

Figure 14.1
Individual differences in distribution parameters predict brain activation. Top left: Conditional accuracy function (CAF) depict accuracy as a function of reaction time (RT) quantile. Top right: Delta plots depict the size of the interference effect as a function of RT quantile. Middle left: Pearson correlations between the slope of the fastest segment of the CAF for noncorresponding trials (y-axis) and the percent signal change (x-axis) in the BOLD signal derived from the pre-SMA. Middle right: Pearson correlations between the slope of the slowest segment of the delta plot (y-axis) and the percent signal change (x-axis) in the BOLD signal derived from the right IFC. Bottom left: BOLD activation of the pre-SMA covaries with the slope of the fastest segment of the CAF for noncorresponding trials. Bottom right: BOLD activation of the right IFG covaries with the slope of the slowest segment of the delta plot. Figure modified after Forstmann et al.[31] with permission.

Animal electrophysiology, human patient studies, transcranial magnetic stimulation (TMS) experiments, and neuroimaging work are beginning to disclose the neurocognitive mechanisms of online action control.[77] Studies that focus on individual differences advance these insights in important ways, as illustrated next.

Insights from Individual-Differences Approaches

To study the neural substrates of impulsive action selection, individual parameter values derived from reaction time distributions (reflecting the tendency to emit fast and impulsive responses that are driven by the irrelevant stimulus dimension) were entered as covariates in the regression model for fMRI-BOLD analyses.[31] Stronger response capture was associated with enhanced activation in the pre-SMA. This pattern indicates that individuals who are highly susceptible to making fast impulsive errors show increased pre-SMA activity, reflecting the elevated need to select a correct response in conflicting situations (see figure 14.1). Notably, the relation between errors and percent signal change derived from the pre-SMA was evident only for the fast RT segment, and was absent for slower responses, a dynamic pattern that is in line with the tenets of the activation-suppression model.

To identify the neurocognitive correlates of selective response inhibition, entering individual delta-slope values into the fMRI regression analyses revealed significant activations in the IFC (BA 44) bordering the right anterior insula[29] (see figure 14.1). This pattern reveals that individuals showing relatively negative-going delta-slope values derived from the slowest segment of the RT distribution present enhanced activation in the IFC.

Anticipatory Regulation of Action Control

The expression of the online action control processes may be modulated by anticipatory adjustments of action-selection priorities. In participating in traffic, for instance, one's responsiveness to action affordances is subject to fluctuations as a function of warnings, changing situations, recent experiences (good or bad), the behavior of others, and so on. Though it may not always be possible to deploy action control processes successfully to completely cancel out the effects of response capture, one may be able to prepare for task-inappropriate action affordances and mitigate their undesired effects by establishing action control. Such anticipatory processes can be described in terms of two orthogonal dimensions: Regulation may be prospective or reactive in nature, and it may take on proactive or preemptive forms.[77]

Anticipatory regulation will often be *reactive*; that is, adjustments of online action control will be contingent on performance errors or internal signals of performance difficulty, such as response conflicts. In other instances, anticipatory regulation will be more *prospective*; for instance, one may slow down when anticipating busy traffic, or make use of explicit cues or instructions to guide adjustments of processing priorities.

Whether prospective or reactive in nature, anticipatory action regulation can be accomplished through either proactive or preemptive adjustments. One may attempt to *proactively* strengthen online action control, for instance, by a priori amplifying those processes that help keep our horses in check when strong response capture is anticipated. Alternatively, one may attempt to *preempt* the need for online action control, for instance, by increasing the focus of selective attention to filter out task-irrelevant stimuli such that these fail to elicit strong response capture in the first place.

Here, we focus on two types of prospective, proactive forms of anticipatory regulation: first, speed-accuracy balance setting and, second, action-rule coordination. Speed-accuracy balance setting and action-rule coordination are typically studied through the reaction-time paradigms of speed-accuracy trade-off (SAT)[15,28,86,107] and task switching,[2,80] respectively. In both cases, action control is modulated by anticipatory regulation of action selection, action shielding, and action priorities. SAT refers to situations in which individuals need to negotiate between the competing demands of response speed and response accuracy. Task switching refers to situations where stimuli that designated one particular action in the past designate another action in the present, requiring a switch of action rule that can be prepared ahead of time. Daily-life examples of SAT dilemmas as well as action-rule switching can be seen in speeded decisions in traffic. For instance, during busy traffic on the highway, if one is late in spotting the exit sign and time to shift to the exit lane is a bit tight, one has to decide whether to go for speed (take the exit now, and accept the risk) or emphasize accuracy (wait for the next exit, and accept a later arrival). In dealing with situation-specific traffic rules, such as having to yield to traffic coming from the right after having had priority at the previous junction, one can use traffic signs to resolve the ambiguity ahead of time and be prepared for the correct action rule before the new situation presents itself.

Speed-Accuracy Balance Setting

One cannot always afford to think long before acting. Information accumulation is a process that increases the probability of making a correct action decision, but that is inherently time-consuming. Several formal models of SAT have been developed in the fields of mathematical psychology and computational neuroscience to predict the speed and error incidence associated with action decisions under time pressure.[64,74,75,98,104] Such models include integrator neurons (or neuron populations) that correspond to particular choice alternatives[88,101] and act as accumulators that gradually accrue noisy sensory input until their firing rate exceeds a certain critical threshold.[14,81] The speed-accuracy balance in such models varies as a function of the distance between the baseline activity of the integrators and the response threshold. A high threshold (relative to baseline) yields accurate but slow action decisions; a low threshold yields decisions that are fast but error prone.

This mechanism provides us with an instrument of anticipatory action regulation: the speed-accuracy balance can be set ahead of time, depending on our current priorities. Model parameters associated with information accumulation (baseline, threshold, drift rate) have been found to correspond to preparatory neural activation in various cortical and subcortical brain areas, including not only premotor cortex but also dorsolateral prefrontal cortex (DLPFC) associated with top-down guidance.[37,43,85] For instance, animal work on the effect of instructed SAT showed an increase in baseline premotor activity prior to actual movement when speed was emphasized over accuracy.[16] fMRI studies in humans showed increased preparatory activity in several frontal and parietal areas, including the DLPFC,[45,103] when speed was emphasized over accuracy. The precise neural mechanisms underlying SAT remain to be determined. Excitation of the subthalamic nucleus (STN) produces slower and more accurate choices,[3,4] and hence might provide a mechanism for emphasizing accuracy.

Insights from Individual-Differences Approaches

Studies of how neural decision circuits in humans implement SAT remain scarce. However, recent studies that focus on individual differences have advanced our understanding of how and where in the brain the SAT is controlled.[8] Forstmann et al.[27,30] used the so-called moving-dots paradigm,[13] in which humans decide whether a dot kinetogram (basically a cloud of moving dots), visually presented in the middle of a computer screen, appears to move to the right or to the left. Since motion direction is coherent for only some proportion of dots, the dominant direction is not immediately obvious. When speed is emphasized over accuracy, information accumulation may be insufficient such that speed is gained at the expense of an increased probability of making an error.

Application of the linear ballistic accumulation model[14] (a mathematical model of speeded decision making, based on the rate of accrual of evidence and response thresholds) to behavioral data confirmed that cueing for speed reduces the distance between baseline and threshold.[30] Individually assessed parameter values were then entered as covariates in subsequent model-based fMRI analyses. This individual-differences approach revealed that cueing for speed activates the pre-SMA and the dorsolateral striatum. Individuals who displayed greater reduction of baseline-to-threshold distance (as estimated through the linear ballistic accumulation model) showed stronger activation of the pre-SMA and striatum. Under the assumption that the observed BOLD signal in the pre-SMA is produced by the activity of integrator neurons, these data suggest that speed instructions implement anticipatory action control by increasing the baseline activity and/or reducing the response threshold of these neurons. Activation in the dorsolateral striatum, presumably through direct excitatory inputs from pre-SMA, is thought to release the motor system from global inhibition, thereby facilitating faster but possibly premature actions. In a follow-up study using covariance-based probabilistic tractography to quantify white-matter connectivity, structural connections between pre-SMA and the dorsal striatum were shown to be crucial for flexibly changing response thresholds.[25]

Task Preparation and Action-Rule Switching

Goal-directed action control requires the ability to maintain task focus and prevent interference from competing task goals (goal shielding[38]) as well as the ability to switch attention flexibly among alternative goals. The concept of preparation incorporates advance selection, activation, and maintenance of task-relevant action rules and the control of interference from task-irrelevant action rules.[47] Action-rule maintenance and switching are typically studied using cued task-switching paradigms, in which task cues allow for advance preparation of the current action rule.

Functional neuroimaging studies of action-rule switching typically report activation in a distributed network encompassing dorsolateral and ventrolateral aspects of the prefrontal cortex (DLPFC, VLPFC), premotor cortex (PMC), pre-SMA, and the posterior parietal cortex (PPC).[12,49,79]

When comparing effectively prepared to less effectively prepared tasks, switch-repeat activation differences were observed during the preparation interval in DLPFC and in task-relevant regions,[108] indicating that preparation served to "pre-activate" task-relevant regions.[110] Likewise, effective preparation was associated with stronger activation of the PPC.[5,11,26,83] By contrast, effective preparation was associated with *weaker* switch-repeat activation differences in VLPFC[5,46] and in PMC/pre-SMA.[9,46,82,91] DLPFC activation appeared to reflect goal-oriented activation during advance preparation, leading to preactivation of task-relevant neural areas and subsequent performance benefits. PPC activation is thought to reflect task-specific preparation. Inefficiently prepared trials, which require greater target-driven control to reduce interference in stimulus processing and response selection, are associated with greater activation in VLPFC and PMC/pre-SMA than well-prepared trials.

Only a few studies report the involvement of the basal ganglia in switch-repeat activation differences.[18] Activation in the STN and striatum was observed to predict the behavioral switch costs of the upcoming trial without showing a significant difference between switch and repeat trials,[60] suggesting that the basal ganglia may be active in preparing for switch and repeat trials alike, which would explain why the basal ganglia have not been prominent in previous neuroimaging studies.

Insights from Individual-Differences Approaches

Findings from the task-switching literature suggest that advance preparation can be conceptualized as a set of processes activated for both switch and repeat trials, but with substantial variability as a function of individual differences. Covariance-based analysis approaches account for such individual differences in preparatory processes by estimating quantitative model parameters that reflect latent psychological processes, allowing us to arrive at meaningful insights regarding *how* advance preparation is accomplished. The association between model parameters that characterize the decision process and neuroscientific measures provides evidence as to the functional and psychological relevance of the latter.

Performance costs associated with advance preparation and target-driven decision processes have been mapped onto different parameters of evidence accumulation models.[50] Nondecision time may provide a measure of how much cue-dependent preparation has occurred in the cue-to-target interval, with an increased nondecision time indicating a greater delay in the initiation of the decision processing once the target appears, because preparation remains to be completed. Indeed, nondecision time was observed to vary as a function of the amount of information afforded by the cue, being highest for noninformative cues.[50] In addition, cues predicting a certain task switch resulted in a higher response threshold than cues predicting task repetition or noninformative cues, suggesting that participants engaged in cue-dependent trial-by-trial adjustment of response thresholds in order to balance demands for both fast and accurate responding. Higher thresholds also resulted in longer decision time.

Accumulator models have, to our knowledge, not yet been used in covariance-based fMRI analyses of task switching. Individual differences in parameters of another quantitative model, the control of associative memory during task switching model, were regressed on fMRI measures of switch-related brain activation.[5] Increased preparation was associated with reduced switch-repeat activation in the VLPFC but increased activation in the PPC, confirming previous conclusions that proactive preparation is supported by PPC, whereas VLPFC comes more into play when advance preparation failed and online control processes are recruited in action-rule switching.

Interfacing Motivation and Action Control

In the preceding sections, we provided brief reviews of the neurocognitive mechanisms of online action control an anticipatory action regulation. Next, we move to the interface question: How can action control be optimized through motivational incentives?

The prospect of obtaining a reward can serve as a potent external motivator of goal-oriented behavior. Rewards come in many guises: bananas, juice drops, sex, status, compliments, money, lottery tickets, and even symbolic tokens (e.g., game points) all are powerful rewards, the prospect of which can serve as a strong motivational incentive. The potential gains (as well as the potential costs) associated with behavioral options are weighed against each other and against the effort associated with each reward,[19,105] a process that is instrumental to efficient behavior.[68,87] Indeed, a growing number of studies have shown that actions are prepared and executed with greater efficiency when animals and humans expect their goals to be rewarded.[22,40,69]

Because anticipatory processes of goal-oriented action regulation require effort, these processes can benefit from energizing by motivational incentives. Indeed, the speed-accuracy balance[7,24,53,61,70,93] as well as action-rule switching[1,84] have been observed to be subject to motivational manipulations.

Reward prospect has been shown to modulate activation in prefrontal and striatal brain areas during action control tasks.[36,57,72,84,89,92,97] Pessoa[71] proposed that motivation serves to recalibrate the allocation of processing resources in order to prioritize those processes that maximize potential reward. In this view, motivation engenders salience processing in the ACC through striatal dopaminergic processes supporting reward anticipation. This motivation-related ACC engagement could trigger subsequent recruitment of action control areas such as dorsolateral PFC (perhaps through phasic locus coeruleus norepinephrine boosts) in ways that optimize reward.

Despite these promising speculations, the neurocognitive mechanisms through which these action control processes interface with motivational influences remain poorly understood to date. In the next section, we approach this interface function from an individual-differences perspective.

Insights from Individual-Differences Approaches

Individual-differences studies of motivational modulation of action control are beginning to emerge. For instance, Locke and Braver[63] observed that individual differences in motivational state and motivation-related personality variables modulated cognitive control through sustained activation of frontostriatal brain circuits associated with reward processing and cognitive control. In briefly reviewing a few illustrations, we hope to convince the reader that such analyses (involving covariance-based or genetic neuroimaging) open up new avenues for exploring the interface between motivation and action control—or at least shed light on the next steps ahead.

Antisaccades are particularly demanding in terms of action preparation, involving the inhibition of eye movements toward a peripheral stimulus and the initiation of eye movements in the opposite direction.[39,66] The dorsomedial striatum (in particular the caudate nucleus) can serve as an important nexus between the neural networks for anticipatory antisaccade programming and for reward-related motivational processes. The dorsomedial striatum can also facilitate or hamper the build-up of activation for a specific saccade in the superior colliculi.[62] but is also responsive to reward prospect.[59,106] Interestingly, dorsomedial striatal neurons whose firing patterns correspond to the speed and accuracy of imminent saccades also respond to reward-prospect cues that announce reward for rapid and accurate saccades.[51,52,95] Hence, the dorsomedial striatum plays a crucial role in transforming cognitive and motivational information into efficient eye movements.[51,52,96,99] Harsay and colleagues focused on individual differences in antisaccade performance to investigate the remedial potential of reward expectations on declining action preparation.[40] The efficiency of preparation is indexed by the antisaccade onset latency.[65] The advantageous effect of reward prospect (versus no-reward prospect) on antisaccade latency was used in covariance-based fMRI analysis to determine which brain regions are involved in interfacing motivational incentives (anticipation of reward) and action control (efficient antisaccades).[41] The dorsomedial striatum, the SMA, and the frontal and parietal eyefields were observed to be engaged more strongly by individuals who showed greater antisaccade benefits from reward-prospect cues. Functional connectivity analysis seeded in the dorsomedial striatum showed greater interregional coupling with the SMA and the eyefields in individuals showing greater reward-prospect benefits.[41] These analyses underline the notion of the dorsomedial striatum as a nexus between reward and oculomotor systems, serving as one potential neural mechanism for interfacing motivation and action control.

The role of (dopaminergic processes in) the dorsomedial striatum in the interaction between motivational and cognitive control was highlighted further in the context of task switching. Aarts et al.[1] used individual differences in a polymorphism of a specific dopamine transporter gene (SLC6A3) for genetic neuroimaging. Specific alleles of this gene correspond to striatal dopamine levels, and also covary with activity in the striatum during reward anticipation.[21,23] Aarts and colleagues observed that carriers of the allele associated with high striatal dopamine exhibited a greater influence of anticipated reward on switch costs. Crucially, these individuals also showed greater activity in the dorsomedial striatum during task switching in anticipation of high reward relative to low reward, confirming the role for (dopaminergic processes in) the dorsal striatum in the modulation of flexible action control by motivational incentives. In a recent fMRI study, Savine and Braver[84] found that individual differences in switch costs were predicted by individual differences in activation of dorsolateral PFC as induced by reward prospects.

Conclusion

These examples illustrate the utility of exploiting individual differences in seeking to further our understanding of how action control is modulated by motivational incentives, which may hopefully render the neurocognitive mechanisms underlying the motivation-cognition interface a little less elusive.

We have focused on how the prospect of reward impacts the anticipatory regulation of action. Initial work on neural networks shows that those individuals who are most proficient in translating the prospect of potential reward into efficient and effective action control were shown to engage stronger activation of, and stronger connectivity among, brain areas central to frontostriatal action control circuits.[41] As a tentative inference, Harsay et al. speculate that functional connectivity between circuits supporting reward anticipation (such as dorsal and ventral striatum and OFC) and (task-specific) circuits supporting action selection and action prioritizing (such as the basal ganglia, DLPFC, and the pre-SMA or eyefields) is key to interfacing motivation to action. Notably, elements that are common to reward and action-control circuits (such as the dorsomedial striatum) might serve as a nexus in the motivation-action interface. The extent to which individuals are able to effectively deploy such a nexus to connect the reward and action circuitries might then predict the extent to which they can translate reward prospect into more efficient anticipatory regulation of action control.[41]

According to an alternative (or perhaps complementary) hypothesis, motivational incentives might serve as salience signals that are picked up and amplified by the so-called salience network (consisting of ACC and anterior insula) in order to allocate additional resources to action-control networks, perhaps at the expense of task-irrelevant neural networks.[71,100] This hypothesis could be examined by entering ACC and anterior insula as seed regions into functional connectivity analyses to evaluate the prediction that individuals who are more proficient in translating reward prospect into anticipatory action regulation are better able to set up the salience network for the recruitment and deactivation of task-relevant and task-irrelevant networks, respectively.

In conclusion, initial individual-differences studies of motivational modulation of action control begin to highlight the interface between motivation and action control. Future studies might adopt this approach to study the interface between motivation beyond reward prospect and control beyond anticipatory action regulation.

Outstanding Questions

• How can individual differences give us more insight into the interface between motivation and control?

• How can we integrate individual differences in genetics, brain structure, brain function, and behavior into a single framework?

Further Reading

Frijda NH. 2010. Impulsive action and motivation. *Biol Psychol* 84: 570–579. This paper explores how emotional events elicit changes in motivational states and as such can cause actions.

Pessoa L. 2009. How do emotion and motivation direct executive control? *Trends Cogn Sci* 13: 160–166. This paper explores the interactions between emotion and cognitive control, arguing that emotions can both enhance and impair behavioral performance depending on how they interact with control functions.

Ridderinkhof KR, Forstmann BU, Wylie SA, Burle B, Van den Wildenberg WPM. in press. Neurocognitive mechanisms of action control: resisting the call of the sirens. *Wylie Interdisciplinary Reviews: Cognitive Science*. An in-depth overview of neurocognitive mechanisms of control in changing environments, includes discussions of individual differences in these mechanisms.

References

1. Aarts E, Roelofs A, Franke B, Rijpkema M, Fernandez G, Helmich RC, Cools R. 2010. Striatal dopamine mediates the interface between motivational and cognitive control in humans: evidence from genetic imaging. *Neuropsychopharmacology* 35: 1943–1951.

2. Allport A, Styles EA, Shieh S. 1994. Shifting intentional set: exploring the dynamic control of tasks. In: Attention & Performance XV: Conscious and Unconscious Information Processing (Umiltà C, Moscovitch M, eds), pp 421–452. Cambridge, MA: MIT Press.

3. Aron AR, Behrens TE, Smith S, Frank MJ, Poldrack RA. 2007. Triangulating a cognitive control network using diffusion-weighted magnetic resonance imaging (MRI) and functional MRI. *J Neurosci* 27: 3743–3752.

4. Aron AR, Poldrack RA. 2006. Cortical and subcortical contributions to Stop signal response inhibition: role of the subthalamic nucleus. *J Neurosci* 26: 2424–2433.

5. Badre D, Wagner AD. 2006. Computational and neurobiological mechanisms underlying cognitive flexibility. *Proc Natl Acad Sci USA* 18: 7186–7191.

6. Baumeister RF, Vohs KD. 2004 Handbook of Self-Regulation: Research, Theory, and Applications. New York: Guilford Press.

7. Bijleveld E, Custers R, Aarts H. 2009. The unconscious eye-opener: pupil size reveals strategic recruitment of resources upon presentation of subliminal reward cues. *Psychol Rev* 20: 1313–1315.

8. Bogacz R, Wagenmakers EJ, Forstmann BU, Nieuwenhuis S. 2010. The neural basis of the speed-accuracy tradeoff. *Trends Neurosci* 33: 10–16.

9. Brass M, Von Cramon DY. 2004. Decomposing components of task preparation with functional magnetic resonance imaging. *J Cogn Neurosci* 16: 609–620.

10. Braver TS, Gray JR, Burgess GC. 2007. Explaining many varieties in working memory variation: dual mechanisms of cognitive control. In: Variation in Working Memory (Conway A, ed), pp 76–106. Oxford: Oxford University Press.

11. Braver TS, Reynolds JR, Donaldson DI. 2003. Neural mechanisms of transient and sustained cognitive control during task switching. *Neuron* 39: 713–726.

12. Braver TS, Ruge H. 2006. Functional neuroimaging of executive function. In: Handbook of Functional Neuroimaging of Cognition (Cabeza R, Kingstone A, eds), pp 307–348. Cambridge, MA: MIT Press.

13. Britten KH, Shadlen MN, Newsome WT, Movshon JA. 1992. The analysis of visual motion: a comparison of neuronal and psychophysical performance. *J Neurosci* 12: 4745–4765.

14. Brown SD, Heathcote A. 2008. The simplest complete model of choice response time: linear ballistic accumulation. *Cognit Psychol* 57: 153–178.

15. Chittka L, Skorupski P, Raine NE. 2009. Speed-accuracy tradeoffs in animal decision making. *Trends Ecol Evol* 24: 400–407.

16. Churchland MM, Santhanam G, Shenoy KV. 2006. Preparatory activity in premotor and motor cortex reflects the speed of the upcoming reach. *J Neurophysiol* 96: 3130–3146.

17. Cohen MX. 2007. Individual differences and the neural representations of reward expectation and reward prediction error. *Soc Cogn Affect Neurosci* 2: 20–30.

18. Crone EA, Wendelken C, Donohue SE, Bunge SA. 2006. Neural evidence for dissociable components of task-switching. *Cereb Cortex* 16: 475–486.

19. Croxson PL, Walton ME, O'Reilly JX, Behrens TE, Rushworth MF. 2009. Effort-based cost-benefit valuation and the human brain. *J Neurosci* 29: 4531–4541.

20. Diserens CM, Vaughn J. 1931. The experimental psychology of motivation. *Psychol Bull* 1: 15–65.

21. Dreher JC, Kohn P, Kolachana B, Weinberger DR, Berman KF. 2009. Variation in dopamine genes influences responsivity of the human reward system. *Proc Natl Acad Sci USA* 106: 617–622.

22. Engelmann JB, Damaraju E, Padmala S, Pessoa L. 2009. Combined effects of attention and motivation on visual task performance: transient and sustained motivational effects. *Front Hum Neurosci* 3: 4.

23. Forbes EE, Brown SM, Kimak M, Ferrell RE, Manuck SB, Hariri AR. 2009. Genetic variation in components of dopamine neurotransmission impacts ventral striatal reactivity associated with impulsivity. *Mol Psychiatry* 14: 60–70.

24. Förster J, Higgins ET, Bianco AT. 2003. Speed/accuracy decisions in task performance. built-in tradeoff or separate strategic concerns? *Organ Behav Hum Decis Process* 90: 148–164.

25. Forstmann BU, Anwander A, Schafer A, Neumann J, Brown S, Wagenmakers EJ, Bogacz R, Turner R. 2010. Cortico-striatal connections predict control over speed and accuracy in perceptual decision making. *Proc Natl Acad Sci USA* 107: 15916–15920.

26. Forstmann BU, Brass M, Koch I, von Cramon DY. 2006. Voluntary selection of task sets revealed by functional magnetic resonance imaging. *J Cogn Neurosci* 18: 388–398.

27. Forstmann BU, Brown S, Dutilh G, Neumann J, Wagenmakers EJ. 2010. The neural substrate of prior information in perceptual decision making: a model-based analysis. *Front Hum Neurosci* 4: 40.

28. Forstmann BU, Dutilh G, Brown S, Neumann J, von Cramon DY, Ridderinkhof KR, Wagenmakers EJ. 2008. Striatum and pre-SMA facilitate decision-making under time pressure. *Proc Natl Acad Sci USA* 105: 17538–17542.

29. Forstmann BU, Jahfari S, Scholte HS, Wolfensteller U, van den Wildenberg WP, Ridderinkhof KR. 2008. Function and structure of the right inferior frontal cortex predict individual differences in response inhibition: a model-based approach. *J Neurosci* 28: 9790–9796.

30. Forstmann BU, Ridderinkhof KR, Kaiser J, Bledowski C. 2007. At your own peril: an ERP study of voluntary task set selection processes in the medial frontal cortex. *Cogn Affect Behav Neurosci* 7: 286–296.

31. Forstmann BU, van den Wildenberg WP, Ridderinkhof KR. 2008. Neural mechanisms, temporal dynamics, and individual differences in interference control. *J Cogn Neurosci* 20: 1854–1865.

32. Ganis G, Morris RR, Kosslyn SM. 2009. Neural processes underlying self- and other-related lies: an individual difference approach using fMRI. *Soc Neurosci* 4: 539–553.

33. Garavan H, Hester R, Murphy KJ, Fassbender C, Kelly C. 2006. Individual differences in the functional neuroanatomy of inhibitory control. *Brain Res* 1105: 130–142.

34. Gates E. 1895. The science of mentation and some new general methods of psychological research. *Monist* 5: 574–597.

35. Gibson JJ. 1979. An Ecological Approach to Visual Perception. Mahwah, NJ: Lauwrence Erlbaum Associates.

36. Gilbert AM, Fiez JA. 2004. Integrating rewards and cognition in the frontal cortex. *Cogn Affect Behav Neurosci* 4: 540–552.

37. Gold JI, Shadlen MN. 2007. The neural basis of decision making. *Annu Rev Neurosci* 30: 535–574.

38. Goschke T, Dreisbach G. 2010. Conflict-triggered goal shielding: response conflicts attenuate background monitoring for prospective memory cues. *Psychol Sci* 19: 25–32.

39. Hallett PE. 1978. Primary and secondary saccades to goals defined by instructions. *Vision Res* 18: 1279–1296.

40. Harsay HA, Buitenweg JIV, Wijnen JG, Guerreiro MJS, Ridderinkhof KR. 2010. Remedial effects of motivational incentive on declining cognitive control in healthy aging and Parkinson's disease. *Front Aging Neurosci* 2: 144.

41. Harsay HA, Cohen MX, Oosterhof NN, Forstmann BU, Mars RB, Ridderinkhof KR (submitted). Functional connectivity of the striatum links motivation to action control in humans.

42. Haruno M, Kawato M. 2006. Different neural correlates of reward expectation and reward expectation error in the putamen and caudate nucleus during stimulus-action reward association learning. *J Neurophysiol* 95: 948–959.

43. Heekeren HR, Marrett S, Ungerleider LG. 2008. The neural systems that mediate human perceptual decision making. *Nat Rev Neurosci* 9: 467–479.

44. Isoda M, Hikosaka O. 2007. Switching from automatic to controlled action by monkey medial frontal cortex. *Nat Neurosci* 10: 240–248.

45. Ivanoff J, Branning P, Marois R. 2008. fMRI evidence for a dual process account of the speed-accuracy tradeoff in decision-making. *PLoS ONE* 3: e2635.

46. Jamadar S, Hughes M, Fulham WR, Michie PT, Karayanidis F. 2010. The spatial and temporal dynamics of anticipatory preparation and response inhibition in task switching. *Neuroimage* 51: 432–449.

47. Jennings JR, Van der Molen MW. 2005. Preparation for speeded action as a psychophysiological concept. *Proc Natl Acad Sci USA* 131: 434–459.

48. Kahnt T, Park SQ, Cohen MX, Beck A, Heinz A, Wrase J. 2009. Dorsal striatal-midbrain connectivity in humans predicts how reinforcements are used to guide decisions. *J Cogn Neurosci* 21: 1332–1345.

49. Karayanidis F, Jamadar S, Ruge H, Phillips N, Heathcote A, Forstmann BU. Advance preparation in task-switching: converging evidence from behavioral, model-based and brain activation approaches. *Front Cogn.* In press.

50. Karayanidis F, Mansfield EL, Galloway KL, Smith J, Provost A, Heathcote A. 2009. Anticipatory reconfiguration elicited by fully and partially informative cues that validly predict a switch in task. *Cogn Affect Behav Neurosci* 9: 202–215.

51. Kawagoe R, Takikawa Y, Hikosaka O. 1998. Expectation of reward modulates cognitive signals in the basal ganglia. *Nat Neurosci* 1: 411–416.

52. Kawagoe R, Takikawa Y, Hikosaka O. 2004. Reward-predicting activity of dopamine and caudate neurons—a possible mechanism of motivational control of saccadic eye movement. *J Neurophysiol* 91: 1013–1024.

53. Kay LM, Beshel J, Martin C. 2006. When good enough is best. *Neuron* 51: 277–278.

54. Kelly AM, Hester R, Foxe JJ, Shpaner M, Garavan H. 2006. Flexible cognitive control: effects of individual differences and brief practice on a complex cognitive task. *Neuroimage* 31: 866–886.

55. Kornblum S, Hasbroucq T, Osman A. 1990. Dimensional overlap: cognitive basis for stimulus response compatibility—a model and taxonomy. *Psychol Rev* 97: 253–270.

56. Kosslyn SM, Cacioppo JT, Davidson RJ, Hugdahl K, Lovallo WR, Spiegel D, Rose R. 2002. Bridging psychology and biology: the analysis of individuals in groups. *Am Psychol* 57: 341–351.

57. Krawczyk DC, Gazzaley A, D'Esposito M. 2007. Reward modulation of prefrontal and visual association cortex during an incentive working memory task. *Brain Res* 1141: 168–177.

58. Kruglanski AW, Shah JY, Fishbach A, Freidman R, Chun WY, Sleeth-Keppler D. 2002. A theory of goal systems. *Adv Exp Soc Psychol* 34: 331–378.

59. Lauwereyns J, Watanabe K, Coe B, Hikosaka O. 2002. A neural correlate of response bias in monkey caudate nucleus. *Nature* 418: 413–417.

60. Leber AB, Turk-Browne NB, Chun MM. 2008. Neural predictors of moment-to-moment fluctuations in cognitive flexibility. *Proc Natl Acad Sci USA* 105: 13592–13597.

61. Leotti LA, Wagner TD. 2010. Motivational influences in response inhibition processes. *J Exp Psychol Hum Percept Perform* 36: 430–447.

62. Lo CC, Wang XJ. 2006. Cortico-basal ganglia circuit mechanism for a decision threshold in reaction time tasks. *Nat Neurosci* 9: 956–963.

63. Locke HS, Braver TS. 2008. Motivational influences on cognitive control: behavior, brain activation, and individual differences. *Cogn Affect Behav Neurosci* 8: 99–112.

64. Luce RD. 1986. Response Times: Their Role in Inferring Elementary Mental Organization. New York: Oxford University Press.

65. Milstein DM, Dorris MC. 2007. The influence of expected value on saccadic preparation. *J Neurosci* 27: 4810–4818.

66. Munoz DP, Everling S. 2004. Look away: the anti-saccade task and the voluntary control of eye movement. *Nat Rev Neurosci* 5: 218–228.

67. Nachev P, Kennard C, Husain M. 2008. Functional role of the supplementary and pre-supplementary motor areas. *Nat Rev Neurosci* 9: 856–869.

68. Opris I, Bruce CJ. 2005. Neural circuitry of judgment and decision mechanisms. *Brain Res* 48: 509–526.

69. Padmala S, Pessoa L. 2010. Interactions between cognition and motivation during response inhibition. *Neuropsychologia* 48: 558–565.

70. Pessiglione M, Schmidt L, Draganski B, Kalisch R, Lau H, Dolan RJ, Frith CD. 2007. How the brain translates money into force: a neuroimaging study of subliminal motivation. *Science* 316: 904–906.

71. Pessoa L. 2009. How do emotion and motivation direct executive control? *Trends Cogn Sci* 13: 160–166.

72. Pochon JB, Levy R, Fossati P, Lehericy S, Poline JB, Pillon B, Le Bihan D, Dubois B. 2002. The neural system that bridges reward and cognition in humans: an fMRI study. *Proc Natl Acad Sci USA* 99: 5669–5674.

73. Rabbitt PMA. 1966. Errors and error correction in choice-response tasks. *J Exp Psychol* 71: 264–272.

74. Ratcliff N, McKoon G. 2008. The diffusion decision model: theory and data for two-choice decision tasks. *Neural Comput* 20: 873–922.

75. Reddi BA, Carpenter RH. 2000. The influence of urgency on decision time. *Nat Neurosci* 3: 827–830.

76. Ridderinkhof KR. 2002. Activation and suppression in conflict tasks: empirical clarification through distributional analyses. In: Attention & Performance XIX: Common Mechanisms in Perception and Action (Prinz W, Hommel B, eds), pp 494–519. Oxford: Oxford University Press.

77. Ridderinkhof KR, Forstmann BU, Wylie SA, Burle B, Van den Wildenberg W. Neurocognitive mechanisms of action control: resisting the call of the Sirens. *WIREs Cogn Sci.* In press.

78. Ridderinkhof KR, Ullsperger M, Crone EA, Nieuwenhuis S. 2004. The role of the medial frontal cortex in cognitive control. *Science* 306: 443–447.

79. Ridderinkhof KR, van den Wildenberg WP, Segalowitz SJ, Carter CS. 2004. Neurocognitive mechanisms of cognitive control: the role of prefrontal cortex in action selection, response inhibition, performance monitoring, and reward-based learning. *Brain Cogn* 56: 129–140.

80. Rogers RD, Monsell S. 1995. Costs of a predictable switch between simple cognitive tasks. *J Exp Psychol Hum Percept Perform* 124: 207–231.

81. Roitman JD, Shadlen MN. 2002. Response of neurons in the lateral intraparietal area during a combined visual discrimination reaction time task. *J Neurosci* 22: 9475–9489.

82. Ruge H, Brass M, Koch I, Rubin O, Meiran N, Von Cramon DY. 2005. Advance preparation and stimulus-induced interference in cued task switching: further insights from BOLD fMRI. *Neuropsychologia* 43: 340–355.

83. Ruge H, Braver T, Meiran N. 2009. Attention, intention, and strategy in preparatory control. *Neuropsychologia* 47: 1670–1685.

84. Savine AC, Beck SM, Edwards BG, Chiew KS, Braver TS. 2010. Enhancement of cognitive control by approach and avoidance motivational states. *Cogn Emotion* 24: 338–356.

85. Schall JD. 2001. Neural basis of deciding, choosing and acting. *Nat Rev Neurosci* 2: 33–42.

86. Schouten JF, Bekker JA. 1967. Reaction time and accuracy. *Acta Psychol (Amst)* 27: 143–153.

87. Schultz W. 2006. Behavioral theories and the neurophysiology of reward. *Annu Rev Psychol* 57: 87–115.

88. Shadlen MN, Newsome WT. 2001. Neural basis of a perceptual decision in the parietal cortex (area LIP) of the rhesus monkey. *J Neurophysiol* 86: 1916–1936.

89. Simões-Franklin C, Hester R, Shpaner M, Foxe JJ, Garavan H. 2010. Executive function and error detection: the effect of motivation on cingulate and ventral striatum activity. *Hum Brain Mapp* 31: 458–469.

90. Simon JR. 1967. Ear preference in a simple reaction-time task. *J Exp Psychol* 75: 49–55.

91. Slagter HA, Weissman DH, Giesbrecht B, Kenemans JL, Mangun GR, Kok A, Woldorff MG. 2006. Brain regions activated by endogenous preparatory set shifting as revealed by fMRI. *Cogn Affect Behav Neurosci* 6: 175–189.

92. Small DM, Gitelman D, Simmons K, Bloise SM, Parrish T, Mesulam MM. 2005. Monetary incentives enhance processing in brain regions mediating top-down control of attention. *Cereb Cortex* 15: 1855–1865.

93. Soukoreff RW, MacKenzie LS. 2009. An informatic rationale for the speed-accuracy tradeoff. In: Proceedings of the IEEE International Conference on Systems, Man, and Cybernetics, pp 2890–2896.

94. Sutton RS, Barto AG. 1998. Reinforcement Learning: An Introduction. Cambridge, MA: MIT Press.

95. Takikawa Y, Kawagoe R, Itoh H, Nakahara H, Hikosaka O. 2002. Modulation of saccadic eye movements by predicted reward outcome. *Exp Brain Res* 142: 284–291.

96. Takikawa Y, Kawagoe R, Itoh H, Nakahara H, Hikosaka O. 2002. Modulation of saccadic eye movements by predicted reward outcome. *Exp Brain Res* 142: 284–291.

97. Taylor SF, Welsh RC, Wagner TD, Phan KL, Fitzgerald KD, Gehring WJ. 2004. A functional neuroimaging study of motivation and executive function. *J Neurosci* 21: 1045–1054.

98. Townsend JT, Ashby FG. 1983. Stochastic Modeling of Elementary Psychological Processes. Cambridge: Cambridge University Press.

99. Tricomi EM, Delgado MR, Fiez JA. 2004. Modulation of caudate activity by action contingency. *Neuron* 41: 281–292.

100. Ullsperger M, Harsay HA, Wessel JR, Ridderinkhof KR. 2010. Conscious perception of errors and its relation to the anterior insula. *Brain Struct Funct* 214: 629–643.

101. Usher M, McClelland JL. 2001. The time course of perceptual choice: the leaky, competing accumulator model. *Psychol Rev* 108: 550–592.

102. Van den Wildenberg WPM, Wylie SA, Forstmann BU, Burle B, Hasbroucq T, Ridderinkhof KR. 2010. To head or to heed: beyond the surface of selective action inhibition. *Front Hum Neurosci* 4: 222.

103. Van Veen V, Krug MK, Carter CS. 2008. The neural and computational basis of controlled speed-accuracy tradeoff during task performance. *J Cogn Neurosci* 20: 1952–1965.

104. Wagenmakers EJ, Ratcliff R, Gomez P, McKoon G. 2008. A diffusion model account of criterion shifts in the lexical decision task. *J Mem Lang* 58: 140–159.

105. Walton ME, Kennerley SW, Bannerman DM, Phillips PE, Rushworth MF. 2006. Weighing up the benefits of work: behavioral and neural analyses of effort-related decision making. *Neural Netw* 19: 1302–1314.

106. Watanabe K, Hikosaka O. 2005. Immediate changes in anticipatory activity of caudate neurons associated with reversal of position-reward contingency. *J Neurophysiol* 94: 1879–1887.

107. Wickelgren WA. 1977. Speed-accuracy tradeoff and information processing dynamics. *Acta Psychol (Amst)* 41: 67–85.

108. Wylie GR, Javitt DC, Foxe JJ. 2006. Jumping the gun: Is effective preparation contingent upon anticipatory activation in task-relevant neural circuitry? *Cereb Cortex* 16: 394–404.

109. Wylie SA, van den Wildenberg WP, Ridderinkhof KR, Bashore TR, Powell VD, Manning CA, Wooten GF. 2009. The effect of Parkinson's disease on interference control during action selection. *Neuropsychologia* 47: 145–157.

110. Yeung N, Nystrom LE, Aronson JA, Cohen JD. 2006. Between-task competition and cognitive control in task switching. *J Neurosci* 26: 1429–1438.

15 Pathological Changes in Performance Monitoring

Ellen R. A. de Bruijn and Markus Ullsperger

Monitoring for deviations of action outcomes from the intended goals and detecting situations requiring adjustments in cognitive control are essential for adaptive, goal-directed behavior. Research in the last two decades has accumulated a large body of evidence on the function of the performance-monitoring system and the implementation of cognitive control in the human brain. The discovery of error-related negativity (ERN) in the early 1990s[32,40] opened a window onto performance-monitoring processes that has been successfully used in healthy participants as well as in patient groups. The ERN is assumed to be generated in the rostral cingulate zone (RCZ; largely overlapping with the dorsal anterior cingulate cortex, ACC) of the posterior medial frontal cortex (pMFC),[22] a region consistently found to be activated in functional neuroimaging of performance monitoring.[89] Current models suggest this region monitors for information that requires an update in action values, to indicate the need for adjustments in other brain regions and be involved in the recruitment of the necessary effort.[89] Errors and unfavorable action outcomes are common sources of updates in action values that require compensatory actions to remedy the failure and/or adjustments to avoid similar problems in the future. Response conflict, that is, the concurrent initiation of competing response tendencies, and decision uncertainty indicate increased likelihood of failure, and thus also call for adjustments and additional recruitment of effort.

Neuroimaging and patient work has revealed that the pMFC is integrated within a complex network of cortical and subcortical structures, many of which are targets of terminals releasing neuromodulators such as dopamine[111] (figure 15.1). Diseases interfering with the integrity of this network affect performance-monitoring functions, leading to varying degrees of impairment in cognitive control, flexibility, and decision making. In this chapter we review impairments of performance-monitoring functions in selected neurological and psychiatric diseases, discuss the impact of these studies on the current understanding of cognitive control and the pathophysiology of the respective disorders, consider the advantages and limitations of studies in clinical groups, and raise questions for ongoing and future research in this field.

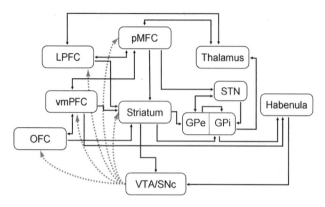

Figure 15.1
Simplified schematic of brain structures involved in performance monitoring and their connectivity. pMFC, posterior medial frontal cortex; LPFC, lateral prefrontal cortex; OFC, orbitofrontal cortex; vmPFC, ventromedial prefrontal cortex; STN, subthalamic nucleus; GPe/GPi, globus pallidus externus/internus; VTA, ventral tegmental area; SNc, substantia nigra pars compacta. Black arrows = information flow (excitatory or inhibitory connections); dashed arrows = dopaminergic axons.

Diagnostics of Performance-Monitoring Impairments

At the single-patient level, no standardized neuropsychological tests specifically tackling performance monitoring are currently available. In group studies in clinical populations, however, a number of behavioral, electrophysiological, and neuroimaging measures have been used that may become the basis of more standardized tests. Classically, speeded choice reaction time tasks (e.g., Stroop, Simon, Eriksen flanker, Go/No-Go tasks) involving interference or the need to overcome prepotent response tendencies have been used to elicit the ERN and to test for post-error adjustments. Moreover, probabilistic learning tasks, reversal learning tasks, and variants of task switching have been used to study flexible adjustments in action selection and learning from feedback. Learning, gambling, and time estimation tasks are well suited to elicit the feedback-related negativity (FRN),[75] a negative deflection typically observed after losses and negative feedback[43] that shares topographical and functional features with the ERN[54] and seems to stem from the same source network.[44] Test-retest reliability of the ERN is rather high, suggesting suitability for repeated measurements in longitudinal studies.[96] The interpretation of ERN amplitude changes associated with clinical conditions may be complicated by concurrent changes in the negative deflection occurring on correct trials at the same response-locked latency, the correct-related negativity (CRN).[35,121] In several patient groups, the CRN amplitude is increased while the ERN amplitude is reduced or unchanged, resulting in a net decrease in the difference of ERP amplitudes for correct and incorrect responses.[42]

At the behavioral level, error correction, error detection/signaling, and posterror slowing are the most widely investigated measures. Error correction does not necessarily require error detection and may thus not be sufficiently sensitive to uncover subtle impairments in performance monitoring.[111,114] Testing conscious error detection raises higher demands on patient cooperation,[112] but simple error signaling may be a good compromise.[111,114] Posterror slowing (PES) has often been interpreted as reflecting adaptation toward a more cautious response mode, allowing improved accuracy in trials subsequent to errors.[89] However, as PES is not necessarily coupled with reduced error likelihood on posterror trials, this view has been challenged.[80] Rather than being a task-specific adjustment, it might reflect a general motor inhibition process[63,113] associated with an orienting response to the salient event of making an error.[80] Therefore, additional forms of adjustments, such as task-specific posterror attentional focusing as reflected in increases in accuracy and/or decreases in interference effects on trials subsequent to errors, may be needed for a complete diagnostic picture.

Performance Monitoring in Patients with Neurological Diseases

Circumscribed Lesions

Ischemic stroke, hemorrhages, tumor excision, vascular malformations, and, to some extent, traumatic brain injury are common causes of circumscribed brain lesions that specifically affect certain areas. Investigating patients suffering from such lesions is an important source of evidence on the necessity of brain structures in cognitive functions. Some limitations of these studies should be considered, however. Most studies are performed in a chronic stage such that compensatory mechanisms are likely to have occurred, and thus no deficits might be found despite an essential role of the lesioned brain structure. Moreover, unilateral lesions may be compensated for by the contralateral side. In contrast, behavioral deficits or changes in neural correlates of performance monitoring provide valuable information on the underlying network. When interpreting the data, connectivities and models need to be taken into account, as some changes in performance monitoring may result from disturbances in upstream processes.[125]

Cortical Lesions

Based on neuroimaging, source localization, and animal studies, the pMFC has been suggested to be essential for performance monitoring and the main generator of the ERN. Isolated, circumscribed lesions of the pMFC, in particular of the ACC, are rare, rendering tests of this region's necessity difficult. Moreover, impairments subsequent to pMFC lesions may be transient and can disappear in chronic stages.[15]

Nevertheless, a series of studies in patients with unilateral focal lesions of the RCZ revealed varying degrees of impairments in posterror and conflict-driven adaptations, accompanied by a reduction of the ERN to the level of the CRN.[24,104–106] In contrast, work by Fellows and colleagues failed to find unequivocal evidence for the necessity of this region in error- and conflict-induced performance adjustments,[33] but demonstrated slowed error corrections in a flanker task.[76] Notably, fast error corrections result from concomitant activation and sequential execution of the incorrect and correct responses.[100,114] Taking into account recent findings that transcranial magnetic stimulation of the presupplementary motor area (pre-SMA) affects processing of competing response tendencies,[107] these findings suggest that lesions in the pMFC interfere with the solution of response conflict. Interestingly, increased false alarm rates in a two-back task were associated with higher subjective confidence in action selection in patients with pMFC lesions,[108] which seems to fit with findings in nonhuman primates with sulcal ACC lesions, suggesting higher impulsivity and less influence of reinforcement history on choice behavior.[60] Taken together, the pMFC appears to be necessary for rapid online adjustments, evaluation of confidence with choice, and between-trial adjustments. Its exact causal role in posterror slowing, attentional focusing, and learning from errors needs to be addressed in the future.

Lesions of the more rostral ACC have been shown to be associated with strongly reduced ERN amplitudes.[102] Consistent with this, patients with lesions of the posterior orbitofrontal cortex (OFC) extending into the subgenual ACC and the ventromedial prefrontal cortex showed severe attenuation of the ERN and error corrections.[110] More anterior OFC and frontopolar lesions did not interfere with performance and ERN generation in a flanker task.[116]

The lateral prefrontal cortex (LPFC) has been implicated in maintaining and updating task representation, goals, and contextual information[8] and in exerting top-down control in mutual interaction with the pMFC.[62,68] Its necessity for performance monitoring is strongly suggested by the fact that ERN generation is impaired in patients with LPFC lesions: no difference in amplitude was found between the waveforms for correct and incorrect responses.[42,115,116] Whereas posterror slowing appeared unaffected, in some patients error corrections were diminished.[42,115] A detailed lesion analysis suggested that error correction was impaired when white matter tracts connecting the LPFC and pMFC to the striatum were disrupted.[115] The strategic importance of the frontal white matter at the base of the middle and inferior frontal gyri was further demonstrated in patients with isolated lesions in that area.[51]

Importantly, even extensive temporal lesions do not seem to affect error monitoring and the generation of the ERN in a flanker task,[116] thereby emphasizing the specificity of the ERN changes for pathologies of the performance monitoring network.

Subcortical Lesions

Both pMFC and LPFC are parts of cortico-striato-thalamic circuits that appear to interact at several levels.[47] Similar to LPFC lesions, focal damage in the striatum disrupts the generation of the ERN.[115] Studies in nonhuman primates suggest that the RCZ receives inputs from the basal ganglia circuitry mostly via the ventral anterior (VA) and ventrolateral anterior (VLa) nuclei of the thalamus.[50,118] This thalamic region also integrates cerebellar circuitries assumed to be involved in motor control.[56] In addition to the VA/VLa nuclei, the mediodorsal thalamus sends ascending fibers to the pMFC.[122] In accordance with these anatomical findings, thalamic lesions impair error signaling and reduce the amplitude of the ERN.[97] When the VA/VLa region is affected, the ERN is completely abolished, suggesting a particularly prominent role of these thalamic nuclei.

Degenerative Diseases of the Basal Ganglia

Parkinson's disease (PD) is characterized by a loss in dopaminergic neurons that, in early stages, leads to a rather selective loss of dopamine (DA) in the dorsal striatum, whereas dopaminergic innervation is preserved longer in the ventral striatum and frontal cortex. This results in an imbalance, reflected in a suboptimal level of DA in dorsal striatum in the unmedicated state or a supraoptimal level of DA in ventral striatum and cortex in the medicated state.[17] As DA appears to be an essential neuromodulator in performance monitoring and adaptation,[58] PD is an interesting model disease for understanding performance monitoring. Indeed, PD patients quite consistently display reduced ERN amplitudes[31,101,124] (but see ref. 55). Surprisingly, no significant effects of medication on the ERN have been observed. While in some studies this may result from incomplete washout of direct DA agonists with long half-lives, it may also hint at a less direct role of DA in generating the ERN than was previously suggested[54] (see also ref. 58). Less is known about the FRN in PD, although behavioral studies show an imbalance of preference versus avoidance learning depending on whether or not the patients are medicated.[36,37] Generally, the FRN might be affected later than the ERN because the ventral striatum, relevant for reward processing, seems to be affected by dopamine depletion only at more severe stages of PD.[17,18] Furthermore, posterror slowing can be hypothesized to be modulated by PD and deep brain stimulation (DBS) in the subthalamic nucleus.[36]

Huntington's disease (HD) is an autosomal dominant neurogenetic disorder characterized by striatal degeneration. In HD patients a consistent reduction of the ERN was found that was related to the genetic mutation (number of CAG repeats) and the reduction of gray matter volume in pMFC.[6,7]

Performance Monitoring in Patients with Psychiatric Diseases

As stated in the introduction of this chapter, continuously monitoring ongoing behavior for possible deviations of action outcomes facilitates flexible online adjustments and learning in goal-directed behavior. Importantly, different psychiatric disorders are characterized by repetitive and inflexible behavioral patterns or a reduced sensitivity to negative feedback for improving performance. These deviant behaviors suggest problems or deficits in performance monitoring and have thus boosted research on these processes in a variety of psychiatric disorders. Following is an overview of the most studied disorders and interesting recent developments in this rapidly expanding research domain.

Obsessive-Compulsive Disorder

Obsessive-compulsive disorder (OCD) was one of the first psychiatric disorders in which possible disturbances in performance monitoring were investigated. Patients with OCD are characterized by repetitive behaviors aimed at neutralizing intrusive thoughts that elicit stress and fear. People with OCD often report feeling that an action was not performed well or incomplete and another action is needed to compensate.[2] These symptoms were arguments for Pitman to presume possible deficits in error-detection processes.[86] He proposed that error signals resulting from an internal comparator mechanism are increased in patients with OCD. These error signals trigger a need for corrective behavior, but complex compulsions can develop when the error signals remain active; thus the adaptive behavior turns out to be repeatedly inadequate. With the discovery of the ERN in the early 1990s, an electrophysiological correlate of these error signals became available to test Pitman's rationale. Also, neuroimaging studies provided support for the involvement of central performance-monitoring brain areas in OCD by showing excessive ACC activation related to the severity of OCD symptoms[90] and abnormal metabolic activity in the pMFC.[45]

The first study to investigate performance monitoring in OCD patients, conducted by Gehring and colleagues,[41] supported Pitman's hypothesis by demonstrating increased ERN amplitudes in the patient group. Over the past 10 years, this initial finding of increased ERN amplitudes in OCD has been replicated by different research groups using various experimental paradigms.[29,30,59,103] Additionally, functional magnetic resonance imaging (fMRI) demonstrated error-related hyperactivity in pMFC areas.[34,69] Increased ERNs have also been demonstrated in healthy volunteers scoring high on OCD symptoms.[46,48] Along with increased ERNs, the CRN amplitude may be enhanced in both nonpatient groups[48] and OCD patients,[29,30] suggesting that OCD is related to excessive monitoring not only on errors, but also on correct trials. This suggestion was further supported by increased pMFC activations on correct high-response conflict trials in OCD patients.[117]

Interestingly, increased error signals have been linked to better learning performance related to avoiding maladaptive behavior in healthy volunteers.[54,64] At first sight, the hyperactive performance-monitoring system found in OCD should thus actually be associated with improved learning and less maladaptive behavior. As Gründler and colleagues[46] rightfully point out, however, the compulsive behaviors associated with OCD are in sharp contrast to any assumed better learning performance. They investigated this intriguing contrast between hyperactive performance monitoring and maladaptive behavior in OCD by directly comparing performance monitoring on two different tasks. As expected from previous work, they found OCD symptoms in nonpatients to be *positively* correlated with ERN amplitude on a standard speeded choice-reaction time task. However, subjects with higher OCD symptom scores had *reduced* ERN amplitudes on a probabilistic-learning paradigm. A later EEG source localization study additionally demonstrated dorsal ACC and ventral ACC activations on the same paradigms to be differently related to OCD symptoms.[12] The authors concluded that obsessive-compulsive symptoms may be dissociated in these neural systems, with hypoactivity in dorsomedial systems that enable learning to avoid maladaptive choices, and hyperactivity in ventromedial systems that enable the same behavior to be repeated and are thus sensitive to maladaptive responses.

Finally, high-frequency DBS can be successful in reducing OCD symptoms in patients unresponsive to pharmacological or any other forms of treatment. The electrodes used for stimulation are usually implanted in the anterior capsula interna or nucleus accumbens.[23,81] A positron emission tomographic (PET) study in six OCD patients that underwent DBS showed that activation differences in rostral ACC was the best predictor for symptom decrease.[119] Interestingly, this area shows a remarkable overlap with the rostral ACC area found to be hyperactive in OCD patients during error trials in previous performance-monitoring research.[34] This might indicate a DBS-induced stabilization of the previously hyperactive performance-monitoring network in these patients. However, evidence for this idea from studies directly comparing these two activation patterns is still missing.

Schizophrenia

Schizophrenia has also received a lot of attention in performance-monitoring research over the past years. One of the authoritative theories on schizophrenia proposes a deficient self-monitoring system as responsible for the positive symptoms often seen in this disorder.[39] This has led to the assumption that patients with schizophrenia may also have problems in performance monitoring. Moreover, an imbalance in frontal and subcortical DA levels has often been reported and both altered pMFC activations and reduced baseline cerebral blood flow have been found.[26,73]

An ERP study by Kopp and Rist[65] showed reduced ERNs in schizophrenia patients, a finding that has been replicated repeatedly in various experimental tasks.[1,4,5,70,77] Along with reduced ERNs, increased CRNs were reported in a number of studies,[35,70,77] but these CRN effects seem not as robust as the ERN findings and more task dependent. In a reinforcement-learning task in schizophrenia patients, both ERN and FRN amplitudes were reduced, suggesting a diminished sensitivity to whether ongoing events are better or worse than expected.[77] Finally, different fMRI studies have also provided evidence of diminished pMFC responses to errors in schizophrenia patients[11,61,67,87] (but see ref. 71).

The question of whether attenuated ERNs reflect state or trait characteristics of the disorder was addressed in a study by Bates and colleagues.[5] The findings demonstrated an increase in ERN amplitude after 6 weeks of treatment with antipsychotics (but see ref. 57). However, despite this increase, ERN amplitudes in the patient group remained reduced compared to healthy controls. So, although ERN amplitude may be modulated by clinical state in schizophrenia, this study suggests that the repeatedly reported reductions in ERN amplitude may reflect an important trait characteristic of schizophrenia. This trait assumption was also supported by the outcomes of a recent study that demonstrated decreased ERN amplitudes even in 9- to 12-year-old children with putative antecedents of schizophrenia.[66]

In sum, it seems appealing to conclude that reduced ERNs may be a useful trait marker for schizophrenia.[5] However, caution is warranted, as it should be noted that ERN reductions are not restricted to schizophrenia and thus far from disorder specific. Attenuated ERNs have, for example, also been demonstrated in borderline personality disorder.[20]

Major Depressive Disorder

Major depressive disorder (MDD) has received increased attention over the past years in performance-monitoring research. It is a common psychiatric disorder characterized by disturbances of mood and affect, but also by a distinct pattern of cognitive, psychomotor, and executive function. Functional imaging studies have demonstrated altered rostral ACC activation in patients with a major depressive episode relative to healthy controls.[3,27,28,72]

In contrast to the findings in OCD and schizophrenia, the results from studies on MDD are less straightforward. Increased performance monitoring and associated brain potentials have been demonstrated in different studies.[13,52,53,109] Parallel to this research, work from Schrijvers and colleagues reported unchanged ERN amplitudes in a severely depressed sample and a clear association between the degree of psychomotor retardation and the level of ERN attenuation.[92,93] The main difference between these two seemingly contradictory findings seems to be related to the nature of the population. Increased error-related brain activations are generally found in patients with mild to moderate depression, whereas more severely depressed patients show unchanged or reduced activations. In line with this, a recent study reported reduced ERNs only for a severely depressed subpopulation of patients.[83]

A possible explanation for these findings is that in mild to moderate depressed patients, heightened levels of anxiety or perfectionism may result in increased error-related activity, while in severely depressed patients the effects of these increased levels may be dampened by the substantial depressive symptoms.[92,93] Also, affective temperament styles and trait features such as negative affect, anxiety, and perfectionism have been documented to enhance ERN amplitudes or ACC activity in nonclinical subjects.[16,82,85] Recent findings supported this explanation by showing that individual differences in error-related brain activations within a group of severely depressed patients were best explained by differences in levels of perfectionism.[94]

At a more general level, the influence of symptoms like anxiety and perfectionism on error-related brain activations highlights the central role these traits play in the involved processes. This was also recently illustrated in a study on error monitoring in alcohol-dependent patients.[91] Whereas drug dependency has previously been linked to reduced performance monitoring and smaller ERN amplitudes,[38,99] the results from the alcohol-dependent patients showed an opposite pattern, that is, larger ERN amplitudes than controls. However, the unexpected finding of increased performance monitoring was driven by heightened levels of anxiety in the dependent patient group: Patients with relatively low levels of anxiety did not show this increase and were comparable to controls.[91] Many psychiatric patient populations are heterogenic and are characterized by individual differences in symptomatology. For example, two different patients with the same diagnosis major depression can have only one overlapping symptom.[2] Identifying these different symptoms and the effects they have on performance-monitoring processes and involved brain structures is thus critical in studying psychiatric disorders. Importantly, a symptom-driven rather than a syndrome-driven approach takes existing individual differences into account and may thus prevent incorrect generalizations.

Psychopathy

Individuals with psychopathy form a particularly interesting population for the investigation of performance monitoring and adaptive behavioral control. Along with the prominent affective problems such as lack of empathy and experiencing no feelings of guilt and remorse, psychopaths are characterized by an inability to adjust behavior following adverse events.[49] This inability is most evident in the repetitive behavioral patterns and the low responsiveness to different forms of treatment. Indeed, previous behavioral work already demonstrated problems in unlearning previously learned associations and a specific problematic response to negative events.[10] Initial ERP research on the relation between error monitoring and psychopathy focused on healthy individuals scoring low on concepts related to psychopathy like socialization[25] and showed that low-scoring individuals had reduced ERN amplitudes, but only in a punishment condition.

More recently, with the introduction of dedicated ERP labs inside forensic psychiatric institutes, performance-monitoring research on incarcerated individuals diagnosed with psychopathy has received an important boost. So far, two studies have demonstrated that psychopaths actually show normal early automatic error processing in a neutral context as reflected by similar ERN amplitudes compared to matched healthy volunteers.[9,78] Munro et al. additionally demonstrated that patients did show reduced monitoring to emotional face stimuli compared to neutral letter stimuli, suggesting that their error-monitoring problems may be especially pronounced in contexts that place a demand on social and emotional processing.

In the study by Brazil and colleagues,[9] a separate condition was introduced in which participants had to signal their erroneous responses by a second button press. The results showed that patients signaled less errors and displayed specific impairments in later, more controlled error-monitoring processes as reflected in reduced error-related positivities (Pe). As the Pe has been linked to more conscious aspects of error processing,[84] the authors concluded that early automatic processing of one's own errors is intact in psychopathic individuals, but the problems arise when they have to consciously use this error information to adapt their behavior. These error-monitoring deficiencies may thus explain why psychopaths have so much difficulty in changing their persistent behavioral patterns.

Indeed, outcomes of a recent study supported this interpretation by showing that individuals with psychopathy learned stimulus-response mappings slower than healthy controls in a reinforcement-learning paradigm.[123] Importantly, the FRN following negative feedback was similar for both the healthy volunteer group as the group with psychopathic individuals. These comparable FRNs were, however, accompanied by reduced ERN amplitudes following incorrect responses for the psychopaths. These findings show that the psychopathic individuals process negative feedback adequately at the neural level, but they have problems in using this error information to learn the correct stimulus-response mappings. As a result, the error cannot effectively be detected at the moment of response and thus response ERNs are reduced.

Obviously, the problems that individuals with psychopathy display are most prominent during social interactions. Effective social interactions, importantly, not only rely on continuous monitoring of one's own actions, but also require monitoring of the actions of the person one is interacting with. Moreover, one needs to adequately and flexibly adjust one's own actions in response to detected errors made by oneself and the other. Recent social neuroscientific research in healthy volunteers has revealed an interesting overlap between performance-monitoring processes in social and in individual settings. For example, an ERN is also elicited when people observe another person making an error[74,120] and participants also show posterror slowing in response to these observed errors.[21,95] These findings suggest involvement of similar brain areas and, indeed, fMRI studies demonstrated pMFC to be significantly more activated for own and observed errors compared to correct actions.[19,98] These recent developments create important new research opportunities within cognitive neuropsychiatry. Many psychiatric disorders are characterized by shallow social interactions or deviant social behavior. Not only does this hold for psychopathy, autism, and schizophrenia, but also for less obvious disorders such as depression and borderline personality. Therefore, investigating these disorders from a social neuroscientific perspective may add significantly to our understanding of disease-related changes in performance monitoring.

Outlook

In sum, the ERN and FRN in combination with behavioral markers of posterror adjustments provide a valuable tool that taps into the function of the performance-monitoring system. Compared to pathological changes of the ERN, the FRN and posterror behavior remain relatively understudied to this date. A complete understanding of possible disturbed performance monitoring requires investigations that include feedback processing and behavioral adjustments as well. Another important goal for the future is to standardize the recording of the ERN such that it can be used for individual diagnostic purposes. Related to this, a symptom-driven approach, rather than a syndrome-driven approach takes individual differences better into account. As a result, incorrect generalizations in often large heterogenic psychiatric patient groups can be better prevented and may thus give us a more refined picture of the various performance deficits in different psychiatric disorders. A focus on symptoms may additionally provide a more reliable reference point for employing the ERN as a biological marker, which may aid future individual diagnostics.

The recent developments in DBS therapy and invasive epilepsy diagnostics have opened a new avenue for performance-monitoring research that allows addressing functional interactions between cortical and subcortical structures. Two approaches are being exploited: (1) Intraoperatively, when—with externalized stimulation cables—the target structures become briefly available for direct electrophysiological recordings.[14,79,88] Simultaneous acquisition of surface electroencephalographic (EEG) and electrical activity from subcortical structures allow to assess the timing of functional interactions. (2) In patients treated with DBS the effect of high-frequency stimulation on performance monitoring can be tested by comparing behavioral measures, EEG, and PET on and off stimulation.

Finally, a social neuroscientific approach in studying pathological changes in performance monitoring will improve our insight in the social impairments known to seriously decrease the quality of life of patients suffering from varying diseases. In this regard, especially the emerging research domain of social cognitive neuropsychiatry may thus crucially advance our understanding of these often still poorly understood psychiatric disorders.

Outstanding Questions

• What trait marker do changes in ERN and FRN reflect? How are pathological symptoms related to this marker across the different psychiatric disorders?

• How do common therapeutic interventions influence performance monitoring?

• What is the relationship between performance monitoring and self-control in social settings, and thus in social interactions?

Further Reading

Gehring WJ, Knight RT. 2000. Prefrontal-cingulate interactions in action monitoring. *Nat Neurosci* 3:516–520. One of the first patient studies investigating the effects of remote focal prefrontal lesions on the generation of the error-related negativity in the posterior medial frontal cortex and on performance monitoring in general.

Ridderinkhof KR, Ullsperger M, Crone EA, Nieuwenhuis S. 2004 The role of the medial frontal cortex in cognitive control. *Science* 306:443–447. Review article discussing theories on the function of the posterior medial frontal cortex in performance monitoring with a specific focus on neuroimaging in healthy participants.

References

1. Alain C, McNeely HE, He Y, Christensen BK, West R. 2002. Neurophysiological evidence of error-monitoring deficits in patients with schizophrenia. *Cereb Cortex* 12: 840–846.

2. American Psychiatric Association. 2000. DSM-IV-TR: Diagnostic and Statistical Manual of Mental Disorders. Arlington, VA: American Psychiatric Publishing.

3. Anand A, Li Y, Wang Y, Wu J, Gao S, Bukhari L, Mathews VP, Kalnin A, Lowe MJ. 2005. Activity and connectivity of brain mood regulating circuit in depression: a functional magnetic resonance study. *Biol Psychiatry* 57: 1079–1088.

4. Bates AT, Kiehl KA, Laurens KR, Liddle PF. 2002. Error-related negativity and correct response negativity in schizophrenia. *Clin Neurophysiol* 113: 1454–1463.

5. Bates AT, Liddle PF, Kiehl KA, Ngan ET. 2004. State dependent changes in error monitoring in schizophrenia. *J Psychiatr Res* 38: 347–356.

6. Beste C, Saft C, Andrich J, Gold R, Falkenstein M. 2006. Error processing in Huntington's disease. *PLoS ONE* 1: e86.

7. Beste C, Saft C, Konrad C, Andrich J, Habbel A, Schepers I, Jansen A, Pfleiderer B, Falkenstein M. 2008. Levels of error processing in Huntington's disease: a combined study using event-related potentials and voxel-based morphometry. *Hum Brain Mapp* 29: 121–130.

8. Brass M, Derrfuss J, Forstmann B, Cramon DY. 2005. The role of the inferior frontal junction area in cognitive control. *Trends Cogn Sci* 9: 314–316.

9. Brazil IA, de Bruijn ER, Bulten BH, von Borries AK, van Lankveld JJ, Buitelaar JK, Verkes RJ. 2009. Early and late components of error monitoring in violent offenders with psychopathy. *Biol Psychiatry* 65: 137–143.

10. Budhani S, Richell RA, Blair RJ. 2006. Impaired reversal but intact acquisition: probabilistic response reversal deficits in adult individuals with psychopathy. *J Abnorm Psychol* 115: 552–558.

11. Carter CS, MacDonald AW, Ross LL, Stenger VA. 2001. Anterior cingulate cortex activity and impaired self-monitoring of performance in patients with schizophrenia: an event-related fMRI study. *Am J Psychiatry* 158: 1423–1428.

12. Cavanagh JF, Gründler TO, Frank MJ, Allen JJ. 2010. Altered cingulate sub-region activation accounts for task-related dissociation in ERN amplitude as a function of obsessive-compulsive symptoms. *Neuropsychologia* 48: 2098–2109.

13. Chiu PH, Deldin PJ. 2007. Neural evidence for enhanced error detection in major depressive disorder. *Am J Psychiatry* 164: 608–616.

14. Cohen MX, Axmacher N, Lenartz D, Elger CE, Sturm V, Schlaepfer TE. 2009. Nuclei accumbens phase synchrony predicts decision-making reversals following negative feedback. *J Neurosci* 29: 7591–7598.

15. Cohen RA, Kaplan RF, Moser DJ, Jenkins MA, Wilkinson H. 1999. Impairments of attention after cingulotomy. *Neurology* 53: 819–824.

16. Compton RJ, Carp J, Chaddock L, Fineman SL, Quandt LC, Ratliff JB. 2007. Anxiety and error monitoring: increased error sensitivity or altered expectations? *Brain Cogn* 64: 247–256.

17. Cools R. 2008. Role of dopamine in the motivational and cognitive control of behavior. *Neuroscientist* 14: 381–395.

18. Cools R, Barker RA, Sahakian BJ, Robbins TW. 2001. Enhanced or impaired cognitive function in Parkinson's disease as a function of dopaminergic medication and task demands. *Cereb Cortex* 11: 1136–1143.

19. De Bruijn ER, De Lange FP, von Cramon DY, Ullsperger M. 2009. When errors are rewarding. *J Neurosci* 29: 12183–12186.

20. De Bruijn ER, Grootens KP, Verkes RJ, Buchholz V, Hummelen JW, Hulstijn W. 2006. Neural correlates of impulsive responding in borderline personality disorder: ERP evidence for reduced action monitoring. *J Psychiatr Res* 40: 428–437.

21. De Bruijn ERA, Mars RB, Bekkering H, Coles MGH. Your mistake is my mistake... or is it? Behavioral adjustments following own and observed actions in cooperative and competitive contexts. *Q J Exp Psychol*. In press.

22. Debener S, Ullsperger M, Siegel M, Fiehler K, von Cramon DY, Engel AK. 2005. Trial-by-trial coupling of concurrent electroencephalogram and functional magnetic resonance imaging identifies the dynamics of performance monitoring. *J Neurosci* 25: 11730–11737.

23. Denys D, Mantione M, Figee M, van den Munckhof P, Koerselman F, Westenberg H, Bosch A, Schuurman R. 2010. Deep brain stimulation of the nucleus accumbens for treatment-refractory obsessive-compulsive disorder. *Arch Gen Psychiatry* 67: 1061–1068.

24. Di Pellegrino G, Ciaramelli E, Ladavas E. 2007. The regulation of cognitive control following rostral anterior cingulate cortex lesion in humans. *J Cogn Neurosci* 19: 275–286.

25. Dikman ZV, Allen JJ. 2000. Error monitoring during reward and avoidance learning in high- and low-socialized individuals. *Psychophysiology* 37: 43–54.

26. Dolan RJ, Fletcher P, Frith CD, Friston KJ, Frackowiak RS, Grasby PM. 1995. Dopaminergic modulation of impaired cognitive activation in the anterior cingulate cortex in schizophrenia. *Nature* 378: 180–182.

27. Drevets WC. 2000. Neuroimaging studies of mood disorders. *Biol Psychiatry* 48: 813–829.

28. Drevets WC, Price JL, Simpson J, Jr, Todd RD, Reich T, Vannier M, Raichle ME. 1997. Subgenual prefrontal cortex abnormalities in mood disorders. *Nature* 386: 824–827.

29. Endrass T, Klawohn J, Schuster F, Kathmann N. 2008. Overactive performance monitoring in obsessive-compulsive disorder: ERP evidence from correct and erroneous reactions. *Neuropsychologia* 46: 1877–1887.

30. Endrass T, Schuermann B, Kaufmann C, Spielberg R, Kniesche R, Kathmann N. 2010. Performance monitoring and error significance in patients with obsessive-compulsive disorder. *Biol Psychol* 84: 257–263.

31. Falkenstein M, Hielscher H, Dziobek I, Schwarzenau P, Hoormann J, Sunderman B, Hohnsbein J. 2001. Action monitoring, error detection, and the basal ganglia: an ERP study. *Neuroreport* 12: 157–161.

32. Falkenstein M, Hohnsbein J, Hoormann J, Blanke L. 1990. Effects of errors in choice reaction tasks on the ERP under focused and divided attention. In: Psychophysiological Brain Research (Brunia CHM, Gaillard AWK, Kok A, eds), pp 192–195. Tilburg: Tilburg University Press.

33. Fellows LK, Farah MJ. 2005. Is anterior cingulate cortex necessary for cognitive control? *Brain* 128: 788–796.

34. Fitzgerald KD, Welsh RC, Gehring WJ, Abelson JL, Himle JA, Liberzon I, Taylor SF. 2005. Error-related hyperactivity of the anterior cingulate cortex in obsessive-compulsive disorder. *Biol Psychiatry* 57: 287–294.

35. Ford JM. 1999. Schizophrenia: the broken P300 and beyond. *Psychophysiology* 36: 667–682.

36. Frank MJ, Samanta J, Moustafa AA, Sherman SJ. 2007. Hold your horses: impulsivity, deep brain stimulation, and medication in parkinsonism. *Science* 318: 1309–1312.

37. Frank MJ, Seeberger LC, O'Reilly RC. 2004. By carrot or by stick: cognitive reinforcement learning in Parkinsonism. *Science* 306: 1940–1943.

38. Franken IH, van Strien JW, Franzek EJ, van de Wetering BJ. 2007. Error-processing deficits in patients with cocaine dependence. *Biol Psychol* 75: 45–51.

39. Frith CD. 1987. The positive and negative symptoms of schizophrenia reflect impairments in the perception and initiation of action. *Psychol Med* 17: 631–648.

40. Gehring WJ, Goss B, Coles MG, Meyer DE, Donchin E. 1993. A neural system for error detection and compensation. *Psychol Sci* 4: 385–390.

41. Gehring WJ, Himle J, Nisenson LG. 2000. Action-monitoring dysfunction in obsessive-compulsive disorder. *Psychol Sci* 11: 1–6.

42. Gehring WJ, Knight RT. 2000. Prefrontal-cingulate interactions in action monitoring. *Nat Neurosci* 3: 516–520.

43. Gehring WJ, Willoughby AR. 2002. The medial frontal cortex and the rapid processing of monetary gains and losses. *Science* 295: 2279–2282.

44. Gentsch A, Ullsperger P, Ullsperger M. 2009. Dissociable medial frontal negativities from a common monitoring system for self- and externally caused failure of goal achievement. *Neuroimage* 47: 2023–2030.

45. Graybiel AM, Rauch SL. 2000. Toward a neurobiology of obsessive-compulsive disorder. *Neuron* 28: 343–347.

46. Gründler TO, Cavanagh JF, Figueroa CM, Frank MJ, Allen JJ. 2009. Task-related dissociation in ERN amplitude as a function of obsessive-compulsive symptoms. *Neuropsychologia* 47: 1978–1987.

47. Haber S. 2003. The primate basal ganglia: parallel and integrative networks. *J Chem Neuroanat* 26: 317–330.

48. Hajcak G, Simons RF. 2002. Error-related brain activity in obsessive-compulsive undergraduates. *Psychiatry Res* 110: 63–72.

49. Hare RD, Hart SD, Harpur TJ. 1991. Psychopathy and the DSM-IV criteria for antisocial personality disorder. *J Abnorm Psychol* 100: 391–398.

50. Hatanaka N, Tokuno H, Hamada I, Inase M, Ito Y, Imanishi M, Hasegawa N, Akazawa T, Nambu A, Takada M. 2003. Thalamocortical and intracortical connections of monkey cingulate motor areas. *J Comp Neurol* 462: 121–138.

51. Hogan AM, Vargha-Khadem F, Saunders DE, Kirkham FJ, Baldeweg T. 2006. Impact of frontal white matter lesions on performance monitoring: ERP evidence for cortical disconnection. *Brain* 129: 2177–2188.

52. Holmes AJ, Pizzagalli DA. 2008. Spatiotemporal dynamics of error processing dysfunctions in major depressive disorder. *Arch Gen Psychiatry* 65: 179–188.

53. Holmes AJ, Pizzagalli DA. 2010. Effects of task-relevant incentives on the electrophysiological correlates of error processing in major depressive disorder. *Cogn Affect Behav Neurosci* 10: 119–128.

54. Holroyd CB, Coles MG. 2002. The neural basis of human error processing: reinforcement learning, dopamine, and the error-related negativity. *Psychol Rev* 109: 679–709.

55. Holroyd CB, Praamstra P, Plat E, Coles MG. 2002. Spared error-related potentials in mild to moderate Parkinson's disease. *Neuropsychologia* 40: 2116–2124.

56. Hoshi E, Tremblay L, Feger J, Carras PL, Strick PL. 2005. The cerebellum communicates with the basal ganglia. *Nat Neurosci* 8: 1491–1493.

57. Houthoofd S, Morrens M, Schrijvers D, Vandendriessche F, Hulstijn W, Sabbe BGC, De Bruijn ERA (submitted). Trait and state aspects of internal and external performance monitoring in schizophrenia: An ERP study on the effects of treatment.

58. Jocham G, Ullsperger M. 2009. Neuropharmacology of performance monitoring. *Neurosci Biobehav Rev* 33: 48–60.

59. Johannes S, Wieringa BM, Nager W, Rada D, Dengler R, Emrich HM, Munte TF, Dietrich DE. 2001. Discrepant target detection and action monitoring in obsessive-compulsive disorder. *Psychiatry Res* 108: 101–110.

60. Kennerley SW, Walton ME, Behrens TE, Buckley MJ, Rushworth MF. 2006. Optimal decision making and the anterior cingulate cortex. *Nat Neurosci* 9: 940–947.

61. Kerns JG, Cohen JD, MacDonald AW, 3rd, Johnson MK, Stenger VA, Aizenstein H, Carter CS. 2005. Decreased conflict- and error-related activity in the anterior cingulate cortex in subjects with schizophrenia. *Am J Psychiatry* 162: 1833–1839.

62. Kerns JG, Cohen JD, MacDonald AW, Cho RY, Stenger VA, Carter CS. 2004. Anterior cingulate conflict monitoring and adjustments in control. *Science* 303: 1023–1026.

63. King JA, Korb FM, Von Cramon DY, Ullsperger M. 2010. Post-error behavioral adjustments are facilitated by activation and suppression of task-relevant and task-irrelevant information processing. *J Neurosci* 30: 12759–12769.

64. Klein TA, Neumann J, Reuter M, Hennig J, von Cramon DY, Ullsperger M. 2007. Genetically determined differences in learning from errors. *Science* 318: 1642–1645.

65. Kopp B, Rist F. 1999. An event-related brain potential substrate of disturbed response monitoring in paranoid schizophrenic patients. *J Abnorm Psychol* 108: 337–346.

66. Laurens KR, Hodgins S, Mould GL, West SA, Schoenberg PL, Murray RM, Taylor EA. 2010. Error-related processing dysfunction in children aged 9 to 12 years presenting putative antecedents of schizophrenia. *Biol Psychiatry* 67: 238–245.

67. Laurens KR, Ngan ET, Bates AT, Kiehl KA, Liddle PF. 2003. Rostral anterior cingulate cortex dysfunction during error processing in schizophrenia. *Brain* 126: 610–622.

68. MacDonald AW, 3rd, Cohen JD, Stenger VA, Carter CS. 2000. Dissociating the role of the dorsolateral prefrontal and anterior cingulate cortex in cognitive control. *Science* 288: 1835–1838.

69. Maltby N, Tolin DF, Worhunsky P, O'Keefe TM, Kiehl KA. 2005. Dysfunctional action monitoring hyperactivates frontal-striatal circuits in obsessive-compulsive disorder: an event-related fMRI study. *Neuroimage* 24: 495–503.

70. Mathalon DH, Fedor M, Faustman WO, Gray M, Askari N, Ford JM. 2002. Response-monitoring dysfunction in schizophrenia: an event-related brain potential study. *J Abnorm Psychol* 111: 22–41.

71. Mathalon DH, Jorgensen KW, Roach BJ, Ford JM. 2009. Error detection failures in schizophrenia: ERPs and FMRI. *Int J Psychophysiol* 73: 109–117.

72. Mayberg HS. 2003. Positron emission tomography imaging in depression: a neural systems perspective. *Neuroimaging Clin N Am* 13: 805–815.

73. Meyer-Lindenberg A, Miletich RS, Kohn PD, Esposito G, Carson RE, Quarantelli M, Weinberger DR, Berman KF. 2002. Reduced prefrontal activity predicts exaggerated striatal dopaminergic function in schizophrenia. *Nat Neurosci* 5: 267–271.

74. Miltner WH, Brauer J, Hecht H, Trippe R, Coles MG. 2004. Parallel brain acitivity for self-generated and observed errors. In: Errors, Conflicts, and the Brain. Current Opinions on Performance Monitoring (Ullsperger M, Falkenstein M, eds), pp 124–129. Leipzig: MPI for Human Cognitive and Brain Sciences.

75. Miltner WHR, Braun CH, Coles MGH. 1997. Event-related brain potentials following incorrect feedback in a time-estimation task: evidence for a "generic" neural system for error detection. *J Cogn Neurosci* 9: 788–798.

76. Modirrousta M, Fellows LK. 2008. Dorsal medial prefrontal cortex plays a necessary role in rapid error prediction in humans. *J Neurosci* 28: 14000–14005.

77. Morris SE, Yee CM, Nuechterlein KH. 2006. Electrophysiological analysis of error monitoring in schizophrenia. *J Abnorm Psychol* 115: 239–250.

78. Munro GE, Dywan J, Harris GT, McKee S, Unsal A, Segalowitz SJ. 2007. ERN varies with degree of psychopathy in an emotion discrimination task. *Biol Psychol* 76: 31–42.

79. Münte TF, Heldmann M, Hinrichs H, Marco-Pallares J, Krämer UM, Sturm V, Heinze HJ. 2008. Contribution of subcortical structures to cognition assessed with invasive electrophysiology in humans. *Front Neurosci* 2: 72–78.

80. Notebaert W, Houtman F, Opstal FV, Gevers W, Fias W, Verguts T. 2009. Post-error slowing: an orienting account. *Cognition* 111: 275–279.

81. Nuttin BJ, Gabriels L, van Kuyck K, Cosyns P. 2003. Electrical stimulation of the anterior limbs of the internal capsules in patients with severe obsessive-compulsive disorder: anecdotal reports. *Neurosurg Clin N Am* 14: 267–274.

82. Olvet DM, Hajcak G. 2008. The error-related negativity (ERN) and psychopathology: toward an endophenotype. *Clin Psychol Rev* 28: 1343–1354.

83. Olvet DM, Klein DN, Hajcak G. 2010. Depression symptom severity and error-related brain activity. *Psychiatry Res* 179: 30–37.

84. Overbeek TJM, Nieuwenhuis S, Ridderinkhof KR. 2005. Dissociable components of error processing: on the functional significance of the Pe vis-à-vis the ERN/Ne. *J Psychophysiol* 19: 319–329.

85. Paulus MP, Feinstein JS, Simmons A, Stein MB. 2004. Anterior cingulate activation in high trait anxious subjects is related to altered error processing during decision making. *Biol Psychiatry* 55: 1179–1187.

86. Pitman RK. 1987. A cybernetic model of obsessive-compulsive psychopathology. *Compr Psychiatry* 28: 334–343.

87. Polli FE, Barton JJ, Thakkar KN, Greve DN, Goff DC, Rauch SL, Manoach DS. 2008. Reduced error-related activation in two anterior cingulate circuits is related to impaired performance in schizophrenia. *Brain* 131: 971–986.

88. Pourtois G, Vocat R, N'Diaye K, Spinelli L, Seeck M, Vuilleumier P. 2010. Errors recruit both cognitive and emotional monitoring systems: simultaneous intracranial recordings in the dorsal anterior cingulate gyrus and amygdala combined with fMRI. *Neuropsychologia* 48: 1144–1159.

89. Ridderinkhof KR, Ullsperger M, Crone EA, Nieuwenhuis S. 2004. The role of the medial frontal cortex in cognitive control. *Science* 306: 443–447.

90. Saxena S, Brody AL, Schwartz JM, Baxter LR. 1998. Neuroimaging and frontal-subcortical circuitry in obsessive-compulsive disorder. *Br J Psychiatry Suppl* 35: 26–37.

91. Schellekens AF, De Bruijn ERA, van Lankveld CA, Hulstijn W, Buitelaar JK, de Jong CA, Verkes RJ. 2010. Alcohol dependence and anxiety increase error-related negativity. *Addiction* 105: 1928–1934.

92. Schrijvers D, de Bruijn ERA, Maas Y, De Grave C, Sabbe BG, Hulstijn W. 2008. Action monitoring in major depressive disorder with psychomotor retardation. *Cortex* 44: 569–579.

93. Schrijvers D, De Bruijn ERA, Maas YJ, Vancoillie P, Hulstijn W, Sabbe BG. 2009. Action monitoring and depressive symptom reduction in major depressive disorder. *Int J Psychophysiol* 71: 218–224.

94. Schrijvers DL, De Bruijn ER, Destoop M, Hulstijn W, Sabbe BG. 2010. The impact of perfectionism and anxiety traits on action monitoring in major depressive disorder. *J Neural Transm* 117: 869–880.

95. Schuch S, Tipper SP. 2007. On observing another person's actions: influences of observed inhibition and errors. *Percept Psychophys* 69: 828–837.

96. Segalowitz SJ, Santesso DL, Murphy TI, Homan D, Chantziantoniou DK, Khan S. 2010. Retest reliability of medial frontal negativities during performance monitoring. *Psychophysiology* 47: 260–270.

97. Seifert S, von Cramon DY, Imperati D, Tittgemeyer M, Ullsperger M (in press). Thalamocingulate interactions in performance monitoring. *J Neurosci*.

98. Shane MS, Stevens M, Harenski CL, Kiehl KA. 2008. Neural correlates of the processing of another's mistakes: a possible underpinning for social and observational learning. *Neuroimage* 42: 450–459.

99. Sokhadze E, Stewart C, Hollifield M, Tasman A. 2008. Event-related potential study of executive dysfunctions in a speeded reaction task in cocaine addiction. *J Neurother* 12: 185–204.

100. Steinhauser M, Maier M, Hubner R. 2008. Modeling behavioral measures of error detection in choice tasks: response monitoring versus conflict monitoring. *J Exp Psychol Hum Percept Perform* 34: 158–176.

101. Stemmer B, Segalowitz SJ, Dywan J, Panisset M, Melmed C. 2007. The error negativity in nonmedicated and medicated patients with Parkinson's disease. *Clin Neurophysiol* 118: 1223–1229.

102. Stemmer B, Segalowitz SJ, Witzke W, Schonle PW. 2004. Error detection in patients with lesions to the medial prefrontal cortex: an ERP study. *Neuropsychologia* 42: 118–130.

103. Stern ER, Liu Y, Gehring WJ, Lister JJ, Yin G, Zhang J, Fitzgerald KD, Himle JA, Abelson JL, Taylor SF. 2010. Chronic medication does not affect hyperactive error responses in obsessive-compulsive disorder. *Psychophysiology* 47: 913–920.

104. Swick D, Jovanovic J. 2002. Anterior cingulate cortex and the Stroop task: neuropsychological evidence for topographic specificity. *Neuropsychologia* 40: 1240–1253.

105. Swick D, Turken AU. 2002. Dissociation between conflict detection and error monitoring in the human anterior cingulate cortex. *Proc Natl Acad Sci USA* 99: 16354–16359.

106. Swick D, Turken AU. 2004. Focusing on the anterior cingulate cortex. Effects of focal lesions on cognitive performance. In: Cognitive Neuroscience of Attention (Posner MI, ed), pp 393–406. New York: The Guilford Press.

107. Taylor PC, Nobre AC, Rushworth MF. 2007. Subsecond changes in top down control exerted by human medial frontal cortex during conflict and action selection: a combined transcranial magnetic stimulation electroencephalography study. *J Neurosci* 27: 11343–11353.

108. Tsuchida A, Fellows LK. 2009. Lesion evidence that two distinct regions within prefrontal cortex are critical for n-back performance in humans. *J Cogn Neurosci* 21: 2263–2275.

109. Tucker DM, Luu P, Frishkoff G, Quiring J, Poulsen C. 2003. Frontolimbic response to negative feedback in clinical depression. *J Abnorm Psychol* 112: 667–678.

110. Turken AU, Swick D. 2008. The effect of orbitofrontal lesions on the error-related negativity. *Neurosci Lett* 441: 7–10.

111. Ullsperger M. 2006. Performance monitoring in neurological and psychiatric patients. *Int J Psychophysiol* 59: 59–69.

112. Ullsperger M, Harsay HA, Wessel JR, Ridderinkhof KR. 2010. Conscious perception of errors and its relation to the anterior insula. *Brain Struct Funct* 214: 629–643.

113. Ullsperger M, King JA. 2010. Proactive and reactive recruitment of cognitive control: comment on Hikosaka and Isoda. *Trends Cogn Sci* 14: 191–192.

114. Ullsperger M, von Cramon DY. 2006. How does error correction differ from error signaling? An event-related potential study. *Brain Res* 1105: 102–109.

115. Ullsperger M, von Cramon DY. 2006. The role of intact frontostriatal circuits in error processing. *J Cogn Neurosci* 18: 651–664.

116. Ullsperger M, von Cramon DY, Muller NG. 2002. Interactions of focal cortical lesions with error processing: evidence from event-related brain potentials. *Neuropsychology* 16: 548–561.

117. Ursu S, Stenger VA, Shear MK, Jones MR, Carter CS. 2003. Overactive action monitoring in obsessive-compulsive disorder: evidence from functional magnetic resonance imaging. *Psychol Sci* 14: 347–353.

118. Van Hoesen GW, Morecraft RJ, Vogt BA. 1993. Connections of the monkey cingulate cortex. In: Neurobiology of Cingulate Cortex and Limbic Thalamus (Vogt BA, Gabriel M, eds), pp 249–284. Boston: Birkhäuser.

119. Van Laere K, Nuttin B, Gabriels L, Dupont P, Rasmussen S, Greenberg BD, Cosyns P. 2006. Metabolic imaging of anterior capsular stimulation in refractory obsessive-compulsive disorder: a key role for the subgenual anterior cingulate and ventral striatum. *J Nucl Med* 47: 740–747.

120. Van Schie HT, Mars RB, Coles MG, Bekkering H. 2004. Modulation of activity in medial frontal and motor cortices during error observation. *Nat Neurosci* 7: 549–554.

121. Vidal F, Burle B, Bonnet M, Grapperon J, Hasbroucq T. 2003. Error negativity on correct trials: a reexamination of available data. Paper presented at the Biological Psychology Meeting.

122. Vogt BA, Sikes RW, Vogt LJ. 1993. Anterior cingulate cortex and the medial pain system. In: Neurobiology of Cingulate Cortex and Limbic Thalamus: A Comprehensive Handbook (Vogt BA, Gabriel M, eds), pp 313–344. Boston: Birkhäuser.

123. Von Borries AK, Brazil IA, Bulten BH, Buitelaar JK, Verkes RJ, de Bruijn ER. 2010. Neural correlates of error-related learning deficits in individuals with psychopathy. *Psychol Med* 40: 1559–1568.

124. Willemssen R, Muller T, Schwarz M, Hohnsbein J, Falkenstein M. 2008. Error processing in patients with Parkinson's disease: the influence of medication state. *J Neural Transm* 115: 461–468.

125. Yeung N, Cohen JD. 2006. The impact of cognitive deficits on conflict monitoring. Predictable dissociations between the error-related negativity and N2. *Psychol Sci* 17: 164–171.

V   COMPUTATIONAL MODELS OF MOTIVATIONAL AND COGNITIVE CONTROL

The chapters in this section review recent developments in the computational modeling of cognitive and motivational control. The importance of computational approaches in this field reflects the unique challenge of "banishing the homunculus" from theories of control[5]: It is all too easy for our theories to rely—sometimes implicitly, sometimes more obviously—on an unspecified intelligent agent for their ability to account for the most interesting aspects of human thought and action. Framing a theory in explicit computational terms thus provides a crucial benchmark of the sufficiency and completeness of any attempt to account for the flexibility and intelligence of human behavior.

Historically, a major focus of research in this area has been on modeling the execution of control, that is, modeling the way in which prefrontal control mechanisms might exert their influence over processing in subcortical and posterior cortical regions. Models of this sort evolved from an established idea in cognitive psychology: that control operates as a supervisory, modulatory influence that serves to bias processing in favor of task-appropriate "schema" as they compete for the control of behavior.[6] Formal computational models have instantiated this idea in terms of "guided activation" of processing by representations of task-relevant information (rules, goals, etc.),[2] a function that is closely associated with regions in lateral prefrontal cortex (PFC).[4,7] The legacy of this work is felt strongly in chapters throughout this volume as researchers in cognitive neuroscience, developmental psychology, psychopathology, and other allied fields, have come to adopt ideas originally pioneered in computational work.

Though hugely influential, the guided activation framework leaves unanswered the crucial question of how lateral PFC might itself "know" at any given moment which task is required, and how strongly control must be exerted. The chapters in this section reflect growing interest in computational answers to this question, a very apt continuation of the research emphasis of the meeting series on which this book is based. The first workshops in this series—held in Jena in 2000 and Dortmund in 2003—saw discussion of two related hypotheses stimulated by discovery of error-related activity in medial PFC: the conflict monitoring theory, which proposes that medial PFC monitors for the occurrence of response conflict to detect the need for controlled interventions by lateral PFC,[1] and a reinforcement learning (RL) account, which suggests error-related activity in medial PFC reflects its role in selecting appropriate behavioral strategies.[3] The third meeting of the series, held in Amsterdam in 2006, saw growing recognition that conflict monitoring and RL approaches may provide complementary perspectives on the optimization of human decision making. The chapters in this section continue this convergence of ideas.

Ribas-Fernandes and colleagues' hierarchical model extends standard RL approaches to address the higher-level organization of behavior in lateral PFC. According to this framework, RL principles operate simultaneously at the levels of temporally extended behavioral sequences (options) and the lower-level actions that make up those sequences. A central claim of this theory is that achieving the subgoal specified by a particular option should act as a reinforcing event even in the absence of explicit reward: Effectively, it is argued that the PFC is able to hijack the brain's basic reward mechanisms to reinforce behaviors consistent with the organism's high-level goals. In support of this view, Ribas-Fernandes and colleagues present new data indicating that setbacks in subgoal attainment elicit error signals in medial PFC that correspond closely to those elicited by withholding primary reinforcement.

This hierarchical framework provides a formal model of the emergence of high-level task structure in lateral PFC through reinforcement learning, but does not directly identify the specific contribution of medial PFC in the RL process. This latter issue is the focus of the chapters by Cockburn and Frank and Holroyd and Yeung. Cockburn and Frank suggest a novel integration of the conflict monitoring and RL approaches, arguing that conflict signals from medial PFC, in particular the anterior cingulate cortex (ACC), may modulate decision processes in the basal ganglia. Their new simulation results from biologically inspired neural network models demonstrate how RL processes in the basal ganglia may conversely induce transient conflict following negative reinforcement, thus providing a conflict-based account of the type of reinforcement-related medial PFC activity studied by Ribas-Fernandes and colleagues. Holroyd and Yeung present a rather different conception of the respective roles of the basal ganglia and ACC, arguing that these structures play parallel roles in selecting and motivating lower-level actions and higher-level options, respectively, as characterized in the hierarchical RL framework.

The chapters by Khamassi and colleagues and Shenoy and Yu focus on the question of "meta-control"—how the high-level parameters of learning and cognitive control are themselves determined. Khamassi and colleagues discuss neural mechanisms that might mediate the critical balance between stability and plasticity in learning, exploration and exploitation in choice behavior, and short- and long-term behavioral goals in action planning. They present a detailed review of evidence suggesting that regions in lateral and medial PFC, and interactions between the two structures, play a crucial role in setting each of these meta-learning parameters. Shenoy and Yu's analyses indicate that human performance in a paradigmatic response inhibition task can be accurately modeled by assuming that human subjects act as rational decision makers who aim to optimize their behavior according to an objective cost-benefit function. Using this approach, Shenoy and Yu demonstrate elegantly that parameters of classical response inhibition models can be derived from a normative model with minimal free parameters.

Collectively, these chapters illustrate some of the principal computational approaches to cognitive and motivational control in current research: seeking neuroscience applications of established formalisms from the machine learning literature, developing detailed biologically inspired neural network models of interacting mechanisms of control, and deriving rational models of decision making and control from optimality constraints. It is hardly a bold prediction to forecast that ideas from the work represented in this section will form the basis for empirical research that we can expect to see in future meetings of the series begun in Jena and continued in Oxford this year.

References

1. Botvinick MM, Braver TS, Barch DM, Carter CS, Cohen JD. 2001. Conflict monitoring and cognitive control. *Psychol Rev* 108: 624–652.

2. Cohen JD, Dunbar K, McClelland JL. 1990. On the control of automatic processes: a parallel distributed processing account of the Stroop effect. *Psychol Rev* 97: 332–361.

3. Holroyd CB, Coles MG. 2002. The neural basis of human error processing: reinforcement learning, dopamine, and the error-related negativity. *Psychol Rev* 109: 679–709.

4. Miller EK, Cohen JD. 2001. An integrative theory of prefrontal cortex function. *Annu Rev Neurosci* 24: 167–202.

5. Monsell S, Driver JS, eds. 2000. Attention and Performance XVIII: Control of Cognitive Processes. Cambridge, MA: MIT Press.

6. Norman DA, Shallice T. 1986. Attention to action: willed and automatic control of behaviour. In: Consciousness and Self-Regulation (Davidson RJ, Schwartz GE, Shapiro D, eds), pp 1–18. New York: Plenum.

7. Sakai K. 2008. Task set and prefrontal cortex. *Annu Rev Neurosci* 31: 219–245.

16 Neural Correlates of Hierarchical Reinforcement Learning

José J. F. Ribas-Fernandes, Yael Niv, and Matthew M. Botvinick

Over the past two decades, ideas from computational reinforcement learning (RL) have had an important and growing effect on neuroscience and psychology. The impact of RL was initially felt in research on classical and instrumental conditioning.[13,104,112] Soon thereafter, its reach extended to research on midbrain dopaminergic function, where the temporal-difference learning paradigm provided a framework for interpreting temporal profiles of dopaminergic activity.[10,51,67,93] Subsequently, actor-critic architectures for RL have inspired new interpretations of functional divisions of labor within the basal ganglia and cerebral cortex[52] (see also chapters 17 and 18, this volume), and RL-based accounts have been advanced to address issues as diverse as motor control,[66] working memory,[74] performance monitoring,[48] and the distinction between habitual and goal-directed behavior.[31]

Despite this widespread absorption of ideas from RL into neurobiology and cognitive science, important questions remain concerning the scope of its relevance. In particular, RL-inspired research has generally focused on highly simplified decision-making situations involving choice among a small set of elementary actions (e.g., left vs. right saccades), or on Pavlovian settings involving no action selection at all. It thus remains uncertain whether RL principles can help us understand learning and action selection in more complex behavioral settings, akin to those arising in everyday life.[30]

In the present chapter, we consider the potential relevance of RL to one particular aspect of complex behavior, namely, its hierarchical structure. Since the inception of cognitive psychology, it has been noted that naturalistic behavior displays a stratified or layered organization.[58,64,89] As stated by Fuster,[38] "Successive units with limited short-term goals make larger and longer units with longer-term objectives. . . . Thus we have a pyramidal hierarchy of structural units of increasing duration and complexity serving a corresponding hierarchy of purposes" (p. 159). A concern with hierarchical action structure has continued to inform behavioral research to the present day,[19,25,91,117] and has figured importantly in neuroscientific research bearing on the prefrontal cortex, where evidence has arisen that representations of successive levels of task structure may map topographically onto the cortical surface.[7,20,27,38,57,114]

Can hierarchical behavior be understood in terms provided by RL, or does it involve fundamentally different computational principles? One lead in pursuing this question can be gleaned from recent RL research. As it turns out, a great deal of recent work in computational RL has focused precisely on the question of how RL methods might be elaborated to accommodate hierarchical behavioral structure. This has given rise to a general framework referred to, aptly enough, as hierarchical reinforcement learning (HRL).[11,34,106] In considering whether RL might be relevant to hierarchical behavior in animals and humans, a natural approach is to evaluate whether the brain might implement anything like the mechanisms stipulated in computational HRL. In recent work, we have undertaken this project.[21,26,82] Our objective in the present chapter is to review the results obtained so far, and to offer an interim evaluation of the HRL hypothesis.

Before getting to neuroscientific data, a number of preliminaries are in order. We begin by reviewing the basics of RL, and in particular temporal-difference learning within the actor-critic architecture. Next, we discuss the computational issues that stimulated the development of HRL, and introduce the fundamental elements of HRL itself. With this foundation in place, we consider potential neuroscientific correlates of HRL, describe results of some initial empirical tests, and finally chart out some directions for further research.

Fundamentals of RL: Temporal Difference Learning in Actor-Critic Models

RL problems comprise four elements: a set of world *states*; a set of *actions* available to the agent in each state; a *transition function,* which specifies the probability of transitioning from one state to another when performing each action; and a *reward function*, which indicates the amount of reward (or cost) associated with each such transition. Given these elements, the objective for learning is to discover a policy, that is, a mapping from states to actions, that maximizes cumulative discounted long-term reward.

There are a variety of specific algorithmic approaches to solving RL problems.[16,105] We focus here on the approach that has arguably had the most direct influence on neuroscientific translations of RL, referred to as the actor-critic paradigm.[10,52] In actor-critic implementations of RL,[14,51,52,103] the learning agent is divided into two parts, an actor and a critic (see figure 16.1a). The *actor* selects actions according to a modifiable policy, $\pi(s)$, which is based on a set of weighted associations from states to actions, often called *action strengths*. The *critic* maintains a *value function*, $V(s)$, associating each state with an estimate of the cumulative, long-term reward that can be expected subsequent to visiting that state. Importantly, both the action strengths

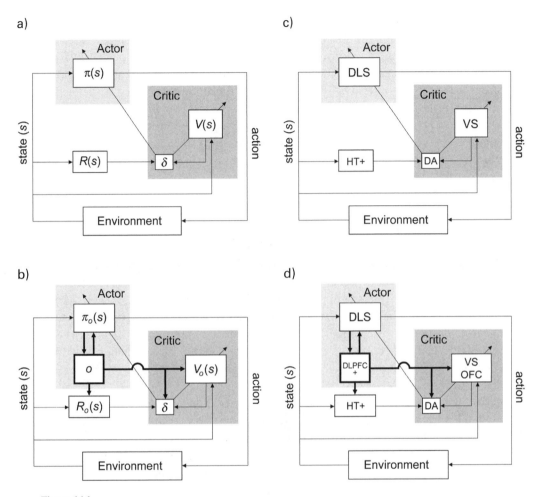

Figure 16.1
An actor-critic implementation. (a) Schematic of the basic actor-critic architecture. (b) An actor-critic implementation of HRL. (c,d) Putative neural correlates of components of elements diagramed in panels a and b. DA, dopamine; DLPFC, dorsolateral prefrontal cortex, plus other frontal structures potentially including premotor, supplementary motor and pre-supplementary motor cortices; DLS, dorsolateral striatum; HT+: hypothalamus and other structures, potentially including the habenula, the pedunculo-pontine nucleus, and the superior colliculus; OFC: orbitofrontal cortex; VS, ventral striatum. Adapted from Botvinick, Niv, and Barto.[21]

and the value function must be learned based on experience with the environment. At the outset of learning, the value function and the actor's action strengths are initialized, for instance, uniformly or randomly, and the agent is placed in some initial state. The actor then selects an action, following a rule that favors high-strength actions but also allows for exploration. Once the resulting state is reached and its associated reward is collected, the critic computes a *temporal-difference prediction error*, δ. Here, the value that was attached to the previous state is treated as a prediction of the reward that would be received in the successor state, $R(s)$, plus the value attached to that successor state. A positive prediction error indicates that this prediction was too low, meaning that things turned out better than expected. Of course, things can also turn out worse than expected, yielding a negative prediction error.

The prediction error is used to update both the value attached to the previous state and the strength of the action that was selected in that state. A positive prediction error leads to an increase in the value of the previous state and the propensity to perform the chosen action at that state. A negative error leads to a reduction in these values. After the appropriate adjustments, the agent selects a new action, a new state is reached, a new prediction error is computed, and so forth. As the agent explores its environment and this procedure is repeated, the critic's value function becomes progressively more accurate, and the actor's action strengths change so as to yield progressive improvements in behavior, in terms of the amount of reward obtained.

The actor-critic architecture, and the temporal-difference learning procedure it implements, have provided a very useful framework for decoding the neural substrates of learning and decision making. Although accounts relating the actor-critic architecture to neural structures do vary,[52] one influential approach has been to identify the actor with the dorsolateral striatum (DLS), and the critic with the ventral striatum (VS) and the mesolimbic dopaminergic system[32,71] (figure 16.1c). Dopamine (DA), in particular, has been associated with the function of conveying reward prediction errors to both actor and critic.[10,67,93] This set of correspondences provides an important backdrop for our later discussion of HRL and its neural correlates.

The Scaling Problem in RL

Even as excitement initially grew concerning potential applications of RL within neuroscience, concerns were already arising in computer science over the limitations of RL. In particular, it became clear very early on in the history of RL research that RL algorithms face a scaling problem: They do not cope well with tasks involving a large space of environmental states or possible actions. It is this scaling problem that immediately stimulated the development of HRL, and it is therefore worth characterizing the problem before turning to the details of HRL itself.

A key source of the scaling problem is the fact that an RL agent can learn to behave adaptively only by exploring its environment, trying out different courses of action in different situations or states of the environment, and sampling their consequences. As a result of this requirement, the time needed to arrive at a stable behavioral policy increases with both the number of different states in the environment and the number of available actions. In most contexts, the relationship between training time and the number of environmental states or actions is a positively accelerating function. Thus, as problem size increases, standard RL eventually becomes infeasible.

Several computational maneuvers have been proposed to address the scaling problem. For example, one important approach is to simplify the state space by treating subsets of environmental states as behaviorally equivalent, a measure referred to as state abstraction.[60] Another approach aims at optimizing the search for an optimal behavioral policy by balancing judiciously between exploration and exploitation of established knowledge.[55]

HRL methods arose as another way of addressing the scaling problem in RL. The key to HRL is the use of *temporal abstraction*.[11,34,77,106] Here, the basic RL framework is expanded to include "temporally abstract" actions, representations that group together a set of interrelated actions (for example, grasping a spoon, using it to scoop up some sugar, moving the spoon into position over a cup, and depositing the sugar), casting them as a single higher-level action or skill ("add sugar"). These new representations are described as temporal abstractions because they abstract over temporally extended, and potentially variable, sequences of lower-level steps. A number of other terms have been used as well, including "skills," "operators," "macro-operators," and "macro-actions." In what follows, we often refer to temporally abstract actions as options.[106]

In most versions of RL that use temporal abstraction, it is assumed that options can be assembled into higher-level skills in a hierarchical arrangement. Thus, for example, an option for adding sugar might form part of other options for making coffee and tea. It is the importance of such hierarchical structures in work using temporal abstraction that gave rise to the moniker HRL.

Adding temporal abstraction to RL can ease the scaling problem in two ways. The first way is through its impact on the exploration process. In order to see how this works, it is useful to picture the agent as searching a tree structure (figure 16.2a). At the apex is a node representing the state occupied by the agent at the outset of exploration. Branching out from this node are links representing primitive actions, each leading to a node representing the state (and, possibly, reward) consequent on that action. Further action links project from each of these nodes, leading to their

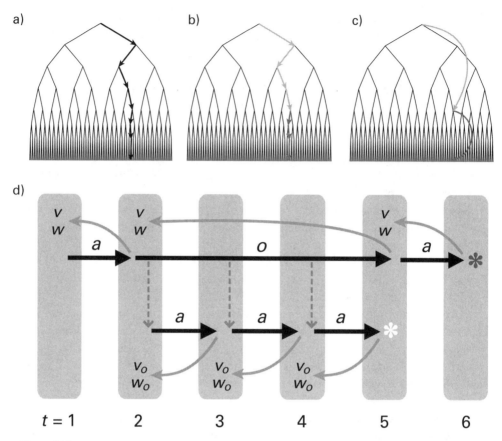

Figure 16.2
The options framework in HRL. (a–c) illustrate how options can facilitate search. (a) A search tree with arrows indicating the pathway to a goal state. A specific sequence of seven independently selected actions is required to reach the goal. (b) The same tree and trajectory, the arrows indicating that the first four and the last three actions have been aggregated into options. Here, the goal state is reached after only two independent choices (option selections). (c) Search using option models allows the consequences options to be forecast without requiring consideration of the lower-level steps involved in executing the option. (d) Schematic illustration of HRL dynamics. a, primitive actions; o, option. On the first time step ($t = 1$), the agent executes a primitive action (forward arrow). Based on the consequent state (i.e., the state at $t = 2$), a prediction error δ is computed (arrow running from $t = 2$ to $t = 1$), and used to update the value (V) and action/option strengths (π) associated with the preceding state. At $t = 2$, the agent selects an option (long forward arrow), which remains active through $t = 5$. During this time, primitive actions are selected according to the option's policy (lower tier of forward arrows), with prediction errors (lower tier of curved arrows) used to update V_o and π_o associated with the preceding state, taking into account pseudo-reward received throughout option execution (lower asterisk). The option is terminated once its subgoal state is reached. Prediction error computed for the entire option (long curved arrow) is used to update the values and option strengths associated with the state in which the option was initiated. The agent then selects a new action at the top level, yielding external reward (higher asterisk). The prediction errors computed at the top level, but not at the level below, take this reward into account. Adapted from Botvinick, Niv, and Barto,[21] with permission.

consequent states, and so forth. The agent's objective is to discover paths through the decision tree that lead to maximal accumulated rewards. However, the set of possible paths increases with the set of actions available to the agent, and the number of reachable states. With increasing numbers of either, it becomes progressively more difficult to discover, through exploration, the specific traversals of the tree that would maximize reward.

Temporally abstract actions can alleviate this problem by introducing *structure* into the exploration process. Specifically, the policies associated with temporally abstract actions can guide exploration down specific partial paths through the search tree, potentially allowing earlier discovery of high-value traversals. The principle is illustrated in figure 16.2. Discovering the pathway illustrated in figure 16.2a, using only primitive, one-step actions, would require a specific sequence of seven independent choices. This changes if the agent has acquired—say, through prior experience with related problems—two options corresponding to the differently colored subsequences in figure 16.2b. Equipped with these, the agent would only need to make two independent decisions to discover the overall trajectory, namely, select the two options. Here, options reduce the effective size of the search space, making it easier for the agent to discover an optimal trajectory.

The second, and closely related, way in which temporally abstract actions can ease the scaling problem is by allowing the agent to learn more efficiently from its experiences. Without temporal abstraction, learning to follow the trajectory illustrated in figure 16.2a would involve adjusting parameters at seven separate decision points. With predefined options (figure 16.2c), policy learning is required at only two decision points, the points at which the two options are to be selected. Thus, temporally abstract actions allow the agent not only to explore more efficiently, but also to make better use of its experiences.

Hierarchical Reinforcement Learning

In order to frame specific hypotheses considering neural correlates of HRL, it is necessary to get into the specifics of how HRL works. In this section we introduce the essentials of HRL, focusing on the options framework[106] as adapted to the actor-critic framework.[21] We focus on aspects of HRL that we believe are potentially most relevant to neuroscience (see ref. 11 for a detailed and comparative discussion of HRL algorithms).

The options framework supplements the set of single-step, primitive actions with a set of temporally abstract actions or options. An option is, in a sense, a "mini-policy." It is defined by an *initiation set*, indicating the states in which the option can be selected; a *termination function,* which specifies a set of states that will trigger termination of the option; and an *option-specific policy,* mapping from states to actions (which now include other options).

Like primitive actions, options are associated with strengths, and on any time step the actor may select either a primitive action or an option. Once an option is selected, actions are selected based on that option's policy until the option terminates. At that point, a prediction error for the option is computed (figure 16.2d). This error is defined as the difference between the value of the state where the option terminated and the value of the state where the option was initiated, plus whatever rewards were accrued during execution of the option. A positive prediction error indicates that things went better than expected since leaving the initiation state, and a negative prediction error means that things went worse. As in the case of primitive actions, the prediction error is used to update the value associated with the initiation state, as well as the action strength associating the option with that state.

Implementing this new functionality requires several extensions to the actor-critic architecture, as illustrated in figure 16.1b. First, the actor must maintain a representation of which option is currently in control of behavior (o) or, in case of options calling other options, of the entire set of active options and their calling relations. Second, because the agent's policy now varies depending on which option is in control, the actor must maintain a separate set of action strengths for each option, $\pi_o(s)$, together with option-dependent reward functions, $R_o(s)$, and value functions, $V_o(s)$. Important changes are also required in the critic. Because prediction errors are computed when options terminate, the critic must receive input from the actor, telling it when such terminations occur (the arrow from o to δ). Finally, to be able to compute the prediction error at these points, the critic must also keep track of the amount of reward accumulated during each option's execution and the identity of the state in which the option was initiated.

Learning Option Policies

The description provided so far explains how the agent learns a top- or root-level policy, which determines what action or option to select when no option is currently in control of behavior. We turn now to the question of how option-specific policies are learned.

In versions of the options framework that address such learning, it is often assumed that options are initially defined in terms of specific *subgoal* states. The question of where these subgoals come from is an important one, to which we will return later. It is further assumed that when an active option reaches its subgoal, the actions leading up to the subgoal are reinforced. To distinguish this reinforcing effect from the one associated with external rewards, subgoal attainment is said to yield *pseudo-reward.*[34]

In order for subgoals and pseudo-reward to shape option policies, the critic in HRL must maintain not only its usual value function, but also a set of option-specific value functions, $V_o(s)$ (see figure 16.1b). As in ordinary RL, these value functions predict the cumulative long-term reward that will be received subsequent to occupation of a particular state. However, they are option-specific in the sense that they take into account the pseudo-reward that is associated with each option's subgoal state. A second reason that option-specific value functions are needed is that the reward (and pseudo-reward) that the agent will receive following any given state depends on the actions it will select. These depend, by definition, on the agent's policy, and under HRL the policy depends on which option is currently in control of behavior. Thus, only an option-specific value function can accurately predict future rewards.

Despite the additions discussed here, option-specific policies are learned in quite the usual way: On each step of an option's execution, a prediction error is computed based on the (option-specific) values of the states visited and the reward received (including pseudo-reward). This prediction error is then used to update the option's action strengths and the values attached to each state visited during the option (figure 16.2d). With repeated cycles through this procedure, the option's policy evolves so as to guide behavior, with increasing directness, toward the option's subgoals.

Potential Neural Correlates

Having laid out the basic mechanisms of HRL, we are now in a position to consider its potential implications for understanding neural function. To make these concrete, we will leverage the actor-critic formulation of HRL[21] presented earlier. As previously noted, existing research has proposed parallels between the elements of the actor-critic framework and specific neuroanatomical structures. Situating HRL within the actor-critic framework thus facilitates the formation of hypotheses concerning how HRL might map onto functional neuroanatomy.

As figure 16.1 makes evident, elaborating the actor-critic architecture for HRL requires only insertion of a very few new elements. The most obvious of these is the component labeled "o" in figure 16.1b. As established previously, the role of this component is to represent the identity of the option currently in control of behavior. From a neuroscientific point of view, this function seems very closely related to those commonly ascribed to the dorsolateral prefrontal cortex (DLPFC). The DLPFC has long been considered to house representations that guide temporally integrated, goal-directed behavior.[38,40,41,78,96,114] Recent work has refined this idea by demonstrating that DLPFC neurons play a direct role in representing *task sets*. Here, a single pattern of DLPFC activation serves to represent an entire mapping from stimuli to responses, that is, a policy.[5,23,50,53,85,99,108,110] According to the guided activation theory,[63] prefrontal representations do not implement policies directly, but instead select among stimulus-response pathways implemented outside the prefrontal cortex. This division of labor fits well with the distinction in HRL between an option's identifier and the policy with which it is associated.

There is evidence that, in addition to the DLPFC, other frontal areas may also carry representations of task set, including presupplementary motor area (pre-SMA)[86] and premotor cortex (PMC).[69,109] Furthermore, like options in HRL, neurons in several frontal areas including DLPFC, pre-SMA, and supplementary motor area (SMA) have been shown to code for particular sequences of low-level actions.[6,17,97,98] Research on frontal cortex also accords well with the stipulation in HRL that temporally abstract actions may organize into hierarchies, with the policy for one option (say, an option for making coffee) calling other, lower-level options (say, options for adding sugar or cream). This fits with numerous accounts suggesting that the frontal cortex serves to represent action at multiple, nested levels of temporal structure,[41,102,114,118] possibly in such a way that higher levels of structure are represented more anteriorly.[20,39,40,46,57]

As reviewed earlier, neuroscientific interpretations of the basic actor-critic architecture generally place policy representations within the DLS. It is thus relevant that such regions as the DLPFC, SMA, pre-SMA, and PMC—areas potentially representing options—all project heavily to the DLS.[4,76] Frank, O'Reilly, and colleagues[36,74,85] (see also chapter 17, this volume) have put forth detailed computational models that show how frontal inputs to the striatum could switch among different stimulus-response pathways. Here, as in guided activation theory, temporally abstract action representations in frontal cortex select among alternative (i.e., option-specific) policies.

In order to support option-specific policies, the DLS would need to integrate information about the currently controlling option with information about the current environmental state, as is indicated by the arrows converging on the policy module in figure 16.1b. This is consistent with neurophysiological data showing that some DLS neurons respond to stimuli in a way that varies with task context.[81,88] Other studies have shown that *action* representations within the DLS can also be task dependent.[2,42,43,59] For example, in rats, different DLS neurons fire in conjunction with simple grooming movements, depending on whether those actions are performed in isolation or as part of a grooming sequence.[1] This is consistent with the idea that option-specific policies (action strengths) might be implemented in the DLS, since this would imply that a particular motor behavior, when performed in different task contexts, would be selected via different neural pathways.

Unlike the selection of primitive actions, the selection of options in HRL involves initiation, maintenance, and termination phases. At the neural level, the maintenance phase would be naturally supported within DLPFC, which has been extensively implicated in working memory function.[27,28,80] With regard to initiation and termination, it is intriguing that phasic activity has been observed, both within the DLS and in several areas of frontal cortex, at the boundaries of temporally extended action sequences.[37,68,116] Since these boundaries correspond to points where new options would be selected, boundary-aligned activity in the DLS and frontal cortex is also consistent with a proposed role of the DLS in gating information into prefrontal working memory circuits.[74,85]

The points considered so far all relate to control, that is, the guidance of action selection. Also critical to HRL is the machinery that drives learning, centering on the temporal-difference prediction error. Here, too, HRL gives us some very specific things to look for in terms of neural correlates. In particular, moving from RL to HRL brings about important alterations in the way the prediction error is computed. One important change is that HRL widens the scope of the events that the prediction error addresses. In standard RL, the prediction error indicates whether things went better or worse than expected since the immediately preceding single-step action. HRL, in addition, evaluates at the completion of an option whether things have gone better or worse than expected since the option was initiated (see figure 16.2d). Thus, unlike standard RL, the prediction errors associated with options in HRL are framed around temporally extended events. Formally speaking, the HRL setting is no longer a Markov decision process, but rather a semi-Markov decision process (SMDP).

The widened scope of the prediction error computation in HRL resonates with work on midbrain DA function. In particular, Daw[29] suggested, based on midbrain responses to delayed rewards, that dopaminergic function is driven by representations that divide event sequences into temporally extended segments. In articulating this account, Daw provided a formal analysis of DA function that draws on precisely the same principles of temporal abstraction that also provide the foundation for HRL, namely, an SMDP framework.

Note that in HRL, in order to compute a prediction error when an option terminates, certain information is needed. In particular, the critic needs access to the reward prediction it made when the option was initially selected, and for purposes of temporal discounting it also needs to know how much time has passed since that prediction was made. These requirements of HRL resonate with data concerning the orbitofrontal cortex (OFC). Neurophysiologic data have shown that within OFC, unlike some other areas, reward-predictive activity tends to be sustained, spanning temporally extended segments of task structure.[94] In addition, in line with the integration of reward and delay information in HRL, the response of OFC neurons to the receipt of primary rewards has been shown to vary depending on the wait time leading up to the reward.[83]

Another difference between HRL and ordinary temporal-difference learning is that prediction errors in HRL occur at all levels of task structure (see figure 16.2d). At the top-most or root level, prediction errors signal unanticipated changes in the prospects for primary reward. However, in addition, once the HRL agent enters a subroutine, separate prediction error signals indicate the degree to which each action has carried the agent toward the currently relevant *subgoal* and its associated pseudo-reward. Note that these subroutine-specific prediction errors are unique to HRL. In what follows, we refer to them as *pseudo-reward prediction errors* (PPE), reserving reward prediction error (RPE) for prediction errors relating to primary reward.

Because the PPE is not found in ordinary RL, it can be considered a functional signature of HRL. If the neural mechanisms underlying hierarchical behavior are related to those found in HRL, it should be possible to uncover a neural correlate of the PPE. On grounds of parsimony, one would expect to find PPE signals in the same structures that have been shown to carry RPE-related signals, in particular targets of midbrain dopaminergic projections including VS[45,71,75] and anterior cingulate cortex,[48,49] as well as other structures including the habenula[62,87,107] and amygdala.[22,115] Unlike some of the other predictions from HRL that we have discussed, for which at least circumstantial evidence can be drawn from the literature, we are aware of no previous work that sheds light on whether anything like the PPE is computed in the brain. Given this, we undertook a set of experiments assaying for neural correlates of the PPE. In the following section, we present an overview of these experiments and their results. (For full details, see ref. 82.)

Testing for the Pseudo-Reward Prediction Error

To ground the distinction between the RPE and PPE, and to set the scene for our experiments, consider the video game illustrated in figure 16.3, which is based on a benchmark task from the computational HRL literature.[33] Only the icon elements in the figure (truck, house, and package) appear in the task display. The overall objective of the game is to complete a "delivery" as quickly as possible, using joystick movements to guide the truck first to the package and from there to the house. The task has a transparent hierarchical structure, with delivery serving as the (externally rewarded) top-level goal and acquisition of the package as an obvious subgoal. For an HRL agent, delivery would be associated with primary reward, and acquisition of the package with pseudo-reward.

Consider now a version of the task in which the package sometimes unexpectedly jumps to a new location before the truck reaches it. According to RL, a jump to point A in the figure, or any location within the ellipse shown, should trigger a positive RPE, because the total distance that must be covered to deliver the package has decreased. We assume temporal discounting or effort costs that imply attaining

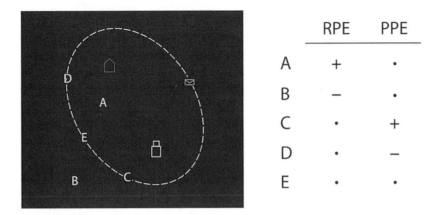

	RPE	PPE
A	+	•
B	−	•
C	•	+
D	•	−
E	•	•

Figure 16.3
Left: Task display and geometry for the delivery task. Right: Prediction errors elicited by the four jump destinations in the task display. + and − indicate positive and negative prediction errors, respectively.

the goal faster is more rewarding. This was enforced by making each movement of the truck effortful. By the same token, a jump to point B (or any other exterior point) should trigger a negative RPE. Cases C through E are quite different. Here, there is no change in the overall distance to the goal, and so no RPE should be triggered. However, in case C, the distance to the subgoal has decreased. According to HRL, a jump to this location should thus trigger a positive PPE. Similarly, a jump to location D should trigger a negative PPE. (Note that location E is special, being the only location that should trigger neither an RPE or a PPE.)

These points translate directly into neuroscientific predictions. As noted earlier, previous research has revealed neural correlates of the RPE in numerous structures.[15,22,45,48,49,73,75,107,115] HRL predicts that neural correlates should also exist for the PPE. To test this, we had normal undergraduate participants perform the delivery task from figure 16.3 while undergoing electroencephalography (EEG) and, in two further experiments, functional magnetic resonance imaging (fMRI).

In our first experiment, participants performed the delivery task while undergoing EEG recording. Over the course of the recording session, one third of trials involved a jump event of type *D* from figure 16.3; these events were intended to elicit a negative pseudo-reward prediction error. Earlier EEG research indicates that ordinary negative reward prediction errors trigger a midline negativity, commonly referred to as the feedback error-related negativity, or fERN[48,49,65] (see also chapters 17 and 18, this volume). Based on HRL, we predicted that a similar negativity would occur following the critical changes in pseudo-reward. To provide a baseline for comparison, another third of trials included jump events of type *E* (following figure 16.3).

a)   b)

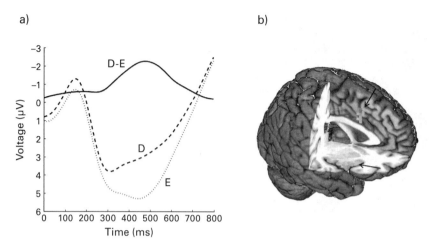

Figure 16.4
(a) Evoked potentials at electrode Cz, aligned to jump events. *D* and *E* refer to jump destinations in figure 16.3. The data-series labeled *D-E* shows the difference between curves *D* and *E*, isolating the pseudo-reward prediction error effect. (b) Regions displaying a positive correlation with the pseudo-reward prediction error (independent of subgoal displacement per se) in the first fMRI experiment. The [x y z] coordinates (Talairach space) of peak statistical significance are, for dorsal anterior cingulate cortex, [0 9 39], left anterior insula [–45 9 –3], right anterior insula [45 12 0], and lingual gyrus [0 –66 0].

Stimulus-aligned EEG averages indicated that class-*D* jump events, which should induce negative pseudo-reward prediction errors, triggered a phasic negativity in the EEG as shown in figure 16.4a. Like the fERN, this negativity was largest in the midline leads, and the time course was consistent with the fERN, as observed in studies where information about the outcome and the appropriate stimulus-response mapping are shown simultaneously.[8]

In a second experiment, we examined neural correlates of the PPE using fMRI. A new group of normal participants underwent fMRI while performing a slightly different version of the delivery task. The task was again designed to elicit negative pseudo-reward prediction errors. As in the EEG experiment, one third of trials included a jump of type *D* (as in figure 16.3) and another third included a jump of type *E*. In contrast to the EEG task, the increase in subgoal distance in this experiment varied in size across trials. By this means, type *D* jumps were intended to induce PPEs that varied in magnitude. Our analyses tested for regions that showed phasic activation correlating with predicted PPE size.

A whole-brain general linear model analysis revealed such a correlation, negative in sign, in the dorsal anterior cingulate cortex (ACC; figure 16.4b). This region is believed to contain the generator of the fERN,[48] and the fMRI result is thus consistent with the result of our EEG experiment. The same parametric fMRI effect was also observed bilaterally in the anterior insula, a region often coactivated with

ACC in the setting of unanticipated negative events.[79] The only other region display-ing the same effect is a small focus within the lingual gyrus.

A set of region-of-interest (ROI) analyses focused in on additional neural struc-tures that, like the ACC, were previously proposed to encode negative reward prediction errors: the habenular complex,[87,107] nucleus accumbens,[95] and amyg-dala.[22,115] The habenular complex was found to display greater activity following type D than type E jumps, consistent with the idea that this structure is also engaged by negative pseudo-reward prediction errors. A comparable effect was also observed in the right, though not the left, amygdala. In the nucleus accumbens (NAcc), where some studies have observed deactivation accompanying negative reward prediction errors,[56] no significant pseudo-reward prediction error effect was observed in this first fMRI study. However, it should be noted that NAcc deactivation with negative reward prediction errors has been an inconsistent finding in previous work.[24,72] More robust is the association between NAcc activation and positive reward prediction errors.[15,45,71,75] With this in mind, we ran a second, smaller ROI fMRI study specifi-cally looking for NAcc activation within a region of interest, with positive pseudo-reward prediction errors. Fourteen participants performed the delivery task, with jumps of type C (in figure 16.3) occurring on one third of trials, and jumps of type E on another third. As described earlier, a positive pseudo-reward prediction error is predicted to occur in association with type C jumps, and in this setting significant activation was observed in the right NAcc, scaling with predicted pseudo-reward prediction error magnitude.

Directions for Further Investigation

Our initial experiments, together with the evidence we have pieced together from the existing literature, suggest that HRL may provide a useful framework for inves-tigating the neural basis of hierarchical behavior. As detailed in our recent work,[21] HRL also gives rise to further testable predictions, each of which presents an oppor-tunity for further research.

To take just one example, HRL predicts that neural correlates should exist for option-specific state-value representations. As explained earlier, in addition to the top-level state-value function, the critic in HRL must also maintain a set of option-specific value functions. This is because the value function indicates how well things are expected to go following arrival at a given state, which obviously depends on which actions the agent will select. Under HRL, the option that is cur-rently in control of behavior determines action selection, and also determines which actions will yield pseudo-reward. Thus, whenever an option is guiding behav-ior, the value attached to a state must take the identity of that option into account.

If there is a neural structure that computes something like option-specific state values, this structure would be expected to communicate closely with the VS, the region typically identified with the locus of state or state-action values in RL. However, the structure would also be expected to receive inputs from the portions of frontal cortex that we have identified as representing options. One brain region that meets both of these criteria is the orbitofrontal cortex (OFC), an area that has strong connections with both VS and DLPFC.[3,84] The idea that the OFC might participate in computing option-specific state values also fits well with the behavior of individual neurons within this cortical region. OFC neurons have been extensively implicated in representing the reward value associated with environmental states.[84,94] However, other data suggest that OFC neurons can also be sensitive to shifts in response policy or task set.[70] Critically, OFC representations of event value have been observed to change in parallel with shifts in strategy,[92] a finding that fits precisely with the idea that the OFC might represent option-specific state values. Although these findings are consistent with an HRL interpretation, further research on OFC directly guided by the relevant predictions from HRL could be quite informative.

Discovering Hierarchical Structure

Another avenue for further research arises from a question we have so far avoided: Where do options come from? Throughout this chapter, we have assumed that the HRL agent simply has a toolbox full of options available for selection. The same assumption is adopted in much purely computational work in HRL. The question inevitably arises, however, of how this toolbox of options is initially assembled. This question, sometimes referred to as the option discovery problem, is obviously relevant to human learning.[21] Indeed, influential behavioral work has characterized childhood development as involving a process of building up a hierarchical set of skills.[35,111] Characterizing this building-up process in specific computational terms turns out to be a challenging task. Indeed, option discovery stands as an open problem in computational HRL.[12,101]

One interesting recent machine-learning proposal for how an HRL agent might discover useful options centers on the notion of *bottleneck* states.[100] These are states that give access to a wide range of subsequent states. As an example, consider a stairwell connecting two floors in a house. To reach any location on one floor from any location on the other, one must pass through the stairwell. The stairwell is, in this sense, a bottleneck location in the house. Both intuitively and formally, such bottleneck locations make good subgoals, around which useful subroutines can be built.

An explicit definition for what makes a state a bottleneck can be derived from graph theory, where the property of being a bottleneck state corresponds to a

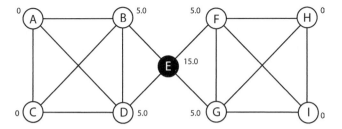

Figure 16.5
Betweenness for states of a graph. Note how state *E* is a clear bottleneck for transitioning from states *A–D* to *F–I*. This is reflected in the value of betweenness, which elects this state as a useful subgoal.

measure called *betweeness centrality*.[100] Figure 16.5 shows a graph with an obvious bottleneck, with each node labeled with its corresponding betweeness value. If this graph represented a behavioral domain, and an agent wanted to carve this domain "at its joints" by identifying useful subgoal states, the node at the center of the graph would make a good candidate, a point that simulation work has borne out.[100]

One may well ask, however, whether human learners identify bottleneck states, and if so whether they use such states as a basis for parsing tasks. Some affirmation of this is provided by Cordova and colleagues.[26] In this study, participants were presented with a set of "landmarks" (e.g., post office, school), and learned their adjacency relations within a fictive town. These adjacencies were based on simple graphs like the one in figure 16.5, each of which included a clear bottleneck (although the graph itself was never shown to the participants). Once the adjacency relations among the town's landmarks had been learned, participants were then asked to make "deliveries" in the town, navigating each time from a specified point of origin to a specified goal, and receiving a reward that varied inversely with the number of steps taken to complete the delivery. Before beginning these deliveries, however, the participant was asked to select one landmark as a location for a "bus stop," understanding that he or she could "jump" to this location from any other during the deliveries, potentially reducing the number of steps taken. Without knowledge of the specific upcoming delivery assignments, the optimal choice for the bus stop location corresponds to the bottleneck location, and participants overwhelmingly selected this location.

In a related experiment, we have shown that human learners not only identify bottleneck states, but also use these as a basis for segmentation.[90] Here, a distinctive visual stimulus was assigned to each vertex of a bottleneck graph (which was itself not shown), and participants viewed these stimuli in sequences generated based on a random walk through the underlying graph. Subjects were then asked to parse a further set of stimulus sequences, generated in the same way, pressing a button when they perceived a transition between subsequences. Participants showed a significant tendency to parse at junctures where the sequence traversed a bottleneck in the underlying graph, consistent with the idea that events or tasks can be decomposed based on a structural analysis of their underlying topological structure. Together, these initial findings suggest that ideas from computational HRL may help answer the question of how humans discover hierarchical structure in the task environment, developing action hierarchies tailored to this structure.

Dual Modes of Control

We believe that further HRL-related research, and indeed all research drawing on RL, must attend to an important but often neglected distinction between two forms of learning or decision making. Work on animal and human behavior suggests that instrumental actions arise from two modes of control, one built on established stimulus-response links or "habits," and the other on prospective planning.[9] Recent work has mapped these modes of control onto RL constructs,[31] characterizing the former as relying on cached action values or strengths and model-free RL, and the latter as looking ahead based on an internal model relating actions to their likely effects, that is, model-based RL.[18] Here, we have cast HRL in terms of the cache-based system, both because this is most representative of existing work on HRL and because the principles of model-based search have not yet been as fully explored, either at the computational level or in terms of neural correlates. However, incorporating temporal abstraction into model-based, prospective control is straightforward. This is accomplished by assuming that each option is associated with an *option model*, a knowledge structure indicating the ultimate outcomes likely to result from selecting the option, the reward or cost likely to be accrued during its execution, and the amount of time this execution is likely to take.[106] Equipped with models of this kind, the agent can use them to look ahead, evaluating potential courses of action. Importantly, the search process can now "skip over" potentially large sequences of primitive actions, effectively reducing the size of the search tree.[47,54,61] This kind of saltatory search process seems to fit well with everyday planning, which introspectively seems to operate at the level of temporally abstract actions ("Perhaps I should buy one of those new cell phones. . . . Well, that would cost me a few hundred dollars. . . . But if I bought one, I could use it to check my email . . ."). The idea of action models, in general, also fits well with work on motor control, which strongly suggests the involvement of predictive models in guiding bodily movements.[113] Because option models encode the consequences of interventions, it is interesting to note that recent neuroimaging work has mapped representations of action outcome information in part to prefrontal cortex,[44] a region whose potential links with HRL we have already considered. Further investigating the potential relevance of model-based HRL to human planning and decision making offers an inviting area for further research.

Conclusion

Computational RL has proved extremely useful in research on behavior and brain function. Our aim here has been to explore whether HRL might prove similarly applicable. An initial motivation for considering this question derives from the fact that HRL addresses an inherent limitation of RL, the scaling problem, which would clearly be relevant to any organism relying on RL-like learning mechanisms. Implementing HRL along the lines of the actor-critic framework, thereby bringing it into alignment with existing mappings between RL and neuroscience, reveals direct parallels between components of HRL and specific functional neuroanatomic structures, including the DLPFC and OFC. HRL suggests new ways of interpreting neural activity in these as well as several other regions. We have reported results from initial experiments prospectively testing predictions from HRL, which provide evidence for a novel form of prediction-error signal. All things considered, HRL appears to offer a potentially useful set of tools for further investigating the computational and neural basis of hierarchical structured behavior.

Acknowledgments

The present work was completed with support from Fundação para a Ciência e Tecnologia (SFRH/BD/33273/2007, J. R-F.), the National Institute of Mental Health (P50 MH062196, M.M.B.), and the James S. McDonnell Foundation (M.M.B.).

Outstanding Questions

• How is hierarchically structured behavior represented at the neural level? Are levels of behavioral structure represented discretely, maximizing compositional flexibility, or in a continuous distributed fashion, maximizing generalization and information sharing? Does the answer to this question differ across decision-making systems (habitual versus goal-directed, for example)?

• How are internal representations of hierarchical behavior learned? How does the brain establish and refine a toolbox of subroutines, skills, subtasks or options, which can be exploited across a wide range of potential future activities? How are useful subgoals discovered, when they are not associated with primary reward?

• Given a set of options, how does learning discover the particular combinations and sequences that solve new task challenges?

• Does the framework of computational reinforcement learning provide a useful heuristic for pursuing the answers to the above questions? In particular, does the resemblance between dopaminergic function and temporal-difference learning extend to the hierarchical case, and does recent evidence concerning hierarchical representation in prefrontal cortex bear any logical relation to hierarchical representation in HRL?

Further Reading

1. Badre D. 2008. Cognitive control, hierarchy, and the rostro-caudal axis of the frontal lobes. *Trends Cogn Sci* 12: 193–200. An excellent brief review of empirical findings concerning hierarchical representation in prefrontal cortex.

2. Badre D, Frank MJ. in press. Mechanisms of hierarchical reinforcement learning in corticostriatal circuits 2: Evidence from fMRI. *Cereb Cortex*. Frank MJ, Badre D. in press. Mechanisms of hierarchical reinforcement learning in corticostriatal circuits 1: Computational analysis. *Cereb Cortex*. Companion empirical and theoretical papers, voicing a different but not incompatible perspective on hierarchical learning mechanisms.

3. Barto AG, Mahadevan S. 2003. Recent advances in hierarchical reinforcement learning. *Discret Event Dyn Syst* 13: 41–77. A review of the HRL framework and its various implementations, from a machine-learning perspective.

4. Botvinick MM. 2008. Hierarchical models of behavior and prefrontal function. *Trends Cogn Sci* 12: 201–208. An overview of computational models that have addressed hierarchical action and its neural underpinnings.

5. Botvinick MM, Niv Y, Barto AC. 2009. Hierarchically organized behavior and its neural foundations: a reinforcement learning perspective. *Cognition* 113: 262–280. An introduction to HRL and its potential neural correlates.

6. Ribas-Fernandes J, Solway A, Diuk C, Barto AG, Niv Y, Botvinick M. in press. A neural signature of hierarchical reinforcement learning. *Neuron*. A set of neuroimaging experiments testing predictions from HRL.

References

1. Aldridge JW, Berridge KC. 1998. Coding of serial order by neostriatal neurons: a "natural action" approach to movement sequence. *J Neurosci* 18: 2777–2787.

2. Aldridge JW, Berridge KC, Rosen AR. 2004. Basal ganglia neural mechanisms of natural movement sequences. *Can J Physiol Pharmacol* 82: 732–739.

3. Alexander GE, Crutcher MD, DeLong MR. 1990. Basal ganglia-thalamocortical circuits: parallel substrates for motor, oculomotor, "prefrontal" and "limbic" functions. *Prog Brain Res* 85: 119–146.

4. Alexander GE, DeLong MR, Strick PL. 1986. Parallel organization of functionally segregated circuits linking basal ganglia and cortex. *Annu Rev Neurosci* 9: 357–381.

5. Asaad WF, Rainer G, Miller EK. 2000. Task-specific neural activity in the primate prefrontal cortex. *J Neurophysiol* 84: 451–459.

6. Averbeck BB, Lee D. 2007. Prefrontal neural correlates of memory for sequences. *J Neurosci* 27: 2204–2211.

7. Badre D. 2008. Cognitive control, hierarchy, and the rostro–caudal organization of the frontal lobes. *Trends Cogn Sci* 12: 193–200.

8. Baker TE, Holroyd CB (in press). Dissociated roles of the anterior cingulate cortex in reward and conflict processing as revealed by the feedback error-related negativity and N200. *Biol Psychol.*

9. Balleine BW, Dickinson A. 1998. Goal-directed instrumental action: contingency and incentive learning and their cortical substrates. *Neuropharmacology* 37: 407–419.

10. Barto AG. 1995. Adaptive critics and the basal ganglia. In: Models of Information Processing in the Basal Ganglia (Houck JC, Davis J, Beiser D, eds), pp 215–232. Cambridge, MA: MIT Press.

11. Barto AG, Mahadevan S. 2003. Recent advances in hierarchical reinforcement learning. *Discret Event Dyn Syst: Theory Appl* 13: 41–77.

12. Barto AG, Singh S, Chentanez N. (2004) Intrinsically motivated learning of hierarchical collections of skills. Proceedings of the 3rd International Conference on Development and Learning.

13. Barto AG, Sutton RS. 1981. Toward a modern theory of adaptive networks: expectation and prediction. *Psychol Rev* 88: 135–170.

14. Barto AG, Sutton RS, Anderson CW. 1983. Neuronlike adaptive elements that can solve difficult learning control problems. *IEEE Trans Syst Man Cybern* 13: 834–846.

15. Berns GS, McClure SM, Pagnoni G, Montague PR. 2001. Predictability modulates human brain response to reward. *J Neurosci* 21: 2793–2798.

16. Bertsekas DP, Tsitsiklis JN. 1996. Neuro-Dynamic Programming. Belmont, MA: Athena Scientific.

17. Bor D, Duncan J, Wiseman RJ, Owen AM. 2003. Encoding strategies dissociate prefrontal activity from working memory demand. *Neuron* 27: 361–367.

18. Botvinick M, An J. 2009. Goal-directed decision making in prefrontal cortex: a computational framework. In: Advances in Neural Information Processing Systems 21 (Koller D, Schuurmans D, Bengio Y, Bottou L, eds). Cambridge, MA: MIT Press.

19. Botvinick M, Plaut DC. 2004. Doing without schema hierarchies: a recurrent connectionist approach to normal and impaired routine sequential action. *Psychol Rev* 111: 395–429.

20. Botvinick MM. 2008. Hierarchical models of behavior and prefrontal function. *Trends Cogn Sci* 12: 201–208.

21. Botvinick MM, Niv Y, Barto AC. 2009. Hierarchically organized behavior and its neural foundations: a reinforcement learning perspective. *Cognition* 113: 262–280.

22. Breiter HC, Aharon I, Kahneman D, Dale A, Shizgal P. 2001. Functional imaging of neural responses to expectancy and experience of monetary gains and losses. *Neuron* 30: 619–639.

23. Bunge SA. 2004. How we use rules to select actions: a review of evidence from cognitive neuroscience. *Cogn Affect Behav Neurosci* 4: 564–579.

24. Cooper JC, Knutson B. 2008. Valence and salience contribute to nucleus accumbens activation. *Neuroimage* 39: 538–547.

25. Cooper RP, Shallice T. 2006. Hierarchical schemas and goals in the control of sequential behavior. *Psychol Rev* 113: 887–916.

26. Cordova N, Diuk C, Niv Y, Botvinick MM (submitted). Discovering hierarchical task structure.

27. Courtney SM, Roth JK, Sala JB. 2007. A hierarchical biased-competition model of domain-dependent working memory maintenance and executive control. In: Working Memory: Behavioural and Neural Correlates (Osaka N, Logie R, D'Esposito M, eds). Oxford: Oxford University Press.

28. D'Esposito M. 2007. From cognitive to neural models of working memory. *Philos Trans R Soc Lond B Biol Sci* 362: 761–772.

29. Daw ND, Courville AC, Touretzky DS. 2003. Timing and partial observability in the dopamine system. In: Advances in Neural Information Processing Systems 15 (Becker S, Thrun S, Obermayer K, eds), pp 99–106. Cambridge, MA: MIT Press.

30. Daw ND, Frank MJ. 2009. Reinforcement learning and higher level cognition: introduction to special issue. *Cognition* 113: 259–261.

31. Daw ND, Niv Y, Dayan P. 2005. Uncertainty-based competition between prefrontal and striatal systems for behavioral control. *Nat Neurosci* 8: 1704–1711.

32. Daw ND, Niv Y, Dayan P. 2006. Actions, policies, values and the basal ganglia. In: Recent Breakthroughs in Basal Ganglia Research (Bezard E, ed), pp 111–130. New York: Nova Science Publishers.

33. Dietterich TG. 1998. The MAXQ method for hierarchical reinforcement learning. In: Proceedings of the Fifteenth International Conference on Machine Learning, pp 118–126. San Francisco: Morgan Kaufmann Publishers.

34. Dietterich TG. 2000. Hierarchical reinforcement learning with the MAXQ value function decomposition. *J Artif Intell Res* 13: 227–303.

35. Fischer KW. 1980. A theory of cognitive development: the control and construction of hierarchies of skills. *Psychol Rev* 87: 477–531.

36. Frank MJ, Claus ED. 2006. Anatomy of a decision: striato-orbitofrontal interactions in reinforcement learning, decision making, and reversal. *Psychol Rev* 113: 300–326.

37. Fujii N, Graybiel AM. 2003. Representation of action sequence boundaries by macaque prefrontal cortical neurons. *Science* 301: 1246–1249.

38. Fuster JM. (1997) The Prefrontal Cortex: Anatomy, Physiology, and Neuropsychology of the Frontal Lobe. Philadelphia: Lippincott-Raven.

39. Fuster JM. 2001. The prefrontal cortex—an update: time is of the essence. *Neuron* 30: 319–333.

40. Fuster JM. 2004. Upper processing stages of the perception-action cycle. *Trends Cogn Sci* 8: 143–145.

41. Grafman J. 2002. The human prefrontal cortex has evolved to represent components of structured event complexes. In: Handbook of Neuropsychology (Grafman J, ed), pp 157–174. Amsterdam: Elsevier.

42. Graybiel AM. 1995. Building action repertoires: memory and learning functions of the basal ganglia. *Curr Opin Neurobiol* 5: 733–741.

43. Graybiel AM. 1998. The basal ganglia and chunking of action repertoires. *Neurobiol Learn Mem* 70: 119–136.

44. Hamilton AFdeC, Grafton ST. 2008. Action outcomes are represented in human inferior frontoparietal cortex. *Cereb Cortex* 18: 1160–1168.

45. Hare TA, O'Doherty J, Camerer CF, Schultz W, Rangel A. 2008. Dissociating the role of the orbitofrontal cortex and the striatum in the computation of goal values and prediction errors. *J Neurosci* 28: 5623–5630.

46. Haruno M, Kawato M. 2006. Heterarchical reinforcement-learning model for integration of multiple cortico-striatal loops: fMRI examination in stimulus-action-reward association learning. *Neural Netw* 19: 1242–1254.

47. Hayes-Roth B, Hayes-Roth F. 1979. A cognitive model of planning. *Cogn Sci* 3: 275–310.

48. Holroyd CB, Coles MG. 2002. The neural basis of human error processing: reinforcement learning, dopamine, and the error-related negativity. *Psychol Rev* 109: 679–709.

49. Holroyd CB, Nieuwenhuis S, Yeung N, Cohen JD. 2003. Errors in reward prediction are reflected in the event-related brain potential. *Neuroreport* 14: 2481–2484.

50. Hoshi E, Shima K, Tanji J. 1998. Task-dependent selectivity of movement-related neuronal activity in the primate prefrontal cortex. *J Neurophysiol* 80: 3392–3397.

51. Houk JC, Adams CM, Barto AG. 1995. A model of how the basal ganglia generate and use neural signals that predict reinforcement. In: Models of Information Processing in the Basal Ganglia (Houk JC, Davis DG, eds), pp 249–270. Cambridge, MA: MIT Press.

52. Joel D, Niv Y, Ruppin E. 2002. Actor-critic models of the basal ganglia: new anatomical and computational perspectives. *Neural Netw* 15: 535–547.

53. Johnston K, Everling S. 2006. Neural activity in monkey prefrontal cortex is modulated by task context and behavioral instruction during delayed-match-to-sample and conditional prosaccade–antisaccade tasks. *J Cogn Neurosci* 18: 749–765.

54. Kambhampati S, Mali AD, Srivastava B. 1998. Hybrid planning for partially hierarchical domains. In: Proceedings of the Fifteenth National Conference on Artificial Intelligence (AAAI-98), pp 882–888. Madison, WI: AAAI Press.

55. Kearns M, Singh S. 2002. Near-optimal reinforcement learning in polynomial time. *Mach Learn* 49: 209–232.

56. Knutson B, Taylor J, Kaufman M, Petersen R, Glover G. 2005. Distributed neural representation of expected value. *J Neurosci* 25: 4806–4812.

57. Koechlin E, Ody C, Kouneiher F. 2003. The architecture of cognitive control in the human prefrontal cortex. *Science* 302: 1181–1185.

58. Lashley KS. 1951 The problem of serial order in behavior. In: Cerebral Mechanisms in Behavior: The Hixon Symposium (Jeffress LA, ed), pp 112–136. New York: Wiley.

59. Lee IH, Seitz AR, Assad JA. 2006. Activity of tonically active neurons in the monkey putamen during initiation and withholding of movement. *J Neurophysiol* 95: 2391–2403.

60. Li L, Walsh TJ. 2006. Towards a unified theory of state abstraction for MDPs. In: Ninth International Symposium on Artificial Intelligence and Mathematics, pp 531–539.

61. Marthi B, Russell SJ, Wolfe J. 2007. Angelic semantics for high-level actions. In: Seventeenth International Conference on Automated Planning and Scheduling (ICAPS 2007).

62. Matsumoto M, Hikosaka O. 2007. Lateral habenula as a source of negative reward signals in dopamine neurons. *Nature* 447: 1111–1115.

63. Miller EK, Cohen JD. 2001. An integrative theory of prefrontal cortex function. *Annu Rev Neurosci* 24: 167–202.

64. Miller GA, Galanter E, Pribram KH. 1960. Plans and the Structure of Behavior. New York: Holt, Rinehart & Winston.

65. Miltner WHR, Braun CH, Coles MGH. 1997. Event-related brain potentials following incorrect feedback in a time-estimation task: evidence for a "generic" neural system for error detection. *J Cogn Neurosci* 9: 788–798.

66. Miyamoto H, Morimoto J, Doya K, Kawato M. 2004. Reinforcement learning with via-point representation. *Neural Netw* 17: 299–305.

67. Montague P, Dayan P, Sejnowski T. 1996. A framework for mesencephalic dopamine systems based on predictive Hebbian learning. *J Neurosci* 16: 1936.

68. Morris G, Arkadir D, Nevet A, Vaadia E, Bergman H. 2004. Coincident but distinct messages of midbrain dopamine and striatal tonically active neurons. *Neuron* 43: 133–143.

69. Muhammad R, Wallis JD, Miller EK. 2006. A comparison of abstract rules in the prefrontal cortex, premotor cortex, inferior temporal cortex, and striatum. *J Cogn Neurosci* 18: 974–989.

70. O'Doherty J, Critchley H, Deichmann R, Dolan RJ. 2003. Dissociating valence of outcome from behavioral control in human orbital and ventral prefrontal cortices. *J Neurosci* 7931: 7931–7939.

71. O'Doherty J, Dayan P, Schultz P, Deischmann J, Friston K, Dolan RJ. 2004. Dissociable roles of ventral and dorsal striatum in instrumental conditioning. *Science* 304: 452–454.

72. O'Doherty JP, Buchanan TW, Seymour B, Dolan R. 2006. Predictive neural coding of reward preference involves dissociable responses in human ventral midbrain and ventral striatum. *Neuron* 49: 157–166.

73. O'Doherty JP, Dayan P, Friston K, Critchley H, Dolan RJ. 2003. Temporal difference models and reward-related learning in the human brain. *Neuron* 38: 329–337.

74. O'Reilly RC, Frank MJ. 2006. Making working memory work: a computational model of learning in the prefrontal cortex and basal ganglia. *Neural Comput* 18: 283–328.

75. Pagnoni G, Zink CF, Montague PR, Berns GS. 2002. Activity in human ventral striatum locked to errors of reward prediction. *Nat Neurosci* 5: 97–98.

76. Parent A, Hazrati LN. 1995. Functional anatomy of the basal ganglia. I. The cortico-basal ganglia-thalamo-cortical loop. *Brain Res Brain Res Rev* 20: 91–127.

77. Parr R, Russell S. 1998. Reinforcement learning with hierarchies of machines. In: Advances in Neural Information Processing Systems 10 (Jordan MI, Kearns MJ, Solla SA, eds), pp 1043–1049. Cambridge, MA: MIT Press.

78. Petrides M. 1995. Impairments on nonspatial self-ordered and externally ordered working memory tasks after lesions to the mid-dorsal part of the lateral frontal cortex in the monkey. *J Neurosci* 15: 359–375.

79. Phan KL, Wager TD, Taylor SF, Liberzon I. 2004. Functional neuroimaging studies of human emotions. *CNS Spectr* 9: 258–266.

80. Postle BR. 2006. Working memory as an emergent property of the mind and brain. *Neuroscience* 139: 23–28.

81. Ravel S, Sardo P, Legallet E, Apicella P. 2006. Influence of spatial information on responses of tonically active neurons in the monkey striatum. *J Neurophysiol* 95: 2975–2986.

82. Ribas-Fernandes JJF, Solway A, Diuk C, McGuire JT, Barto AG, Niv Y, Botvinick MM (under review). A neural signature of hierarchical reinforcement learning.

83. Roesch MR, Taylor AR, Schoenbaum G. 2006. Encoding of time-discounted rewards in orbitofrontal cortex is independent of value representation. *Neuron* 51: 509–520.

84. Rolls ET. 2004. The functions of the orbitofrontal cortex. *Brain Cogn* 55: 11–29.

85. Rougier NP, Noell DC, Braver TS, Cohen JD, O'Reilly RC. 2005. Prefrontal cortex and flexible cognitive control: rules without symbols. *Proc Natl Acad Sci USA* 102: 7338–7343.

86. Rushworth MF, Walton ME, Kennerley SW, Bannerman DM. 2004. Action sets and decisions in the medial frontal cortex. *Trends Cogn Sci* 8: 410–417.

87. Salas R, Baldwin P, de Biasi M, Montague PR. 2010. BOLD responses to negative reward prediction errors in human habenula. *Front Hum Neurosci* 4: 36.

88. Salinas E. 2004. Fast remapping of sensory stimuli onto motor actions on the basis of contextual modulation. *J Neurosci* 24: 1113–1118.

89. Schank RC, Abelson RP. 1977. Scripts, Plans, Goals and Understanding. Hillside, NJ: Erlbaum.

90. Schapiro A, Rogers T, Botvinick MM. 2010. Beyond uncertainty: behavioral and computational investigations of the structure of event representations. Paper presented at the Annual Meeting of the Cognitive Science Society.

91. Schneider DW, Logan GD. 2006. Hierarchical control of cognitive processes: switching tasks in sequences. *J Exp Psychol Gen* 135: 623–640.

92. Schoenbaum G, Chiba AA, Gallagher M. 1999. Neural encoding in orbitofrontal cortex and basolateral amygdala during olfactory discrimination learning. *J Neurosci* 19: 1876–1884.

93. Schultz W, Dayan P, Montague P. 1997. A neural substrate of prediction and reward. *Science* 275: 1593.

94. Schultz W, Tremblay KL, Hollerman JR. 2000. Reward processing in primate orbitofrontal cortex and basal ganglia. *Cereb Cortex* 10: 272–283.

95. Seymour B, Daw ND, Dayan P, Singer T, Dolan RJ. 2007. Differential encoding of losses and gains in the human striatum. *J Neurosci* 27: 4826–4831.

96. Shallice T, Burgess PW. 1991. Deficits in strategy application following frontal lobe damage in man. *Brain* 114: 727–741.

97. Shima K, Isoda M, Mushiake H, Tanji J. 2007. Categorization of behavioural sequences in the prefrontal cortex. *Nature* 445: 315–318.

98. Shima K, Tanji J. 2000. Neuronal activity in the supplementary and presupplementary motor areas for temporal organization of multiple movements. *J Neurophysiol* 84: 2148–2160.

99. Shimamura AP. 2000. The role of the prefrontal cortex in dynamic filtering. *Psychobiology* 28: 207–218.

100. Şimşek Ö, Wolfe A, Barto A. 2005. Identifying useful subgoals in reinforcement learning by local graph partitioning. In: Proceedings of the 22nd International Conference on Machine Learning, pp 816–823. New York: ACM.

101. Singh S, Barto AG, Chentanez N. 2005. Intrinsically motivated reinforcement learning. In: Advances in Neural Information Processing Systems 17: Proceedings of the 2004 Conference (Saul LK, Weiss Y, Bottou L, eds), pp 1281–1288. Cambridge, MA: MIT Press.

102. Sirigu A, Zalla T, Pillon B, Dubois B, Grafman J, Agid Y. 1995. Selective impairments in managerial knowledge in patients with pre-frontal cortex lesions. *Cortex* 31: 301–316.

103. Suri RE, Bargas J, Arbib MA. 2001. Modeling functions of striatal dopamine modulation in learning and planning. *Neuroscience* 103: 65–85.

104. Sutton RS, Barto AG. 1990. Time-derivative models of pavlovian reinforcement. In: Learning and Computational Neuroscience: Foundations of Adaptive Networks (Gabriel M, Moore J, eds), pp 497–537. Cambridge, MA: MIT Press.

105. Sutton RS, Barto AG. 1998. Reinforcement Learning: An Introduction. Cambridge, MA: MIT Press.

106. Sutton RS, Precup D, Singh S. 1999. Between MDPs and semi-MDPs: a framework for temporal abstraction in reinforcement learning. *Artif Intell* 112: 181–211.

107. Ullsperger M, von Cramon DY. 2003. Error monitoring using external feedback: specific roles of the habenular complex, the reward system, and the cingulate motor area revealed by functional magnetic resonance imaging. *J Neurosci* 23: 4308–4314.

108. Wallis JD, Anderson KC, Miller EK. 2001. Single neurons in prefrontal cortex encode abstract rules. *Nature* 411: 953–956.

109. Wallis JD, Miller EK. 2003. From rule to response: neuronal processes in the premotor and prefrontal cortex. *J Neurophysiol* 90: 1790–1806.

110. White IM, Wise SP. 1999. Rule-dependent neuronal activity in the prefrontal cortex. *Exp Brain Res* 126: 315–335.

111. White RW. 1959. Motivation reconsidered: the concept of competence. *Psychol Rev* 66: 297–333.

112. Wickens J, Kotter R, Houk JC. 1995. Cellular models of reinforcement. In: Models of Information Processing in the Basal Ganglia (Davis JL, Beiser DG, eds), pp 187–214. Cambridge, MA: MIT Press.

113. Wolpert D, Flanagan J. 2001. Motor prediction. *Curr Biol* 18: R729–R732.

114. Wood JN, Grafman J. 2003. Human prefrontal cortex: processing and representational perspectives. *Nat Rev Neurosci* 4: 139–147.

115. Yacubian J, Gläscher J, Schroeder K, Sommer T, Braus DF, Büchel C. 2006. Dissociable systems for gain- and loss-related value predictions and errors of prediction in the human brain. *J Neurosci* 26: 9530–9537.

116. Zacks JM, Braver TS, Sheridan MA, Donaldson DI, Snyder AZ, Ollinger JM, Buckner RL, Raichle ME. 2001. Human brain activity time-locked to perceptual event boundaries. *Nat Neurosci* 4: 651–655.

117. Zacks JM, Speer NK, Swallow KM, Braver TS, Reynolds JR. 2007. Event perception: a mind/brain perspective. *Psychol Bull* 133: 273–293.

118. Zalla T, Pradat-Diehl P, Sirigu A. 2003. Perception of action boundaries in patients with frontal lobe damage. *Neuropsychologia* 41: 1619–1627.

17 Reinforcement Learning, Conflict Monitoring, and Cognitive Control: An Integrative Model of Cingulate-Striatal Interactions and the ERN

Jeffrey Cockburn and Michael Frank

Fortune favors those who are able to align their plans and goals to accord with the constraints imposed on them by an intricate and dynamic world. However, this presents an exceedingly difficult assignment, since the constraints pressed on an organism are typically complex, uncertain, and even paradoxical. When foodstuffs run low in the fall, should a hungry forager explore new and unfamiliar territory, or should it conserve energy and wait for something to turn up? The situation may appear dire and warrant the hazards of straying from routine, yet knowledge built up over years of experience may suggest that patience will be rewarded.

Flexible goal-directed behavior demands an adaptive system capable of selecting behavior appropriate for a given context. Evidence spanning a range of methodologies suggests that the anterior cingulate cortex (ACC) and the basal ganglia (BG) are two of the core brain structures involved in cognitive control, both contributing to pathways critical for learning and decision making (see also chapters 2, 9, 17, and 18, this volume). At an abstract level of description, the ACC is generally thought to be involved in monitoring performance and instigating rapid behavioral adjustments when required, whereas the BG is thought to facilitate and suppress behavior based on more stable environmental statistics. Both of these functions have been simulated in separate computational models of the ACC[5] and BG.[14] Although considerable debate still surrounds the unique function each system serves, here we take the approach that a better understanding may also emerge from considering the interaction between the ACC and the BG.

We propose a model in which ACC activity is modulated in part by reinforcement learning processes in the BG. In particular, we focus on how this relationship between the ACC and the BG may help clarify our understanding of the error-related negativity (ERN), a component of the event-related potential (ERP) thought to be generated in the ACC. We begin with a brief overview of the two dominant theories explaining the ERN: the reinforcement learning hypothesis advanced by Holroyd, Coles, and colleagues, and the conflict monitoring hypothesis advocated by Botvinick, Yeung, and colleagues. This overview is followed by a sketch of the core BG model and its role in reinforcement learning and action selection. We then include a novel extension incorporating the ACC into the BG model, using simulated ACC activity to quantify the ERN as response conflict driven by reinforcement learning processes in the BG as a function of feedback processing. We conclude with a discussion of how this model may advance our understanding of both the ACC and the BG, in addition to resolving an ongoing debate between the two dominant models of the ERN.

The Error-Related Negativity

The term error-related negativity (ERN) is most commonly associated with incorrect responses (response ERN or rERN) and incorrect feedback (feedback ERN or fERN). The rERN is typically observed 0 to 150 msec following overt incorrect responses in speeded-response tasks, exhibiting a frontocentral distribution symmetrical about the midline.[24] The fERN is typically observed 200 to 350 msec following unexpected incorrect feedback and has a scalp topography nearly identical to that of the rERN.[33] Dipole modeling has consistently located the neural source of both the rERN and the fERN to be within the medial frontal cortex, most likely in the ACC.[10] However, despite nearly two decades of research on the topic, the cognitive processes that give rise to the ERN are still under debate. In the following, we briefly outline two dominant theories, one relating the ERN to reinforcement learning processes, and the other linking the ERN to performance monitoring (see also chapter 18, this volume).

The Reinforcement Learning Theory of the ERN

An influential theory proposed by Holroyd and Coles has linked the ERN to reinforcement learning processes in the brain.[28] Rooted in a temporal difference reinforcement learning framework, the rERN and fERN are integrated as indices of phasic dopamine signals impacting the ACC. The ACC, in turn, was proposed to use these signals to learn which action should be executed given the current context and goal.

Based on a wealth of behavioral, neurological, and theoretical evidence, the midbrain dopamine system has been shown to encode a powerful reinforcement learning signal referred to as a reward prediction error.[35,45] Within the framework of temporal-difference (TD) reinforcement learning, a prediction error signal provides a mechanism through which actions and events are linked to their outcomes, even when outcomes are temporally distal from their antecedent cause. In short, the goal of a TD learning agent can be reduced to making decisions that maximize its opportunity to encounter rewards in the future. This is achieved by ascribing values to actions and/or states that reflect the expected value of future rewards. At the heart of this value learning process is the reward prediction error, which quantifies the discrepancy between the expected and actual outcomes of an action or state. This learning signal is used to adjust the agent's expectations such that they accurately predict actual outcomes. By propagating reward values back to the actions and/or states that reliably precede them, the agent learns to accurately predict future outcomes and can therefore make decisions that maximize future rewards.

If the ERN is associated with the arrival of phasic dopamine signals in the ACC, then the characteristics of the ERN should conform to predictions from normative reinforcement learning theory. Critically, TD reinforcement learning theory states that reward prediction error signals propagate back from reward delivery to preceding actions and cues as predictive values are learned. Holroyd and Coles, demonstrated that the ERN exhibits precisely this signature by employing a probabilistic learning task.[28] Early in learning, before reward feedback could be predicted, ERN amplitude was larger following feedback and smaller following responses. Later in learning, once the reward contingencies had been learned, ERN amplitude was smaller following reward feedback and larger following response. These results were extended to show that simply presenting a stimulus predictive of reward also modulated ERN amplitude in correspondence with learning.[1] Subsequent work has also correlated fERN variance with reward expectancy violations. In accordance with normative TD learning, unexpected outcomes elicit larger fERNs than expected outcomes.[29] Together, these results, alongside those from numerous additional studies, suggest that the ERN is indeed related to reinforcement learning processes in the brain, linking the rERN and fERN as indices of the ACC's response to the arrival of phasic dopamine signals. However, a theory has also been proposed that likens the ERN to a response monitoring processes, which we outline here.

The Conflict Monitoring Theory of the ERN

In a model-based investigation of ACC function, Botvinick et al.[5] proposed that the ERN is a product of conflict monitoring processes in the ACC. The authors argued that the ACC is a response conflict monitor, a system that tracks the coactivation of mutually exclusive responses as an indication that additional cognitive resources may be required to help perform the task at hand. As conflict increases, the ACC can engage additional control processes to assist in guiding performance.

Various experimental methodologies have demonstrated that ACC activity increases when a prepotent response must be overridden, when one of several equally permissible responses must be selected, or when errors are made. Botvinick and colleagues hypothesized that response conflict is common to all three of these scenarios.[5] This hypothesis was tested by applying a connectionist model to simulated tasks known to engage the ACC, most notably a version of the Eriksen flanker task used to investigate the ERN.[5] During the flanker task, subjects are asked to identify the central character in a multiletter array, which can be either congruent (>>>) or incongruent (><). Modeling results demonstrated that simulated conflict was greater and more sustained on incorrect trials, which were overwhelmingly associated with incongruent trials. On incorrect incongruent trials, flanker information initially drove activation of the incorrect response unit, which was sufficient to generate the incorrect response. Hence, prior to the central character gaining control of response units, both responses exhibited some degree of activation, which is quantified as an increase in response conflict. Simulated response times revealed that incorrect responses were typically associated with faster response times, replicating human performance. An investigation into the model's activation dynamics demonstrated that the probability of eliciting the correct response increased when extra processing time allowed response conflict to resolve before a response was made. Critically, this finding predicted that conflict should be present prior to responses on difficult (incongruent) correct trials.

If the ERN is generated by ACC activation associated with response conflict, then an ERN-like signature should be observed before correct responses on high conflict trials. Yeung and colleagues confirmed this prediction in a detailed investigation of ERPs recorded during a variant of the Eriksen flanker task.[54] As predicted, their results revealed a large rERN following incorrect responses. In addition, their results also revealed modulation of the N2 prior to correct responses. A large negative deflection was observed prior to correct response on high-conflict trials (incongruent, ><) but not on low-conflict trials (congruent, >>>). Scalp topography and dipole source localization suggested that N2 modulation prior to response shared the same neural generator as the rERN following incorrect responses. Additionally, simulations demonstrated that conflict detection can provide a simple yet reliable mechanism for error detection, thus linking the ERN to conflict monitoring and error detection processes.

In summary, two theories have come to provide the dominant explanations of the ERN: one proposing that the ERN is an index of reinforcement learning processes, and the other positing that the ERN is an index of conflict monitoring. Although these theories are commonly understood to be mutually exclusive, the abundance of data supporting each theory argues against the tenability of rejecting one theory in favor of the other. In the following, we outline preliminary results suggesting that both theories of the ERN may be unified by considering the activation dynamics of the BG in relation to the ACC. However, we first visit evidence for a functional link between the BG and the ACC.

The Basal Ganglia

The basal ganglia (BG) are composed of an anatomically and functionally linked group of subcortical nuclei located at the base of the forebrain[34] (see also chapter 2, this volume). The BG are thought to facilitate a wide range of faculties, including motor, motivational, and cognitive processes. Such breadth could be interpreted as an indication that multiple disparate roles are subsumed by the BG; however, a more unified and integrative functional role has been suggested by recent model-based investigations of the BG.

In much the same way that discovering the viral source of the common cold unified seemingly unrelated coughing, sneezing, fatigue, and feverish symptoms; broadly speaking, the BG's function can be conceptualized as a system that dynamically and adaptively gates the flow of information among cortical regions via cortico–basal ganglia–thalamocortical loops. Anatomically, the BG is well suited for this role, serving as a central way station where projections from numerous cortical structures converge, including prefrontal cortex, sensory cortex, hippocampus, and amygdala. Hence, the BG is positioned to integrate information from multiple systems, including the candidate motor or cognitive actions represented in frontal cortex, and to gate the most adaptive of these actions to be carried out while suppressing the execution of competing actions.

But how do the BG "know" which action plans should be facilitated and which should be suppressed? Any plausible model of such functionality should avoid appealing to what amounts to a homunculus in the BG, demanding a priori knowledge and pulling the levers as necessary. Following is a high-level overview of a biologically constrained neural-network model of the BG. This model has accounted for a variety of seemingly disparate behaviors, and has led to novel predictions that have been confirmed, as a result of medication, diseases, neuroimaging, and genetics.[14,15] By encapsulating the BG's core structure and activation dynamics, the model explicitly specifies the mechanisms though which the BG learns to integrate and gate information.

Neural-Network Model of the Basal Ganglia

The neural-network model described here strikes a balance between biological realism and conceptual clarity. Low-level details such as cell geometry are abstracted away, while other critical biological details such as the temporal dynamics of membrane potentials, the divergent firing properties of neurons in distinct brain regions, and anatomical connectivity are captured. The result is a model with both biologically and functionally oriented constraints, positioning the model between detailed biophysical models and traditional connectionist models. Although the models described in this chapter focus on the mechanisms of basic action selection, the same core circuitry has been extended to model cognitive functions such as working memory,[36] the role of instructions,[12] and the complementary roles of orbitofrontal representations of reward value and their influence on the BG.[16]

Model Structure and Dynamics   The BG model consists of several layers that comprise the core structures associated with the BG (see figure 17.1): the striatum, globus pallidus (internal and external segments, GPi, and GPe), substantia nigra pars compacta (SNc), thalamus, and subthalamic nucleus (STN). When a stimulus is represented in sensory cortex, candidate actions are generated in premotor cortex, with both of these cortical regions projecting to the striatum. Columns of striatal units then encode information related to a particular candidate action in the context of the sensory stimulus.

The BG's core gating function emerges as activity from "direct" and "indirect" pathways converges on the thalamus, resulting in either the facilitation or suppression of cortical activations due to recurrent connectivity between thalamus and cortex.[34] The direct pathway originates in striatal D1-receptor–expressing units that

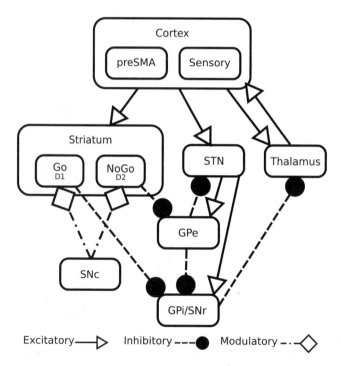

Figure 17.1
Functional anatomy of the BG circuit.

provide focused inhibitory input to the GPi. The GPi is tonically active in the absence of synaptic input and sends inhibitory projections to the thalamus, preventing it from facilitating any cortical response representations. When striatal units in the direct pathway fire, they inhibit the GPi, and remove tonic inhibition of the thalamus. This "disinhibition" process allows premotor representation of the candidate action in question to excite the corresponding column of thalamus, which reciprocally amplifies the cortical activity via recurrent thalamocortical activity. Once a given action is amplified by striatal disinhibition of the thalamus, the competing candidate actions are immediately suppressed due to lateral inhibition in cortex. Thus, we refer to activity in the direct pathway as "Go" signals, which facilitate the selection of particular cortical actions.

Note that, critically, disinhibiting thalamic units only permits those units to become active if those same units also receive top-down excitation from cortex. Hence, the BG is not directly responsible for determining which actions are selected; rather, it modulates the activity of candidate representations already present in cortex. This conceptualization implies that cortex implements its own action-selection process to determine the appropriate candidate actions, which in our models is based on the prior probability of having selected these actions in the context of the current stimulus.

The indirect pathway, so labeled due to its additional synapse passing through the GPe, provides an oppositional force to the direct pathway. Originating in striatal D2 receptor–expressing units, the indirect pathway provides direct and focused inhibitory input to the GPe, which in the absence of input is also tonically active and sends focused inhibitory input to the GPi. We refer to activity in this pathway as "No-Go" signals since these striatal columns inhibit GPe, which transitively disinhibit their respective columns in the GPi further, ultimately preventing the flow of thalamocortical activity. Together, the balance between activity in the direct and in the indirect pathways for each action determines the probability that the action in question is gated.

In addition to the direct and indirect pathways, the model also includes a "hyperdirect" pathway through the STN, so named because this pathway originates in cortex and bypasses the striatum entirely. Like the striatum, the STN receives excitatory input from cortex; however, the STN projects excitatory input to the GPi, which further inhibits thalamocortical activity. Unlike the indirect pathway, STN projections to the GPi are diffuse, and therefore STN activity provides a "global No-Go" signal preventing any response from being gated (see also chapter 11, this volume). Further differentiating the hyperdirect pathway from the striatum, overall STN activity is dynamically regulated over the course of a trial: When a stimulus is presented, an initial STN surge is observed that sends a transient global No-Go signal preventing any response from being selected. When STN activity subsides (due to feedback inhibition from GPe and neural accommodation), the effective threshold to gate a response declines.[15] Notably, the initial STN surge is amplified when several candidate actions are coactivated in cortex. Thus, the global No-Go signal is adaptively modulated by the degree of response coactivation (response conflict). This self-regulatory mechanism helps prevent premature response selection when multiple actions appear appropriate by allowing the striatum more time to integrate the information provided to it.

Model Plasticity   As previously discussed, dopamine is central to reinforcement learning processes in the brain. Although our discussion of the reinforcement learning theory of the ERN focused on dopamine signals in the ACC, the relationship between dopamine and learning is perhaps best characterized in the BG. Evidence from patient studies and pharmacological manipulations that primarily affect and target the BG[38,43] suggest that DA processes in the BG are critically involved in reinforcement learning and action selection.[4,7,20,21,37,51] These human studies are complemented by optogenetic manipulations, voltammetry, synaptic plasticity, and single-cell recordings in nonhuman animal studies demonstrating that synaptic plasticity in the striatum depends on phasic dopamine signals.[39,41,42,44,46,48]

Correspondingly, dopamine plays a critical role in the BG model, allowing it to learn which cortical representation should be facilitated and which should be suppressed. Dopamine's impact depends on both the receptor type and the state of the target unit. In Go units, dopamine has a D1 receptor–mediated contrast-enhancing effect by further increasing activity in highly active units while simultaneously decreasing activity in less active units.[14] Thus, only those Go units that have the strongest activity, due to strong weights associated with the stimulus-action conjunction in question, are amplified. In No-Go units, dopamine has a D2 receptor–mediated inhibitory effect, such that greater levels of dopamine inhibit No-Go cells, whereas these cells are more excitable when DA levels are low.[9,53]

The net result is that increased dopamine levels facilitate Go activity while suppressing No-Go activity. Conversely, by reducing inhibition of D2-expressing units, decreased dopamine levels increase the activity of No-Go units while simultaneously reducing activity in Go units. Hence, variation in dopamine levels has differential effects on Go and No-Go signals projected by striatum. In the context of this model, dopaminergic effects play a critical role in both modulating the overall propensity for responding (by modulating Go relative to No-Go activity), and (by modulating activity-dependent plasticity) also allowing the model to learn which representations should be facilitated and which should be suppressed.

The model learns by dynamically changing the connections strength between units over time and experience, according to Hebbian principles. Weights between units that are strongly and repeatedly coactivated are strengthened, simulating long-term potentiation (LTP), whereas weights between units that do not reliably coactivate are weakened, simulating long-term depression (LTD). Both LTP and LTD processes are strongly modulated by dopamine[46] in a manner that is adaptive in the BG model based on principles of reinforcement learning,[14] as described next.

Dopamine activity in the SNc shows properties consistent with that required by reinforcement learning.[35,45] Specifically, dopamine neurons in the SNc fire in a phasic burst when unexpected rewards are encountered, whereas activity in these same neurons falls below tonic baseline firing rates when expected rewards are not delivered. In the model, phasic DA bursts are simulated by the SNc layer to encode reward feedback following correct responses. Following a phasic SNc burst, activity is increased in Go units associated with the action selected in the current stimulus context, while activity in other Go units and No-Go units declines. Driven by activity-dependent Hebbian learning principles, the weights between representative Go units and active cortical units (sensory and motor) are strengthened, while all other weights are weakened. Thus, Go learning to choose a particular action in the context of a given stimuli is supported by phasic dopamine bursts.

Conversely, dopamine dips are simulated by the SNc layer to encode error feedback following incorrect responses. D2-expressing striatal units in the No-Go pathway, which are typically inhibited by baseline dopamine activity, are disinhibited following a phasic SNc dip, thereby increasing No-Go unit activity driven by excitatory cortical input. This increased activity strengthens the weights between active cortical and No-Go units. Hence, phasic dips of dopamine support learning to avoid certain actions given a particular stimulus.

By coupling simple Hebbian-learning principles with reinforcement learning signals projected to striatal units, the BG comes to reliably facilitate actions that have the highest probability of yielding a positive outcome, and to avoid those actions leading to negative outcomes. In addition, as stimulus-response representations in sensory cortex and pre-SMA coactivate, the connection strengths between these active units increase. As such, the pre-SMA eventually learns to refine its selection of candidate actions based on the probability of having selected these actions in the past for a given context. This slower form of learning ingrains repeated actions as "habits," enabling action selection to become increasingly independent of BG activity over time.

In summary, the model presented here encapsulates several of the BG's key structures and the activation dynamics among them. Direct Go and indirect No-Go pathways, differentially modulated by dopamine, allow the model to learn not only what it should do, but what it should not do in particular stimulus contexts. Additionally, the hyperdirect pathway through the STN modulates the within-trial action selection dynamics by preventing premature decisions when a number of potential candidates seem appropriate, thereby allowing striatal units more time to settle on the most appropriate course of action. Eventually, once reward contingencies are well learned and intercortical connections have been sufficiently strengthened, action selection no longer depends on bottom-up support from the BG. Hence, alongside a wealth of neurological and behavioral evidence, and supported by several empirically confirmed model-based predictions, the model presented here links processes within the BG to action selection, reinforcement learning, and the development of direct intercortical connections. In the following, we investigate an extension of this model aimed at exploring the relationship between the BG and the ACC, with an emphasis on the BG's role in the emergence of the ERN. However, we first consider empirical evidence for a functional relationship between the BG and the ACC.

Evidence of a Functional Link between the BG and the ACC

The ACC is thought to play a critical role in executive control. ACC activation has been noted in tasks involving learning and memory, language, perception, and motor control, which suggests that like the BG, the ACC subserves a relatively general cognitive function. A unifying hypothesis conceptualizes the ACC as monitoring performance with respect to anticipated rewards.[40] Within this framework, the ACC monitors for signals indicating that events are not going as well or as smoothly as expected, and engages additional adaptive control processes when they are required. Thus, broadly speaking, the BG and the ACC appear to share functional concerns as both structures contribute to optimizing performance with respect to anticipated rewards.

A relationship between the BG and the ACC is supported by research spanning multiple methodologies including functional imaging (fMRI), event-related potentials (ERP), genetics, and lesions studies. First and foremost, the BG and the ACC share rich reciprocal connectivity that constitutes a major component of the limbic loop, and are thus thought to play a major role in motivation. Limbic pathways originating in orbitofrontal cortex and ACC pass through the BG and back to the ACC via the thalamus to complete the loop. In addition to thalamic input, the ACC receives input from a number of cortical structures, including prefrontal and motor cortex.[11,13] Pyramidal cells in ACC project to numerous regions involved in motor control, including the BG as well as supplementary and primary motor areas.[50] Hence, in addition to the reciprocal neural connectivity between the BG and the ACC, these two systems also share indirect projections through intermediary structures such as motor cortex.

Empirical support for a functional link between the BG and the ACC is found in a study investigating the ERN in patients with BG lesions.[49] The ERN was significantly reduced in lesion patients compared to age-matched controls, demonstrating that damage to the BG alters activity in the ACC. Further evidence linking ACC and BG activity has emerged from predictions based on the BG model discussed here. Frank and colleagues found that individuals that learn better from negative feedback exhibited a larger rERN and a larger fERN,[23] with similar effects found in subsequent studies.[6,17,26] Findings across several methodologies, including fMRI,[52] PET,[8] genetics,[19] and targeted genetic engineering manipulations of striatal direct and indirect pathways[27] have all demonstrated that ones' ability to learn from positive and negative feedback is determined by the capacity for reinforcement learning signals to shape activity in the Go and No-Go pathways, respectively.

These studies suggest that either ACC activity that produces the ERN is associated with learning from feedback independent of activity in the BG, or variance in BG activity associated with learning from feedback is correlated with variance in the ERN due to corticostriatal loops driving activity in the ACC. Evidence for the latter hypothesis comes from an experiment combining fMRI and genetics, in which a genetic variation known to affect striatal D2 receptor density predicted ACC activity.[32] Using a variant of the probabilistic learning task applied in Frank et al.,[14] Klein and colleagues grouped subjects according to genetic polymorphisms associated with D2 receptor expression.[32] They found that subjects with the A1 allele (A1+ group), which is associated with a 30% reduction of striatal D2 receptor density, were significantly worse at learning from negative feedback, replicating the findings reported with another D2 polymorphism.[19] Furthermore, they found that the A1+ group exhibited a significantly smaller change in ACC activation following error feedback compared to the A1– group (those without the A1 allele). Since D2 receptors are predominantly expressed by striatal No-Go pathway neurons,[25] and this same genetic variation affects striatal activity during negative outcomes,[31] this result provides further support for a functional link between activity in the BG and the ACC. Similarly, a recent study showed that D2 receptor genetic variation impacts D2 receptor binding in the striatum, which in turn, correlates with prefrontal cortical activity.[3]

BG Model of the ERN

Although the reinforcement learning and conflict monitoring theories of the ERN are both supported by a wealth of empirical data, neither theory explains all ERN phenomenology. The reinforcement learning theory provides an account of the rERN and the fERN but omits the N2, whereas the conflict monitoring theory explains the N2 and rERN but neglects the fERN. Here, we propose an initial step toward a unified theory of the ERN by linking conflict in the ACC with striatal activation dynamics following reinforcement learning signals that encode reward feedback. In doing so, the model provides a means of quantifying the fERN in terms of conflict, allowing for precise predictions regarding variance in the fERN, and also integrates the well-studied functions of the BG and their implications for ACC function.

Given that the conflict monitoring theory of the ERN outlined by Yeung and colleagues has already demonstrated that variance in the N2 and rERN can be predicted by response conflict,[54] here we focus exclusively on activity following feedback. More specifically, the model presented here demonstrates that conflict in the ACC depends in part on the strength of bottom-up projections from the BG. Since thalamic output to cortical response representations is governed in part by dopaminergic modulation of striatal activity, the model specifies a mechanistic link between reinforcement learning signals and conflict in the ACC.

We augmented the core BG model discussed at the beginning of the chapter with a simple ACC layer (figure 17.2). The ACC layer consists of units representing each response available to the model, with each ACC unit receiving excitatory input from units in the pre-SMA layer encoding the equivalent response. The ACC monitors activity in the pre-SMA layer such that, for example, increased activity in pre-SMA units representing response "A" will drive a corresponding increase in the response

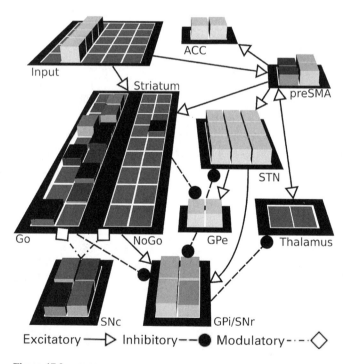

Figure 17.2
Neural network model of the BG circuit, with two different responses represented by two columns of units in each of the Go, No-Go, GPe, GPi/SNr, thalamus, pre-SMA, and ACC layers.

"A" unit of the ACC layer. In accordance with previous formalizations of conflict, we quantify conflict as the Hopfield energy[30] in the ACC layer. However, since there are only two possible responses in the current model, and two units in the ACC layer, the energy calculation reduces to

$$\text{Conflict} = -a_1 a_2 \qquad\qquad (17.1)$$

where a_1 and a_2 represent the activity in each unit of the ACC layer.

We applied the model to a simulation of a probabilistic selection task.[15,22] In this task, stimuli are probabilistically associated with reward and punishment, with some stimuli delivering rewards more reliably than others. On each trial, the model is forced to choose one of two stimuli, each response followed immediately by reward feedback. In order to provide a clear description of the mechanisms under investigation, we prevent the model from learning the task's reward contingencies. Thus, response selection is random and all reward feedback is unpredictable throughout the task.

At the start of each simulated trial, units in the input layer representing the trial stimuli are activated and the network is allowed to freely settle on a response. Since the network has no experience with any of the stimuli or their associated rewards, response selection depends on random activity in the Go and No-Go pathways together with noise in pre-SMA. As outlined earlier, one response is selected via gating mechanisms of the BG and thalamus, and lateral inhibition between mutually exclusive response units in the pre-SMA. This ensures that a response will always be selected: Even a relatively subtle bottom-up bias for one response over the other (due to random initial weights and/or noise in activation dynamics) will be sufficient to select that response once the thalamus is disinhibited. Once a unit in the pre-SMA layer surpasses a threshold of 95% activation, a response is elicited. Feedback is then provided by the SNc layer in the form of a reinforcement learning signal encoded as a phasic burst or dip in activity. Finally, having delivered its phasic learning signal, the SNc returns to baseline activation levels and the network continues to settle until the end of the trial.

As illustrated in figure 17.3b, the activation dynamics of conflict in the ACC following feedback bear a striking resemblance to the temporal signature of the fERN, with conflict rapidly increasing following negative feedback, and returning to baseline levels once the reinforcement learning signal was processed. As discussed previously, input from the SNc differentially modulates activity in the Go and No-Go pathways. Correct feedback, encoded as a burst of output from the SNc, simultaneously strengthens the Go signal and weakens the No-Go signal projected to the thalamus (figure 17.3a). Thus, following correct feedback, bottom-up support for the selected response will increase, and in turn, lateral inhibition of the alternative response will also increase. Hence, should any response coactivation remain in the pre-SMA following response selection, a phasic dopamine burst will tend to facilitate the activation of a single response representation. As the ACC layer monitors activity in the pre-SMA layer following feedback, any remaining conflict is correspondingly reduced. When SNc activity returns to baseline levels, Go signal strength is reduced and conflict returns to normal levels.

Conversely, incorrect feedback, encoded as a dip in SNc activity, increases the No-Go signal projecting to the thalamus (figure 17.3a). Hence, following incorrect feedback, increased No-Go activity counteracts the original Go pathway activity, and the thalamus is no longer disinhibited. As a result, bottom-up support for the selected response in the pre-SMA layer is reduced, as is lateral inhibition of the response that was not selected. Consequently, pre-SMA layer activity reflects only the relatively weak influences of sensory cortical activation and noise, which are incapable of inducing activation of a single response in the absence of substantial prior corticocortical learning. Thus, conflict increases as the ACC layer monitors the activity of response representations in the pre-SMA layer. When SNc activity is restored to baseline levels, No-Go signal strength is reduced and Go signals are able to bias response representations once more. As the Go signal gains footing, facilitating the previously selected response in the pre-SMA, activity in the ACC comes to uniquely represent the biased response and conflict returns to baseline levels. Thus, much like the model of the rERN described by Yeung et al.,[54] an increase in ACC conflict provides an account of the fERN, where conflict is driven by negative reinforcement learning signals that induce NoGo signals in the BG.

We detail the emergence of conflict further by manipulating the capacity for information to pass through BG and cortical pathways into the pre-SMA. As was just discussed, conflict in the ACC layer is driven by the relative strength of Go and No-Go signals, which were themselves modulated by SNc activity. Given the current model structure, variance in the amount of conflict was dominated by activity in the No-Go pathway following errors.* This suggests that altering the potency of reinforcement learning signals in the No-Go pathway (as would be expected due to D2 receptor genetic variation[18]) should impact conflict in the ACC. We investigated this by varying the duration of the phasic pause in SNc activity during negative outcomes. We note that this approach to manipulating dopamine efficacy in the No-Go pathway encompasses variation in the dopamine signal itself (the magnitude of negative prediction errors has been shown to be reflected in the duration of dopamine pauses[2]), and in turn the ability of the No-Go pathway to react to these signals

---

* Given the model's response threshold of 95% activation, the Go pathway was unable to significantly reduce conflict following phasic dopamine bursts due to a ceiling effect. However, it is possible for the Go pathway to play a more prominent role in the fERN if responses were elicited at a lower threshold, allowing increased Go pathway activation to further excite the selected response, thereby reducing conflict in the ACC.

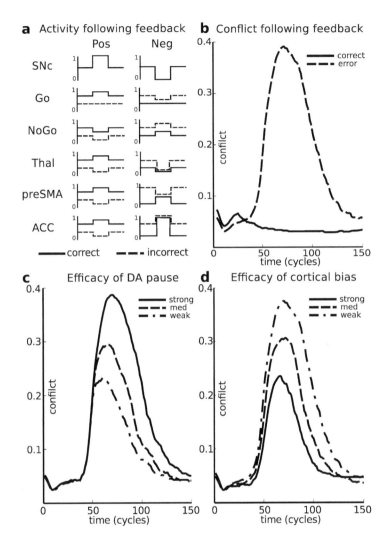

Figure 17.3
(a) Network activity associated with the correct (solid line) and incorrect (dashed line) response representations in each layer following correct (Pos) and incorrect (Neg) feedback. (b) Measure of conflict in the ACC layer following correct (solid line) and incorrect (dashed line) feedback. (c) Measure of conflict following incorrect feedback as a result of varying the efficacy of negative prediction errors from highly effective (solid line) to weakly effective (dash-dot line). (d) Measure of conflict following incorrect feedback as a result of varying the strength of cortical bias weights projecting to the pre-SMA layer from strong (solid line) to weak (dash-dot line).

(sufficient pause durations are necessary to disinhibit No-Go cells). Figure 17.3c illustrates that as pause duration is progressively reduced and dopamine efficacy is weakened, the duration and magnitude of conflict in the ACC is correspondingly reduced. Thus, our model suggests that variation in the No-Go signal should correlate with conflict in the ACC, and therefore predict the strength of the fERN signal.

We also investigated the relationship between top-down cortical information projected into the pre-SMA and the emergence of conflict in the ACC. Numerous cortical systems influence activity in the pre-SMA, including the ACC, sensory cortex, and prefrontal cortex. Thus, to avoid overcomplicating the model, we simulate top-down input as an excitatory bias weight projecting onto units in the pre-SMA layer, thus simulating aggregate input from all cortical structures signaling the response. Following response selection, the bias weights were applied to the pre-SMA units that encode the selected response for the remainder of the trial. Just as increasing bottom-up response facilitation reduced conflict in the ACC, increasing the top-down bias on response representations in the pre-SMA produced a corresponding reduction in conflict (figure 17.3d). Although a temporary reduction in thalamic facilitation following negative feedback remains as the primary factor contributing to the emergence of conflict, top-down bias weights were able to dampen the amount of activity in the ACC layer when thalamic input was removed. Thus, as the top-down bias weights were strengthened, the modulatory potency of thalamic input into pre-SMA was reduced as was the amount of conflict following negative feedback signals encoded by the SNc.

Discussion

The model presented here provides preliminary evidence linking the fERN to a conflict-detection mechanism in the ACC. Critically, the model demonstrated that reinforcement learning signals encoded by phasic SNc activity differentially modulated the Go and No-Go signals responsible for facilitating response representations in the pre-SMA. When bottom-up support was removed due to increased No-Go signal strength following negative feedback, response coactivation increased and emerged as conflict in the ACC layer. It was further demonstrated that top-down biasing also played a role in the dynamics of conflict in the ACC. As cortical input to the pre-SMA layer increased, units there were less dependent on thalamic support to maintain activation of a single response representation, thus reducing conflict in the ACC.

As previously discussed, subjects with reduced striatal D2 receptor expression have been found to exhibit a diminished change in ACC activity following negative feedback.[32] Since D2 receptors are predominantly expressed by cells in the No-Go pathway, this finding suggests that the No-Go pathway plays a critical role in modulating activity in the ACC. In addition, subjects that did not learn well from negative feedback were found to exhibit smaller fERNs.[6,23] Given that learning from negative feedback was also found to depend on activity in the No-Go pathway,[19,27] this further supports a functional link between the No-Go pathway and activity in the ACC responsible for generating the fERN. In line with these findings, our model demonstrated that the manifestation of conflict depends on the efficacy of reinforcement leaning signals in the No-Go pathway (see figure 17.3c). When the No-Go pathway's response to negative outcomes was blunted, as would be the case in populations with impaired D2 receptor function, the No-Go pathway's capacity to withhold thalamic support to the pre-SMA was reduced. This, we suggest, would emerge as a reduction in the fERN (with the critical assumption that the groups in question differ in striatal function but not in cortical measures).

Normative learning theory states that the magnitude of the reward prediction error is correlated with the severity of the prediction violation.[47] Results reported by Holroyd and Krigolson[29] show that the fERN correlates with violation of expectation, suggesting that the fERN is modulated by reward prediction errors encoded by the midbrain dopamine system. Although the reinforcement learning theory of the ERN argued that this correlation is driven by dopamine's arrival in the ACC, the model presented here demonstrates that dopaminergic modulation of striatal activity predicts the same correlation between dopamine signals and conflict in the ACC. Longer phasic pauses in dopamine activity induced greater NoGo signals that withheld bottom-up support more effectively, leading to more conflict in the ACC layer and a larger fERN (see figure 17.3c).

Our understanding of the rERN may benefit from the observation that cortical input to response representations in the pre-SMA also regulated conflict in the ACC layer. This suggests that as cortical projections to the pre-SMA are strengthened, conflict will be progressively less sensitive to influences of the BG. In the model presented here, input representations were externally clamped; however, a more realistic approach would allow these representations to emerge as stimuli are processed and differentially attended. The stability and veridicality of the stimulus representation would likely be determined by biological constraints and attentional processes. As such, activation patterns associated with the stimulus representation would be expected to waver, leading to fluctuations in the response representations with which they are associated. When response selection is more challenging (e.g., incongruent trials in the flanker task), increased levels of conflict would develop as stimulus representations compete for control. A correct response would be more probable on trials when this conflict was allowed to resolve prior to response, whereas an incorrect response would be more probable on trials when a response was elicited prior to conflict resolution. Thus, N2-like modulation of

ACC activity prior to response selection, and a rERN-like increase in conflict following incorrect responses will emerge in the absence of bottom-up conflict-inducing mechanisms.

Although the model presented here specified a mechanism that linked reinforcement learning to conflict monitoring in the ACC, this preliminary model has yet to ascribe a particular function to conflict detection in the ACC: Although conflict detection may provide a simple means of error detection,[54] this cannot be so in the case of conflict associated with the fERN. For the fERN to emerge, the error must first be detected and encoded as a phasic pause in SNc activity. Additionally, the astute reader may have noticed that the hyperdirect pathway through the STN is also monitoring conflict in cortical layers[15]; thus, it may initially appear that including a conflict monitor in the ACC does no more than add redundancy to the model. First, we note that the STN modulates activity in accordance with *instantaneous* conflict in a given trial; however, by itself, the STN is incapable of accumulating information across trials in order to adjust performance to meet more global task demands. Though purely speculative at this point in our research, we suggest that the ACC may provide a means of accumulating task performance over time (e.g., adjusting response caution in proportion to integrated conflict over trials, as proposed by Botvinick and colleagues[5]), allowing the ACC to modify behavior so as to meet more global task demands. By integrating pre-SMA conflict across trials, the ACC would be in a position to regulate behavioral control as a function of global task demands, a process that may be embodied by projecting this integrated signal to the STN as a means of blending global and local task demands. Alternatively (or in addition), the ACC may regulate trial-to-trial behavioral adjustments as a function of negative outcomes ("lose-switch") as individuals acquire reinforcement contingencies (see Cavanagh et al.[6] for EEG data), in contrast to the BG, which integrates reinforcement probabilities across a longer time horizon.[19]

Conclusion

We have outlined a biologically inspired and constrained neural network model aimed at investigating the functional relationship between the ACC and the BG. The model defined mechanisms through which dopamine-induced modulation of striatal activation patterns emerged as variance in ACC activity, which we quantified as conflict. By coupling reinforcement learning processes in the BG with activity in the ACC, the model provides a means of quantifying the fERN as an index of conflict-monitoring processes in the ACC. Although much work remains, this model provides preliminary evidence for a unified account of the ERN by including both reinforcement learning and conflict monitoring mechanisms within a single model.

Outstanding Questions

• If conflict monitoring does indeed provide a means of error detection, as proposed by Yeung et al.,[54] could the phasic reinforcement learning signals encoded by the dopamine system that train the BG be driven in part by conflict processes associated with the ERN?

• How might the learning embodied by the BG and the ACC be differentially specialized, and how might the roles of each system differ with respect to guiding behavior?

• What experiment could be used to shed light on the proposed interactive model (e.g., simultaneous model-based fMRI and EEG to explore the relationship between striatal prediction errors and the ERN on a trial-by-trial basis)?

Further Reading

Hazy TE, Frank MJ, O'Reilly RC. 2010. Neural mechanisms of acquired phasic dopamine responses in learning. *Neurosci Biobehav Rev* 34: 701–720. An overview and discussion of the biological mechanisms that underlie reward-predictive firing properties of midbrain dopamine neurons. Discusses specifically their relationship to learning.

Houk JC, Davis JL, Beiser DG (eds). 1995. Models of Information Processing in the Basal Ganglia. Cambridge, MA: MIT Press. The largest overview of models of the basal ganglia available. Although written quite some time ago, it is still extremely relevant today.

References

1. Baker TE, Holroyd CB. 2009. Which way do I go? Neural activation in response to feedback and spatial processing in a virtual T-maze. *Cereb Cortex* 19: 1708.

2. Bayer HM, Lau B, Glimcher PW. 2007. Statistics of midbrain dopamine neuron spike trains in the awake primate. *J Neurophysiol* 98: 1428.

3. Bertolino A, Taurisano P, Pisciotta NM, Blasi G, Fazio L, Romano R, Gelao B, et al. 2010. Genetically determined measures of striatal D2 signaling predict prefrontal activity during working memory performance. *PLoS ONE* 5: e9348.

4. Bodi N, Keri S, Nagy H, Moustafa A, Myers CE, Daw N, Dibo G, Takats A, Bereczki D, Gluck MA. 2009. Reward-learning and the novelty-seeking personality: a between-and within-subjects study of the effects of dopamine agonists on young Parkinson's patients. *Brain* 132: 2385.

5. Botvinick MM, Braver TS, Barch DM, Carter CS, Cohen JD. 2001. Conflict monitoring and cognitive control. *Psychol Rev* 108: 624–652.

6. Cavanagh JF, Frank MJ, Allen JJB. Social stress reactivity alters reward and punishment learning. *Soc Cogn Affect Neurosci*. In press.

7. Cools R, Altamirano L, D'Esposito M. 2006. Reversal learning in Parkinson's disease depends on medication status and outcome valence. *Neuropsychologia* 44: 1663–1673.

8. Cools R, Frank MJ, Gibbs SE, Miyakawa A, Jagust W, D'Esposito M. 2009. Striatal dopamine predicts outcome-specific reversal learning and its sensitivity to dopaminergic drug administration. *J Neurosci* 29: 1538.

9. Day M, Wokosin D, Plotkin JL, Tian X, Surmeier DJ. 2008. Differential excitability and modulation of striatal medium spiny neuron dendrites. *J Neurosci* 28: 11603.

10. Debener S, Ullsperger M, Siegel M, Fiehler K, Von Cramon D, Engel A. 2005. Trial-by-trial coupling of concurrent electroencephalogram and functional magnetic resonance imaging identifies the dynamics of performance monitoring. *J Neurosci* 25: 11730.

11. Devinsky O, Morrell M, Vogt B. 1995. Contributions of anterior cingulate cortex to behaviour. *Brain* 118: 279–306.

12. Doll BB, Jacobs WJ, Sanfey AG, Frank MJ. 2009. Instructional control of reinforcement learning: a behavioral and neurocomputational investigation. *Brain Res* 1299: 74–94.

13. Dum RP, Strick PL. 1993. Cingulate motor areas. In: Neurobiology of Cingulate Cortex and Limbic Thalamus: A Comprehensive Handbook (Vogt BA, Gabriel M, eds), pp 415–441. Cambridge, MA: Birkhaeuser.

14. Frank MJ. 2005. Dynamic dopamine modulation in the basal ganglia: a neurocomputational account of cognitive deficits in medicated and nonmedicated Parkinsonism. *J Cogn Neurosci* 17: 51–72.

15. Frank MJ. 2006. Hold your horses: a dynamic computational role for the subthalamic nucleus in decision making. *Neural Netw* 19: 1120–1136.

16. Frank MJ, Claus ED. 2006. Anatomy of a decision: striato-orbitofrontal interactions in reinforcement learning, decision making, and reversal. *Psychol Rev* 113: 300–326.

17. Frank MJ, D'Lauro C, Curran T. 2007. Cross-task individual differences in error processing: neural, electrophysiological, and genetic components. *Cogn Affect Behav Neurosci* 7: 297–308.

18. Frank MJ, Hutchison K. 2009. Genetic contributions to avoidance-based decisions: striatal D2 receptor polymorphisms. *Neuroscience* 164: 131–140.

19. Frank MJ, Moustafa AA, Haughey HM, Curran T, Hutchison KE. 2007. Genetic triple dissociation reveals multiple roles for dopamine in reinforcement learning. *Proc Natl Acad Sci USA* 104: 16311–16316.

20. Frank MJ, O'Reilly RC. 2006. A mechanistic account of striatal dopamine function in human cognition: psychopharmacological studies with cabergoline and haloperidol. *Behav Neurosci* 120: 497–517.

21. Frank MJ, Samanta J, Moustafa AA, Sherman SJ. 2007. Hold your horses: impulsivity, deep brain stimulation, and medication in parkinsonism. *Science* 318: 1309–1312.

22. Frank MJ, Seeberger LC, O'Reilly RC. 2004. By carrot or by stick: cognitive reinforcement learning in Parkinsonism. *Science* 306: 1940–1943.

23. Frank MJ, Woroch BS, Curran T. 2005. Error-related negativity predicts reinforcement learning and conflict biases. *Neuron* 47: 495–501.

24. Gehring WJ, Goss B, Coles MG, Meyer DE, Donchin E. 1993. A neural system for error detection and compensation. *Psychol Sci* 4: 385–390.

25. Gerfen CR, Engber TM, Mahan LC, Susel Z, Chase TN, Monsma FJ, Jr, Sibley DR. 1990. D1 and D2 dopamine receptor-regulated gene expression of striatonigral and striatopallidal neurons. *Science* 250: 1429.

26. Hewig J, Trippe R, Hecht H, Coles MGH, Holroyd CB, Miltner WHR. 2007. Decision-making in blackjack: an electrophysiological analysis. *Cereb Cortex* 17: 865–877.

27. Hikida T, Kimura K, Wada N, Funabiki K, Nakanishi S. 2010. Distinct roles of synaptic transmission in direct and indirect striatal pathways to reward and aversive behavior. *Neuron* 66: 896–907.

28. Holroyd CB, Coles MG. 2002. The neural basis of human error processing: reinforcement learning, dopamine, and the error-related negativity. *Psychol Rev* 109: 679–709.

29. Holroyd CB, Krigolson OE. 2007. Reward prediction error signals associated with a modified time estimation task. *Psychophysiology* 44: 913–917.

30. Hopfield JJ. 1982. Neural networks and physical systems with emergent collective computational abilities. *Proc Natl Acad Sci USA* 79: 2554.

31. Jocham G, Klein TA, Neumann J, von Cramon DY, Reuter M, Ullsperger M. 2009. Dopamine DRD2 polymorphism alters reversal learning and associated neural activity. *J Neurosci* 29: 3695–3704.

32. Klein TA, Neumann J, Reuter M, Hennig J, von Cramon DY, Ullsperger M. 2007. Genetically determined differences in learning from errors. *Science* 318: 1642–1645.

33. Miltner WHR, Braun CH, Coles MGH. 1997. Event-related brain potentials following incorrect feedback in a time-estimation task: evidence for a "generic" neural system for error detection. *J Cogn Neurosci* 9: 788–798.

34. Mink J. 1996. The basal ganglia: focused selection and inhibition of competing motor programs. *Prog Neurobiol* 50: 381–425.

35. Montague P, Dayan P, Sejnowski T. 1996. A framework for mesencephalic dopamine systems based on predictive Hebbian learning. *J Neurosci* 16: 1936.

36. O'Reilly RC, Frank MJ. 2006. Making working memory work: a computational model of learning in the prefrontal cortex and basal ganglia. *Neural Comput* 18: 283–328.

37. Palminteri S, Lebreton M, Worbe Y, Grabli D, Hartmann A, Pessiglione M. 2009. Pharmacological modulation of subliminal learning in Parkinson's and Tourette's syndromes. *Proc Natl Acad Sci USA* 106: 19179.

38. Pavese N, Evans AH, Tai YF, Hotton G, Brooks DJ, Lees AJ, Piccini P. 2006. Clinical correlates of levodopa-induced dopamine release in Parkinson disease: a PET study. *Neurology* 67: 1612.

39. Reynolds JN, Hyland BI, Wickens JR. 2001. A cellular mechanism of reward-related learning. *Nature* 413: 67–70.

40. Ridderinkhof KR, Ullsperger M, Crone EA, Nieuwenhuis S. 2004. The role of the medial frontal cortex in cognitive control. *Science* 306: 443–447.

41. Roesch MR, Calu DJ, Schoenbaum G. 2007. Dopamine neurons encode the better option in rats deciding between differently delayed or sized rewards. *Nat Neurosci* 10: 1615–1624.

42. Samejima K, Ueda Y, Doya K, Kimura M. 2005. Representation of action-specific reward values in the striatum. *Science* 310: 1337–1340.

43. Sawamoto N, Piccini P, Hotton G, Pavese N, Thielemans K, Brooks DJ. 2008. Cognitive deficits and striato-frontal dopamine release in Parkinson's disease. *Brain* 131: 1294–1302.

44. Schultz W. 2002. Getting formal with dopamine and reward. *Neuron* 36: 241–263.

45. Schultz W, Dayan P, Montague P. 1997. A neural substrate of prediction and reward. *Science* 275: 1593.

46. Shen W, Flajolet M, Greengard P, Surmeier DJ. 2008. Dichotomous dopaminergic control of striatal synaptic plasticity. *Science* 321: 848.

47. Sutton RS, Barto AG. 1998. Reinforcement Learning: An Introduction. Cambridge, MA: MIT Press.

48. Tsai H, Zhang F, Adamantidis A, Stuber G, Bonci A, de Lecea L, Deisseroth K. 2009. Phasic firing in dopaminergic neurons is sufficient for behavioral conditioning. *Science* 324: 1080.

49. Ullsperger M, von Cramon DY. 2006. The role of intact frontostriatal circuits in error processing. *J Cogn Neurosci* 18: 651–664.

50. Van Hoesen GW, Morecraft RJ, Vogt BA. 1993. Connections of the monkey cingulate cortex. In: Neurobiology of Cingulate Cortex and Limbic Thalamus (Vogt BA, Gabriel M, eds), pp 249–284. Cambridge, MA: Birkhäuser.

51. Volkow ND, Wang G-J, Fowler JS, Telang F, Maynard L, Logan J, Gatley SJ, et al. 2004. Evidence that methylphenidate enhances the saliency of a mathematical task by increasing dopamine in the human brain. *Am J Psychiatry* 161: 1173–1180.

52. Voon V, Pessiglione M, Brezing C, Gallea C, Fernandez HH, Dolan RJ, Hallett M. 2010. Mechanisms underlying dopamine-mediated reward bias in compulsive behaviors. *Neuron* 65: 135–142.

53. Wiecki TV, Frank MJ. 2010. Neurocomputational models of motor and cognitive deficits in Parkinson's disease. *Prog Brain Res* 183: 275–297.

54. Yeung N, Botvinick MM, Cohen JD. 2004. The neural basis of error detection: conflict monitoring and the error-related negativity. *Psychol Rev* 111: 931–959.

18 An Integrative Theory of Anterior Cingulate Cortex Function: Option Selection in Hierarchical Reinforcement Learning

Clay B. Holroyd and Nick Yeung

The anterior cingulate cortex (ACC), a region on the medial surface of the frontal lobes, has received substantial research attention in recent years as a key neural substrate of cognitive control. In part this interest derives from neuroanatomical evidence that ACC is uniquely well positioned to collate information about the motivational significance of ongoing events—based on its inputs from the limbic system, orbitofrontal cortex (OFC), and midbrain dopamine system—and to use this information to guide behavior via its dense interconnections with primary motor, premotor, and lateral prefrontal cortex.[41] In accord with the idea that ACC plays this central role in behavioral control, human neuroimaging studies have shown that the area consistently coactivates with regions in the lateral prefrontal and parietal cortex as part of an "executive" network responding to a diverse range of cognitive demands.[19] However, although there is widespread agreement that ACC plays an important role in motivational and cognitive control, far less agreement exists as to what that role might be.

Theories of ACC function fall into four main categories: *Performance monitoring* theories emphasize its role in evaluating ongoing behavior, detecting errors or conflicts in response execution, and implementing remedial actions as appropriate.[9,44] *Action selection* theories focus on the contribution of ACC to the internal, willful generation of behavior.[18,41] *Reinforcement learning* (RL) theories propose a role for ACC in learning action values that can be used to select appropriate goal-directed behaviors.[25,45] Finally, *motivational* theories underscore the sensitivity of ACC to affect, effort, and costs.[52,56] These theoretical frameworks are not mutually exclusive and in key respects share important claims. For example, performance monitoring and RL theories agree that ACC is sensitive to the efficiency and effectiveness of chosen actions (see also chapter 17, this volume), while both action selection and motivational theories emphasize the contribution of ACC to the willed generation of behavior. Nevertheless, despite this overlap, a unifying theory that spans the wealth of existing anatomical, neurophysiological, neuroimaging, and lesion data has yet to be developed.

In this chapter we propose a new account of ACC function that integrates several salient features of existing theories while aiming to reconcile their inconsistencies. Our account focuses specifically on the dorsal region of ACC believed to be involved in cognitive control, rather than on the rostral-ventral subdivision that is more involved in emotional processing.[16] We propose that dorsal ACC supports the selection and execution of coherent behaviors over extended periods, an idea we formalize in terms of recent advances in the theory of RL that use a hierarchical mechanism for action selection to choose between *options*—sequences of primitive actions associated with particular goals.[7] This proposal builds on existing theories rather than representing a radical departure from them. We therefore begin with a review of these theories.

Current Theories of ACC Function

Performance Monitoring

An influential hypothesis within the human neuroimaging literature is that ACC monitors for signs of inefficient or suboptimal performance to signal when increased cognitive control is required.[6,9,44] Initial evidence for this view came from primate neurophysiology[22] and human electroencephalographic[20] evidence of ACC activity following errors. In the scalp-recorded electroencephalogram (EEG), for example, a component labeled the error-related negativity (ERN or Ne) is elicited by errors in speeded decision-making tasks,[20] while a related feedback ERN (fERN) is seen following error feedback in trial-and-error learning tasks.[33] Converging evidence from dipole modeling, EEG-informed fMRI, and intracranial recording studies indicates that the ERN and fERN are generated in ACC.

However, ACC activity is also apparent in conditions of increased cognitive demand in the absence of errors.[9] For example, increased ACC activity is observed in the Stroop task when the presented word is incongruent with the required color-naming response, even when participants ultimately respond correctly. Although such findings do not rule out that ACC is involved in error processing—for example, ACC may predict error likelihood rather than specifically detect errors as they occur[8]—they have nevertheless motivated a prominent alternative account of ACC function. According to this view, ACC monitors for occurrences of conflict between incompatible actions, such as the competing responses cued by color and word information in the Stroop task, to signal the need for increased cognitive control by dorsolateral prefrontal cortex (DLPFC).[6] Formal computational models have shown this theory to account for a range of findings regarding conflict- and error-related activity in ACC. Subsequent neuroimaging studies have confirmed key predictions of the theory. For example, in the Stroop task, high levels of conflict-related

ACC activity on one trial are predictive of increased DLPFC activity on the next trial, leading to reduced conflict and improved performance on that trial, consistent with the notion that ACC and DLPFC form a regulatory feedback loop in cognitive control.[28]

These successes notwithstanding, conflict monitoring has been challenged as a comprehensive account of ACC function. First, human neuroimaging evidence indicates that ACC not only shows transient responses to experienced conflict as predicted by the theory, but also shows sustained activation during task preparation and execution.[17] This finding suggests that ACC plays a broader role in cognitive control than the conflict-monitoring theory proposes. Second, although some patients with ACC lesions exhibit deficits in Stroop task performance and impaired conflict adaptation,[53] these effects are far less consistently observed than the conflict-monitoring theory predicts.[21] Finally, single-unit recording studies in monkeys have failed to find convincing evidence of conflict-related activity in ACC.[36] Instead, it has been suggested that conflict modulates movement-specific neural activity and that conflict-related activity seen in human neuroimaging studies may be an artifact created by averaging activity across populations of neurons that selectively code for the conflicting responses.

Action Selection

Whereas performance monitoring accounts suggest that ACC plays a primarily evaluative role, an alternative class of theories suggests that ACC contributes directly to the generation and control of behavior. In support of this view, neuroanatomical evidence indicates that ACC comprises several distinct premotor areas,[18] while human neuroimaging studies demonstrate functional specialization within ACC for movements of different effectors.[43] Single-unit recordings in monkeys indicate that neuronal firing in ACC may precede overt movements by several hundred milliseconds.[48] Converging evidence from this primate work and from human neuroimaging indicates that this movement-related activity increases when actions are internally selected rather than externally instructed.[15,48] Further, patients with cingulate lesions exhibit characteristic reductions in their spontaneous speech and movement.[13] These deficits in self-initiated movements are seen in extreme form in akinetic mutism following bilateral damage to ACC and surrounding cortex, in which the awake patient remains immobile and unresponsive to external stimuli beyond simple eye movements.[37] Taken together, these findings are suggestive of a role for ACC in voluntary, or "willed," action selection.[41]

However, despite compelling evidence that ACC is involved in the generation of voluntary actions, the precise functional role of the region remains unclear: whether ACC selects particular actions or provides a generalized motivating arousal signal; what specific computations ACC might perform in order to drive or guide behavior;

and how the role of ACC complements the operations of other motor regions such as the supplementary motor area (SMA) and basal ganglia. Moreover, the role of ACC does not appear to be limited to voluntary action selection: As reviewed in the preceding section, ACC activity is robustly observed during performance of stimulus-driven as well as self-initiated actions,[9] and in association with the evaluation (e.g., through feedback) as well as the selection of actions.[33]

Reinforcement Learning

RL theories agree that ACC plays an important role in action selection, but propose a computationally specific account of this role that explains its sensitivity to performance feedback and action outcomes. According to RL approaches, actions are selected on the basis of stored values derived from their past association with positive and negative outcomes.[11,34,38] ACC has been proposed to play a pivotal role in linking actions and their outcomes according to RL principles.[25,45] Consistent with this view, ACC neurons in primates are sensitive to the degree and magnitude of expected rewards,[2,47] code for reward prediction errors associated with action selection,[29] and fire in relation to both actions and rewards in a manner that appears to link these events.[24] Disturbances of normal ACC function impair animals' ability to switch to alternative behaviors following the reduction of an expected reward,[49] and disrupt the utilization of outcome information for learning about action-reward relationships.[23,27,58]

Human functional neuroimaging studies also suggest that ACC learns about the consequences of internally generated actions.[26,55] These learning-related changes appear to be instigated by the activity of the midbrain dopamine system, which projects to, and reaches its highest density over, medial regions of the frontal cortex,[57] and which conveys so-called reward prediction error signals to its neural targets.[46] It has been proposed that ACC uses these signals in adaptive decision making, and further, that this learning process elicits the ERN and fERN.[25]

As with performance monitoring theories, however, lesion studies in animals and patients provide only partial support for RL accounts. Thus, whereas some lesion studies in animals indicate deficits related to fast trial-to-trial learning,[49] others suggest that the deficits relate to integration of reward information across multiple trials.[27] More troubling still, ACC damage in humans appears to spare feedback-based learning in the Wisconsin Card Sort Test (WCST) despite disrupting spontaneous movement production.[13] Human neuroimaging evidence that ACC activity is consistently observed in tasks such as the Stroop task—in which no reward is provided and responses are instructed rather than learned—is likewise problematic for RL theories: This evidence suggests that ACC implements a specific computational function beyond simply associating actions with outcomes. A similar conclusion follows from an important conceptual challenge to RL theories: that the function ascribed to ACC by these theories is more commonly attributed to the basal ganglia.[39] The fact that human behavior in standard decision-making tasks can be accounted for without recourse to simulating ACC[11] suggests strongly that ACC implements a function that is not exploited by these tasks (see also chapter 17, this volume).

Motivation and Effort

ACC has been associated with motivation and emotion since Papez first identified this structure within the limbic circuit.[40] Subsequent articulations of this idea held that ACC monitors the motivational significance of stimuli and events[31] and integrates hedonic value with action plans,[52] positions that have been supported by observations of converging limbic connections onto the cingulate motor areas.[35] Such considerations have led to the view that ACC does not directly mediate performance monitoring or action selection, but may instead produce affective responses and concurrent autonomic activity to salient events as they take place.[14] Likewise, ACC may contribute to motivational control during task execution by supplying a "global energizing factor" that facilitates neural processes underlying decision making.[50] According to this view, akinetic mutism results from the withdrawal of this energizing factor.

A specific role for ACC in effort-related decision making is suggested by evidence that rats with ACC lesions tend to shift from selecting effortful actions that yield large rewards to choices that yield less reward but require less effort.[54] It has further been shown that dopaminergic input to ACC is essential for this function, apparently by facilitating response selection based on the relative values associated with different actions.[3] These observations parallel reports that human akinetic mutism is ameliorated by administration of dopamine agonists.[1]

However, a criticism of motivational theories is that they lack computational specificity[59]: It remains to be demonstrated how ACC computes qualities such as affect and effort and how these constructs mediate action production and selection. Potentially instructive in this regard are theories of dopamine function that emphasize its role in carrying "incentive salience" signals that are said to "transform the neural representation of a stimulus into an object of attraction that animals will work to acquire."[4] This idea has been formalized using computational RL models in which dopaminergic signaling of action values serves to boost the probability of those actions being selected.[30] In the following, we suggest that these ideas might provide a framework for understanding the dual role of ACC in learning and motivation.

Evaluation of Current Theories

Current theories of ACC function therefore emphasize its role in four key aspects of behavior: monitoring ongoing performance, selecting and initiating voluntary actions, learning about the consequences of actions, and motivating effortful behavior. Crucially, however, no single theory seems capable of explaining the full range of existing findings. Thus, performance monitoring theories cannot easily explain ACC activity observed as people prepare to act, while action selection accounts provide no ready explanation of ACC activity observed following delivery of reward and feedback. Conversely, both RL and motivational theories struggle to account for ACC activity in stimulus-driven cognitive tasks that have little direct affective significance or motivational content.

Moreover, a deeper concern with all current theories is that they seemingly fail to capture adequately the unique contribution of ACC to behavior. As a striking illustration of this point, each of the theories ascribes to ACC a function that seems vital to normal cognitive processing; yet, aside from rare reports of akinetic mutism, the deficits induced by ACC lesions tend to be subtle and limited. For example, ACC-lesioned patients often show broadly intact executive functioning and learning from feedback,[13] and deficits in conflict paradigms such as the Stroop task are not universally observed even in patients with large bilateral lesions.[21] Interpretation of this neuropsychological evidence is complicated by the heterogeneity of function within ACC, variability in lesion extent and location across patients, and effects of neural reorganization and behavioral compensation. Nevertheless, taken with the limitations in existing theories noted earlier, this evidence suggests that current theories and the experimental paradigms used to test them may not effectively capture the core functions of ACC.

In the second part of this chapter, we therefore outline a new theory that aims to reconcile the central claims of existing theories while addressing their principal weaknesses. The starting point for our proposal is a desire to provide an integrative account of the key findings already discussed. To account for this range of findings, we extend previous RL theories by proposing that ACC contributes specifically to reinforcement learning of high-level, temporally extended behaviors. In so doing, we hope to explain why, despite its apparently central role in motivational and cognitive control, lesions to ACC tend to have rather subtle behavioral consequences, and thereby begin to outline new tasks that might more accurately target the proposed functions of ACC.

ACC and the Hierarchical Control of Action

Option Selection in ACC

Drawing on recent advances in RL theory[7] (see also chapter 16, this volume), we propose that ACC implements a mechanism for selecting high-level behavioral plans, or *options*, that comprise structured sequences of actions directed toward specified subgoals. Within this framework, options are defined in terms of *initiation sets* specifying states of the world in which they can be selected, option-specific *policies* specifying the individual actions they comprise, and *termination functions* specifying when option execution has been completed. Options are learned and selected according to established RL principles. In turn, completion of an option serves as a "pseudo-reward" that reinforces preceding lower-level actions according to those same principles. This hierarchical formulation of the RL problem (hierarchical reinforcement learning, or HRL) can increase computational efficiency in situations in which multiple permutations of potential courses of action can lead to a combinatorial explosion.

We specifically frame the role of ACC in HRL within an extension of the well-known actor-critic architecture, in which an actor component selects and executes behaviors and a critic evaluates the appropriateness of those actions.[51] Neurally, the actor is typically associated with the dorsolateral striatum (DLS) and the critic with the ventral striatum (VS).[39] Recent conceptualizations of HRL have extended the domains of the actor and critic to include DLPFC and OFC, respectively.[7] Our proposal extends this framework further by placing ACC at the apex of the actor (figure 18.1). We suggest that ACC stores (or has access to) the option-specific policies, their initiation states, and their termination functions, and uses this information in the probabilistic selection of options. The output of the option selection process is then mediated by two primary routes: via the actor (consisting of DLPFC and DLS) and the critic (consisting of OFC and VS), as detailed in the following.

According to this proposal, ACC supports the selection and execution of high-level, temporally extended sequences of responses underpinning complex, long-term behaviors. As an everyday example, ACC might be responsible for a jogger's decision to run up a mountain and for seeing that this goal is ultimately fulfilled, rather than, say, the would-be jogger staying home to watch TV. Lesions to ACC would result in behavior characterized by immediate reactions to external events rather than by extended, internally driven actions (e.g., the decision to watch TV rather than run). By contrast, ACC should be less important in standard laboratory paradigms that require learning about simple stimulus-response contingencies (such as the WCST) or that involve instructed stimulus-driven responding (such as the Stroop task). Yet even in these stimulus-dependent tasks, ACC may be responsible for compliance with experimental instructions to ensure that task performance is fast and accurate.

Interactions Involving ACC

Our HRL account suggests that ACC performs complementary functions in learning, selecting, and motivating high-level behavioral options. These functions depend in turn on its interactions with other core components of the actor-critic architecture (figure 18.1). First, by way of the actor route, options selected by ACC provide

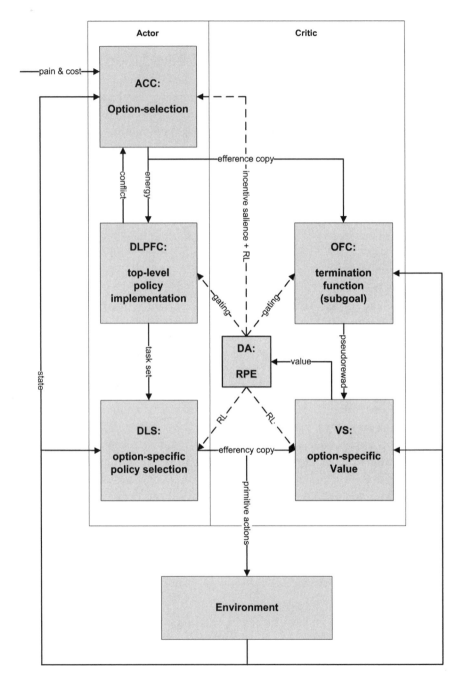

Figure 18.1

Schematic illustration of the proposed role of ACC in the hierarchical actor-critic reinforcement learning architecture. ACC, anterior cingulate cortex; DLPFC, dorsolateral prefrontal cortex; OFC, orbitofrontal cortex; DA, dopamine; RPE, reward prediction error; DLS, dorsolateral striatum; VS, ventral striatum.

excitatory input to the DLPFC, which in turn implements option-specific policies (i.e., sets or sequences of lower-level actions) via its connections with the DLS and other motor structures. In the example of our would-be jogger, ACC would be responsible for the decision to run up the mountain, whereas DLPFC and DLS would be responsible for implementing this decision as a specific sequence of actions. This excitatory effect of ACC option selection on DLPFC policy implementation provides one important route by which ACC can be said to energize or motivate behavior.

By way of the critic route, the OFC receives information about and assigns value to options received as "efference copy" from ACC.[12] Value signals from OFC serve three important functions. First, they facilitate option selection and implementation by acting as an incentive salience signal that communicates whether the option under consideration is a good one (e.g., "Yes, you should jog up the mountain"). Second, these signals provide context to the VS during option execution ("All behaviors consistent with jogging up the mountain are good"). Third, they serve as a "pseudo-reward" once the termination function has been satisfied, indicating that the goal has been achieved ("You made it to the top—good for you!"). In turn, the VS maintains a separate set of values for each option based on external state input, efference copy from the DLS, and contextual input from the OFC. For example, if contextual information from OFC indicates that the task is to jog up the hill, then the VS evaluates individual steps in that direction as being good.

The midbrain dopamine system is the lynchpin of this HRL system. First, dopaminergic signals communicate reward prediction errors, defined as instantaneous changes in value plus pseudo-reward, to induce synaptic plasticity in target structures according to RL principles.[34,38] This learning serves to optimize evaluative predictions of the critic (OFC and VS) and option/action selection processes of the actor (ACC, DLS). In this way, successfully completed action plans (which elicit pseudo-reward on goal obtainment) will be more likely to be selected again in the future. Second, dopaminergic projections provide incentive salience signals that facilitate option selection by ACC and policy (task-set) implementation by DLPFC: During option selection, value signals that are generated by OFC and signaled via the dopamine system cause the specifics of the associated policy to be coordinated across multiple neural structures (especially ACC, DLPFC, and OFC) by gating relevant information into working memory.[10] This incentive salience mechanism provides a second key route by which option selection in ACC can be said to motivate or energize behavior.

Comparison with Existing Theories

We next outline how our theory explains key empirical findings previously taken to support the four main accounts of ACC function discussed earlier, while drawing out important differences in how our theory accounts for these results.

Performance Monitoring

Our proposal shares with performance monitoring accounts an emphasis on the sensitivity of ACC to suboptimal task performance, and on the importance of its interactions with DLPFC.[32] However, our theory recasts ACC primarily as a recipient rather than source of monitoring signals, and suggests that ACC directly guides behavior through selecting options that DLPFC translates into specific sets of actions. This framework provides two ways to explain neuroimaging evidence of conflict-related activity in ACC.[9] First, ACC might monitor for conflict between options just as it has been proposed to monitor conflict between individual actions.[5] According to the HRL framework,[7] task sets studied in the laboratory (e.g., the set of stimulus-response mappings employed in the Stroop task) are a special case of options wherein individual actions are deployed in an entirely stimulus-driven manner. Given this identity between options and task sets, it follows that ACC might be sensitive to the performance costs associated with option-level conflict—the simultaneous activation of incompatible task sets in DLPFC—a process that could lead to stronger policy implementation.

However, our framework is also consistent with the view that conflict-related activity is simply an epiphenomenon of ACC's primary role in action selection[36]: This activity may reflect the summed activation of multiple options in the presence of incongruent stimulus information. Alternatively, ACC may be active in high-conflict conditions because, by definition, the required response is only weakly cued by the stimulus, leading to greater or more prolonged involvement of high-level energizing input from ACC. In either view, conflict adaptation (i.e., increased control following conflict) could reflect the benefit of repeated option selection: Executing the correct task and response in the face of conflict would lead to strengthening of task-relevant associations such that the option would subsequently be executed more efficiently. This increase in efficiency would result in reduced ACC activity (reflecting the reduced need to constrain action by option context) and perhaps also increased DLPFC activity (reflecting increased effectiveness of imposing the option).

Action Selection

According to the HRL theory, ACC input is required primarily when behavior is guided by high-level, internal constraints rather than directly cued by the environment. This interpretation provides a straightforward account of ACC activity in voluntary action selection tasks requiring unpredictable or irregular movement sequences[15]: Such sequences are, by definition, unconstrained with respect to environmental stimuli, precisely the conditions that demand option selection from among the many potential option-specific policies afforded. In contrast, ACC should be less important, and less active, when the range of possible behaviors is strongly constrained (e.g., because of experimental instruction). In such situations, options and actions essentially become preselected, rendering ACC less important for effective behavior. As a consequence, standard stimulus-driven laboratory tasks (such as the Stroop task) may be relatively insensitive to ACC lesions, whereas underconstrained real-world tasks dependent on longer-term courses of action (such as jogging up a mountain) would rely on ACC to a greater extent.

Nevertheless, even for instructed tasks, ACC may (via its interactions with DLPFC) play a facilitatory role when the task has hierarchical structure, for example, by linking successive actions or by providing contextual input that weakens selection of task-irrelevant actions in the DLS. In this view, sustained ACC activity during task selection and execution[17] reflects its role in selecting, maintaining, and evaluating behavioral options. This process is enforced through a division of labor between ACC and DLPFC, with the former being responsible for selecting and energizing task-relevant representations, and the latter implementing those representations by providing top-down biasing signals that facilitate execution of appropriate stimulus-response mappings in lower-level structures in motor cortex and the basal ganglia.

Reinforcement Learning

The present theory extends previous RL accounts to propose that ACC and the DLS play complementary roles in learning and selecting high-level options and individual actions, respectively. Our theory thus inherits from these accounts its explanation of ACC sensitivity to reward (primarily via dopaminergic input) and pain and costs (perhaps via input from the cingulate gyrus and insula[42]). However, it is distinguished by its emphasis on reinforcement of options by goal achievement (pseudo-reward) rather than of individual actions by primary reward. Learning by ACC is thus related mainly to sequences of actions (i.e., which options to choose) as opposed to the primitive actions that comprise the option: ACC learns whether to run up the mountain, not how to put one foot in front of the other. Performance feedback may therefore elicit ACC activity even in the absence of task-related behavior, because dopaminergic signals can reinforce the option itself (e.g., the decision to participate in the task) in addition to the primitive actions that comprise the task sequence.[60]

This reasoning implies that behavior following ACC lesions should be driven primarily by outcomes of individual actions rather than by temporally extended behavioral strategies. This prediction provides a straightforward account of primate work showing that ACC lesions cause responding to become fragmented and reliant on recent reward history rather than on rewards integrated over longer behavioral sequences.[27] Disruption of ACC function should similarly reduce animals' ability to represent transitions between individual actions, and hence impair their ability to switch plans flexibly when reduced reward indicates the need to change strategy[49]:

Without higher-level structure, new actions will not be attempted (and learned) until previous contingencies are largely extinguished. However, because ACC primarily cares about the value of actions, lesions to this region should have much less impact in stimulus-driven tasks for which contingencies reflect the value or relevance of particular stimulus attributes, as is the case for the WCST in human neuropsychology.[13]

Motivation and Effort

Our theory suggests that ACC contributes to motivation and effort in two principal ways. First, options selected in ACC provide excitatory input to DLPFC, energizing the adoption of particular behavioral policies (task sets). Second, efference copy of selected options elicits value signals in OFC that are broadcast via the midbrain dopamine system to facilitate option selection by ACC and policy implementation by the DLPFC and DLS. These ACC contributions are important when goal-oriented actions are not strongly driven by the environment, thus capturing the essence of motivation and effort in a variety of contexts: when no stimuli are provided and action must be internally generated (as in voluntary selection paradigms), when stimuli are presented but strongly cue a different response from the one required (as in conflict paradigms), and when the value of the current option does not outweigh that of competing options (as when the desire to reach the top of the hill matches the desire to rest one's aching legs and lungs).

According to HRL theory, then, ACC lesions should result in biases away from extended action sequences accruing long-term reward, toward less effortful but more immediately rewarding actions. Corresponding deficits in incentive salience will cause a shift toward overall behavioral inhibition. Thus, in contrast to other formulations,[5] our hypothesis does not imply that ACC specifically codes for effort. If this were the case, one might expect ACC-lesioned animals to be insensitive to effort (i.e., factoring this cost poorly into their action choices). Instead, these animals show hypersensitivity and aversion to effortful options. Human patients with ACC lesions exhibit similar reductions in spontaneous speech and behavior.

Future Directions

The option-selection theory provides a unified account of the role of ACC in performance monitoring, selecting and initiating action, learning about the consequences of actions, and motivating effortful behavior. It extends previous RL accounts[25] to attribute a specific computational function to ACC that distinguishes it from other neural systems—such as the basal ganglia and DLPFC—that are likewise integral to adaptive decision making.

Unsurprisingly, the theory raises as many questions as it answers. Foremost among these is how to test it: What types of task might probe the proposed functions of ACC? We have argued that many existing paradigms rely too heavily on stimulus-dependent tasks that can be solved without the advantages of HRL,[11] thus explaining why patients with ACC lesions show only mild and subtle deficits. Our theory allows us to sketch the outlines of a task that might be more sensitive to the contributions of ACC: The crucial elements are that responding should be underconstrained by the stimuli presented and that the task should have a hierarchical structure in which the reinforcement value of individual actions provides a weak, or even misleading, guide to the appropriate overall strategy. A valuable approach in future research would be to develop HRL-based computational models to identify appropriate task designs and to predict human performance, ACC activity, and ACC lesion effects in these contexts.

A second question concerns how the dual-level neural architecture we propose (figure 18.1) might deal with real-world problems that typically involve multiple embedded goals. For example, the desire to lead a long, healthy life might encompass as a subgoal the intent to exercise regularly, which itself might contain the subgoal of running up a mountain on a particular day, which in turn would depend on a subgoal of placing one foot in front of the other, and so on. We suggest that in practice these multilevel problems are translated into series of two-level problems, the top level of which at any given moment is mediated by the contents of working memory. For example, our jogger might one morning choose between running and relaxing, but executing the former option itself entails choosing among suboptions (e.g., regarding which route to run). During this choice, the highest-level option (the decision to run) might be temporarily cleared from working memory, to be reinstated later on completion of the lower-level decision.

A third question concerns the implications of the proposal that action selection can be shaped by the pseudo-reward associated with each option's termination function. Specifically, departing somewhat from standard treatments of HRL, our framework allows the possibility that failure to achieve the termination state of an option may reduce the strength of that option, implying a reduced preference for its corresponding subgoal. This implication seems antithetical to the fundamental assumption in the artificial intelligence approach to RL that the values of rewards are intrinsic and immutable.[51] But perhaps this flexibility is in fact a lineament of human behavior. In Aesop's fable, the hungry fox is unable to jump high enough to reach some grapes hanging high on the vine. Turning away in disgust, the fox grumbles: "You aren't even ripe yet! I don't need any sour grapes!" This fable serves as an apposite reminder that human goals change in response to our evolving beliefs about what we can and cannot achieve. In this way, ACC may provide the impetus for the seemingly infinite variety of individual preferences that characterizes human culture, including the pursuits of music, science, art, and sport.

Outstanding Questions

• What kind of experimental task will best test the role played by ACC in option selection?

• How does the brain carry out multilevel HRL problems? Must hierarchical task structure be replicated in a hierarchical neural architecture, or can multilevel problems be solved using flexible switching within a dual-level architecture as outlined here?

• How are option strengths initialized and modified?

Further Reading

Botvinick MM, Niv Y, Barto AC. 2009. Hierarchically organized behavior and its neural foundations: a reinforcement learning perspective. *Cognition* 113: 262–280. This paper provides the conceptual foundations of the present chapter, laying out the computational framework of HRL and suggesting a possible neural implementation.

Paus T. 2001. Primate anterior cingulate cortex: where motor control, drive and cognition interface. *Nat Rev Neurosci* 2: 417–424. An influential review of anatomical and functional evidence that ACC plays a pivotal role in the motivational control of behavior.

Vogt BA. 2009. Cingulate Neurobiology and Disease. Oxford: Oxford University Press. A comprehensive handbook on the functional neuroanatomy of cingulate cortex, with an emphasis on its cytoarchitecture and connectivity.

References

1. Alexander MP. 2001. Chronic akinetic mutism after mesencephalic-diencephalic infarction: remediated with dopaminergic medications. *Neurorehabil Neural Repair* 15: 151–156.

2. Amiez C, Joseph J-P, Procyk E. 2005. Anterior cingulate error related activity is modulated by predicted reward. *Eur J Neurosci* 21: 3447–3452.

3. Assadi SM, Yucel M, Pantelis C. 2009. Dopamine modulates neural networks involved in effort-based decision-making. *Neurosci Biobehav Rev* 33: 383–393.

4. Berridge KC, Robinson TE. 1998. What is the role of dopamine in reward: hedonic impact, reward learning, or incentive salience? *Brain Res Brain Res Rev* 28: 309–369.

5. Botvinick MM. 2007. Conflict monitoring and decision making: reconciling two perspectives on anterior cingulate function. *Cogn Affect Behav Neurosci* 7: 356–366.

6. Botvinick MM, Braver TS, Carter CS, Barch DM, Cohen JD. 2001. Conflict monitoring and cognitive control. *Psychol Rev* 108: 624–652.

7. Botvinick MM, Niv Y, Barto AC. 2009. Hierarchically organized behavior and its neural foundations: a reinforcement learning perspective. *Cognition* 113: 262–280.

8. Brown JW, Braver TS. 2005. Learned predictions of error likelihood in the anterior cingulate cortex. *Science* 307: 1118–1121.

9. Carter CS, Braver TS, Barch DM, Botvinick MM, Noll D, Cohen JD. 1998. Anterior cingulate cortex, error detection, and the online monitoring of performance. *Science* 280: 747–749.

10. Cohen JD, Braver TS, Brown JW. 2002. Computational perspectives on dopamine function in prefrontal cortex. *Curr Opin Neurobiol* 12: 223–229.

11. Cohen MX, Frank M. 2008. Neurocomputational models of basal ganglia function in learning, memory and choice. *Behav Brain Res* 199: 141–156.

12. Cohen MX, Heller AS, Ranganath C. 2005. Functional connectivity with anterior cingulate and orbitofrontal cortices during decision-making. *Brain Res Cogn Brain Res* 23: 61–70.

13. Cohen RA, Kaplan RF, Zuffante P, Moser DJ, Jenkins MA, Salloway S, Wilkinson H. 1999. Alteration of intention and self-initiated action associated with bilateral anterior cingulotomy. *J Neuropsychiatry Clin Neurosci* 11: 444–453.

14. Critchley HD, Mathias CJ, Josephs O, O'Doherty J, Zanini S, Dewar BK, Cipolotti L, Shallice T, Dolan RJ. 2003. Human cingulate cortex and autonomic control: converging neuroimaging and clinical evidence. *Brain* 126: 2139–2152.

15. Deiber M-P, Honda M, Ibanez V, Sadato N, Hallett M. 1999. Mesial motor areas in self-initiated versus externally triggered movements examined with fMRI: effect of movement type and rate. *J Neurophysiol* 81: 3065–3077.

16. Devinsky O, Morrell MJ, Vogt BA. 1995. Contributions of anterior cingulate cortex to behaviour. *Brain* 118: 279–306.

17. Dosenbach NUF, Visscher KM, Palmer ED, Miezin FM, Wenger KK, Kang HSC, Burgund ED, Grimes AL, Schlaggar BL, Petersen SE. 2006. A core system for the implementation of task sets. *Neuron* 50: 799–812.

18. Dum RP, Strick PL. 1993. Cingulate motor areas. In: Neurobiology of Cingulate Cortex and Limbic Thalamus: A Comprehensive Handbook (Vogt BA, Gabriel M, eds), pp 415–441. Boston: Birkhauser.

19. Duncan J, Owen AM. 2000. Common regions of the human frontal lobe recruited by diverse cognitive demands. *Trends Neurosci* 23: 475–483.

20. Falkenstein M, Hohnsbein J, Hoorman J, Blanke L. 1990. Effects of errors in choice reaction tasks on the ERP under focused and divided attention. In: Psychophysiological Brain Research (Brunia CHM, Gaillard AWK, Kok A, eds), pp 192–195. Tilburg, Netherlands: Tilburg University Press.

21. Fellows LK, Farah MJ. 2005. Is anterior cingulate cortex necessary for cognitive control? *Brain* 128: 788–796.

22. Gemba H, Sasaki K, Brooks VB. 1986. "Error" potentials in limbic cortex (anterior cingulate area 24) of monkeys during motor learning. *Neurosci Lett* 70: 223–227.

23. Hadland KA, Rushworth MFS, Gaffan D, Passingham RE. 2003. The anterior cingulate and reward-guided selection of actions. *J Neurophysiol* 89: 1161–1164.

24. Hayden BY, Platt ML. 2010. Neurons in anterior cingulate cortex multiplex information about reward and action. *J Neurosci* 30: 3339–3346.

25. Holroyd CB, Coles MGH. 2002. The neural basis of human error processing: reinforcement learning, dopamine, and the error-related negativity. *Psychol Rev* 109: 679–709.

26. Holroyd CB, Nieuwenhuis S, Yeung N, Nystrom LE, Mars RB, Coles MGH, Cohen JD. 2004. Dorsal anterior cingulate cortex shows fMRI response to internal and external error signals. *Nat Neurosci* 7: 497–498.

27. Kennerley SW, Walton ME, Behrens TE, Buckley MJ, Rushworth MF. 2006. Optimal decision making and the anterior cingulate cortex. *Nat Neurosci* 9: 940–947.

28. Kerns JG, Cohen JD, MacDonald AW, 3rd, Cho RY, Stenger VA, Carter CS. 2004. Anterior cingulate conflict monitoring and adjustments in control. *Science* 303: 1023–1026.

29. Matsumoto M, Matsumoto K, Abe H, Tanaka K. 2007. Medial prefrontal cell activity signaling prediction errors of action values. *Nat Neurosci* 10: 647–656.

30. McClure SM, Daw ND, Montague PR. 2003. A computational substrate for incentive salience. *Trends Neurosci* 26: 423–428.

31. Mesulam M. 1981. A cortical network for directed attention and unilateral neglect. *Ann Neurol* 10: 309–325.

32. Miller EK, Cohen JD. 2001. An integrative theory of prefrontal cortex function. *Annu Rev Neurosci* 24: 167–202.

33. Miltner WHR, Braun CH, Coles MGH. 1997. Event-related potentials following incorrect feedback in a time-estimation task: evidence for a "generic" neural system for error detection. *J Cogn Neurosci* 9: 788–798.

34. Montague PR, Hyman SE, Cohen JD. 2004. Computational roles for dopamine in behavioral control. *Nature* 431: 760–767.

35. Morecraft RJ, van Hoesen GW. 1998. Convergence of limbic input to the cingulate motor cortex in the rhesus monkey. *Brain Res Bull* 45: 209–232.

36. Nakamura K, Roesch MR, Olson CR. 2005. Neuronal activity in macaque SEF and ACC during performance of tasks involving conflict. *J Neurophysiol* 93: 884–908.

37. Nemeth G, Hegedus K, Molnar L. 1988. Akinetic mutism associated with bicingular lesions: clinico-pathological and functional anatomical correlates. *Arch Psychiatry Clin Neurosci* 237: 218–222.

38. Niv Y. 2009. Reinforcement learning in the brain. *J Math Psychol* 53: 139–154.

39. O'Doherty J, Dayan P, Schultz J, Deichmann R, Friston K, Dolan RJ. 2004. Dissociable roles of ventral and dorsal striatum in instrumental conditioning. *Science* 304: 452–454.

40. Papez JW. 1937. A proposed mechanism of emotion. *Arch Neurol Psychiatry* 38: 725–743.

41. Paus T. 2001. Primate anterior cingulate cortex: where motor control, drive and cognition interface. *Nat Rev Neurosci* 2: 417–424.

42. Peyron R, Laurent B, Garcia-Larrea L. 2000. Functional imaging of brain responses to pain. a review and meta-analysis. *Neurophysiol Clin* 30: 263–288.

43. Picard N, Strick PL. 1996. Motor areas of the medial wall: a review of their location and functional activation. *Cereb Cortex* 6: 342–353.

44. Ridderinkhof KR, Ullsperger M, Crone EA, Nieuwenhuis S. 2004. The role of medial frontal cortex in cognitive control. *Science* 306: 443–447.

45. Rushworth MFS, Behrens TE, Rudebeck PH, Walton ME. 2007. Contrasting roles for cingulate and orbitofrontal cortex in decisions and social behaviour. *Trends Cogn Sci* 11: 168–176.

46. Schultz W. 2002. Getting formal with dopamine and reward. *Neuron* 36: 241–263.

47. Shidara M, Richmond BJ. 2002. Anterior cingulate: single neuronal signals related to degree of reward expectancy. *Science* 31: 1709–1711.

48. Shima K, Aya K, Mushiake H, Inase M, Aizawa H, Tanji J. 1991. Two movement-related foci in primate cingulate cortex observed in signal-triggered and self-paced forelimb movements. *J Neurophysiol* 65: 188–202.

49. Shima K, Tanji J. 1998. Role for cingulate motor area cells in voluntary movement selection based on reward. *Science* 282: 1335–1338.

50. Stuss DT, Alexander MP, Shallice T, Picton TW, Binns MA, Macdonald R, Borowiec A, Katz DI. 2005. Multiple frontal systems controlling response speed. *Neuropsychologia* 43: 396–417.

51. Sutton RS, Barto AG. 1998. Reinforcement Learning: An Introduction. Cambridge, MA: MIT Press.

52. Tucker DM, Luu P, Pribram KH. 1995. Social and emotional self-regulation. *Ann N Y Acad Sci* 769: 213–239.

53. Turken AU, Swick D. 1999. Response selection in the human anterior cingulate cortex. *Nat Neurosci* 2: 920–924.

54. Walton ME, Bannerman DM, Alterescu K, Rushworth MF. 2003. Functional specialization within medial frontal cortex of the anterior cingulate for evaluating effort-related decisions. *J Neurosci* 23: 6475–6479.

55. Walton ME, Devlin JT, Rushworth MF. 2004. Interactions between decision making and performance monitoring within prefrontal cortex. *Nat Neurosci* 7: 1259–1265.

56. Walton ME, Kennerley SW, Bannerman DM, Phillips PEM, Rushworth MFS. 2006. Weighing up the benefits of work: behavioral and neural analyses of effort-related decision making. *Neural Netw* 19: 1302–1314.

57. Williams SM, Goldman-Rakic PS. 1993. Characterization of the dopaminergic innervation of the primate frontal cortex using a dopamine-specific antibody. *Cereb Cortex* 3: 199–222.

58. Williams ZM, Bush G, Rauch SL, Cosgrove GR, Eskandar EN. 2004. Human anterior cingulate neurons and the integration of monetary reward with motor responses. *Nat Neurosci* 7: 1370–1375.

59. Yeung N. 2004. Relating cognitive and affective theories of the error-related negativity. In: Errors, Conflicts, and the Brain. Current Opinions on Performance Monitoring (Ullsperger M, Falkenstein M, eds), pp 63–70. Leipzig, Germany: Max Planck Institute of Cognitive Neuroscience.

60. Yeung N, Holroyd CB, Cohen JD. 2005. ERP correlates of feedback and reward processing in the presence and absence of response choice. *Cereb Cortex* 15: 535–544.

19 Meta-Learning, Cognitive Control, and Physiological Interactions between Medial and Lateral Prefrontal Cortex

Mehdi Khamassi, Charles R. E. Wilson, Marie Rothé, René Quilodran, Peter F. Dominey, and Emmanuel Procyk

Reacting to errors and adapting choices to achieve long-term goals are fundamental abilities used in reasoning and problem solving. These abilities require the proper operation of executive functions to support decision making and the organization of behavior in new and challenging situations. Several theoretical models propose that this involves high-level cognitive control of action, in particular when routines need to be modified or reorganized.[20,64,74] There is evidence for a range of subcomponent processes in cognitive control, including selection, active maintenance and use of information for planning (working memory), inhibition, and performance monitoring.[51] In problematic situations, automatic responding becomes inefficient or suboptimal, and so cognitive control must be triggered in order to promote the selection of appropriate actions, given the circumstances. It is clear that the proper functioning of these processes does not depend on the integrity of one particular brain structure but on a specific distributed network. Converging evidence suggests that subdivisions of the prefrontal cortex house an important part of this network, but the mechanisms used to implement these processes remain unclear.

In the past 15 years, the reinforcement learning (RL) theory has been used successfully to describe neural mechanisms of decision making based on action valuation, and learning of action values based on reward prediction and reward prediction errors[29,79] (see also chapters 16 and 17, this volume). Its extensive use in the computational neuroscience literature is grounded in the observation that dopaminergic neurons respond according to reward prediction error,[70] that dopamine strongly innervates the prefrontal cortex and striatum and there modifies synaptic plasticity,[30,63] and that prefrontal cortical and striatal neurons encode a variety of RL-consistent information.[19,36,69,78]

However, RL models rely on crucial meta-parameters (e.g., learning rate, exploration rate, temporal discount factor) that need to be dynamically tuned to cope with variations in the environment. If one postulates that the brain implements RL-like decision-making mechanisms, one needs to understand how the brain regulates such mechanisms, in other words how it "tunes meta-parameters." Regulation of decision making has been largely studied in terms of "cognitive control," and is hypothesized to involve interactions between subdivisions of the prefrontal cortex (PFC), especially the medial and lateral PFC. We argue here that neural data concerning such interactions can be interpreted within the meta-learning theoretical framework proposed by Kenji Doya to synthesize computational principles for regulating RL meta-parameters.[21]

Theoretical Bases of Meta-Learning

RL is a research field within computer science that studies how an agent can appropriately adapt its behavioral policy so as to reach a particular goal in a given environment.[79] Here, we assume this goal to be maximizing the amount of reward obtained by the agent. RL methods rely on Markov decision processes. This is a mathematical framework for studying decision making which supposes that the agent is situated in a stochastic or deterministic environment, that it has a certain representation of its state (e.g., its location in the environment, the presence of stimuli or rewards, its motivational state), and that future states depend on the performance of particular actions in the current state. Thus, the objective of the agent is to learn the value associated with performance of each possible action, a, in each possible state, s, in terms of the amount of reward that they provide: $Q(s,a)$. In a popular class of RL algorithms called temporal-difference learning, which has shown strong resemblance to dopaminergic signaling,[70] the agent iteratively performs actions and updates action values based on a reward prediction error (RPE), δ:

$$\delta_t = r_t + \gamma . \max_a Q(s_t, a) - Q(s_{t-1}, a_{t-1}) \tag{19.1}$$

where r_t is the reward obtained at time t, $Q(s_{t-1}, a_{t-1})$ is the value of action a_{t-1} performed in state s_{t-1} at time $t-1$, which leads to the current state s_t, and $\gamma . \max_a Q(s_t, a)$ is the quality of the new state s_t; that is, the maximal value that can be expected from performing any action a. The latter term is weighted by a meta-parameter γ ($0 \leq \gamma < 1$) called the discount factor, which gives the temporal horizon of reward expectations. If γ is tuned to a high value, the agent has a behavior oriented toward long-term rewards. If γ is tuned to a value close to 0, the agent focuses on immediate rewards.

The RPE, δ_t, constitutes a reinforcement signal based on the unpredictability of rewards (e.g., unpredicted reward will lead to a positive RPE and thus to a reinforcement[79]). Action values are then updated with this RPE term:

$$Q(a_{t-1}, s_{t-1}) \leftarrow Q(a_{t-1}, s_{t-1}) + \alpha . \delta_t \tag{19.2}$$

where α is a second meta-parameter called the learning rate ($0 \leq \alpha \leq 1$). Tuning α will determine whether new reinforcement will drastically change the representation of action values, or if instead an action should be repeated several times before its value is significantly changed.

Once action values are updated, an action selection process enables a certain exploration-exploitation trade-off: The agent should most of the time select the action with the highest value (*exploitation*) but should also sometimes select other actions (*exploration*) to possibly gather new information, especially when the agent detects that the environment might have changed.[32] This can be done by transforming each action value into a probability of performing the associated action, a, in the considered state, s, with a Boltzmann softmax equation:

$$P(a/s) = \frac{\exp(\beta.Q(a,s))}{\sum_i \exp(\beta.Q(a_i,s))} \tag{19.3}$$

where β is a third meta-parameter called the exploration rate ($0 \le \beta$). Although it is always the case that the action with the highest value has a higher probability of being performed, exploration is further regulated in the following way: When β is set to a small value, action probabilities are close to each other so that there is a high probability of selecting an action whose action value is not the greatest (exploration). When β is high, the difference between action probabilities is increased so that the action with the highest action value is almost always selected (exploitation).

Clearly, these equations devoted to action value learning and action selection rely on crucial meta-parameters: α, β, γ. Most computational models use fixed meta-parameters, hand-tuned for a given task or problem. However, animals face a variety of tasks and deal with continuously varying conditions. If animal learning does rely on RL as suggested,[45,69] there must exist some brain mechanisms to decide, in each particular situation, which set of meta-parameters is appropriate (e.g., when an animal performs stereotypical behavior in its nest, or repetitive food gathering behavior in an habitual place, learning rate and exploration rate should not be the same as those used when the animal discovers a new place). Moreover, within a given task or problem, it is more efficient to dynamically regulate these meta-parameters, so as to optimize performance (e.g., it is appropriate to initially explore more in a new task environment while the rule for obtaining rewards is not yet known, to explore less when the rule has been found and the environment is stable, and to reexplore more when a rule change is detected).

The dynamic regulation of meta-parameters has been called *meta-learning*.[21] Meta-learning is a general principle that allows us to solve problems of nonstationary systems in machine learning, but the principle does not assume specific methods for the regulation itself. We invite readers interested in particular solutions to refer to methods such as "ε-greedy," which chooses the action believed to be best most of the time, but occasionally (with probability ε) substitutes a random action[79];

upper-confidence bound policies, which select actions based on their associated reward averages and the number of times they were selected so far[6]; EXP3-S for Exponential-weight algorithm for Exploration and Exploitation, which is also based on a Boltzmann softmax function[14]; uncertainty-based methods awarding bonuses to actions whose consequences are uncertain[19]; and reviews of these methods applied to abruptly changing environments.[23,27]

Although mathematically different, these methods stand on common principles to regulate action selection. Most are based on estimations of the agent's performance, which we will refer to as *performance monitoring*, and on estimations of the stability of the environment across time or its variance when abrupt environmental changes occur, which we will refer to as *task monitoring*. The former employs measures such as the average reward measured with the history of feedback obtained by the agent, or the number of times a given action has already been performed. The latter often considers the environment's uncertainty, which in economic terms refers to the risk (the known probability of a given reward source), and the volatility (variance) over time of this risk.

A simple example of implementation of a meta-learning algorithm has been proposed in which an agent has to solve a nonstationary Markov decision task.[71,80] In this task, the agent has two possible actions (pressing one of two buttons). The task is decomposed into two conditions: a short-term condition where one button is associated with a small positive reward and the other button with a small negative reward; and a long-term condition such that a button with small negative rewards has to be pressed on a number of steps in order to obtain a much larger positive reward in a subsequent step. The authors used an RL algorithm in which meta-parameters were subject to automatic dynamic regulation. The general principle of the algorithm is to operate such regulation based on variations in the average reward obtained by the agent. Figure 19.1 shows a sample simulation. The agent learned the short-term condition, starting with a small meta-parameter β (i.e., high exploration rate), which progressively increased and produced less exploration as the average reward increased. At mid-session, the task condition was changed from short-term condition to long-term condition, resulting in a drop in the average reward obtained by the agent. As a consequence, meta-parameters varied allowing more randomness in the agent's actions (due to a small β), and leading the agent to focus on immediate reward (due to a small γ), which is more appropriate when the environment is unstable. After some time, the agent learns the new task condition and converges to a more exploitative behavior (high β value) combined with a more long-term oriented behavioral policy (large γ) appropriate for this new task condition.

This type of computational process appears suitably robust to account for animal behavioral adaptation. The meta-learning framework has been formalized with neural mechanisms in mind. Doya proposed that the level of different neuromodula-

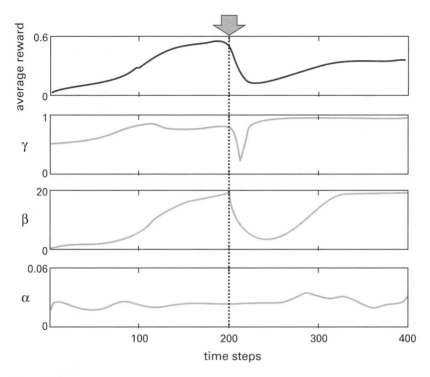

Figure 19.1
Simulation of a meta-learning algorithm. Adapted from Schweighofer and Doya.[71] A change in the task condition from short-term reward to long-term reward at time-step #200 produces an adaptation of meta-parameter values.

tors in the prefrontal cortex and striatum might operate the tuning of specific meta-parameters for learning and action selection.[21]

We argue in the following sections that the meta-learning framework indeed offers valuable tools to study neural mechanisms of decision making and learning, especially within the medial and lateral prefrontal cortex. This framework offers formal descriptions of the functional biases observed in each structure and also provides explanatory principles for their interaction and role in the regulation of behavior. In order to describe how meta-learning can improve the functional descriptions of prefrontal areas, we first present a short neurobiological overview.

Anatomy, Physiology, and Function of PFC Areas

The PFC is a large area of cortex, and there have been several attempts to subdivide it on both anatomical and functional lines. It seems clear now that the PFC has not only an overall functional role that is not localized within its subdivisions, but also significant differences in function between those regions.[84] The prefrontal cortex's anatomical heterogeneity, observed in its local cytoarchitectonic organization and in the connectivity pattern of areas, reveals a functional heterogeneity (see also chapter 1, this volume). PFC areas are highly interconnected, but each seems to contribute to specific functions of the prefrontal cortex as a whole.[41] One standard functional high-order grouping of PFC areas defines lateral (LPFC), orbital, and medial subdivisions. The PFC is the target of multiple neuromodulatory afferents (including strong dopaminergic inputs), and it appears that impaired functioning of these systems results in numerous psychiatric and neurological disorders (see also chapters 3 and 15, this volume).

Several theories have been proposed regarding the function of LPFC.[22,26,51,56] Most theories are based on the fact that LPFC neural activity participates in bridging cues and responses separated in time and space by actively representing task-relevant information (i.e., information relative to targets, responses, and goals). Debates on functional dissociations within LPFC are intense, but most admit that active representation of information is a key feature of LPFC function. Active maintenance and the ability to link information across time delays are at the core of the role of LPFC in the control and sequential organization of behavior. Although this is still under investigation, it has been proposed that the maintenance and control of information involve several mechanisms, somewhat dependent on dopaminergic input, and related to recurrent excitation within LPFC and between LPFC and distant areas.[17,51,52] The coding properties of LPFC tonic activity are modified between routine and nonroutine or exploratory behaviors,[57] suggesting a neurophysiological correlate of cognitive control and a modulation predicted by theories.

Crucial information required for action planning during adaptive behaviors is also encoded within LPFC activity. LPFC neurons encode information about the animal's responses as well as states of the environment.[25,83] LPFC neurons represent the sequence of steps and state transitions that lead from the present to the desired goal,[7,54] which is reminiscent of goal-oriented action planning, also referred to as model-based RL.[18] The quality and quantity of expected or obtained reward influence prefrontal delay activities.[1,42,82] Several lines of evidence suggest that the LPFC does not simply sum task-relevant information, but rather integrates reward-related information into knowledge about spatial location.[39,42] Simultaneous information coding related to spatial location and reward takes place in this region as well as in the caudate nucleus.[39] Although spatial selectivity relates well to the role of LPFC in action selection, these hypotheses fail to provide a functional explanation for observed variations in spatial selectivity in LPFC. Spatial selectivity variations were observed depending on task phases and independent of the actual selection.[58] As we will see later, consistent with previous computational models describing the effect of average reward on variation in exploration rate within the LPFC,[49] meta-learning principles enable good predictions of variations in spatial selectivity in LPFC between exploration and exploitation phases.[38]

Within the medial frontal cortex, the anterior cingulate cortex (ACC), and in particular area 24c, has an intermediate position between limbic, prefrontal, and premotor systems[3,55] (see also chapter 18, this volume). ACC neuronal activity tracks task events and encodes reinforcement-related information.[3,59,75] Muscimol injections in dorsal ACC induce strong deficits in finding the best behavioral option in a probabilistic learning task and in shifting responses based on reward changes.[4,75] Dorsal ACC lesions induce failures in integrating reinforcement history to guide future choices.[34] These data converge toward describing a major role of ACC in integrating reward information over time, which is confirmed by single-unit recordings,[72] and thereby in decision making based on action-reward associations. This function contrasts with that of the orbitofrontal cortex, which is necessary for stimulus-reward associations[65] (see also chapter 4, this volume).

In addition, the ACC certainly has a related function in detecting and valuing unexpected but behaviorally relevant events. This notably includes the presence or absence of reward outcomes and failure in action production, and has been largely studied using event-related potentials in humans and unit recordings in monkeys. The modulation of phasic ACC signals by prediction errors, as defined in the RL framework, supports the existence of a key functional relationship with the dopaminergic system.[2,28] In the dopamine system, the same cells encode positive and negative RPE by a phasic increase and a decrease in firing, respectively.[9,53,70] By contrast, in the ACC, different populations of cells encode positive and negative prediction errors, and both types of error result in an increase in firing.[48,62,68] Moreover, ACC neurons are able to discriminate choice errors (choice-related RPE) from execution errors (motor-related RPE, such as a break of eye fixation).[62] These two error types should be treated differently because they lead to different posterior adaptations. This suggests that, although the dopaminergic RPE signal could be directly used for adapting action values, ACC RPE signals also relate to a higher level of abstraction of information, like *feedback categorization*.

A third important aspect of ACC function was revealed by the discovery of changes in neural activity between exploratory and exploitative trials,[60,62] or between volatile and stable rewarding schedules.[10] This suggests a more general involvement of ACC in translating results of performance monitoring and task monitoring into a regulatory level.

From this short review, clear functional dissociations appear between ACC and LPFC. However, we shall see later that a fine description of dissociations and interactions is required for a good functional description of these two regions.

Dissociations and Interactions between ACC and LPFC

Dissociations

Studies on ACC-LPFC coactivations in various cognitive tasks significantly helped to dissociate their specific roles or describe their interactions.[35,46,50,76] An influential proposal is that ACC and LPFC are involved, respectively, in detection/monitoring of response conflict and implementing cognitive control to cope with it[35,46] (see also chapters 17 and 18, this volume). The dissociation is supported by evidence for correlations between sustained LPFC activation and the level of cognitive control on the one hand, and rapid changes in ACC activation during task practice on the other.[50]

Overall, ACC appears to be important when a task requires behavioral adaptation. In an fMRI study involving task shifts, the ACC was active especially after cues that were informative regarding behavioral adaptation whereas LPFC was activated even after noninformative cues.[44] Other fMRI studies pointed to a general role for ACC in assigning motivational priorities to task sets at any time, as opposed to a role for LPFC of dealing with interference arising from recently used task sets.[31] This last view is highly consistent with the theory according to which ACC has a major role in decision making by relating actions to their outcomes.[67]

Comparative electrophysiological studies show a certain level of redundancy of coding and similar response patterns in ACC and LPFC, but also stress the complementary properties of activity from the two structures. For instance, differential activations related to reward encoding have been shown in ACC and LPFC.[43] In this study, ACC neurons encoded both reward and the behavioral response, whereas LPFC neurons mostly coded for the response. Matsumoto et al. have reported that ACC neurons were more likely to encode response-outcome associations, whereas LPFC neurons encoded stimulus–response associations.[47] Seo and Lee used a dynamic binary choice task to show that more LPFC than ACC unit activity correlates with the difference between the reward values of two alternative choices. That is, LPFC seems to indicate the best option to a greater degree, whereas there is more evidence in ACC for encoding reinforcement history.[73] Importantly, this study showed that both structures share some aspects of reinforcement-related computation. Overall, these data converge toward a bias for ACC to encode performance monitoring signals, whereas LPFC neurons show a bias toward properties reflecting action selection. Note, however, that when one considers the overall properties of encoding by single units, the dissociation is not absolute.

Interactions

Although ACC and LPFC have been mainly highlighted in the literature in terms of their respective functions, their contribution to cognitive control might be fully realized in their interaction. The typology and function of these interactions are still unclear and are the topic of ongoing investigations.

The study of the dynamic of conflict resolution appears to show correlated increases of ACC and LPFC activations in the face of conflict.[8,35] In the context of the cognitive control loop scheme, this has been interpreted as a sequential and directed involvement of ACC and LPFC in the response to and resolution of conflict. However, the occurrence of ACC-LPFC interaction only in situations involving conflict resolution is debated.[31] Koechlin and colleagues have, instead, proposed that ACC might regulate the level or rate of cognitive control in LPFC as a function of motivation based on action cost-benefit estimations.[40]

By means of electrophysiological recordings in the monkey, Tsujimoto and colleagues have shown synchronous local field potentials (LFP) between areas 9 and 32, homologous to subparts of LPFC and ACC regions in humans, during a variety of cognitive tasks.[81] Similar results have been found in electroencephalograms (EEGs) in humans with the Eriksen flanker task,[13] where oscillatory activity in the theta band (4–8 Hz) in the medial prefrontal cortex was enhanced after errors, associated with transient synchronization with LPFC, and followed by a behavioral adjustment. Gehring and Knight showed that, in patients with an LPFC lesion, the well-studied medial frontal error-related negative potential, putatively produced from ACC, was still present but no longer discriminated between errors and correct trials.[24] At the behavioral level, the same patients showed difficulties in adapting responses following errors. These data bring into question the direction of influence between ACC and LFPC, although the effect could also be explained by an increased detection of response conflicts under abnormal cognitive control.[16]

The temporality of activations of the two structures appears to be consistent with the hypothesis that at times of instructive events, performance monitoring (mainly ACC) is followed by adjustment in control and selection (in LFPC). Temporality was studied both by unit recordings in nonhuman primates[33] and by EEG studies in humans.[76] The former study showed that the effect of task switching appear earlier in ACC than in LFPC.[33] The EEG study revealed phasic and early nonselective activations in ACC as opposed to a late LPFC activation correlated with performance. However, Silton and colleagues underlined that when task-relevant information is taken into account, late ACC activity appears to be influenced by earlier activation in LPFC. Data from our laboratory show that after relevant feedback leading to adaptation, advanced activation is seen in ACC before activation of LPFC at the population level, for both unit activity and high gamma power of LFP (figure 19.2).

PFC and the Regulation of Cognitive Control

The functions of prefrontal areas have been widely studied within a framework that strongly echoes meta-learning principles: the cognitive control loop theory.[11,15]

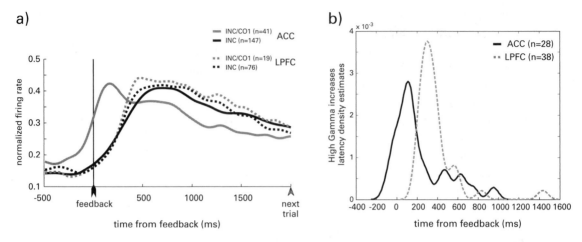

Figure 19.2
Latencies of neural responses after feedback in ACC and LPFC. (a) From unit activity recorded in the
PST task[62]: Neurons selective to incorrect feedbacks (INC, after an incorrect choice) discharge at comparable latencies in ACC and LPFC (black curves). However, neurons responding to salient feedbacks
(first correct CO1 and INC feedbacks after incorrect choice and after the first reward delivery; gray)
have a shorter latency in ACC than in LPFC. (b) Latencies of significant high gamma power increase in
LFP after incorrect feedbacks in ACC (black) and LPFC (gray).

The cognitive control loop describes the modulation of the control level in order
to adapt to immediate needs imposed by the environment. It also enables a shift
from routine behaviors in a known context requiring little attention and concentration, to more flexible behaviors involving rapid and active control. Two main phases
are necessary for the regulation and implementation of cognitive control. The
first consists of the systematic detection and evaluation of the relevance of performed actions. This information is used, in a second phase, to regulate cognitive
control and to potentiate appropriate action selection to reach a particular goal.
Norman and Shallice had formalized such a system with two components: an entity
for automatic action selection and an attentional supervisory/control system.[74]
The more familiar the environment and the more stably rewarded the actions are,
the more the system tends toward automatic functioning. In contrast, complex situations impose an active recovery of control to deal with new contexts and select
appropriate actions. Botvinick and colleagues followed the same perspective by
proposing conflict detection as a central mechanism to regulate cognitive control.[11]
The neural substrates proposed to support the mechanisms described by these
theories largely involve interactions between prefrontal areas,[11,51] in particular the
medial prefrontal cortex, including the ACC for its role in performance and task
monitoring and the LPFC for its role in action planning and the implementation of
cognitive control.

Several computational models have been developed to describe functioning of the cognitive control loop, and explicitly referring to ACC and LPFC. The respective roles attributed to these two structures are always based on the canonical view that ACC processes errors and monitors performance to regulate control in LPFC where action selection is implemented. The "global workspace" model explains how control is resumed in situations where routines get interrupted, where errors are made, or where an environmental change is detected. This model is composed of separate specialized modules regulated by a global workspace. The postulate here is that, considering functions attributed to ACC and LPFC, these two structures are perfectly appropriate to accomplish regulation.[20]

Cohen and colleagues describe an auto-regulated system responding to the demands of control by adjusting the exploration-exploitation trade-off.[15] In this model, ACC detects action consequences and attributes to them a value. This information is then used to modulate the cognitive control rate in LPFC via the locus coeruleus (see also chapter 12, this volume). Their model explicitly mentions noradrenergic innervation of the LPFC as a possible intermediate substrate to translate ACC modulation. The resulting increased cognitive control will facilitate behavioral adaptation in an appropriate way in associative areas. In a later version of the model, ACC is dedicated to conflict monitoring while the orbitofrontal cortex (OFC) monitors performance by estimating the reward average.[49] ACC and OFC would exert a systematic regulation of LC, which in turn modulates the level of exploration in the LPFC. Although the model fails to take into account ACC's involvement in RL mechanisms such as RPE signaling and action value updating, it has the merit of implicitly echoing the meta-learning framework by proposing a regulation of exploration based on reward average. Moreover, the model proposes a neural implementation of exploration regulation by varying the contrast between neural activities associated with competing actions, similar to the effect of the Boltzmann softmax function presented earlier (eq. 19.3). Our recent work using the meta-learning framework helped reconcile and integrate ACC mechanisms related to RL and mechanisms related to performance monitoring. Moreover, as described in the next section, it predicted formal variations of influence on LPFC mediated by ACC functions, which were verified by simultaneous recordings of the two structures.[38]

Neural Correlates of Meta-Parameter Regulation

Rushworth and colleagues recently highlighted the presence, at the level of ACC activity, of information relevant to the modulation of one of the RL metaparameters: the learning rate α.[10] Their study is grounded in theoretical accounts, suggesting that feedback information from the environment does not have the same uncertainty and will be treated differently depending on whether the environment is stable or unstable. In unstable and constantly changing ("volatile") environments, rapid behavioral adaptation is required in response to new outcomes, and so a higher learning rate is required. In contrast, the more stable the environment, the less RPEs should influence future actions. In the latter situation, more weight should be attributed to previous outcomes and the learning rate should remain small. These crucial variables of volatility and uncertainty correlate with the blood oxygen level–dependent response in the ACC at the time of outcomes.[10] Experimental controls in these studies allowed these signals influencing the learning rate to be identified independently from signals representing the prediction error.

This suggests that variations in ACC activity reflect the flexible adaptation of meta-parameter α (i.e., the learning rate) based on task requirements, and that previous reports of ACC activity encoding RPEs might be a consequence of such a meta-learning function.[48,62] This hypothesis can also explain differences in the time window over which previous reward information is encoded in ACC and related structures, as measured in different protocols involving different volatilities: A low learning rate produces a slow integration of reward information and thus preserves previous reward information over a large time window. In contrast, a high learning rate quickly erases information about previous rewards. Consistent with this interpretation, Sugrue et al. found that reward contingencies remained stable for hundreds of trials, which allowed outcomes from more than 30 trials ago to still have some influence over the values of choice options.[77] In Kennerley et al., the monkeys experienced a more volatile environment that switched approximately every 25 trials.[34] As a consequence, a much shorter reward integration period was reported in this study. In an adaptation of the matching pennies game, Seo and Lee showed that monkeys' choice in a given trial was potentially influenced by the choice outcomes in multiple previous trials, as expressed by a slow updating (low learning rate $\alpha = 0.24$) of action value functions, and ACC unit activity reflected the persistence of reward information across trials.[72]

Quilodran et al. used a very volatile environment (problem-solving task, or PST) where the action-reward contingency could be obtained from one single outcome and the task rule shifted after fewer than 10 trials on average.[62] This task enabled us to clearly dissociate exploratory and exploitative trials. Animals had to find which target presented in a set of four is rewarded. In each block (problem) the animal can explore targets until discovering the rewarded one, and then exploit (repeat) its choice for at least four trials. The target was then changed to initiate a new problem. This produced a complete reset of monkeys' action values at each new problem, independent of the previous problem.[37] Consistent with the theoretical relationship between volatility and learning rate, we found that monkey behavior in the PST is best fit with a RL model using a very high learning rate ($\alpha = 0.9$). In this task, the learning rate is not expected to change over time, reflecting a high but somewhat stable volatility. However, the exploratory rate should be varied to optimally regulate decision stochasticity. Previous recordings of either ACC or LFPC neurons in this task revealed strong firing rate variations between exploratory (uncertain) trials and repetitive trials.[58,62]

Recent investigations in our laboratory using the PST showed neural correlates of regulation of meta-parameter β (i.e., exploration rate) using recordings from both ACC and LPFC. We developed a computational model providing a formal description of ACC-LPFC interactions to allow experimental predictions to be drawn.[37] The model integrates ACC's role in adapting action values based on dopaminergic reward-prediction errors and reward history,[28,66] its function in performance monitoring through feedback categorization mechanisms,[62] and its role in regulating LPFC's function.[5] Finally, we integrated Cohen and Aston-Jones's proposal that the exploration rate is regulated within the LPFC based on performance monitoring.[15,49] To do so, our LPFC part filters action values sent by the ACC with eq. 19.3, where β is regulated by feedback history measured in ACC (figure 19.3a). Simulation of the model led to a set of experimental predictions that were verified by analyses of recordings from ACC and LPFC in the PST: (1) An overall decrease of activity during repetition trials was observed only in the LPFC; (2) target selectivity was globally higher in LPFC than in ACC; and (3) an increase of target selectivity was observed during repetition trials, consistent with the hypothesized exploitative mode of the system (figure 19.3b). Analysis of single-unit activity in this protocol also revealed correlates of information related to different variables in the model and confirmed the hypothesized function of ACC-LPFC interactions in this task.

Conclusion

The cognitive control theory previously stressed the importance of performance monitoring and task monitoring in ACC to regulate the level of control within LPFC. It appears that the meta-learning framework can complete this picture by providing testable computational principles that could formally underlie the regulation of such control. This framework explains the finding of a diversity of performance-monitoring processes previously associated with ACC function, such as estimations of error likelihood.[12] It also supports the previously highlighted fundamental role of this structure in relating actions to outcomes.[67] Recent investigations have explicitly referred to the involvement of the ACC in the regulation of RL meta-parameters.[10] This and our studies suggest that ACC might contribute to adapting the learning rate based on estimations of the environment's volatility, and the exploration rate based on feedback history and reward average.

However, the current picture drawn from the dissociation between ACC and LPFC function is not yet complete. Recent findings, including our own analyses,

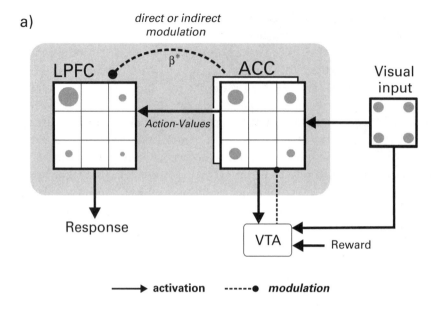

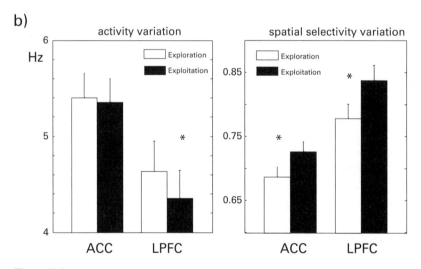

Figure 19.3
(a) Theoretical scheme of the hypothesized respective roles of ACC and LPFC in action value learning and exploration regulation (β^*) in the PST task. The interaction of these structures with the striatum through cortico-basal ganglia–thalamocortical anatomical loops is not represented here. (b) Global physiological tendencies measured in ACC and LPFC consistent with the theoretical scheme.

suggest that function is somewhat distributed over ACC and LPFC and that they both contain information related to action valuation, action selection, and their regulation. Also, while most theoretical approaches focused on ACC's influence over the LPFC, the opposite has to be considered. As mentioned earlier, Gehring and Knight showed that in patients with LPFC lesion, the medial frontal error-related negative potential, associated to ACC, was still present but no longer discriminated between errors and correct trials.[24] Moreover, anatomical data suggest that connections exist in both directions and have different patterns, suggesting different functional effects[61] (see also chapter 1, this volume). Thus, information flow from LPFC to ACC appears to be important and has to be taken into account to better understand ACC-LPFC interactions. Further investigations will be required to understand how ACC and LPFC share information, interact, and still show dissociable contributions to specific functions. The combinations of neurophysiological, interruptive, and computational approaches will be essential to answer such complex questions.

Outstanding Questions

• What are the neurophysiological substrates of communication between ACC and LPFC?

• How do ACC and LPFC, embedded in frontostriatal loops, form interacting dynamical systems whose configuration is influenced by neuromodulators?

• How do ACC-LPFC interactions impact on processing in posterior brain regions?

• How is the information required to tune different meta-learning parameters extracted?

Further Reading

Buzsaki G. 2006. Rhythms of the Brain. Oxford: Oxford University Press. A very comprehensive book on the nature and role of oscillations in brain computation on multiple spatial and temporal scales. A must for those interested in large-scale networks and their dynamics during cognition.

Glimcher PW, Camerer CF, Fehr E, Poldrack RA (eds). 2009. Neuroeconomics: Decision Making and the Brain. Amsterdam: Academic Press. The first complete handbook on neuroeconomics, in which top scientists joined to provide a clear description of this multidisciplinary approach to decision making.

References

1. Amemori K, Sawaguchi T. 2006. Contrasting effects of reward expectation on sensory and motor memories in primate prefrontal neurons. *Cereb Cortex* 16: 1002–1015.

2. Amiez C, Joseph JP, Procyk E. 2005. Anterior cingulate error-related activity is modulated by predicted reward. *Eur J Neurosci* 21: 3447–3452.

3. Amiez C, Joseph JP, Procyk E. 2005. Primate anterior cingulate cortex and adaptation of behaviour. In: From Monkey Brain to Human Brain (Dehaene S, Duhamel JR, Hauser MD, Rizzolatti G, eds), pp 315–336. Cambridge, MA: MIT Press.

4. Amiez C, Joseph JP, Procyk E. 2006. Reward encoding in the monkey anterior cingulate cortex. *Cereb Cortex* 16: 1040–1055.

5. Aston-Jones G, Cohen JD. 2005. An integrative theory of locus coeruleus-norepinephrine function: adaptive gain and optimal performance. *Annu Rev Neurosci* 28: 403–450.

6. Auer P, Cesa-Bianchi N, Fischer P. 2002. Finite-time analysis of the multiarmed bandit. *Mach Learn* 47: 235–256.

7. Averbeck BB, Sohn JW, Lee D. 2006. Activity in prefrontal cortex during dynamic selection of action sequences. *Nat Neurosci* 9: 276–282.

8. Badre D, Wagner AD. 2004. Selection, integration, and conflict monitoring; assessing the nature and generality of prefrontal cognitive control mechanisms. *Neuron* 41: 473–487.

9. Bayer HM, Glimcher PW. 2005. Midbrain dopamine neurons encode a quantitative reward prediction error signal. *Neuron* 47: 129–141.

10. Behrens TE, Woolrich MW, Walton ME, Rushworth MF. 2007. Learning the value of information in an uncertain world. *Nat Neurosci* 10: 1214–1221.

11. Botvinick MM, Braver TS, Barch DM, Carter CS, Cohen JD. 2001. Conflict monitoring and cognitive control. *Psychol Rev* 108: 624–652.

12. Brown JW, Braver TS. 2005. Learned predictions of error likelihood in the anterior cingulate cortex. *Science* 307: 1118–1121.

13. Cavanagh JF, Cohen MX, Allen JJ. 2009. Prelude to and resolution of an error: EEG phase synchrony reveals cognitive control dynamics during action monitoring. *J Neurosci* 29: 98–105.

14. Cesa-Bianchi N, Gabor L, Stoltz G. 2006. Regret minimization under partial monitoring. *Math Oper Res* 31: 562–580..

15. Cohen JD, Aston-Jones G, Gilzenrat MS. 2004. A systems-level perspective on attention and cognitive control. In: Cognitive Neuroscience of Attention (Posner MI, ed), pp 71–90. New York: Guilford.

16. Cohen JD, Botvinick M, Carter CS. 2000. Anterior cingulate and prefrontal cortex: who's in control? *Nat Neurosci* 3: 421–423.

17. Constantinidis C, Procyk E. 2004. The primate working memory networks. *Cogn Affect Behav Neurosci* 4: 444–465.

18. Daw ND, Niv Y, Dayan P. 2005. Uncertainty-based competition between prefrontal and dorsolateral striatal systems for behavioral control. *Nat Neurosci* 8: 1704–1711.

19. Daw ND, O'Doherty JP, Dayan P, Seymour B, Dolan RJ. 2006. Cortical substrates for exploratory decisions in humans. *Nature* 441: 876–879.

20. Dehaene S, Kerszberg M, Changeux JP. 1998. A neuronal model of a global workspace in effortful cognitive tasks. *Proc Natl Acad Sci USA* 95: 14529–14534.

21. Doya K. 2002. Metalearning and neuromodulation. *Neural Netw* 15: 495–506.

22. Fuster JM. 1997. The Prefrontal Cortex. Anatomy, Physiology and Neuropsychology of the Frontal Lobe, 3rd Ed. Philadelphia: Lippincott-Raven.

23. Garivier A, Moulines E. 2008. On upper-confidence bound policies for nonstationary bandit problems. Arxiv preprint arXiv:0805.3415.

24. Gehring WJ, Knight RT. 2000. Prefrontal-cingulate interactions in action monitoring. *Nat Neurosci* 3: 516–520.

25. Genovesio A, Brasted PJ, Wise SP. 2006. Representation of future and previous spatial goals by separate neural populations in prefrontal cortex. *J Neurosci* 26: 7305–7316.

26. Goldman-Rakic PS. 1987. Circuity of primate prefrontal cortex and regulation of behavior by representational memory. In: Higher Functions of the Brain (Plum F, ed), pp 373–414. Bethesda, MD: American Physiological Society.

27. Hartland C, Gelly S, Baskiotis N, Teytaud OMS. 2006. Multi-armed bandit, dynamic environments and meta-bandits. Paper presented at the NIPS-2006 workshop: Online trading between exploration and exploitation.

28. Holroyd CB, Coles MG. 2002. The neural basis of human error processing: reinforcement learning, dopamine, and the error-related negativity. *Psychol Rev* 109: 679–709.

29. Houk JC, Adams J, Barto AG, eds. 1995. A model of how the basal ganglia generate and use neural signals that predict reinforcement. In: Models of Information Processing in the Basal Ganglia, pp 249–270. Cambridge, MA: MIT Press.

30. Humphries MD, Prescott TJ. 2010. The ventral basal ganglia, a selection mechanism at the crossroads of space, strategy, and reward. *Prog Neurobiol* 90: 385–417.

31. Hyafil A, Summerfield C, Koechlin E. 2009. Two mechanisms for task switching in the prefrontal cortex. *J Neurosci* 29: 5135–5142.

32. Ishii S, Yoshida W, Yoshimoto J. 2002. Control of exploitation-exploration meta-parameter in reinforcement learning. *Neural Netw* 15: 665–687.

33. Johnston K, Levin HM, Koval MJ, Everling S. 2007. Top-down control-signal dynamics in anterior cingulate and prefrontal cortex neurons following task switching. *Neuron* 53: 453–462.

34. Kennerley SW, Walton ME, Behrens TE, Buckley MJ, Rushworth MF. 2006. Optimal decision making and the anterior cingulate cortex. *Nat Neurosci* 9: 940–947.

35. Kerns JG, Cohen JD, MacDonald AW, 3rd, Cho RY, Stenger VA, Carter CS. 2004. Anterior cingulate conflict monitoring and adjustments in control. *Science* 303: 1023–1026.

36. Khamassi M, Mulder AB, Tabuchi E, Douchamps V, Wiener SI. 2008. Anticipatory reward signals in ventral striatal neurons of behaving rats. *Eur J Neurosci* 28: 1849–1866.

37. Khamassi M, Quilodran R, Enel P, Procyk E, Dominey P. 2010. A computational model of integration between reinforcement learning and task monitoring in the prefrontal cortex. In From Animals to Animats 11: Lecture Notes in Computer Science (S. Doncieux et al., eds.), pp 424–434. Berlin: Springer-Verlag.

38. Khamassi M, Quilodran R, Procyk E, Dominey PF. 2009. Anterior cingulate cortex integrates reinforcement learning and task monitoring. Paper presented at the Annual Meeting of the Society for Neuroscience.

39. Kobayashi S, Kawagoe R, Takikawa Y, Koizumi M, Sakagami M, Hikosaka O. 2007. Functional differences between macaque prefrontal cortex and caudate nucleus during eye movements with and without reward. *Exp Brain Res* 176: 341–355.

40. Kouneiher F, Charron S, Koechlin E. 2009. Motivation and cognitive control in the human prefrontal cortex. *Nat Neurosci* 12: 939–945.

41. Lee D, Rushworth MF, Walton ME, Watanabe M, Sakagami M. 2007. Functional specialization of the primate frontal cortex during decision making. *J Neurosci* 27: 8170–8173.

42. Leon MI, Shadlen MN. 1999. Effect of expected reward magnitude on the response of neurons in the dorsolateral prefrontal cortex of the macaque. *Neuron* 24: 415–425.

43. Luk CH, Wallis JD. 2009. Dynamic encoding of responses and outcomes by neurons in medial prefrontal cortex. *J Neurosci* 29: 7526–7539.

44. Luks TL, Simpson GV, Feiwell RJ, Miller WL. 2002. Evidence for anterior cingulate cortex involvement in monitoring preparatory attentional set. *Neuroimage* 17: 792–802.

45. Luksys G, Gerstner W, Sandi C. 2009. Stress, genotype and norepinephrine in the prediction of mouse behavior using reinforcement learning. *Nat Neurosci* 12: 1180–1186.

46. MacDonald AW, 3rd, Cohen JD, Stenger VA, Carter CS. 2000. Dissociating the role of the dorsolateral prefrontal and anterior cingulate cortex in cognitive control. *Science* 288: 1835–1838.

47. Matsumoto K, Suzuki W, Tanaka K. 2003. Neuronal correlates of goal-based motor selection in the prefrontal cortex. *Science* 301: 229–232.

48. Matsumoto M, Matsumoto K, Abe H, Tanaka K. 2007. Medial prefrontal cell activity signaling prediction errors of action values. *Nat Neurosci* 10: 647–656.

49. McClure SM, Gilzenrat MS, Cohen JD. 2006. An exploration–exploitation model based on norepinephrine and dopamine activity. In: Advances in Neural Information Processing Systems (Weiss Y, Sholkopf B, Platt J, eds), pp 867–874. Cambridge, MA: MIT Press.

50. Milham MP, Banich MT, Claus ED, Cohen NJ. 2003. Practice-related effects demonstrate complementary roles of anterior cingulate and prefrontal cortices in attentional control. *Neuroimage* 18: 483–493.

51. Miller EK, Cohen JD. 2001. An integrative theory of prefrontal cortex function. *Annu Rev Neurosci* 24: 167–202.

52. Montague PR, Hyman SE, Cohen JD. 2004. Computational roles for dopamine in behavioural control. *Nature* 431: 760–767.

53. Morris G, Nevet A, Arkadir D, Vaadia E, Bergman H. 2006. Midbrain dopamine neurons encode decisions for future action. *Nat Neurosci* 9: 1057–1063.

54. Mushiake H, Saito N, Sakamoto K, Itoyama Y, Tanji J. 2006. Activity in the lateral prefrontal cortex reflects multiple steps of future events in action plans. *Neuron* 50: 631–641.

55. Paus T. 2001. Primate anterior cingulate cortex: where motor control, drive and cognition interface. *Nat Rev Neurosci* 2: 417–424.

56. Petrides M. 1998. Specialized systems for the processing of mnemonic information within the primate frontal cortex. In: The Prefrontal Cortex. Executive and Cognitive Functions (Roberts AC, Robbins TW, Weiskrantz L, eds), pp 103–116. Oxford: Oxford University Press.

57. Procyk E, Gao WJ, Goldman-Rakic PS. 2001. Prefrontal unit activity during delayed response and self-initiated performance. Paper presented at the Annual Meeting of the Society for Neuroscience.

58. Procyk E, Goldman-Rakic PS. 2006. Modulation of dorsolateral prefrontal delay activity during self-organized behavior. *J Neurosci* 26: 11313–11323.

59. Procyk E, Joseph JP. 2001. Characterization of serial order encoding in the monkey anterior cingulate sulcus. *Eur J Neurosci* 14: 1041–1046.

60. Procyk E, Tanaka YL, Joseph JP. 2000. Anterior cingulate activity during routine and non-routine sequential behaviors in macaques. *Nat Neurosci* 3: 502–508.

61. Quilodran R. 2009. Réseaux corticaux préfrontaux et adaptation du comportement: Physiologie et anatomie quantitative chez le singe. PhD thesis: Université Claude Bernard Lyon I.

62. Quilodran R, Rothé M, Procyk E. 2008. Behavioral shifts and action valuation in the anterior cingulate cortex. *Neuron* 57: 314–325.

63. Reynolds JN, Hyland BI, Wickens JR. 2001. A cellular mechanism of reward-related learning. *Nature* 413: 67–70.

64. Robbins TW. 1998. Dissociating executive functions of the prefrontal cortex. In: The Prefrontal Cortex. Executive and Cognitive Functions (Roberts AC, Robbins TW, Weiskrantz L, eds), pp 117–130. New York: Oxford University Press.

65. Rudebeck PH, Behrens TE, Kennerley SW, Baxter MG, Buckley MJ, Walton ME, Rushworth MF. 2008. Frontal cortex subregions play distinct roles in choices between actions and stimuli. *J Neurosci* 28: 13775–13785.

66. Rushworth MF, Behrens TE, Rudebeck PH, Walton ME. 2007. Contrasting roles for cingulate and orbitofrontal cortex in decisions and social behaviour. *Trends Cogn Sci* 11: 168–176.

67. Rushworth MF, Walton ME, Kennerley SW, Bannerman DM. 2004. Action sets and decisions in the medial frontal cortex. *Trends Cogn Sci* 8: 410–417.

68. Sallet J, Quilodran R, Rothé M, Vezoli J, Joseph JP, Procyk E. 2007. Expectations, gains, and losses in the anterior cingulate cortex. *Cogn Affect Behav Neurosci* 7: 327–336.

69. Samejima K, Ueda Y, Doya K, Kimura M. 2005. Representation of action-specific reward values in the striatum. *Science* 310: 1337–1340.

70. Schultz W, Dayan P, Montague PR. 1997. A neural substrate of prediction and reward. *Science* 275: 1593–1599.

71. Schweighofer N, Doya K. 2003. Meta-learning in reinforcement learning. *Neural Netw* 16: 5–9.

72. Seo H, Lee D. 2007. Temporal filtering of reward signals in the dorsal anterior cingulate cortex during a mixed-strategy game. *J Neurosci* 27: 8366–8377.

73. Seo H, Lee D. 2008. Cortical mechanisms for reinforcement learning in competitive games. *Philos Trans R Soc Lond B Biol Sci* 363: 3845–3857.

74. Shallice T. 1988. From Neuropsychology to Mental Structure. Cambridge: Cambridge University Press.

75. Shima K, Tanji J. 1998. Role for cingulate motor area cells in voluntary movement selection based on reward. *Science* 282: 1335–1338.

76. Silton RL, Heller W, Towers DN, Engels AS, Spielberg JM, Edgar JC, Sass SM, Stewart JL, Sutton BP, Banich MT, Miller GA. 2010. The time course of activity in dorsolateral prefrontal cortex and anterior cingulate cortex during top-down attentional control. *Neuroimage* 50: 1292–1302.

77. Sugrue LP, Corrado GS, Newsome WT. 2004. Matching behavior and the representation of value in the parietal cortex. *Science* 304: 1782–1787.

78. Sul JH, Kim H, Huh N, Lee D, Jung MW. 2010. Distinct roles of rodent orbitofrontal and medial prefrontal cortex in decision making. *Neuron* 66: 449–460.

79. Sutton RS, Barto AG. 1998. Reinforcement Learning: An Introduction. Cambridge, MA: MIT Press.

80. Tanaka SC, Doya K, Okada G, Ueda K, Okamoto Y, Yamawaki S. 2004. Prediction of immediate and future rewards differentially recruits cortico-basal ganglia loops. *Nat Neurosci* 7: 887–893.

81. Tsujimoto T, Shimazu H, Isomura Y, Sasaki K. 2010. Theta oscillations in primate prefrontal and anterior cingulate cortices in forewarned reaction time tasks. *J Neurophysiol* 103: 827–843.

82. Watanabe M. 1996. Reward expectancy in primate prefrontal neurons. *Nature* 382: 629–632.

83. Watanabe M, Sakagami M. 2007. Integration of cognitive and motivational context information in the primate prefrontal cortex. *Cereb Cortex* 17(Suppl 1): i101–i109.

84. Wilson CR, Gaffan D, Browning PG, Baxter MG. 2010. Functional localization within the prefrontal cortex: missing the forest for the trees? *Trends Neurosci* 33: 533–540.

20 Wherefore a Horse Race: Inhibitory Control as Rational Decision Making

Pradeep Shenoy and Angela J. Yu

Humans and animals often face the need to choose among actions with uncertain consequences, and to modify those choices according to ongoing sensory information and changing task demands. The requisite ability to dynamically modify or cancel planned actions, termed inhibitory control, is considered a fundamental element of flexible cognitive control.[6,33] Experimentally, inhibitory control is often studied using the stop signal paradigm.[28] In this task, subjects' primary task is to perform detection[25] or discrimination (two-alternative forced choice or 2AFC)[29] on an imperative "go" stimulus. In a small fraction of trials, a stop signal appears after some delay, termed the stop signal delay (SSD), instructing the subject to withhold the go response. Characteristically, subjects' ability to inhibit the go response decreases as the stop signal arrives later[28] (see also chapters 7 and 11, this volume).

The classical model for the stop signal task is the race model,[28] which posits the behavioral output on each trial, go or stop, to be the outcome of two competing, independent go and stop processes, respectively. The go process has a finishing time with stochasticity assumed to be due to noise or other sources independent of the stop process. The stop process has a finishing time of SSD + SSRT, where the stop signal reaction time (SSRT) is a subject-specific stopping latency. A stop trial ends in an error response (stop error, SE) if the go process finishes before the stop process (go RT < SSD + SSRT) or a correct cancellation otherwise (go RT ≥ SSD + SSRT). Thus, the cumulative distribution of go RT, up to SSD + SSRT, determines the error rate at each SSD. Conversely, given the observed go RT distribution and inhibition function, as well as the experimentally imposed SSD, an estimate of SSRT can be formed for each subject. Importantly, it is assumed that the go finishing time distribution is identical across go and stop trials. Given the race model assumptions, the shorter the SSRT, the fewer error responses in stop trials. Consequently, SSRT is often seen as an index of inhibitory ability, and indeed appears to be longer in populations with presumed inhibitory deficits, such as attention-deficit hyperactivity disorder,[2] substance abuse,[34] and obsessive-compulsive disorder.[32]

Despite its elegant simplicity and ability to explain a number of classical behavioral results, the race model by itself is fundamentally descriptive, without addressing how the go and stop processes arise from underlying cognitive goals and constraints. As such, the race model is generally silent on how the stop and go processes might be altered in response to changing task demands. For example, it has been shown that, when the cost associated with making a stop error is increased, not only do subjects make fewer stop errors, but their estimated SSRT also decreases.[26] The race model can be modified to include this SSRT decrease in a post hoc manner, but as it makes no claims on the computational provenance of the go and stop processes, it cannot predict a priori how the SSRT would or should change according to task demands. Likewise, the global frequency of stop signal trials, as well as local trial history (in terms of the prevalence of stop trials), has systematic effects on stopping behavior: As the fraction of stop trials is increased, go RT slows down, stop error rate decreases, and SSRT decreases.[15,26] Again, an increasing delay to the go process or a decreasing SSRT can be imposed in an ad hoc manner, but the race model cannot predict a priori which model parameters should be affected or how they should change as a function of stop signal frequency or local trial history.

In this chapter, we review a rational decision-making framework for inhibitory control in the stop signal task, which optimizes sensory processing and action choice relative to a quantitative, global behavioral objective function that takes into account the costs associated with go errors, stop errors, and response delay.[39] Specifically, optimal decision making in this task involves precisely specified interactions among several cognitive processes: the continual monitoring of noisy sensory information, the integration of sensory inputs with top-down expectations, and the assessment of the relative values of potential actions. We show that classical behavioral results in the stop signal task are natural consequences of rational decision making in the task. Moreover, the model can quantitatively predict how more subtle manipulations in task demands should affect stopping behavior, since its normative foundation enables it to distinguish the individual contributions of the various cognitive factors to the observed behavior. In particular, we show that the rational model[39] can explain the effects of manipulating reward structure[26] and prevalence of stop signals[15,26,48] on stopping behavior, as well as sequential effects due to recent trial history.[15] We also discuss the relationship between the race model and the rational decision-making model, specifically envisaging the former as a computationally simpler, neurally plausible approximation to the latter. Altogether, the work suggests that multiple, interactive cognitive processes underlie stopping behavior, and that the brain implements optimal or near-optimal decision making, possibly via a race-model-like process, in an adaptive and context-dependent manner.

A Rational Decision-Making Framework for the Stop Signal Task

In recent years, much progress has been made in understanding how noisy sensory inputs lead to simple perceptual decisions, such as in two-alternative forced choice (2AFC) motion discrimination tasks.[19,41] This is a notable area of cognitive neuroscience, where a simple theoretical framework contributed much to facilitate an elegant conceptual link between behavior and neurobiology. In the 2AFC reaction time task, subjects choose not only which of two responses to make, based on two types of stimuli, but also when to respond. In several implementations of the 2AFC task, such as the random-dot coherent motion paradigm, humans and animals appear to accumulate information and make perceptual decisions close to optimally,[9,30,37,38] where the optimal strategy (known as sequential probability ratio test, or SPRT), minimizing a combination of error probability and decision delay, requires the accumulation of sensory evidence until a decision threshold is breached. Moreover, neurons in the parietal cortex (specifically lateral intraparietal sulcus, or LIP) exhibit response dynamics similar to what can be expected of neural evidence integrators as prescribed by the optimal algorithm.[19,31,38]

The success of the rational decision-making framework in providing a common conceptual understanding for behavioral and neural data motivates our approach to use a similar framework in understanding the psychology and neurobiology of inhibitory control. Based on observed behavioral modifications in response to a range of subtle variations of the stop signal task, we hypothesize that the brain implements optimal or near-optimal behavior in an adaptive, context-sensitive manner. We formalize this hypothesis using Bayesian statistical inference and stochastic control theory, which together provide an optimal framework for specifying the various uncertainties and deriving the interactions among them, in the context of optimizing a quantitative, global objective function. Specifically, in the stop signal task, a rational agent must be able to cope with the following: sensory uncertainty associated with the presence and properties of the stop and go stimuli, cognitive uncertainty associated with prior beliefs about the frequency and timing of stimuli (especially the stop signal), and action uncertainty in terms of how each decision to go or stop would affect overall expected reward or cost. Conceptually, the model has two major components: (1) a monitoring process that uses Bayesian statistical inference to make inferences about the identity of the go stimulus and the presence of the stop signal, and (2) a decision process, formalized in terms of stochastic control theory, that translates the current expectations based on sensory evidence into a decision of whether to choose one of the two go responses or to wait at least one more time step for more observation. The decision to stop, in our model, emerges from a series of decisions to wait.

The monitoring process in our model tracks sensory information about the go and stop stimuli during each trial, integrating it with prior belief about the distribution of go stimulus identity, and prevalence and timing of the stop signal. This moment-by-moment summary of available information is represented as a two-dimensional belief state, consisting of the probability of the go stimulus being one of two alternatives (we focus on the discrimination[27] version of the stop signal task in this chapter, but the adaptation to the detection version[25] is straightforward) and the probability that the current trial is a stop trial. Using a simple application of Bayes's rule,[7] computing the belief state based on prior expectations and the continuous stream of noisy sensory inputs, each of which only weakly favors one hypothesis over another, is straighforward. We assume that subjects have veridical priors for go stimulus identity and stop signal frequency, reflecting the true experimental design.

Figure 20.1A shows the average trajectories of belief states, along with their standard errors of mean in simulations, in different types of trials: go trials (GO), successful stop trials (SS), and error (SE) stop trials. Over time, the iteratively updated belief corresponding to the identity of the go stimulus, $P(r)$, increases as sensory evidence accumulates. Sensory noise drives individual trajectories to rise faster or slower. Note that stop error trials (noncanceled trials) are those on which the go stimulus belief state happens to be rising fast, whereas successful stop trials show the opposite trend. Also shown is the probability of a stop trial, $P(s)$, on the three trial types. $P(s)$ initially rises on all trials, due to prior expectation of a stop signal arriving, at a time drawn from a known temporal distribution. In go trials, $P(s)$ eventually drops to zero when the stop signal fails to appear. In stop trials, $P(s)$ rises subsequent to stop signal onset (dashed black line). Due to sensory noise, $P(s)$ can be at a different baseline when the stop signal appears, and also rises faster or slower subsequent to the stop signal onset. As shown in figure 20.1A, successful stop trials are those in which both $P(s)$ happens to be at a higher baseline and the subsequent rise happens to be faster; vice versa for error stop trials.

The decision process in our model makes a moment-by-moment choice between going and waiting, as a function of the continually updated belief state. One could imagine a decision policy that chooses to go after the total probability of the go stimulus being one or the other possibility exceeds a threshold (say 0.95), not to go if the probability of there being a stop signal exceeds some threshold (say 0.8), or to go at 400 msec into the trial if the probability of a stop signal does not exceed some value (say 0.3), or the policy could even be stochastic as in choosing to go on 80% of the trials regardless of observations. The set of possible decision policies is literally infinite. So how do we begin to guess which one might be employed by subjects?

To determine a plausible decision policy, we hypothesize subjects to be rational decision makers, in terms of minimizing a global behavioral cost function

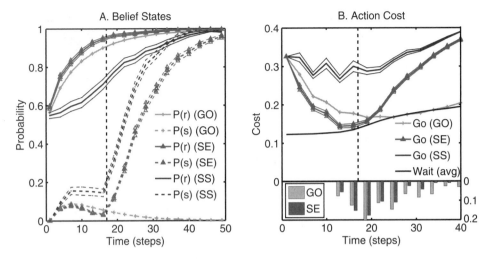

Figure 20.1
Inference and action selection in the stop signal task. (A) Evolution of the belief state over time, on go trials (gray diamond), successful stop trials (SS; black), and error stop trials (SE; black triangle). Solid lines represent the posterior probabilities assigned to the true identity of the go stimulus (one of two possibilities) for the three types of trials: They all rise steadily toward the value 1 as sensory evidence accumulates. The vertical dashed black line represents the onset of the stop signal on stop trials. The probability of a stop signal being present (dashed lines) rises initially in a manner dependent on prior expectations of frequency and timing of the stop signal, and subsequently rises farther toward the value 1 (stop trials) or drops to zero (go trials) based on sensory evidence. (B) Average action costs corresponding to going and waiting, using the same sets of trials as (A). The black dashed vertical line denotes the onset of the stop signal. A response is initiated when the cost of going drops below the cost of waiting. The RT histograms for go and error stop trials (bottom) indicate the spread of when the go action is chosen in each of those cases. Each data point is an average of 10,000 simulated trials. Error bars: SEM.

consisting of a combination of various types of costs: response delay, stop errors, and go errors:

$$\text{Expected cost} = c \cdot (\text{mean RT}) + c_s \cdot P(\text{stop error}) + P(\text{go error}) \qquad (20.1)$$

whereby a stop error is a noncanceled response to the stop signal, and a go error can be either a wrong discrimination response or exceeding the go response deadline (note that, in practice, a deadline for go response is typically explicitly or implicitly imposed, since without that incentive subjects tend to wait for the stop signal). The parameter c specifies the cost of speed versus accuracy. We assume it to be the subjects' actual reward rate in the experiment, P(correct)/(mean RT + mean RSI), based on the notion that the value of time relative to accuracy should be measured in terms of how many correct trials can be expected per unit of time. The parameter c_s specifies how much stop errors matter relative to go errors, and is also determined by actual experimental design (so 1 if the two types of errors are punished equally).

Given the globally specified cost function, we use the dynamic programming principle[8] to compute the optimal decision policy (up to discretization of the belief state), without any assumptions with respect to the form of the policy. The dynamic program computes the expected costs of going and waiting at each moment in time, as a function of the current belief state, and determines which action to take depending on which is less costly at each instant in time. Note, we are not proposing that the brain necessarily implements dynamic programming, which for now is merely a computationally efficient algorithm to compute and visualize the optimal decision policy. If we find subjects' behavior closely tracks predictions made by the optimal policy, it implies that the brain has found some means of implementing or approximating the optimal decision process in the task. Understanding the nature of the computations leading to the observed behavior can shed light on the cognitive and neural processes that underlie inhibitory control. Exactly how the brain discovers that optimal policy, whether in a manner similar to or very different from dynamic programming, and whether via evolutionary or developmental mechanisms, is beyond the scope of this chapter.

Figure 20.2 shows a visualization of the decision policy at one point in time. The policy transforms the two-dimensional belief state into an action choice (go or wait) based on the delineated regions in the belief space. A higher degree of certainty with respect to the go stimulus tends to result in a go response, whereas greater certainty of a stop trial results in a choice of waiting. Notably, the choice of going versus waiting is jointly dependent on beliefs about both the go stimulus and the

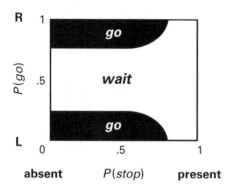

Figure 20.2
Schematic illustration of the optimal decision policy. At each time step, the two-dimensional belief state is divided into go and wait regions, corresponding to the two available actions. Increased certainty about the identity of the go stimulus induces a go action choice, whereas increased certainty about the trial being a stop trial results in a wait action. Notably, the ultimate decision is jointly dependent on the two: Only when stop trial probability is low and go stimulus identity is well determined would the go action be chosen. The figure shows the decision boundaries for one time step; the oncoming deadline and the temporal distribution of stop signals can affect the size and shape of the boundaries at each time step.

stop signal, as a go action is issued only when there is high confidence about the go stimulus identity and the probability of a stop trial is low. The exact size and shape of the go and wait regions are different at different points in the trial, depending on factors such as the proximity of an impending deadline or the temporal distribution of stop signal arrival times. Figure 20.1B illustrates the action costs associated with go and stop actions for different types of trials: go (GO) trials, error stop (SE) trials, and successful stop (SS) trials. As the probability associated with the (correct) go stimulus identity increases with accumulating sensory evidence, the cost of going drops, eventually crossing the cost of waiting and triggering a go response. On stop trials, the onset of the stop signal initiates an increase in the cost of going. In stop error trials, the go cost crosses the wait cost before the stop stimulus is fully processed. In successful stop trials, the go cost never dips below the wait cost. The RT histograms for go and error stop trials illustrate that, although the average go cost trajectories do not cross the cost of waiting, the individual trajectories all cross over at various points. (For full details of the model and the simulations, see ref. 39.)

Stopping Behavior as a Natural Consequence of Rational Decision Making

Two classic results in the stop signal task are the increase in stop error rate with increasing SSD, known as the inhibition function, and the faster RT on stop error trials compared to go trials.[15,47] These characteristics have been observed in a large number of studies in humans and animals.[14,22,28] We show that these basic results arise in our model as a natural consequence of rational decision making in the task. Figure 20.3 compares our model predictions to data from human subjects performing a version of the stop signal task.[15] Error rate increases as SSD increases, in both behavioral data (figure 20.3A) and the model (figure 20.3B). Figure 20.3C and D show that the RTs on stop error trials are, on average, faster than go trials, both in behavior data (figure 20.3C) and in our model (figure 20.3D). Intuitively, a longer SSD should increase the likelihood of the go cost dipping below the wait cost before the stop signal is detected sufficiently to increase the go cost. The faster RT on stop error trials is related to the SSD and the stochasticity in the sensory processing of go and stop stimuli: As figure 20.1 indicates, stop error trials are those in which the go stimulus is processed faster than average (and the stop stimulus slower than average). This difference gives rise to the observed faster RT (see figure 20.1B).

The race model explains these results as well, using a similar proximate explanation: Later initiation of the stop process allows more go processes to "escape," giving rise to the form of the inhibition function; stochasticity in the go process allows the go process to sometimes escape the stop process, and those that do happen to escape have shorter finishing times.[28] However, the race model does not attempt to explain the computational provenance of the parameters of the stop and go processes, and

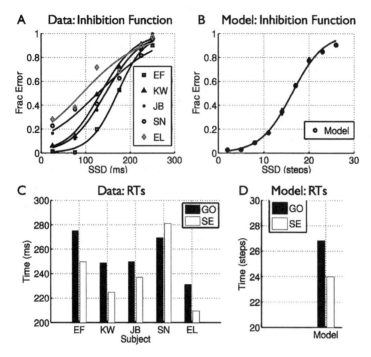

Figure 20.3
Classical stopping behavior arises naturally from rational decision making. (A) Inhibition function:
Errors on stop trials increase as a function of SSD. (B) Similar inhibition function seen for the model.
(C) Discrimination RT is generally faster on stop error trials than on go trials. (D) Similar results seen
in the model. (A, C) Data adapted from Emeric et al.[15]

therefore cannot predict a priori how parameters of the processes should change
according to task demands. In the following, we describe how experimental manipulations of the prevalence of stop trials and reward structure automatically translate
into changes in the parameters of the rational decision-making model, resulting in
predictions that correspond excellently with behavioral data. Moreover, we discuss
how parameters of the race model, such as SSRT, can be viewed as emergent properties of optimal stopping behavior, and should therefore change in predictable ways
under subtle manipulations of experimental design.

Influence of Reward Structure on Stopping

Leotti and Wager[26] showed that subjects can be biased toward stopping or going
when the relative penalties associated with go and stop errors are experimentally
manipulated. Their experiments associated a reward with fast go response times and
penalty with stop errors, and manipulated these values in an iterative fashion to
induce a particular degree of bias in each subject, as measured by the fraction of

stop errors committed. As subjects are biased toward stopping, they make fewer stop errors and have slower go responses. Critically, the SSRT also decreases with increasing bias toward stopping. As a descriptive model, the race model cannot predict or explain a priori why the SSRT should change according to the reward structure of the task.

In contrast, our model explicitly represents task parameters such as the relative costs of go and stop errors (parameterized by c_s the expected cost function), from which we can predict the effects of modifying these relative costs on the optimal decision policy, and consequently on behavioral measures. Increasing the cost of a stop error induces an increase in go RT, a decrease in stop errors, and a decrease in SSRT (although SSRT is not an explicit component of the rational model, the same procedure used to estimate SSRT from experimental data can nevertheless be used to estimate it for our model). Overall, when stop errors are more expensive, there is an incentive to delay the go response in order to minimize the possibility of missing a stop signal. Moreover, as stop errors become more costly, the cost of going should increase more rapidly after stop signal onset, making the stop signal more effective and faster at canceling the go response. We would therefore expect the SSRT also to reduce with greater stop error cost, similar to what is observed in human subjects. The process of adjusting the relative balance between going and stopping automatically changes the measured SSRT in our model in a manner similar to that in human subjects. This suggests that SSRT can be viewed as an emergent property of a rational decision process that dynamically and optimally chooses between going and stopping.

Influence of Global Stop-Trial Prevalence on Stopping Behavior

In addition to reward manipulation, the global frequency of stop signal trials has systematic effects on stopping behavior.[15,26] As the fraction of stop trials is increased, go RT slows down and the stop error rate deceases.[15] This can be explained by the rational decision model as follows. The model's belief about stop signal frequency, r, influences the speed with which a stop signal is detected: Larger r leads to greater prior belief, thus posterior belief, in stop signal presence, and also greater confidence in a stop signal appearing later in the trial if it has not already. It therefore controls the trade-off between going and stopping in the optimal policy. When stop signals are more prevalent, the optimal decision policy can use that information to make fewer errors on stop trials by delaying the go response. A more subtle prediction of the optimal model, as the assumed prevalence of stop signal (r) is increased, is that the SSRT also decreases. Again, SSRT is not an explicit component of the optimal model, but can be estimated for each condition based on inhibition function and go RT distribution produced by the optimal model. This SSRT prediction is confirmed by experimental data.[26]

Influence of Local Stop-Trial Prevalence on Stopping Behavior

Even in experiments where the fraction of stop trials is held constant, chance runs of stop or go trials may result in fluctuating local frequency of stop trials, which in turn may lead to trial-by-trial behavioral adjustments due to subjects' fluctuating estimate of r. Indeed, subjects speed up after a chance run of go trials and slow down following a sequence of stop trials.[15] We modeled these effects by assuming that subjects track the local stop signal frequency, $\hat{r}$, on a trial-to-trial basis, in a manner similar to sequential effects often observed in simple 2AFC tasks.[12,24,42] Previously, we modeled such sequential effects as Bayes-optimal inference about an unknown Bernoulli parameter that controls the frequency of repetition versus alternation trials, where the Bernoulli parameter is assumed to change over time with probability $1 - \alpha$ in each trial.[50] We showed that Bayesian inference in this hidden Markov model is well-approximated by a leaky accumulator process, in which the "leakiness" of the memory is controlled by α: Large α corresponds to a world that rarely changes and necessitates small leakiness in memory, whereas small α corresponds to one that frequently changes and necessitates large leakiness in memory. The adaptation of this sequential effects model to the stop signal task is straightforward: The critical underlying Bernoulli rate parameter is now r, the frequency of stop signal trials, and α specifies subjects' assumptions about how stable r is over time. Using this approach, our model can successfully explain observed sequential effects in behavioral data, with go RT decreasing after sequences of go trials of increasing length, and slowing following longer sequences of stop trials.[39]

Race Model Approximation to Rational Decision Making

Although the race model and the optimal decision-making model are grounded in fundamentally different levels of analysis, we can nevertheless think of the race model as a computationally simpler, and potentially neurally more plausible, approximation to the optimal decision-making algorithm. As we saw in the previous section, although SSRT is not an explicit component of the optimal model, it can nevertheless be estimated from the optimal model's simulated "behavior" such as the inhibition function and the go RT distribution. In this light, SSRT can be seen as an emergent property of the interactive decision process negotiating going and stopping, and the race model as an approximation to the optimal model. In fact, we can make the connection more explicit by considering a more concrete implementation of the race model as a diffusion model, which has a long history of being used to model reaction times,[9,19,23,24,30,31,36,43] and more recently has been applied specifically to the stop signal task.[20,48]

Typically, the diffusion model consists of a constant drift process corrupted by additive, cumulative white noise, whereby a response is initiated by the process crossing a threshold. In addition to the drift rate and threshold, a third parameter is a constant offset or nondecision time added to the diffusion process. Here, we propose an augmented diffusion model containing a fourth parameter—namely, SSRT—in order to model both go RT and the inhibition function. In this diffusion model, a response is produced when the drift-diffusion go process crosses the threshold, unless it is at a time exceeding SSD + SSRT, which is the finishing time of the stop process. In the latter case, no response is produced. Our version differs from the Verbruggen and Logan[48] diffusion model of the stop signal task in two ways: (1) Our model simultaneously fits both reaction time and accuracy data instead of only reaction time, and (2) the fit is to the output of the optimal decision-making model and not directly to the experimental data. The diffusion model we suggest also differs from the LATER model, which is not technically a diffusion model, since it does not have diffusive noise corrupting the drift process, but instead posits stochasticity only in the drift magnitude across trials.[20]

We propose to examine how parameters of the best-fitting diffusion model vary as experimental parameters of the task, such as the reward structure or the stop signal frequency, are manipulated (c_s takes on different values), where the fitting procedure minimizes the KL divergence between the output distribution of the race model and the optimal model, or, equivalently, maximizes the log likelihood of observing the optimal model output given parameters of the race model. The diffusion model has four parameters: drift rate, response threshold, offset, and SSRT. For each reward condition, these parameters can be adjusted to produce the best-fitting approximation to the optimal model. We expect there to be systematic changes in one or more of the diffusion model parameters as task parameters are manipulated, thus providing an a priori procedure for predicting how the race-diffusion model parameters should change under these task manipulations.

Discussion

In this chapter, we presented a rational decision-making framework for inhibitory control in the stop signal task. Our framework optimizes sensory processing and action choice relative to a quantitative, global behavioral objective function that explicitly takes into account the experimental costs associated with go errors, stop errors, and response delay.[39] We show that classical behavioral results in the stop signal task are natural consequences of rational decision making in the task. Moreover, the model can quantitatively predict the influence of subtle manipulations of task parameters, such as reward structure[26] and prevalence of stop signals,[15,26,48] on stopping behavior, as well as sequential effects in RT due to recent trial history.[15]

The optimal model and the race model are motivated by fundamentally different levels of analysis, akin to that between proximate and ultimate causes in ethology, respectively.[1] Despite its elegant simplicity and ability to explain a number of classical behavioral results, the race model by itself is fundamentally descriptive, without addressing how the go and stop processes arise from underlying cognitive goals and constraints, which is precisely the purview of the optimal model. On the other hand, the optimal model requires complex computations, and even if subjects' behavior is similar to model predictions, the brain may well implement a simpler approximation to the optimal algorithm. For example, we used dynamic programming to compute the optimal policy for each set of task parameters, but the brain is unlikely to implement the computationally intense algorithm of dynamic programming exactly. Instead, it may opt for an approximate solution, such as the race model. If that is the case, however, the race model will need its parameters, such as SSRT, to be carefully adjusted in different task conditions, in order to best approximate the optimal model and account for experimental data.[15,26] Exactly how the brain manages to modify the neural implementation of the race model just right to approach optimal behavior in each task condition is an interesting question. In any case, our results imply that SSRT should not be viewed as a unique, invariant measure of stopping ability for each subject, but rather as an emergent property sensitive to a number of cognitive factors.

Another key assumption of the race model, the independence between go and stop processes, also requires more nuanced analysis. Our optimal decision-making framework suggests that go and stop processes are fundamentally intertwined, since the continual choice between go and wait always pits the two options directly against each other, and many underlying cognitive factors can affect this competition. This is supported by experimental data and model simulation results that manipulations of reward structure[26] and stop signal frequency[15] can systematically affect stopping behavior, including the go RT latency and the estimated SSRT—suggesting that go and stop processes are fundamentally interactive.

A notable feature of the optimal model is that, although it is computationally complex, it has very few free parameters. Almost all of the model parameters, such as the fraction of stop trials, the SSD distribution, stop error cost, and go response deadline are set directly by the experimental design. The only exceptions are parameters corresponding to the sensory noise corrupting the go stimulus and stop signal processing, but even these two trade off with the step size in the discretization of time in the model. The absence of a large number of free parameters is a hallmark of normative Bayesian statistical models, which enables complex cognitive and neural modeling without the typical problems associated with too many parameters in a model: overfitting, local minima, arbitrary fitting criteria, and limited capacity to generalize across tasks and contexts. What allows a Bayesian model to capture complex neural computation without the need for many free parameters is the assumption of optimality, which strongly constrains the form of the necessary computations. The assumption of optimality is justified if it is a behavioral context for which brain functioning is naturally suited—this is independently a scientifically desirable criterion for experimental design. If we find that subjects' behavior closely tracks predictions made by the optimal model in a task, it implies that the brain has found some means of implementing or approximating the optimal computations. The optimal algorithm then guides the search for the cognitive and neural processes that underlie the behavior in question—inhibitory control in this particular case.

An important question is how the brain might implement or approximate the computations required by the optimal decision-making model. Recent studies suggest that the activity of neurons in the frontal eye fields (FEF[21]) and superior colliculus[35] of monkeys could be implementing a version of the race model. Specifically, movement and fixation neurons in the FEF show responses that diverge on go and correct stop trials, indicating that they may encode computations leading to the execution or cancellation of movement. The point of divergence is closely related to the behaviorally estimated SSRT. Various diffusion-race models have been proposed to explain FEF neural activities.[10,21,49] Also, recent data show that supplementary eye field may encode the local frequency of stop trials and influence stopping behavior in a statistically appropriate manner.[45,46] In addition to the results from monkey neurophysiology, we wish to take into account recent results in human imaging studies: The right inferior frontal gyrus, the subthalamic nucleus, and the prefrontal cortex all appear to play important roles in stopping behavior.[4,11] One hypothesis, supported by functional magnetic resonance imaging (fMRI) and diffusion tractography data, is that the inferior frontal gyrus may directly activate the subthalamic nucleus, via a hyperdirect pathway, inducing strong overall inhibition of the motor cortex[4] (see also chapters 11 and 17, this volume).

One major aim of our work is to understand how stopping ability and SSRT arise from various cognitive factors. Our work points to the significance of a number of contributing elements including reward/penalty sensitivity and memory or learning capacity related to the estimation of stop signal frequency. Elsewhere, we showed that it may also depend on sensory processing abilities.[39] This more nuanced view of stopping ability and SSRT may aid in the understanding and differentiation of the cognitive and neural factors underlying inhibitory ability. Impaired stopping ability, particularly longer SSRT, has been observed in a number of psychiatric and neurological conditions, such as substance abuse,[34] attention deficit–hyperactivity disorder (ADHD),[2] schizophrenia,[5] obsessive-compulsive disorder (OCD),[32] Parkinson's disease,[18] Alzheimer's disease,[3] and others. Yet it is unlikely that these varied conditions share an identical set of underlying neural and cognitive deficits. One of our goals for future research is to map group differences in stopping behavior to the parameters of our model, thus gaining insight into exactly which cognitive components go awry in each dysfunctional state.

So far, our model does not incorporate a specific stop action: A stop decision is a consequence of a serial decision to wait. Neurophysiological evidence from monkeys[21] and humans[4] suggests that successfully stopped actions may involve increased activity in certain neural populations such as the fixation neurons of the FEF, or cortical regions such as the inferior frontal gyrus and subthalamic nucleus. One important and planned line of inquiry for our work is to consider a rational model with an explicit stop action, in order to better account for what is known about the neurophysiology of stopping.

Inhibitory control has been studied extensively using a variety of behavioral tasks.[13,16,28,40,44] Sometimes, a distinction is made[33] between behavioral inhibition as exemplified by the stop signal task and the go/no-go task,[13] and cognitive inhibition in tasks such as the Stroop and Eriksen tasks.[16,44] Our model of rational decision making in the stop signal task, along with the excellent correspondence between model predictions and experimental data, demonstrates that the stop signal task also probes important elements of cognitive processing: establishment of prior expectations about stimulus identity and frequency, integration of immediate sensory inputs with top-down expectations, and strategic, continual decision making among available actions in a reward-sensitive manner. Previously, we showed that Bayesian statistical inference can account for behavior in the Eriksen task.[51] An interesting challenge for future work is to examine whether and how performance measures in these inhibitory control tasks may relate to each other in a within-subjects design.[17]

Outstanding Questions

• How is an optimal decision policy derived in the stop signal task: Is there an implementation of the race model with parameters that are dynamically tuned to approximate the optimal model?

• What is the neural basis of the optimal model (or its approximation)? Can the present approach be reconciled with neurophysiological evidence that the stop process is explicitly represented?

• The rational decision-making model explains stopping behavior as emerging from a confluence of cognitive factors. How does this complex machinery go awry, presumably distinctly, in each of ADHD, OCD, drug abuse, and other conditions with hypothesized inhibitory deficits?

• Can rational decision-making models provide an integrated account of inhibitory control across task domains?

Further Reading

Verbruggen F, Logan GD. 2009. Models of response inhibition in the stop-signal and stop-change para-digms. *Neurosci Biobehav Rev* 33: 647–661. A comprehensive recent review of key empirical findings and standard theoretical models of inhibitory control in the stop signal task.

Yu AJ, Cohen JD. 2009. Sequential effects: superstition or rational behavior? In: Advances in Neural Information Processing Systems 21 (Koller D, Schuurmans D, Bengio Y, Bottou L, eds), pp 1873–1880. Cambridge, MA: MIT Press. A Bayesian model of sequential effects and its equivalence to a leaky memory filter. We assume similar computations and mechanisms are at play to give rise to sequential effects in the stop signal task.

Frazier P, Yu AJ. 2008. Sequential hypothesis testing under stochastic deadlines. In: Advances in Neural Information Processing Systems 20 (Platt JC, Koller D, Singer Y, Roweis S, eds), pp 465–72. Cambridge, MA: MIT Press. A theoretical analysis of speed-accuracy trade-off in binary decision-making tasks when there is an impending, possibly stochastic, deadline. The rational model for the stop signal task is an extension of this model.

Yu AJ, Dayan P, Cohen JD. 2009. Dynamics of attentional selection under conflict: toward a rational Bayesian account. *J Exp Psychol Hum Percept Perform* 35: 700–717. An application of the rational decision-making approach to another important class of cognitive control tasks: those involving selection of stimuli and responses in situations of conflict.

References

1. Alcock J, Sherman P. 1994. The utility of the proximate-ultimate dichotomy in ethology. *Ethology* 86: 58–62.

2. Alderson R, Rapport M, Kofler M. 2007. Attention-deficit/hyperactivity disorder and behavioral inhibition: a meta-analytic review of the stop-signal paradigm. *J Abnorm Child Psychol* 35: 745–758.

3. Amieva H, Lafont S, Auriacombe S, Le Carret N, Dartigues JF, Orgogozo JM, Colette F. 1992. Inhibitory breakdown and dementia of the Alzheimer type: a general phenomenon? *J Clin Exp Neuropsychol* 24: 503–516.

4. Aron AR, Durston S, Eagle DM, Logan GD, Stinear CM, Stuphorn V. 2007. Converging evidence for a fronto-basal-ganglia network for inhibitory control of action and cognition. *J Neurosci* 27: 11860–11864.

5. Badcock JC, Michie PT, Johnson L, Combrinck J. 2002. Acts of control in schizophrenia: dissociating the components of inhibition. *Psychol Med* 32: 287–297.

6. Barkley R. 1997. Behavioral inhibition, sustained attention, and executive functions: constructing a unifying theory of ADHD. *Psychol Med* 121: 65–94.

7. Bayes T. 1763. An essay toward solving a problem in the doctrine of chances. *Phil Trans R Soc* 53: 370–418.

8. Bellman R. 1952. On the theory of dynamic programming. *Proc Natl Acad Sci USA* 38: 716–719.

9. Bogacz R, Brown E, Moehlis J, Holmes P, Cohen JD. 2006. The physics of optimal decision making: a formal analysis of models of performance in two-alternative forced-choice tasks. *Psychol Rev* 113: 700–765.

10. Boucher L, Palmeri T, Logan G, Schall J. 2007. Inhibitory control in mind and brain: an interactive race model of countermanding saccades. *Psychol Rev* 114: 376–397.

11. Chambers CD, Garavan H, Bellgrove MA. 2009. Insights into the neural basis of response inhibition from cognitive and clinical neuroscience. *Neurosci Biobehav Rev* 33: 631–646.

12. Cho RY, Nystrom LE, Brown ET, Jones AD, Braver TS, Holmes PJ, Cohen JD. 2002. Mechanisms underlying dependencies of performance on stimulus history in a two-alternative forced choice-task. *Cogn Affect Behav Neurosci* 2: 283–299.

13. Donders F. 1969. On the speed of mental processes. *Acta Psychol (Amst)* 30: 412.

14. Eagle DM, Robbins T. 2003. Inhibitory control in rats performing a stop-signal reaction-time task: effects of lesions of the medial striatum and d-amphetamine. *Behav Neurosci* 117: 1302–1317.

15. Emeric E, Brown J, Boucher L, Carpenter RH, Hanes D, Harris RL, Logan GD, et al. 2007. Influence of history on saccade countermanding performance in humans and macaque monkeys. *Vision Res* 47: 35–49.

16. Eriksen BA, Eriksen CW. 1974. Effects of noise letters upon identification of a target letter in a nonsearch task. *Percept Psychophys* 16: 143–149.

17. Friedman N, Miyake A. 2004. The relations among inhibition and interference control functions: a latent-variable analysis. *J Exp Psychol Gen* 133: 101–135.

18. Gauggel S, Rieger M, Feghoff TA. 2004. Inhibition of ongoing responses in patients with Parkinson's disease. *J Neurol Neurosurg Psychiatry* 75: 539–544.

19. Gold JI, Shadlen MN. 2002. Banburismus and the brain: decoding the relationship between sensory stimuli, decisions, and reward. *Neuron* 36: 299–308.

20. Hanes DP, Carpenter RH. 1999. Countermanding saccades in humans. *Vision Res* 39: 2777–2791.

21. Hanes DP, Patterson WF, II, Schall JD. 1998. Role of frontal eye fields in countermanding saccades: visual, movement, and fixation activity. *J Neurophysiol* 79: 817–834.

22. Hanes DP, Schall JD. 1995. Countermanding saccades in macaque. *Vis Neurosci* 12: 929–937.

23. Hanes DP, Shall J. 1996. Neural control of voluntary movement initiation. *Science* 274: 427–430.

24. Laming DRJ. 1968. Information Theory of Choice Reaction Times. London: Academic Press.

25. Lappin JS, Eriksen CW. 1966. Use of a delayed signal to stop a visual reaction-time response. *J Exp Psychol* 72: 805–811.

26. Leotti LA, Wager TD. 2010. Motivational influences in response inhibition processes. *J Exp Psychol Hum Percept Perform* 36: 430–447.

27. Logan GD. 1983. On the ability to inhibit simple thoughts and actions: I. Stop-signal studies of decision and memory. *J Exp Psychol Learn Mem Cogn* 9: 585–606.

28. Logan GD, Cowan WB. 1984. On the ability to inhibit thought and action: a theory of an act of control. *Psychol Rev* 91: 295–327.

29. Logan GD, Zbrodoff NJ, Fostey AR. 1983. Costs and benefits of strategy construction in a speeded discrimination task. *Mem Cognit* 11: 485–493.

30. Luce RD. 1986. Response Times: Their Role in Inferring Elementary Mental Organization. New York: Oxford University Press.

31. Mazurek ME, Roiman JD, Ditterich J, Shadlen MN. 2003. A role for neural integrators in perceptual decision making. *Cereb Cortex* 13: 1257–1269.

32. Menzies L, Achard S, Chamberlain SR, Fineberg N, Chen CH, Del Campo N, Sahakian BJ, Robbins TW, Bullmore E. 2007. Neurocognitive endophenotypes of obsessive-compulsive disorder. *Brain* 130: 3223–3236.

33. Nigg JT. 2000. On inhibition/disinhibition in developmental psychopathology: views from cognitive and personality psychology and a working inhibition taxonomy. *Psychol Bull* 126: 220–246.

34. Nigg JT, Wong MM, Martel MM, Jester JM, Puttler LI, Glass JM, Adams KM, Fitzgerald HE, Zucker RA. 2006. Poor response inhibition as a predictor of problem drinking and illicit drug use in adolescents at risk for alcoholism and other substance use disorders. *J Am Acad Child Adolesc Psychiatry* 45: 468–475.

35. Pare M, Hanes DP. 2003. Controlled movement processing: superior colliculus activity associated with countermanded saccades. *J Neurosci* 23: 6480–6489.

36. Ratcliff R. 1978. A theory of memory retrieval. *Psychol Rev* 85: 59–108.

37. Ratcliff R, Rouder JN. 1998. Modeling response times for two-choice decisions. *Psychol Sci* 9: 347–356.

38. Roitman JD, Shadlen MN. 2002. Response of neurons in the lateral intraparietal area during a combined visual discrimination reaction time task. *J Neurosci* 22: 9475–9489.

39. Shenoy R, Rao R, Yu AJ. (in press). A rational decision-making framework for inhibitory control. In: Advances in Neural Information Processing Systems 23 (Lafferty J, Williams CKI, Shawe-Taylor J, Zemel RS, Culotta A, eds). Cambridge, MA: MIT Press.

40. Simon JR. 1967. Ear preference in a simple reaction-time task. *J Exp Psychol* 75: 49–55.

41. Smith PL, Ratcliff R. 2004. Psychology and neurobiology of simple decisions. *Trends Neurosci* 27: 161–168.

42. Soetens E, Boer LC, Heuting JE. 1985. Expectancy or automatic facilitation? Separating sequential effects in two-choice reaction time. *J Exp Psychol Hum Percept Perform* 11: 598–616.

43. Stone M. 1960. Models for choice reaction time. *Psychometrika* 25: 251–260.

44. Stroop J. 1935. Studies of interference in serial verbal reactions. *J Exp Psychol Gen* 18: 643–662.

45. Stuphorn V, Brown JW, Schall JD. 2010. Role of supplementary eye field in saccade initiation: executive, not direct, control. *J Neurophysiol* 103: 801–816.

46. Stuphorn V, Schall JD. 2006. Executive control of countermanding saccades by the supplementary eye field. *Nat Neurosci* 9: 925–931.

47. Verbruggen F, Logan GD. 2009. Models of response inhibition in the stop-signal and stop-change paradigms. *Neurosci Biobehav Rev* 33: 647–661.

48. Verbruggen F, Logan GD. 2009. Proactive adjustments of response strategies in the stop-signal paradigm. *J Exp Psychol Hum Percept Perform* 35: 835–854.

49. Wong-Lin K, Eckhoff P, Holmes P, Cohen JD. 2009. Optimal performance in a countermanding saccade task. *Brain Res* 1318: 178–187.

50. Yu AJ, Cohen JD. 2009. Sequential effects: superstition or rational behavior? In: Advances in Neural Information Processing Systems 21 (Koller D, Schuurmans D, Bengio Y, Bottou L, eds), pp 1873–1880. Cambridge, MA: MIT Press.

51. Yu AJ, Dayan P, Cohen JD. 2009. Dynamics of attentional selection under conflict: toward a rational Bayesian account. *J Exp Psychol Hum Percept Perform* 35: 700–717.

VI PERSPECTIVES

The chapters in this final section bring to the foreground an important trend apparent throughout this edited volume: that the borders between different sub-fields in psychology and neuroscience have become increasingly blurred. In the past, researchers studying the influence of reward and reinforcement on choice behavior in animals were isolated from psychologists studying human performance in choice reaction time tasks, and both of these groups were in turn isolated from computer scientists and economists working on optimality in decision making and learning. In contrast, recent years have seen the study of the neural basis of motivational and cognitive control attract researchers from psychology, zoology, medical sciences, anatomy, social science, economics, and computer science, among other disciplines; and this research has come to span converging work on humans and nonhuman animals, healthy populations and patients, comparison across stages of development in ontogeny, and the integration of empirical methods with formal computational and mathematical models. The last three chapters of this volume explore these trends.

Economics is one field of science whose influence on the study of the neural basis of control is being increasingly felt. Functional imaging studies applying paradigms originally developed in behavioral economics are now commonplace and, as discussed in the chapter by Chierchia and Coricelli, the terminology of economics has become mainstream in cognitive neuroscience and vice versa. Indeed, the integration between economic thinking and cognitive neuroscience has given rise to a whole subfield that goes by the name of neuroeconomics, which is now spawning its own departments, conferences, and journals.[6]

Research on the error-related negativity, a component of the human event-related brain potential elicited following errors in choice reaction time tasks,[4,5] provides another compelling illustration of the integration of different research fields. As described by Cockburn and Frank (chapter 17) and Holroyd and Yeung (chapter 18), recent computational models have integrated research on the error-related negativity, one of the core signatures of performance monitoring, with reinforcement learning models from computer science. This work has found tremendous application in clinical neuroscience, where deficits of performance monitoring are associated with a number of neurological and psychiatric disorders, as described by De Bruijn and Ullsperger (chapter 15). Recently, a number of groups have extended the application of the ERN even further, into the domain of social decision making. Miltner, Coles, Van Schie, and colleagues have shown that a similar potential is elicited when people observe others making errors,[7,8] with corresponding results now observed using functional magnetic resonance imaging (fMRI).[3] Meanwhile, as Ribas-Fernandes and colleagues (chapter 16) discuss, hierarchical models are beginning to forge direct links between these models of reinforcement learning and classical theories of cognitive control in the prefrontal cortex of the kind discussed by Mars and colleagues (chapter 7).

A similar trend is apparent in research beyond the ERN. For instance, Behrens and colleagues have employed computational principles originally studied in the context of reward-based decision making in choice tasks[2] and applied them to complex decision making in the social context.[1] In their chapter, Hunt and Behrens develop this theme to consider the challenges for the study of the neural basis of social decision making. Their chapter dovetails with that of Van den Bos and Crone (chapter 13), who considered the developmental trends involved in these processes.

The chapters in section V illustrate how computational models can provide a very important tool for studying control. The chapter by Bestmann and Mars illustrates how computational models developed in a variety of fields, including models from foraging theory, machine learning, and economics, can be applied to interrogate neuroimaging data. They focus specifically on methods for integrating the results from computational modeling with the data obtained from neuroimaging experiments, thus drawing out and making explicit a methodological theme running through many of the chapters in this volume. Collectively, the chapters in this section highlight important developments across a range of fields that extend beyond the traditional boundaries of cognitive neuroscience.

The work reviewed in this concluding section illustrates once again the importance of considering together the "motivational" and "cognitive" aspects of control that are emphasized in our title. These complementary aspects of control have often been dealt with rather separately: Studies of cognitive control have traditionally focused on the question of how control is exerted by mechanisms in prefrontal and parietal cortex, but have paid less attention to the motivational forces driving that control. Similarly, studies of motivational control have made considerable progress in understanding how behavior is shaped by reward and punishment, while having rather less to say about the resulting high-level structure of complex human and animal behavior. As illustrated by the chapters in this volume, and by the broader picture of research presented in talks and posters at the Oxford meeting in June 2010 that inspired them, it is increasingly obvious that research in the two areas has been addressing the same computational mechanisms and the same underlying neural structures all along. Thus, we began with an apparently simple question: How does the brain choose efficiently and adaptively among available options to ensure coherent, goal-directed behavior? The emerging answers to this question from a range of theoretical perspectives have homed in on a consistent set of key computational principles—which emphasize the shaping of behavior at different levels of organization by reward and reinforcement—and their implementation in a core set of neural structures that support the valuation, comparison, and selection of behavioral options. In this way, the present collection illustrates both the current achievements and the future promise of the integrated study of the neural basis of motivational and cognitive control.

References

1. Behrens TE, Hunt LT, Woolrich MW, Rushworth MF. 2008. Associative learning of social value. *Nature* 456: 245–249.

2. Behrens TE, Woolrich MW, Walton ME, Rushworth MF. 2007. Learning the value of information in an uncertain world. *Nat Neurosci* 10: 1214–1221.

3. De Bruijn ER, De Lange FP, von Cramon DY, Ullsperger M. 2009. When errors are rewarding. *J Neurosci* 29: 12183–12186.

4. Falkenstein M, Hohnsbein J, Hoormann J, Blanke L. 1990. Effects of errors in choice reaction tasks on the ERP under focused and divided attention. In: Psychophysiological Brain Research (Brunia CHM, Gaillard AWK, Kok A, eds), pp 192–195. Tilburg: Tilburg University Press.

5. Gehring WJ, Goss B, Coles MG, Meyer DE, Donchin E. 1993. A neural system for error detection and compensation. *Psychol Sci* 4: 385–390.

6. Glimcher PW, Camerer CF, Fehr E, Poldrack RA, eds. 2009. Neuroeconomics: Decision Making and the Brain. Amsterdam: Academic Press.

7. Miltner WH, Brauer J, Hecht H, Trippe R, Coles MG. 2004. Parallel brain acitivity for self-generated and observed errors. In: Errors, Conflicts, and the Brain. Current Opinions on Performance Monitoring (Ullsperger M, Falkenstein M, eds), pp 124–129. Leipzig: MPI for Human Cognitive and Brain Sciences.

8. Van Schie HT, Mars RB, Coles MG, Bekkering H. 2004. Modulation of activity in medial frontal and motor cortices during error observation. *Nat Neurosci* 7: 549–554.

21 The Neuroeconomics of Cognitive Control

Gabriele Chierchia and Giorgio Coricelli

In cognitive (neuro)science cognitive control broadly refers to our capacity to go beyond relatively reflexive reactions to salient stimuli in accordance to internal often far-removed goals.[39] This idea is of interest to economics: even economist Vilfredo Pareto, among the first and strongest advocates of the separation of economics and psychology (a position similar to that held today by many economists with regard to neuroscience[25]), felt the need to distinguish between choice-guided versus routine-guided behaviors, such as "a man removing his hat whenever he enters a drawing room or (perhaps provocatively) a Catholic who regularly attends mass."[6]

Indeed, cognitive control is deeply connected to decision making, and at least three related lines of evidence suggest this: (1) The factors that are held to trigger cognitive control are also implicated in the economic notion of *utility*; (2) cognitive skills correlate with decision-making tendencies; and (3) cognitive "loads" can impact on decision making. Let us briefly illustrate these points separately.

1. There are many ways to think of and subdivide the environmental or cognitive factors that recruit cognitive control. Norman and Shallice[42] propose that there are five general classes of them; among which are novelty or complexity of the environments or tasks, performance errors, and uncertainty and conflict. Ridderinkhof[45] synthesizes these well as situations in which actions need to be adjusted to goals. In what follows we give some examples of why the same factors are fundamental in decision-making and how, in particular, they appear to be connected to the economic notion of utility.

For instance, regarding conflict and uncertainty, imagine we were offered to choose between the following options: a) $10 dollars for sure, or b) a bet on a fair coin flip such that you win $11 for "heads" and $0 otherwise. It probably wouldn't take us much to decide and our responses would be rather automatic (fast) and stereotyped (constant in time, within and between subjects). However, imagine now that we changed the value of the uncertain payoff to $21, keeping the sure payoff fixed at $10, This would probably elicit much more variability in responses and slower response times, which are some of the behavioral signs of cognitive control. Specifically, what happened between the two decision proposals is that we modulated the desirability, henceforth, the *utility*, of one of the options, thus generating higher conflict and uncertainty; two factors, which in turn, signal that higher cognitive control is required.

Similar reasoning holds for other factors proposed by Norman and Shallice, such as complexity. To give one example of a topic that will be treated later in this chapter, economists have shown that if an option is presented in an ambiguous manner this will decrease its perceived utility (see Theme 4). To keep the example above, in which we win $21 if heads comes out on a coin flip, let's imagine now that we were offered the same option but we are also told that the coin actually isn't fair but is unbalanced toward either heads or tails. Though it is intuitive how this might decrease the appeal of the coin-flip bet, relative to the 10$ sure payoff, it isn't clear that committing to this impression would be the best choice. Indeed, from what we know, the coin has equal chances to be unbalanced toward the winning outcome (heads) as it does toward the losing one. Thus, ultimately, the expected value of the betting option is the same as before, when we knew the outcome probabilities. What changed is the fact that resolving ambiguity requires second-order probability estimations (inferring the probability of outcome probabilities), which are clearly more complex than reasoning on established outcome probabilities. Thus, aversion to ambiguity in economic decision making could easily have to do with the fact that increased complexity of ambiguously described options requires more cognitive control, which is costly, and subjects might then avoid ambiguity to not incur such costs.

Though we don't go over all of Norman and Shallice's factors for reasons of space, the above examples should give an idea of how such factors share intricate connections with those thought to shape the utility of options. The following two points provide two general lines of empirical support for this idea.

2. There is behavioral evidence linking cognitive skills to decision preferences. For instance, early studies showed that children who are better at postponing an immediate gratification for a later larger one (Theme 3) are more likely to develop better social and cognitive competences as adolescents.[40] Along the same line, adults who obtain higher scores on IQ tests are also less susceptible to risk when deciding in uncertain contexts[2] where, on average, it has been shown that risk affects people more than it should[4] (Theme 2). Subjects with higher IQ scores are also more patient in postponing gratification and, in *social* decision contexts, are

more generous and cooperative, as well as readier to retaliate if counterparts fail to reciprocate.[46]

3. Another eloquent example of how (value-unrelated) cognitive processes are linked to decision preferences is given in "cake versus fruit experiments."[50] In such experiments, subjects were divided into two groups, one of which was asked to remember seven digits, the other only two. Both groups were subsequently asked to choose between a slice of chocolate cake and a bowl of fruit (both equally priced). The "seven-digit group" was shown to more frequently choose the unhealthier but probably more gratifying chocolate cake. These data were taken to suggest that memorization and decisions tap related cognitive processes. In other words, the seven-digit group had to process a larger "cognitive load," leaving it with less cognitive resources to resist the more tempting option.

In summary, cognitive control and decision-making processes are deeply entangled areas of cognition, thus one way to recruit, and study, cognitive control is to make decisions harder, or as some say more interesting.[46] To do so, in turn, we need to manipulate the *factors* that determine the utility of options. In what follows we illustrate several of them in respective themes (Themes 1–5), first giving an example and then a definition. We will then proceed by attempting to draw the borders between broad opposing tendencies in the neurocognitive explanations of cognitive control in decision making. In particular, we focus on a dual versus unitary framework,[46] which has been very prevalent in neuroeconomic research. The "battlegrounds" of such opposing views are the neuroeconomic data, which we illustrate using the factors mentioned in Themes 1 through 5. Throughout, we will argue that, at present, none of such broad models fully accounts for the growing corpus of neuroeconomic data. Finally, we discuss recent neuroeconomic studies that stress a more interdependent nature of controlled and controlling processes in the brain.

Themes

Theme 1: Loss Aversion[31]

Imagine you are invited to either accept or reject the following coin flip bet: heads you win $50, tails you lose $30. If you feel some struggle, that's the grip of loss aversion. Theoretically, winning $50 should attract you more than losing the same amount scares you. However, in a number of experimental settings, people (as well as young children[27] and nonhuman primates[10]) tend to refuse similarly structured bets. Normally, they require that potential gains nearly double potential losses to take the risk. To account for this, it has thus been proposed that losses are weighted differently from gains.

Theme 2: Risk Aversion[3]

Imagine being proposed the following choice between (a) $100 for sure, or (b) $200 if heads comes up on a fair coin flip. If you choose b, you are susceptible to risk. One definition of risk is variance of outcomes; the two gambles here, indeed, have the same mean, or expected value, but different variance. On average, people are risk averse[4] (they tend to go for option a); however, there is much interindividual variability.

Theme 3: Temporal Discounting[47]

Do you prefer (a) $10 right now or (b) $11 next month? If you chose b, that is you are patient, try increasing the time of payoff receipt in b by, say, an extra month. If you keep repeating this, at some point you are likely to pick option a, no matter how patient you are. Indeed, even though we may expect different people to give different answers on options with specific values, the tendency remains: people (and nonhuman animals, from pigeons to macaques), appear to discount the value of goods, in our case money, as the time to their receipt increases. Much of this behavior can be accounted for by exponential discounting, which decreases the value of goods constantly across time. However, choose between the following: (c) $10 in 12 months, or (d) $11 in 13 months. This choice should be similar to the former, as we only added one year to both options a and b. However, subjects tend to switch their preferences, from the nearer payoff to the farther one when both far and near payoffs are delayed. If we were to discount goods in a constant fashion (e.g., exponentially), such reversals shouldn't occur. One way to account for this behavior is to hypothesize that discounting is stronger when immediate payoffs are involved, whereas it decreases when there is no possibility to act immediately.

Theme 4: Ambiguity Effect[18]

Imagine a game host offers you two extraction-type lotteries, presented as two boxes, to bet on. For either box, you win $50 if a red ball is extracted. In box 1 is one red ball and one blue ball. In box 2, the game host initially put two red balls and two blue balls and subsequently extracted two balls but didn't show their colors. Thus, in box 2 there could be either two balls of the same color (either red or blue) or one ball of each color. Which box do you prefer to bet on? If you choose box 1 you are susceptible to ambiguity. Indeed, the two boxes offer the same chances of winning (the same expected value). The simplest definition of ambiguity is that outcome probabilities are unknown to the subject.

Theme 5: Framing Effects[31,58]

You are offered 100 euros to make two separate choices, 50 prior to each: in choice 1, you are offered to decide between (A) keeping 20 of your 50 euros and (B) betting everything on a "wheel of fortune" type lottery with a 65% chance to keep all and a 35% chance to lose all. Now, suppose you are offered decision 2, between (C) *losing* 30 of your 50 euros and (D) betting everything on the same lottery above. If you chose A and D, you are in line with the majority of subjects; alternatively, you might have realized that the two decisions are equivalent. In fact, B = D, but also A = C, since in one case you keep 20, in the other you lose 30 from the originally endowed 50 euros. Indeed, it all boils down to preferring a half empty glass or a half full one: the two glasses refer to the same object, that is, they are extensionally equivalent, as are the preceding prospects; however, subjects tend to reverse their choices according to how the options are framed.

Cognitive Control and Emotions in Economic Decision Making

Let us think in extremes: perhaps the largest doubt one can have about cognitive control is whether it *exists* at all as a dissociable anatomical and functional system. At the opposite extreme, cognitive control could be completely integrated with other structures/functions unrelated to control, perhaps functionally emerging from a more distributed network. This schematization lends itself to a very broad and yet open-ended debate in cognitive (neuro)science regarding the relatively dualistic or unitary nature of decision processes. This issue is more specific to economics and decision making, as similar debates in economics (i.e., regarding the impact of emotions on decisions) predate brain studies, to the point that some hope that neuroscience could help resolve some of the lingering problems of economics.[7]

Dual models stress the relative "independence" of "decision subsystems," that is, systems that can *independently* generate a decision, "as if" we had different "selves" competing for different options.[36] The unitary approach, on the other hand, also predicts the involvement of a number of "subsystems," however, none of these can generate an independent decision. From a neuroscientific viewpoint, dual models predict that a dissociable neuroanatomical network subserves cognitive control, whereas in a unitary framework there is no need for a functionally or anatomically distinguishable control system.

The distinction between different subsystems apparent in the dual models often runs parallel to the one between emotional and deliberative processes[43] (or between variously labeled fast and frugal, automatic/effortless, intuitive, experiential or hot processes, on one hand, versus effortful, analytic, rule-based, verbal, cool, or rational processes, on the other).[41]

Broadly speaking, both unitary and dual frameworks have apparent strong and weak points. For instance, it is nearly a truism that the unitary approach is simpler, as it explains decision phenomena with one rather than two systems. The dual system on the other hand appears particularly appealing for explaining "inconsistencies" observed in decision behavior. In what follows, we explain why this is so, reviewing the neuroeconomic literature that has focused on a number of such behavioral inconsistencies (see Themes). We show, however, that in many cases unitary frameworks can also accommodate the data. Throughout, we argue that both models fail to capture some important aspects of how the brain processes decisions.

Loss Aversion (Theme 1)

There is an intuitive appeal in hypothesizing that the different impacts that gains and losses have on behavior could be explained by different underlying neurocognitive systems. In particular, it would be consistent with a dual approach to predict that losses might have a greater impact on behavior as a result of their being processed in more emotion-related cortical regions. An alternative explanation more consistent with the unitary approach, however, is that the same neural network is *differentially* recruited by the processing of both gains and losses.

Neuroimaging evidence on healthy decision makers appeared to support the dual systems hypothesis, as the anticipation and experience of economic losses has been repeatedly associated with activity in structures strongly associated with affective and autonomic processing, such as the amygdala and the anterior insula.[35] With some exceptions,[52,61] the same regions were not sensitive to gains, which have instead been shown to recruit a system centered on the midbrain and the striatum, branching to various regions of the prefrontal cortex (PFC).[48] Only one study, by Tom and colleagues,[57] showed that increasing potential losses and gains recruited a same network, which was activated by gains and deactivated by losses. However, a study that included a task very similar to that used by Tom and colleagues was unable to replicate their results.[9] Recently, De Martino and colleagues[14] showed that patients with circumscribed damage to the amygdala clearly dissociated from their matched controls, as they didn't exhibit loss aversion. Overall, though studies employing different tasks show that the amygdala is sensitive to both positively and negatively valenced cue,[26] studies specifically focusing on loss aversion seem to tilt in the direction of a dual view.

Risk (Theme 2)

In a dual view, risk attitudes could be the result of emotions (and emotion-related cortices), which would be modulated by cognitive control in risk-neutral subjects. There is evidence that corroborates this hypothesis. Patients with lesions in areas thought to integrate emotion and cognition, such as the orbitofrontal cortex (OFC),[13] exhibit risk-neutral behavior,[30] paradoxically, as do high-scoring subjects on IQ tests.[2] Moreover, imaging studies revealed that areas previously associated with cognitive control, such as the lateral prefrontal cortex lPFC[56] (in particular, the ventrolateral PFC) play a role in mediating aversion to risk.[55] These findings are consistent with transcranial magnetic stimulation (TMS) studies showing the causal regulatory link between the inferior frontal gyrus (IFG) and risky behavior, by which interference with IFG activity using repetitive TMS (rTMS) decreases risk aversion.[34] The authors of the latter study propose that, when facing choices between options with different levels of risk (i.e., choose between (a) winning $20 with an 80% chance or lose -$20 otherwise, and (b) winning $80 with a 20% chance or lose -$80 otherwise), the risky option is more salient and attractive, as it usually features a greater outcome. This automatic attraction toward higher-paying outcomes would require the intervention of control processes, which, in turn, would support a more analytical assessment of the options, that is, enabling one to weigh the higher-paying option by its probability, making it overall *less* attractive. However, Rustichini[46] stresses that the same data are compatible with a unitary view, as the IFG may subserve general information processing, thus its disruption leads to the failure of integrating reward magnitude and probability. Moreover, although some subcortical and PFC regions appear to code risk and expected value separately,[44,49] others dissociate between the measures through distinct *temporal dynamics*, rather than regional segregation (such as dopamine neurons[22]).

Temporal Discounting (Theme 3)

Models to account for preference reversals have been proposed within both (a) dual and (b) unitary models.[46] Dual type explanations hinge on the idea that competition for guiding behavior occurs between an "impulsive" and a "patient" system. To represent this, Phelps and Pollak proposed[44] a model that employs two parameters in a temporal discounting function. One, "delta," discounts evenly across different time points—and is consistent with the previous exponential discounting (see Theme 3)—the other, "beta," gives the function a steep curvature for immediate rewards. In contrast to this, supporters of the unitary view have often taken from psychophysics, stressing parallelisms with better-understood perceptual systems.[46] A third line of research has proposed that hyperbolic discounting (i.e., preference reversals) can be explained by a logarithmic perception of time and exponential time discounting.[54] Incidentally, this seems to be supported by a neuropsychological study showing that ventromedial PFC (vmPFC) patients behaved comparably to controls on intertemporal decisions but were impaired in a task that assessed their ability to consistently focus on different time horizons.[20] Therefore, even if discounting behaviors can be described as a result of two processes (i.e., patient vs. impatient), they seem to presently leave open a number of possible subfunction combinations.

Taking the "unitary versus dual" dispute into the brain doesn't simplify the scenario foreshadowed by the preceding behavioral debates. A first study by McClure and colleagues[38] was able to dissociate between beta- and delta-pliant systems; a second study by Kable and Glimcher,[30] however, showed a unitary set of reward-related regions modulated by near and far rewards, and a third one by Ballard and Knutson[1] was partially consistent with both studies. Overall, while there appear to be some "dualisms" in the brain, they don't align well to those of a typical dual model. For instance, dual models predict that a neural system would be preferentially activated by immediate as opposed to future rewards; however, Ballard and Knutson's study suggests that a key dissociation might be between reward magnitude and reward delay, which is compatible with Kable and Glimcher's results. Overall, the most consistent result appears that of an lPFC involvement in the processing of the delay of rewards, as this is confirmed by two of the preceding studies,[1,38] an electrophysiological study on monkeys,[32] and several patient and imaging studies in different but related tasks.[33] Moreover, this idea is not in conflict with Kable and Glimcher's findings, as this could not differentiate well between reward magnitude and delay.[1] The lPFC's involvement for processing rewards that are delayed in time is consistent with the notion that this region is needed to override prepotent responses such as those that could derive from the temptation to accept immediate payoffs.

Decisions under Ambiguity (Theme 4)

It could be tempting to explain ambiguity aversion within a dual framework. Not knowing the contingencies of our decision environments could easily "frighten" us, perhaps so quickly and automatically that we don't give ourselves the time to consider the possible situations and make a balanced choice. The first neuroimaging research by Huettel and colleagues[29] to directly confront neural responses to risk versus ambiguity showed that subjects that chose the ambiguous lotteries more often (see Theme 4) exhibited enhanced inferior frontal gyrus (IFG) activity in response to ambiguity. Such activity was interpreted to be a signature of cognitive control, which could override the impulsive decision of automatically avoiding ambiguity and plausibly mobilize cognitive resources to explore the ambiguous scenario (i.e., considering the various alternatives underlying the ambiguously described probabilities). A second study, by Hsu et al.,[28] was particularly consistent with dual models, as it showed that emotion-related cortices, among which, the amygdala and the OFC, responded preferentially to ambiguity and that striatal responses were more sensitive to risk. The two types of responses also differed in timing, as the amygdala was activated seconds earlier than the striatum. Moreover, the causal role of the OFC in ambiguity processing was demonstrated by the observation that patients with lesions in this area were less sensitive, and even became prone to both ambiguity and risk, relative to their matched controls. Together, the functional magnetic resonance imaging (fMRI) and lesion data leaded the authors to speak of an amygdala-OFC centered *vigilance-evaluation* system (requiring regulation, via the dorsomedial PFC, or dmPFC) that quickly tracks salient aspects of the stimuli that carry uncertainty-related information (i.e., signaling that information is missing).

Though Hsu and colleagues' results seem to support the idea that risk and ambiguity are processed by distinct mechanisms in the brain, their neuropsychological results also suggested that ambiguity and risk tendencies are connected, as they seemed to correlate in both the control and patient samples (which is consistent with a previous study linking ambiguity and risk in healthy subjects[5]). In line with this, and closer to a unitary perspective, a study by Levy et al.[37] found that the activity in the set of regions, including the medial PFC, striatum, amygdala, and posterior cingulate cortex (PCC) covaried with subjective value in both risky and ambiguous decisions. There was moreover evidence for differential activation patterns (rather than segregation), as connectivity analysis suggested that connection "weights" are stronger between the amygdala and the striatum under ambiguous than risky choices.

It is hard to argue that these results answer the question of whether dual or unitary systems underlie ambiguity.

Framing Effects (Theme 5)

Consistently with a dual systems approach, it has been proposed that emotional processes may underlie subjects' susceptibility to choices framed either as losses or gains. Such a model would predict that frame-driven behavior would correlate with activity in emotion-related regions and that behavioral consistency across frames (the "rational" behavior) would elicit activity in areas associated with cognitive control, since consistent behavior across different contexts is costly. In line with this, a study by De Martino and colleagues[16] showed that amygdala activity correlated with risk-averse behavior in "gain frames" and risk-seeking behavior in games framed negatively, which is consistent with the idea that this limbic structure amplifies risk-related biases by processing contextual cues. In contrast, when subjects "resisted" frames, the anterior cingulate cortex (ACC) was preferentially recruited in a subregion later associated with strategic control.[60] Moreover, the authors obtained individual "rationality" indexes from behavior (a measure of their subjects' degree of susceptibility to frames) that correlated with medial OFC (mOFC) activity. The OFC is considered to integrate emotional valence and goal-oriented behavior,[13] and as such the authors suggested that subjects who chose more "rationally" had richer representations of their own emotional biases, enabling them to better modify their behavior.

Interplay between Emotions and Cognitive Control: A Paradigmatic Example

Coricelli et al.[12] measured brain activity using fMRI while subjects participated in a simple gambling task. The experimental task required subjects to choose between two gambles, each having different probabilities and different expected outcomes. Regret was induced by providing information regarding the outcome of the unchosen gamble. Increasing regret was correlated with enhanced activity in the medial orbitofrontal region, the dorsal ACC and anterior hippocampus. This hippocampal activity is consistent with the idea that a cognitive-based declarative process of regret is engaged by the task. This supports a modulation of declarative (consciously accessible) memory[17,53] such that after a bad outcome the lesson to be learned is: "In the future pay more attention to the potential consequences of your choice." Furthermore, Coricelli et al.[12] showed that activity in response to experiencing regret (OFC/ACC/medial temporal cortex) is distinct from activity seen with mere outcome evaluation (ventral striatum), and in response to disappointment elicited by the mismatch between actual and expected outcome of choice. Indeed, the magnitude of disappointment correlated with enhanced activity in middle temporal gyrus and dorsal brainstem, including periaqueductal gray matter, a region implicated in processing aversive signal such as pain. This suggests distinctive neural substrates in reward processing, and that the OFC and medial temporal cortex areas can bias basic dopamine-mediated reward responses.[17]

Coricelli et al.[12] reported that, across their fMRI experiment subjects became increasingly regret aversive, a cumulative effect reflected in enhanced activity within ventromedial orbitofrontal cortex and amygdala. Under these circumstances, the same pattern of activity that was expressed with the experience of regret was also expressed just prior to choice, suggesting the same neural circuitry mediates both direct experience of regret and its anticipation. Thus, the OFC and the amygdala contribute to this form of high-level learning based on past emotional experience, in a manner that mirrors the role of these structures in acquisition of value in low-level learning contexts.[23]

Moreover, and of particular interest for our current discussion, affective consequences of choice can induce specific mechanisms of cognitive control.[62] Coricelli et al.[12] observed enhanced responses in right dorsolateral prefrontal cortex, right lateral OFC, and inferior parietal lobule during a choice phase after the experience of regret,[12] where subsequent choice processes induced reinforcement, or avoidance of, the experienced behavior.[11] Corroborating results from Simon-Thomas et al.[51] show that negative emotions can recruit "cognitive" right hemisphere responses. Thus, negative affective consequences (regret) induce specific mechanisms of cognitive control on subsequent choices. These data suggest a mechanism through which comparing choice outcome with its alternatives (fictive error), and the associated feeling of regret, promotes behavioral flexibility and exploratory strategies in dynamic environments so as to minimize the likelihood of emotionally negative outcomes. These studies stress a more interdependent nature of controlled and controlling processes in the brain.

Brief Discussion and Synthesis

One of the problems with treating cognitive control in economic decision making is that there is a resilient idea that control makes behavior rational and that emotions make it irrational. A line of literature coming from neuropsychological observations supports this idea: Patients with lesions in the amygdala do not exhibit loss aversion,[14] patients with lesions in the OFC/vmPFC are less risk and ambiguity averse, and are close to neutrality in both domains,[28] they are also utilitarian in moral decision making[24] and are less influenced by regret in economic decisions[8]; similarly, subjects with autistic syndromes are less susceptible to framing effects.[15] All these pathologies are thus associated with *increased* "economic rationality" in a number of contexts.

This interpretation, however, ignores the most prominent and consequential behavioral feature of these patients; that is, they are also severely impaired in everyday decision making. In experimental tasks, this is suggested by vmPFC/OFC patients' inability to learn from negative decision outcomes,[13] their impairments in reversal learning,[19] their violations of preference transitivity[21] (i.e., they are more likely to exhibit inconsistent preferences of the type A > B, B > C, but A < C) and abnormal decision making in a number of interactive choice contexts.[59] Thus, overall, emotions take part in inconsistent *and* consistent/adaptive decisions.

This has implications for the dual versus unitary discussion. We suggest that there is a "strong" interpretation of dual models and a "weaker" one. The weak version makes only the first of the following two claims, the strong one makes both: (1) that there are two relatively distinct broad systems in the brain, one that preferentially takes part in fast, effortless, emotional, and context-related processes, another that is preferentially activated in situations requiring control and deliberation; and (2) that these two systems make separate contributions to, respectively, "rational" and "irrational" economic decision making. The stronger version appears at odds with current neuroscientific evidence. Our review of neuroimaging evidence further stresses and complicates this point: Even *within* economic categorizations of behavior, which depend on the factors manipulated in the decision environment (Themes 1–5), the brain is capable of responding either as a unitary or as a dual system, plausibly according to specific differences in task designs that should gradually be disentangled. In none of the individual factors we examined do imaging studies uniquely support either a unitary or dual view: in some designs, the two putative neural systems do not dissociate whereas in others they do. Thus, under a strict falsificationism, both theories are falsified.

Our impression is that the reviewed results appear less odd outside a strict opposition between a dual and unitary framework; although it is hard to deny that there are cortices more related to bodily/emotional processes and others more related to analytical ones (something close to the weaker claim above), results ultimately stress the flexibility with which the two systems seem to interact, thus the different effects cognitive control and emotions can have on behavior.

Outstanding Questions

• What is the relationship between cognitive control and the reward system?

• What is the role of cognitive control in the computations underlying social interaction?

• To what extent do we need cognitive control to behave optimally?

Further Reading

Koechlin E, Hyafil A. 2007. Anterior prefrontal function and the limits of human decision-making. *Science* 318: 594–598. In scenarios in which goals do not match expectations, one of the big problems a cognitive agent faces is that of analyzing and confronting a number of possible plans of actions. However, the lPFC is functionally limited, and only serially represented plans can be processed, as in a bottleneck. The authors suggest that "branching" is the function that counters the bottleneck problem in the lPFC. It is attributed to the FPC (frontopolar cortex, BA 10) and would enable the exploration/execution of a target task, while maintaining a previously selected task in a pending state for subsequent automatic retrieval and execution.

Venkatraman V, Alexandra GR, Taran AA, Huettel SA. 2009. Resolving response, decision, and strategic control: Evidence for a functional topography in dorsomedial prefrontal cortex. *J Neurosci* 29: 13158–13164. Several studies have investigated further functional dissociations within the pmPFC, reporting a ventral-dorsal gradient for emotional versus more cognitive processes as well social relevance. This recent fMRI study further qualifies anatomofunctional specialization of cognitive control in the mPFC.

References

1. Ballard K, Knutson B. 2009. Dissociable neural representations of future reward magnitude and delay during temporal discounting. *Neuroimage* 45: 143–150.

2. Benjamin DJ, Brown SA, Shapiro JM. 2006. Who is "behavioral"? Cognitive ability and anomalous preferences. Unpublished working paper.

3. Bernoulli D. 1954; 1738. Exposition of a new theory on the measurement of risk (Translation of Speciment theoriae novae de mensura sortis). *Econometrica* 22: 23–36.

4. Binswager HP. 1980. Attitudes toward risk: experimental measurement in rural India. *Am J Agric Econ* 62: 395–407.

5. Bossaerts P, Ghirardato P, Guarnaschelli S, Zame WR. 2010. Ambiguity in asset markets: theory and experiment. *Rev Financ Stud* 23: 1325–1359.

6. Bruni L, Sugden R. 2007. The road not taken: how psychology was removed from economics, and how it might be brought back. *Econ J* 117: 146–173.

7. Camerer CF, Loewenstein G, Prelec D. 2005. Neuroeconomics: how neuroscience can inform economics. *J Econ Lit* 34: 9–64.

8. Camille N, Coricelli G, Sallet J, Pradat-Diehl P, Duhamel JR, Sirigu A. 2004. The involvement of the orbitofrontal cortex in the experience of regret. *Science* 304: 1167–1170.

9. Canessa N, Chierchia G, Motterlini M, Baud-Bovy G, Tettamanti M, Cappa S. (in preparation). Distinct neural correlates for the processing of magnitude, probability and uncertainty of potential monetary wins and losses.

10. Chen MK, Lakshminaryanan V, Santos LR. 2006. The evolution of our preferences: evidence from capuchin monkey trading behavior. *J Polit Econ* 114: 517–537.

11. Clark L, Cools R, Robbins TW. 2004. The neuropsychology of ventral prefrontal cortex: decision-making and reversal learning. *Brain Cogn* 55: 41–53.

12. Coricelli G, Critchley HD, Joffily M, O'Doherty JP, Sirigu A, Dolan RJ. 2005. Regret and its avoidance: a neuroimaging study of choice behavior. *Nat Neurosci* 8: 1255–1262.

13. Damasio AR. 1994. Decartes' Error: Emotion, Reason, and the Human Brain. New York: Putnam Publishing.

14. De Martino B, Camerer CF, Adolphs R. 2010. Amygdala damage eliminates monetary loss aversion. *Proc Natl Acad Sci USA* 107: 3788–3792.

15. De Martino B, Harrison NA, Knafo S, Bird G, Dolan RJ. 2007. Explaining enhanced logical consistency during decision making in autism. *J Neurosci* 28: 10746–10750.

16. De Martino B, Kumaran D, Seymour B, Dolan RJ. 2006. Frames, biases, and rational decision-making in the human brain. *Science* 313: 684–687.

17. Eichenbaum H. 2004. Hippocampus: cognitive processes and neural representations that underlie declarative memory. *Neuron* 44: 109–120.

18. Ellsberg D. 1961. Risk, ambiguity, and the savage axioms. *Q J Econ* 75: 643–699.

19. Fellows LK, Farah MJ. 2005. Different underlying impairments in decision-making following ventromedial and dorsolateral frontal lobe damage in humans. *Cereb Cortex* 15: 58–63.

20. Fellows LK, Farah MJ. 2005. Dissociable elements of human foresight: a role for the ventromedial frontal lobes in framing the future, but not in discounting future rewards. *Neuropsychologia* 43: 1214–1221.

21. Fellows LK, Farah MJ. 2007. The role of ventromedial prefrontal cortex in decision making: judgment under uncertainty or judgment per se? *Cereb Cortex* 17: 2669–2674.

22. Fiorillo CD, Tobler PN, Schultz W. 2003. Discrete coding of reward probability and uncertainty by dopamine neurons. *Science* 299: 1898–1902.

23. Gottfried JA, O'Doherty J, Dolan RJ. 2003. Encoding predictive reward value in human amygdala and orbitofrontal cortex. *Science* 301: 1104–1107.

24. Greene JD. 2007. Why are VMPFC patients more utilitarian? A dual-process theory of moral judgment explains. *Trends Cogn Sci* 11: 322–323.

25. Gul F, Pesendorfer W. 2007. The case for mindless economics. In: Handbook of Economic Methodologies (Caplin A, Schotter A, eds). New York: Oxford University Press.

26. Hamann S, Mao H. 2002. Positive and negative emotional verbal stimuli elicit activity in the left amygdala. *Neuroreport* 13: 15–19.

27. Harbaugh WT, Krause K, Vesterlund L. 2001. Are adults better behaved than children? Age, experience, and the endowment effect. *Econ Lett* 70: 175–181.

28. Hsu M, Bhatt M, Adolphs R, Tranel D, Camerer CF. 2005. Neural systems responding to degrees of uncertainty in human decision-making. *Science* 310: 1680–1683.

29. Huettel SA, Stowe CJ, Gordon EM, Warner BT, Platt ML. 2006. Neural signatures of economic preferences for risk and ambiguity. *Neuron* 49: 765–775.

30. Kable JW, Glimcher PW. 2007. The neural correlates of subjective value during intertemporal choice. *Nat Neurosci* 10: 1625–1633.

31. Kahneman D, Tversky A. 1979. Prospect theory: an analysis of decision under risk. *Econometrica* 47: 263–291.

32. Kim S, Hwang J, Lee D. 2008. Prefrontal coding of temporally discounted values during intertemporal choice. *Neuron* 59: 161–172.

33. Knoch D, Fehr E. 2007. Resisting the power of temptations: the right prefrontal cortex and self-control. *Ann N Y Acad Sci* 1104: 123–134.

34. Knoch D, Gianotti LR, Pascual-Leone A, Treyer V, Regard M, Hohmann M, Brugger P. 2006. Disruption of right prefrontal cortex by low-frequency repetitive transcranial magnetic stimulation induces risk-taking behavior. *J Neurosci* 26: 6469–6472.

35. Knutson B, Bossaerts P. 2007. Neural antecedents of financial decisions. *J Neurosci* 27: 8174–8177.

36. Laibson D. 1997. Golden eggs and hyperbolic discounting. *Q J Econ* 112: 443–477.

37. Levy I, Snell J, Nelson A, Rustichini A, Glimcher P. 2010. Neural representation of subjective value under risk and ambiguity. *J Neurophysiol* 103: 1036–1047.

38. McClure SM, Laibson DI, Loewenstein G, Cohen JD. 2004. Separate neural systems value immediate and delayed monetary rewards. *Science* 306: 503–507.

39. Miller EK. 2000. The prefrontal cortex and cognitive control. *Nat Rev Neurosci* 1: 59–65.

40. Mischel W, Shoda Y, Rodriguez MI. 1989. Delay of gratification in children. *Science* 244: 933–938.

41. Mukherjee A. 2010. Dual system model of preferences under risk. *Psychol Rev* 117: 243–255.

42. Norman DA, Shallice T. 2000. Attention to action: willed and automatic control of behaviour. In: CHIP Report 99. San Diego: University of California.

43. Ochsner KN, Gross JJ. 2005. The cognitive control of emotion. *Trends Cogn Sci* 9: 242–249.

44. Phelps ES, Pollak RA. 1968. On second-best national saving and game-equilibrium growth. *Rev Econ Stud* 35: 185–199.

45. Ridderinkhof KR, Ullsperger M, Crone EA, Nieuwenhuis S. 2004. The role of the medial frontal cortex in cognitive control. *Science* 306: 443–447.

46. Rustichini A. 2008. Dual or unitary system? Two alternative models of decision making. *Cogn Affect Behav Neurosci* 8: 355–362.

47. Samuelson PA. 1937. A note on measurement of utility. *Rev Econ Stud* 4: 155–161.

48. Schultz W. 2006. Behavioral theories and the neurophysiology of reward. *Annu Rev Psychol* 57: 87–115.

49. Seymour B, Daw ND, Dayan P, Singer T, Dolan RJ. 2007. Differential encoding of losses and gains in the human striatum. *J Neurosci* 27: 4826–4831.

50. Shiv B, Fedorkhin A. 1999. Heart and mind in conflict: the interplay of affect and cognition in consumer decision making. *J Consum Res* 26: 278–292.

51. Simon-Thomas ER, Role KO, Knight RT. 2005. Behavioral and electrophysiological evidence of a right hemisphere bias for the influence of negative emotion on higher cognition. *J Cogn Neurosci* 17: 518–529.

52. Smith BW, Mitchell DG, Hardin MG, Jazbec S, Fridberg D, Blair RJ, Ernst M. 2009. Neural substrates of reward magnitude, probability, and risk during a wheel of fortune decision-making task. *Neuroimage* 44: 600–609.

53. Steidl S, Mohi-uddin S, Anderson AK. 2006. Effects of emotional arousal on multiple memory systems: evidence from declarative and procedural learning. *Learn Mem* 13: 650–658.

54. Takahashi T. 2005. Loss of self-control in intertemporal choice may be attributable to logarithmic time perception. *Med Hypotheses* 65: 691–693.

55. Tobler PN, Christopoulos GI, O'Doherty JP, Dolan RJ, Schultz W. 2009. Risk-dependent reward value signal in human prefrontal cortex. *Proc Natl Acad Sci USA* 106: 7185–7190.

56. Tobler PN, O'Doherty JP, Dolan RJ, Schultz W. 2007. Reward value coding distinct from risk attitude-related uncertainty coding in human reward systems. *J Neurophysiol* 97: 1621–1632.

57. Tom SM, Fox CR, Trepel C, Poldrack RA. 2007. The neural basis of loss aversion in decision-making under risk. *Science* 315: 515–518.

58. Tversky A, Kahneman D. 1981. The framing of decisions and the psychology of choice. *Science* 211: 453–458.

59. Van den Bos W, Güroglu B. 2009. The role of the ventral medial prefrontal cortex in social decision making. *J Neurosci* 29: 7631–7632.

60. Venkatraman V, Alexandra GR, Taran AA, Huettel SA. 2009. Resolving response, decision, and strategic control: evidence for a functional topography in dorsomedial prefrontal cortex. *J Neurosci* 29: 13158–13164.

61. Yacubian J, Gläscher J, Schroeder K, Sommer T, Braus DF, Büchel C. 2006. Dissociable systems for gain- and loss-related value predictions and errors of prediction in the human brain. *J Neurosci* 26: 9530–9537.

62. Yarkoni T, Gray JR, Chrastil ER, Brach DM, Green L, Braver TS. 2005. Sustained neural activity associated with cognitive control during temporally extended decision making. *Brain Res Cogn Brain Res* 23: 71–84.

22 Frames of Reference in Human Social Decision Making

Laurence T. Hunt and Timothy E. J. Behrens

The ability to place the study of the neural basis of motivational and cognitive control in its full social context could be considered a fairly recent one. Because the number and complexity of human social interactions is unique,[17] it is only with the advent of neuroimaging tools that we have begun to understand the physiological correlates of human social behavior in the brain. The field of social cognitive neuroscience has grown rapidly, and many studies have begun to investigate human subjects' brain activity while they choose how to behave in a given social context.

In this chapter, we argue that understanding the *frame of reference* in which neural activity changes in these studies is fundamental to understanding the function of that activity. This point has long been appreciated in brain regions that are involved in sensorimotor integration,[12,38] the challenge here being to elucidate the intermediate transformations between neural activity in one frame of reference (sensation) as they are transformed into activity in an entirely different one (motor control). We contend that it is equally important to establish the frame of reference in which neural activity varies during a social interaction. Similar transformations, from the observation of a social partner's behavior to the inference of intention and then to the eventual modification of one's own actions, must be performed by the brain to elicit successful social behavior. Although the discrimination made here may be rather more blunt, two broad categories of activations can be delineated from functional magnetic resonance imaging (fMRI) studies of social interaction conducted thus far.

First, a particular social setting will often cause adaption of behavior in a particular way. This influence of others on one's own behavior affects activity in a network of brain regions associated with reward and selecting one's *own* actions. Second, social interactions also require inference of another individual's intentions, so as to adapt one's own behavior accordingly. Importantly, this process of mental inference, or *mentalizing*, engages a quite distinct set of brain regions. It is useful to think of this activity as being in the frame of reference of the *other* person's actions. Successful social behavior requires *both* inference of other individuals' thoughts *and* adaptation of one's own behavior accordingly, and several recent studies have investigated activity during tasks in which both processes are required, but the two vary *independently* of one another. By ensuring that task variables in the two frames of reference remain independent, variance in neural activity can be ascribed to one, the other, or both frames of reference.

Socially Derived Reward

It has long been argued that social exchanges can be described in terms of costs and benefits to the individual,[27] and so might be valued against other (nonsocial) costs and rewards. Socially rewarding or aversive stimuli might therefore need to be translated into the same neural "common currency" as other (nonsocial) stimuli, within which currency their value can be compared. Evidence for this exists at the level of single neurons; macaques will forgo a juice reward to view a photograph of certain conspecifics,[15] and the subjective value of this viewing is reflected in the firing rate of neurons in the lateral intraparietal area at the time of choice.[32]

In human subjects, primary rewards and decision values are frequently found to activate portions of ventral striatum and ventromedial prefrontal cortex. Evidence has recently been found for common activations in these regions for reward derived from a social interaction.

Ventral Striatum Activates for Reward Derived from a Social Interaction

Izuma and colleagues[29] used fMRI to scan human volunteers as they received appraisals from social partners on their moral character, and (in a separate condition) as they performed a monetary gambling task. Both monetary rewards and positive social appraisals were found to activate an overlapping portion of the striatum. It may also be rewarding to cooperate with other individuals or conform to the opinion of experts; the striatum is again active in both cases.[11,42]

A rewarding stimulus, by definition, is one that increases (or reinforces) behavior that elicits the stimulus. For example, the potential value of social conformity can reinforce behaviors that comply with a social norm. Subjects who adjust their behavior to comply with others have greater activation in the striatum than those who leave their behavior unchanged.[11] This striatal activation occurs at the time when the discrepancy between one's own behavior and other individuals' behavior is revealed, even if norm compliance is measured at a much later time point in the experiment.[33] Activations in striatum can therefore be related not only to reward, but also to signals observed in paradigms of reinforcement learning, where an error in prediction of reward is frequently witnessed in the striatum,[39] and is thought to cause an adaptation of one's future behavior. The concept of a socially derived reward prediction error has been examined more explicitly in the case of a trust game, in which the striatum is more active on trials where donations from a partner induce an increase in trusting behavior.[31] Similarly to the reward prediction error in dopamine cells,[45] striatal signals in this study were found to transfer back in time from the time point of the rewarding stimulus (trusting behavior from the partner) to the time point of trial onset. Importantly, the prediction error in these studies are "egocentric"—in the *self* frame of reference—in that they reflect a change in one's own behavior, rather than a perceived change in the behavior of other individuals.

Ventral Striatal Activations for Other-Regarding Preferences

Human actions in a social environment are not only guided by self-interest, but may also be influenced by the impact of these actions on the behavior of others. Altruistic behavior such as charitable donation has provided a puzzle for pure "self-interest" economic theories that view donation as giving away a good for no direct gain for oneself in terms of material wealth or reputation. However, such behavior can be explained by economic models that include terms incorporating a value for "other-regarding" preferences.[20] These values show a common neural substrate to that of self-regarding preferences, as indicated by the value of a charitable donation being reflected by blood oxygen level–dependent (BOLD) fMRI responses in ventral striatum and ventromedial prefrontal cortex.[25,26,36]

A direct measure of altruistic tendencies can be obtained by studying the behavior of individuals participating in collaborative (or competitive) games. Such games may be designed so that certain actions can be interpreted only in terms of their impact on other players, rather than on oneself. By making the games single-shot and anonymous, the potential confounds of later reciprocation and the desire to build a reputation with the social partner are also removed, and so the behavior of subjects (and their brain activity) can be explained only by appealing to subjects' other-regarding preferences. In one such game,[14] subjects could punish unfair behavior in social partners who retained an unfair share of money with which the subject had entrusted them. The striatum was found to be more active when this punishment was costly to the partner rather than symbolic, and was particularly active in subjects who invested a greater amount of their own money in punishing their partner. This set of activations may appeal to the idea that humans punish unfair behavior *because* they find it rewarding to do so—in other words, the subjects place a higher value on delivering a punishment than on keeping monetary reward to themselves. A similar conclusion can be drawn from the finding that male subjects have a greater striatal activation when they observe an unfair player receiving an electric shock than a fair player receiving the same treatment.[47]

Behavior in these games can be captured by several quantitative economic models, including those featuring a term that factors in aversion for inequality between participants,[21] or those that assume subjects act in response to fair (or unfair) behavior with reciprocation.[19] Neural evidence for the former has come from a recent study,[51] that splits subjects into unequal starting positions ("rich" or "poor"). Activation in striatum was stronger for rewards delivered to the *partner* in subjects who were in an initial position of being richer than their partner, but stronger for rewards delivered to the *subject* in subjects who were in an initial position of being poorer. The findings might be taken as neural evidence that subjects find a reduction in inequality rewarding.

The Pitfalls (or Promises?) of Reverse Inference

Does the increased activity in striatum truly reflect the rewarding properties of other-regarding preferences? Striatal activations can also be found for noxious stimuli[3] or monetary losses.[46] This highlights the danger of making a "reverse inference" about the psychological process being recruited by a given task.[40] We should not leap to the conclusion that, because a region is activated in a task (e.g., a behavior in a social setting) and that region is also known to respond to a particular psychological state (e.g., reward), this implies the task must engage that state (i.e., the prosocial behavior *must be* rewarding). This conclusion would be valid only if the region *solely* responded to reward; in the case of the ventral striatum, this is not the case.

On the other hand, there are cases where reverse inference *has*, apparently, been of use, as in a recent study of why subjects overbid in auctions.[16] When subjects participated in a socially competitive auction, the ventral striatum showed a different pattern of activity compared to a formally identical (but nonsocially competitive) lottery. *Winning* in the auction elicited the same striatal response as winning in the lottery, but *losing* elicited deactivation selectively in the competitive auction. The authors interpreted this finding as subjects showing a particular *aversion to losing to others* in the competitive environment of an auction. Crucially, they then used this reverse inference to design a further behavioral experiment; subjects were found to further increase their overbidding if the auction was framed in terms of losing a certain amount that had already been given to the subject, as opposed to winning the same quantity at the end of the auction.

So, a reverse inference may be a valid tool if it used to generate a novel hypothesis that can then be tested behaviorally. It is important to bear in mind that without subsequent testing of the generated hypotheses, it is dangerous to leap to conclusions about why a region is found to be more active in a given task.

Socially Derived Reward and Other-Regarding Preferences Have Been Studied in the "Self" Frame of Reference

Whether or not we can make inferences about reward, it is clear that social preferences activate a common set of regions as those engaged in processing more basic rewards. Clearly, this activity is an important aspect of how social influences modify behavior. Importantly, however, all of the reviewed findings can be considered as reflecting one's *own* utility function for a particular outcome or behavior, and so are egocentric in nature. Activity in striatum (and other regions that respond to reward or decision value) may represent a "final output" of social influences on one's own behavior, but this need not imply that the striatum is involved in the *computation* of these social influences in the first place. The key test would be to devise a way to manipulate the factors that *lead* to a particular social influence being expressed, without manipulating the *value* of that social influence to one's own actions.

Action Selection and Cognitive Control in a Social Environment

Other-regarding and self-regarding preferences often come into conflict. A network of brain regions encompassing anterior cingulate cortex (ACC) and dorsolateral prefrontal cortex (DLPFC) has been isolated to show increased activity when task demands are heightened or one must select between competing action plans[18,41] (see chapter 1, this volume, for a discussion). This same network of regions has also been found to be active during tasks where subjects must weigh the benefits to themselves with the impact their actions will have on another individual.

DLPFC, ACC, and "Self-Control" in Social Interactions

Competing motives for self and other have been captured in several economic games.[9] One such game is the ultimatum game, in which two subjects undergo a one-shot interaction in which a pot of money provided by the experimenter must be divided. One subject, the "proposer," makes an offer of how the pot should be split between the two players, and the second player, the "responder," decides either to accept this offer (in which case the players receive this split) or to reject it (in which case both players leave with nothing). The rational strategy (assuming both players act in their own self-interest) is for the proposer to make the minimum possible offer (an "unfair" split of the pot), and for the responder to accept this. In practice, modal behavior is for proposers to offer a fair (50-50%) split of the pot, and unfair offers (e.g., 20-80%) are frequently punished by the responder with rejection.[50] In rejecting an unfair offer, the responder sacrifices his own earnings to ensure that the proposer walks away with nothing, which again can be explained by appealing to an aversion to inequality[21] or a desire for reciprocity[19] (but see ref. 54 for evidence of an additional, non-other–regarding explanation of this behavior).

Sanfey and colleagues[44] measured BOLD fMRI in subjects playing the role of responder in several one-shot trials of the ultimatum game, with interleaved trials played with either a human or computer partner. Unfair offers from human partners were typically equally likely to be accepted or rejected, whereas fair offers (or any offer from the computer, fair or unfair) were invariably accepted. DLPFC, ACC, and insular cortex were all found to be more active when responders were faced with an unfair proposal than a fair one, and specifically when receiving this unfair proposal from a human. Activity in these areas was therefore greater on trials where subjects were equally likely to accept or reject the offer (that is, when self-regarding and other-regarding preferences came into conflict) than when they were certain to accept the offer (when no such conflict existed).

The importance of DLPFC in balancing prosocial and selfish behavior has been further emphasized by studies in which its activity has been temporarily disrupted using repetitive transcranial magnetic stimulation (rTMS). After receiving 15 minutes of rTMS to the right (but not the left) DLPFC, subjects show a reduced tendency to reject unfair offers in the ultimatum game.[34] The right DLPFC, it is argued, appears critical in overriding the "selfish" desire to keep an unfair offer when weighing this against an other-regarding rejection. This has been further investigated in a related game, the trust game, in which subjects choose whether to return or keep money with which their partners have entrusted them. rTMS to right DLPFC does not affect subjects' willingness to return the money in a condition where they are doing so anonymously (and where return rates are relatively low). However, whereas most subjects increase their rate of return when their returns are made public, subjects who have received TMS keep the same rate of return as in the anonymous condition.[35] The key difference in the latter condition is that subjects have an opportunity to build a reputation for being trustworthy; subjects who have undergone TMS give the appearance of neglecting this opportunity and taking into account only their own short-term self-interest in making their choices.

Self and Other Frames of Reference in Ultimatum and Trust Games

What aspect of behavior has changed in these subjects? It might be that they are no longer able to infer the impact that their actions will have on the behavior of other individuals, or what the prevailing norm for fair behavior is. Alternatively, it might be that these functions are perfectly intact, but the *implementation* of this knowledge in modifying their *own* behavior has changed. In fact, in both studies there was clear evidence for the latter. In the ultimatum game, rDLPFC TMS subjects would still report an offer of an 80%-20% split as being highly unfair, in line with reports of control subjects—but would nevertheless go on to accept it.[34] Similarly, in the trust game, the subjects' reports of what constituted fair behavior remained in line with those who had not received rTMS to the rDLPFC.[35] Impairing the function of rDLPFC does not appear to change one's perception of other individuals, or the impact of one's own behavior on other individuals; it instead changes the use of this knowledge in guiding one's own behavior.

This leaves open the possibility that another brain region, or set of regions, performs the "allocentric" computations necessary to infer the impact of one's own behavior on others. A hint toward which regions might be important in this process was provided by a recent manipulation of the trust game by van den Bos and colleagues.[52] In this game, an *investor* chooses whether to entrust the subject being scanned (the *trustee*) with some money. This money is multiplied by the experimenter; the trustee must then decide how to split it between the two players. In one manipulation, the actions of the investor were made to be particularly beneficial to the trustee, but not to himself. This created more conflict for the trustee (in his *own* frame of reference), who is inclined to be fair as he has done better out of the situation. The trustee's rDLPFC is found to be more active. In another manipulation, the actions of the investor were made to be particularly beneficial to *himself*. This changes the inferred *intention* of the investor in sending the money—he is doing so in order to obtain more money for himself—and so is in the frame of reference of *his* actions. This manipulation affected BOLD fMRI responses at another region, which has been emphasized by a complementary literature in social interactions—the right temporoparietal junction.

In the next section, we introduce this region as one of several whose activity may vary as a function of the inferred behavior of other individuals in a social interaction.

Inferring the Intentions of Others in Social Interactions

Much work has gone into studying regions of the brain that support the ability to infer the intentions of other individuals, or to possess a *theory of mind*. One hypothesis[7] argues that there might be a specialized set of brain regions devoted to social cognitive functions including theory of mind. The research effort in this field has been intense, in part spurred on by the finding that autistic patients have a specific deficit in understanding other's intentions, as demonstrated by the "false belief" task.[1] A dorsomedial portion of prefrontal cortex and portions of the superior temporal sulcus and temporoparietal junction are both more active during tasks requiring inference of false beliefs,[22,23,53] and these regions show altered activity in autistic subjects.[2]

What metric is coded in these regions that causes them to be important in intentional inference? While it has been established that these regions are typically more active when performing an interactive game with a human partner as opposed to a computer,[43] several recent studies have investigated these regions' activity in more detail, investigating the precise computations that they perform during a social interaction.[4]

Dorsomedial PFC Activity Reflects Both the Depth of Strategic Inference and Learning about This Quantity

While in the trust and ultimatum games decisions can be based purely on reaction to the partner's behavior, other games have been devised that require careful consideration of how the partner is *likely* to behave in order to devise one's own strategy. Such thinking can become "hierarchical" or "higher order"—as my strategy will depend on what my partner is thinking, but this will depend on what he thinks I am thinking, and so on. Three recent studies have measured neural activity in games requiring this strategic inference.

In one study,[6] subjects were shown goods of which only they were told the value, and had the opportunity to buy these from social partners. Buyers were given the opportunity to suggest a price to their partners, but a deal was only made if the seller offered a price less then the true value of the goods. A good deal for the buyer is therefore one where the price offered is far lower than the true value of the goods. The key feature of this task is that the "suggestion" forms the only social exchange between buyer and seller, and the buyer can determine the relationship between this suggestion and the true value. Machiavellian subjects will try to throw sellers off the scent by pretending high value goods are worth little, but low value goods are very valuable. If sellers follow their suggestions, they will never obtain the low value goods, but will get the high value goods at a cheap price. Buyers who perform in this Machiavellian way show particular activation in a region of the theory of mind network, the right temporoparietal junction (rTPJ), on the trials where they are presented with high value goods (which they attempt to buy at a low price).

An elegant means of measuring strategic inference is to make use of a game from experimental economics known as the "beauty contest."[37] In this game, a group of subjects have to pick a number between 0 and 100, but the winner is selected by picking the subject who is closest to a fraction M (e.g., 4/5) of all other players' selections. If a subject assumes everyone else is naïve and chooses 50 on average, then it makes sense to select 4/5 of 50, 40 ("first-order" theory of mind). A more sophisticated subject might realize that this is what everyone else will think, and so select 32 ("second-order" theory of mind). Yet more sophistication will yield an answer of 26, 21, 17, and so on. Across multiple rounds of the game with varying values of M, subjects tend to show a consistent level of strategic inference, but there is considerable interindividual variability in the strategy chosen. Coricelli and colleagues[13] exploited this to investigate which brain structures showed differential brain activity across subjects with different levels of strategic sophistication. When contrasting trials in which the game was played with human (as opposed to computer) partners, subjects with higher-level reasoning showed more activity in another region in the theory of mind network, the dorsomedial prefrontal cortex (DMPFC).

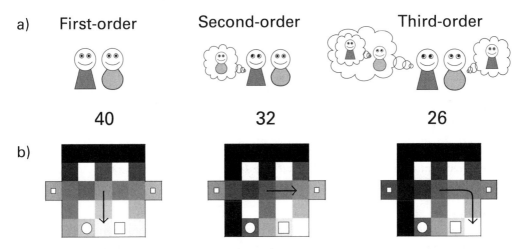

Figure 22.1
Different levels of strategic inference yield different strategies in experimental games. (a) In the beauty contest game,[13] subjects select a number between 1 and 100, aiming for a fixed proportion of the selections of other players of the game (in this case, 4/5). Assuming other players are naïve (a first-order strategy) yields an optimal guess of 40; assuming other players are first-order yields an optimal "second-order" strategy (32), and so on. (b) In the stag hunt game, subjects either hunt a stationary rabbit (small squares) or cooperate with a partner (circle) to hunt a moving stag (large square). The color intensity of each of the squares shows the *value function* for each position on the board, derived from the computational model devised by Yoshida and colleagues.[55] Adopting a first-, second-, or third-order strategy yields different value functions, and so different movements from the center of the board (arrows). Fitting the model to real subjects' behavior allows inference of which strategy best describes subjects' current play.

The level of strategic inference has typically been found to be quite limited in the beauty contest game (the median level being either first- or second-order inference[10]). However, this may be because such calculations must be performed explicitly as opposed to implicitly in this task, and critically, because there is no opportunity to adapt one's strategy in light of witnessing social partners' recent behavior. Yoshida and colleagues have recently developed a paradigm that allows for precisely this (figure 22.1). The task is based on the "stag hunt" game,[48] in which players must choose whether to act in a cooperative manner with their partner. Cooperative behavior from both players is more rewarding than noncooperative play, but unreciprocated cooperative play is least rewarding of all. One therefore needs to infer that the partner is likely to cooperate before deciding that cooperation is worthwhile.

In the version of the stag hunt presented by Yoshida et al., subjects played iteratively with a computer player who adopted a strategy with a particular level of inference. The authors had previously constructed a model[55] that attempts to infer this strategy from the behavior of the partner. Human subjects were found to be successful in tracking the level of inference of quite sophisticated computer agents (such as a computer playing a fifth-order strategy). Moreover, when witnessing the partner's behavior, the dorsomedial prefrontal cortex was found to correlate with a model parameter that described the entropy of the distribution over possible values that the partner's strategy might take.[56] By finding a correlate of this term, which is critical for updating the likely future behavior of the partner, in DMPFC, we can conclude that DMPFC may play an important role in *learning* about sophisticated aspects of the future behavior of other individuals.

Regions Implicated in Theory of Mind Are Implicated in Learning via Reinforcement about Other Agents' Behavior

Two further studies have used the strategy of applying a reinforcement learning (RL) model to tracking the behavior of a partner in a socially interactive setting. In one study,[5] subjects had to simultaneously learn about which of two options was likely to be rewarded, but had the advice of a confederate at each trial, who had the option of providing the subject with the correct (or incorrect) answer (figure 22.2). The confederate was motivated such that he might provide helpful or unhelpful advice, but the subject could learn this motive only by carefully observing how often the confederate was helpful. This learning could be tracked using an RL model, which contained separable terms for the *prediction error* and *learning rate* of the confederate's intentions. At the time point critical for learning, the DMPFC, right TPJ, and superior temporal sulcus were found to correlate with the prediction error term, which was not in the traditional frame of reference of reward to oneself, but instead in the frame of reference of the *other individual's actions*. A gyral portion of anterior cingulate cortex correlated with the learning rate in this frame of reference.

Another study employed an iterated inspection game, in which an "inspector" chooses whether or not to monitor the behavior of a "worker."[24] Inspecting is costly if the worker is already working, whereas working is costly if the inspector fails to inspect. If both players were to play the task optimally, the best strategy would be to adopt a mixed strategy of assigning a certain probability to each action, and selecting from these probabilities at random. However, if either player is suboptimal, human subjects might track the *previous* behavior of the partner, and use this to *infer* a strategy that exploits the other subject's behavior. A yet more sophisticated strategy would incorporate the *influence* of each player's current action on the next move that the partner would take. Quantitative RL models can be built that deploy each of these strategies; both superior temporal sulcus and DMPFC signal the "influence update term" at the time critical for learning, and activity in DMPFC correlates with the likelihood that the sophisticated influence model is being used.

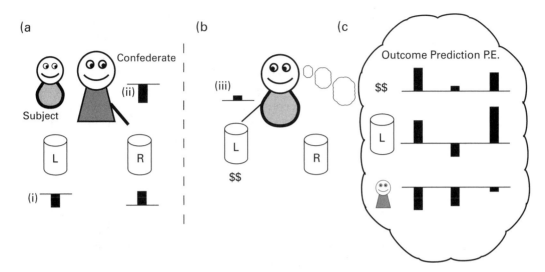

Figure 22.2
Different prediction errors in dissociable frames of reference. The figure depicts an example trial from the study by Behrens and colleagues.[5] (a) The subject aims to maximize reward obtained by choosing which cup (left or right) contains money. From previous trials, he has learned a prediction that the right cup is slightly more likely to yield reward than left (i). However, he also observes advice from a confederate who *knows* which cup contains reward, and who he has learned is very likely to give him misleading advice (ii). The confederate advises him to choose the right cup. (b) Combining these two probabilities convinces the subject that the left cup is more likely to be rewarding (iii). He chooses this cup, and discovers that he has won on this trial. (c) This yields dissociable prediction errors in three distinct frames of reference: first, in the traditional frame of reference of reward on one's own actions; second, in the frame of reference of which cup is likely to yield reward; and third, in the frame of reference of the *intentions* of the other player—how likely he is to be helpful or otherwise in the future.

The Frame of Reference Has Been Established, But the Computations Performed Remain Unclear

While the use of reinforcement learning models in tracking the value of one's own possible behaviors has now become commonplace, these studies argue that the neural mechanisms supporting the tracking of other's behavior may require similar computations, but implemented in parallel in discrete neural structures, and discrete frames of reference. While they all agree that the computation performed in DMPFC is critical for inference about the intention of a social partner, already some differences can be seen between the terms in the model used to describe activity in this region. For instance, DMPFC activity in the study by Behrens et al.[5] reflected a *signed* prediction on the probability of the social partner *lying*, whereas activity in the study by Hampton[24] reflected an *unsigned* prediction error, that is activity was greatest when the partner's behavior was most *surprising*. In the Yoshida et al.[56] study, the *entropy* of the distribution over possible partner strategies should determine how important each new partner move is for updating future estimates of partner behavior, and this term is reflected in the DMPFC; in study by Behrens et al.,[5] however, the analogous metric that is important for learning (the *volatility* of subject behavior) was reflected in the gyral portion of ACC, not DMPFC. Careful dissection and examination of the differences between the tasks and the models that are used to explain these data and to capture the dynamics of the task are needed. This may be achieved by designing tasks in which computational models of activity in these regions can be directly pitted against one another.[49]

What about Striatal Activations for Social Prediction Errors?

Here it is worth briefly revisiting studies that have found signals that resemble prediction errors in a socially interactive setting, but have found these in striatum rather than the theory of mind network. King-Casas and colleagues[30,31] have carefully examined data collected from subjects interacting in an iterated version of the trust game, that allows for the building of a reputation between investor and trustee. In the trustee's brain, they find increased activity in the head of the caudate nucleus when the investor reciprocates their past behavior in a generous fashion (benevolent reciprocity) compared to trials when they fail to do so (malevolent reciprocity). This activity could be a prediction error in the frame of reference of the *investor's* future behavior—an adjustment of the trustee's expectations of the investor—or alternatively a prediction error in the frame of reference of the *trustee's* future behavior—as benevolent reciprocity is more likely to induce an increase in trust. King-Casas et al. show clear evidence for the latter proposition—the activity in striatum is increased selectively on trials in which the trustee is to increase his *own* level of trusting behavior in future rounds.

Klucharev and colleagues[33] scanned subjects as they rated the attractiveness of photographs of individuals in a "hot or not"-style task; they then presented the average rating of a group of other individuals who had rated the picture. As expected, later ratings of the same photographs were highly influenced by what others thought of the photo, and the striatum and ACC were both found to be influenced by conflict between one's own opinions and that of others. Again, however, this signal (likened by the authors to a prediction error) is in the frame of reference of one's own behavior, as evidenced by the fact that it is stronger when one's own behavior is modified by the conflict than when it is not.

Finally, two recent studies have focused on prediction errors witnessed during learning by observation, in which two subjects perform the same task in parallel. In this situation, information useful for the subject can be gleaned from the outcomes experienced by the other player. In one study,[28] the subject and social partner were placed in direct competition, and the prediction error in the ventral striatum for the other player was found to be negatively signed—thus, it reflected a reward prediction error from the player's own egocentric perspective, rather than that of the other player. In another study,[8] subjects received varying levels of information about the performance of another player—they either received no information, were able to observe the other player's actions, or were able observe both their actions and their payoff at each trial. In the last condition, even though the payoffs for the subjects meant they were not placed in direct competition, the ventral striatum still signaled a negative reward prediction error for the outcomes of the other player (while also signaling a positive reward prediction error for one's own outcomes).

Conclusions

There is a rapidly expanding literature on decision making, or the use of motivational and cognitive control, in a social setting. Socially derived reward and conflict appear to activate similar networks to those found in nonsocial settings. The formal, quantitative models derived from game theory allow close measurement of the impact that others' presence or behavior has on one's own actions. Recent studies have begun to tease apart networks where the social preferences expressed in these games might be computed. Regions of the theory of mind network perform computations in the frame of reference of a social partner's intentions. The right DLPFC appears particularly important in balancing conflict between the inferred intentions of other individuals and one's own goals. By being precise and formal about the metrics that vary within a task and their frame of reference, we should achieve a much more rigorous and precise understanding of the underlying computations that these regions perform.

Outstanding Questions

• How can the frame of reference in which neural activity varies be refined to accurately reflect neural activity? How do computations in subregions of the theory of mind network differ from each? Do they vary in discrete frames of reference?

• How is information in discrete frames of reference combined to support action selection? Can we distinguish competing accounts of activity within the same region?

• What happens at the single cell, rather than the metabolic level? What are the computations instantiated at the neural network level that underlie the observed phenomena in the BOLD fMRI signal? Are these computations uniquely human or do they also take place in other organisms?

Further Reading

Behrens TEJ, Hunt LT, Rushworth MFS. 2009. The computation of social behavior. *Science* 324: 1160–1164. Describes some of the first applications of reinforcement learning models to studies of human social interaction, with particular reference to neuroimaging data and distinctions between the theory of mind network and other brain regions.

Fehr E, Camerer CF. 2007. Social neuroeconomics: the neural circuitry of social preference. *Trends Cogn Sci* 11: 419–427. Reviews in detail some of the paradigms from experimental economics that have been used to demonstrate other-regarding preferences, and their effects on regions associated with motivational and cognitive control.

Yoshida W, Seymour B, Friston KJ, Dolan RJ. 2010. Neural mechanisms of belief inference during cooperative games. *J Neurosci* 30: 10744–10751. An elegant study in which the authors used a reinforcement learning model to track the level of strategic inference used by players in a stag hunt game, and found neural correlates of dissociable model parameters in regions associated with reward (striatum) and mentalizing (paracingulate cortex)

References

1. Baron-Cohen S, Leslie AM, Frith U. 1985. Does the autistic child have a "theory of mind"? *Cognition* 21: 37–46.

2. Baron-Cohen S, Ring HA, Wheelright S, Bullmore ET, Brammer MJ, Simmons A, Williams SCR. 1999. Social intelligence in the normal and autistic brain: an fMRI study. *Eur J Neurosci* 11: 1891–1898.

3. Becerra L, Breiter HC, Wise R, Gonzalez RG, Borsook D. 2001. Reward circuitry activation by noxious thermal stimuli. *Neuron* 32: 927–946.

4. Behrens TE, Hunt LT, Rushworth MF. 2009. The computation of social behavior. *Science* 324: 1160–1164.

5. Behrens TE, Hunt LT, Woolrich MW, Rushworth MF. 2008. Associative learning of social value. *Nature* 456: 245–249.

6. Bhatt MA, Lohrenz T, Camerer CF, Montague PR. 2010. Neural signatures of strategic types in a two-person bargaining game. *Proc Natl Acad Sci USA* 107: 19720–19725.

7. Brothers L. 1990. The social brain: a project for integrating primate behavior and neurophysiology in a new domain. *Concepts Neurosci* 1: 27–51.

8. Burke CJ, Tobler PN, Baddeley M, Schultz W. 2010. Neural mechanisms of observational learning. *Proc Natl Acad Sci USA* 107: 14431–14436.

9. Camerer CF. 2003. Behavioral Game Theory: Experiments in Strategic Interaction. Princeton, NJ: Princeton University Press.

10. Camerer CF, Ho T-H, Chong J-K. 2004. A cognitive hierarchy model of games. *Q J Econ* 119: 861–898.

11. Campbell-Meiklejohn DK, Bach DR, Roepstorff A, Dolan RJ, Frith C. 2010. How the opinion of others affects our valuation of objects. *Curr Biol* 20: 1165–1170.

12. Cohen YE, Andersen RA. 2002. A common reference frame for movement plans in the posterior parietal cortex. *Nat Rev Neurosci* 3: 553–562.

13. Coricelli G, Nagel R. 2009. Neural correlates of depth of strategic reasoning in medial prefrontal cortex. *Proc Natl Acad Sci USA* 106: 9163–9168.

14. De Quervain DJ, Fischbacher U, Treyer V, Schellhammer M, Schnyder U, Buck A, Fehr E. 2004. The neural basis of altruistic punishment. *Science* 305: 1254–1258.

15. Deaner RO, Khera AV, Platt ML. 2005. Monkeys pay per view: adaptive valuation of social images by rhesus macaques. *Curr Biol* 15: 543–548.

16. Delgado MR, Schotter A, Ozbay EY, Phelps EA. 2008. Understanding overbidding: using the neural circuitry of reward to design economic auctions. *Science* 321: 1849–1852.

17. Dunbar R. 1993. Coevolution of neocortex size, group size and language in humans. *Behav Brain Sci* 16: 681–735.

18. Duncan J, Owen AM. 2000. Common regions of the human frontal lobe recruited by diverse cognitive demands. *Trends Neurosci* 23: 475–483.

19. Falk A, Fischbacher U. 2006. A theory of reciprocity. *Games Econ Behav* 54: 293–315.

20. Fehr E, Fischbacher U. 2003. The nature of human altruism. *Nature* 425: 785–791.

21. Fehr E, Schmidt KM. 1999. A theory of fairness, competition and cooperation. *Q J Econ* 114: 817–868.

22. Fletcher PC, Happe F, Frith U, Baker SC, Dolan RJ, Frackowiak RS, Frith CD. 1995. Other minds in the brain: a functional imaging study of "theory of mind" in story comprehension. *Cognition* 57: 109–128.

23. Gallagher HL, Happé F, Brunswick N, Fletcher PC, Frith U, Frith C. 2000. Reading the mind in cartoons and stories: an fMRI study of "theory of mind" in verbal and nonverbal tasks. *Neuropsycholgia* 38: 11–21.

24. Hampton AN, Bossaerts P, O'Doherty JP. 2008. Neural correlates of mentalizing-related computations during strategic interactions in humans. *Proc Natl Acad Sci USA* 105: 6741–6746.

25. Harbaugh WT, Mayr U, Burghart DR. 2007. Neural responses to taxation and voluntary giving reveal motives for charitable donations. *Science* 316: 1622–1625.

26. Hare TA, Camerer CF, Knoepfle DT, O'Doherty JP, Rangel A. 2010. Value computations in ventral medial prefrontal cortex during charitable decision making incorporate input from regions involved in social cognition. *J Neurosci* 30: 583–590.

27. Homans G. 1958. Social behavior as exchange. *Am J Sociol* 62: 597–606.

28. Howard-Jones PA, Bogacz R, Yoo JH, Leonards U, Demetriou S. 2010. The neural mechanisms of learning from competitors. *Neuroimage* 53: 790–799.

29. Izuma K, Saito DN, Sadato N. 2008. Processing of social and monetary rewards in the human striatum. *Neuron* 58: 284–294.

30. King-Casas B, Sharp C, Lomax-Bream L, Lohrenz T, Fonagy P, Montague PR. 2008. The rupture and repair of cooperation in borderline personality disorder. *Science* 321: 806–810.

31. King-Casas B, Tomlin D, Anen C, Camerer CF, Quartz SR, Montague PR. 2005. Getting to know you: reputation and trust in a two-person economic exchange. *Science* 308: 78–83.

32. Klein JT, Deaner RO, Platt ML. 2008. Neural correlates of social target value in macaque parietal cortex. *Curr Biol* 18: 419–424.

33. Klucharev V, Hytonen K, Rijpkema M, Smidts A, Fernadez G. 2009. Reinforcement learning signal predicts social conformity. *Neuron* 61: 140–151.

34. Knoch D, Gianotti LR, Pascual-Leone A, Treyer V, Regard M, Hohmann M, Brugger P. 2006. Disruption of right prefrontal cortex by low-frequency repetitive transcranial magnetic stimulation induces risk-taking behavior. *J Neurosci* 26: 6469–6472.

35. Knoch D, Schneider F, Schunk D, Hohmann M, Fehr E. 2009. Disrupting the prefrontal cortex diminishes the human ability to build a good reputation. *Proc Natl Acad Sci USA* 106: 20895–20899.

36. Moll J, Krueger F, Zahn R, Pardini M, de Oliveira-Souza R, Grafman J. 2006. Human fronto-mesolimbic networks guide decisions about charitable donation. *Proc Natl Acad Sci USA* 103: 15623–15628.

37. Nagel R. 1995. Unravelling in guessing games: an experimental study. *Am Econ Rev* 85: 1313–1326.

38. Nitz DA. 2009. Parietal cortex, navigation and the construction of arbitrary reference frames for spatial navigation. *Neurobiol Learn Mem* 91: 179–185.

39. O'Doherty JP, Dayan P, Friston KJ, Critchley H, Dolan RJ. 2003. Temporal difference models and reward-related learning in the human brain. *Neuron* 38: 329–337.

40. Poldrack RA. 2006. Can cognitive processes be inferred from neuroimaging data? *Trends Cogn Sci* 10: 59–63.

41. Ridderinkhof KR, Ullsperger M, Crone EA, Nieuwenhuis S. 2004. The role of the medial frontal cortex in cognitive control. *Science* 306: 443–447.

42. Rilling J, Gutman D, Zeh T, Pagnoni G, Berns G, Kilts C. 2002. A neural basis for social cooperation. *Neuron* 35: 395–405.

43. Rilling JK, Sanfey AG, Aronson JA, Nystrom LE, Cohen JD. 2004. The neural correlates of theory of mind within interpersonal interactions. *Neuroimage* 22: 1694–1703.

44. Sanfey AG, Rilling JK, Aronson JA, Nystrom LE, Cohen JD. 2003. The neural basis of economic decision-making in the Ultimatum Game. *Science* 300: 1755–1758.

45. Schultz W, Dayan P, Montague PR. 1997. A neural substrate of prediction and reward. *Science* 275: 1593–1599.

46. Seymour B, Daw ND, Dayan P, Singer T, Dolan RJ. 2007. Differential encoding of losses and gains in the human striatum. *J Neurosci* 27: 4826–4831.

47. Singer T, Seymour B, O'Doherty JP, Stephan KE, Dolan RJ, Frith CD. 2006. Empathic neural responses are modulated by the perceived fairness of others. *Nature* 439: 466–469.

48. Skyrms B. 2004. The Stag Hunt and Evolution of Social Structure. Cambridge: Cambridge University Press.

49. Stephan KE, Penny WD, Daunizeau J, Moran RJ, Friston KJ. 2009. Bayesian model selection for group studies. *Neuroimage* 46: 1004–1017.

50. Thaler RH. 1988. Anomalies: the ultimatum game. *J Econ Perspect* 2: 195–206.

51. Tricomi E, Rangel A, Camerer CF, O'Doherty JP. 2010. Neural evidence for inequality-averse social preferences. *Nature* 463: 1089–1091.

52. Van den Bos W, van Dijk E, Westenberg M, Rombouts S, Crone EA. 2009. What motivates repayment? Neural correlates of reciprocity in the Trust Game. *Soc Cogn Affect Neurosci* 4: 294–304.

53. Van Overwalle F. 2009. Social cognition and the brain: a meta-analysis. *Hum Brain Mapp* 30: 829–858.

54. Yamagishi T, Horita Y, Takagishi H, Shinada M, Tanida S, Cook KS. 2009. The private rejection of unfair offers and emotional commitment. *Proc Natl Acad Sci USA* 106: 11520–11523.

55. Yoshida W, Dolan RJ, Friston KJ. 2008. Game theory of mind. *PLOS Comput Biol* 4: e1000254.

56. Yoshida W, Seymour B, Friston KJ, Dolan RJ. 2010. Neural mechanisms of belief inference during cooperative games. *J Neurosci* 30: 10744–10751.

23 Model-Based Approaches to the Study of the Neural Basis of Cognitive Control

Sven Bestmann and Rogier B. Mars

Our brains have been formed by evolution to optimize action selection and execution in order to promote our survival. This requires the processing of incoming sensory information, weighing its contextual relevance based on both the external environment and our internal state, deciding between alternative actions, selecting the appropriate movement, and evaluating the executed behavior for its result. Often, these processes rely on internal variables that are not directly observable to an experimenter, such as motivation, homeostasis, and decision history. A complete, ecologically valid approach for studying the neural processes underlying cognitive control necessitates taking these variables into account.

The question, then, is how to study these context-specific, dynamic, and interacting processes. Functional imaging studies have traditionally used an approach based on identifying brain regions that show a change in activity during an experimental condition compared to an appropriate control condition (e.g., rest). Rather than asking for the presence or absence of activity changes due to changes in an experimental variable, however, understanding the neural activity changes underlying processes as diverse as action preparation, probabilistic learning, or contextual updating requires formal models that provide access to the "hidden states" in the neural data that may underlie action selection (figure 23.1a, b).

Computationally informed models can capture these hidden states or internal variables that the brain needs to represent, and one can then use these models to interrogate the behavioral and neural data. Types of models that have been employed include optimal foraging models describing animal's decisions in finding food[43] and in social interaction[21] in zoology, game theory in economics,[8] and also reinforcement learning models developed in machine learning.[46] More recently, such models have found increased employment in the study of the neural basis of cognitive control and decision making.[19,33]

In the present chapter we aim to first illustrate how model-based approaches can provide accurate mechanistic descriptions of behavioral and neural data. Second, we use examples from functional magnetic resonance imaging (fMRI),

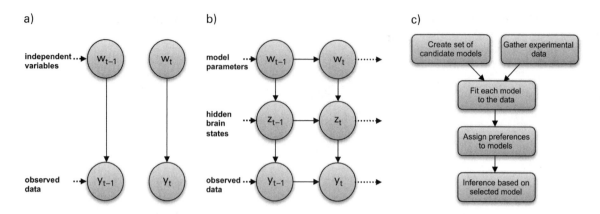

Figure 23.1
(a) Schematic representation of the traditional approach to analysis of neural data. The presence or absence of a certain condition, *w*, on each trial is correlated directly with neural activity, *y*, for instance, the amplitude of an event-related potential or BOLD. (b) The model-based approach suggests that we employ computational models to estimate the relations between trials and the value of the hidden, not directly observable, states, *z*, that mediate the transfer from the specific stimulus input on a given trial and the neural data. (c) Stages involved in the model-based approach, as suggested by MacKay.[30]

electroencephalography (EEG), and transcranial magnetic stimulation (TMS) studies that demonstrate the type of inferences arising from computational models and model comparison that in the future will become more and more essential to address topical questions about cognitive control.

Model-Based Analyses

Model-based approaches provide quantitative predictions about the hidden states, *z*, that our brain is likely to encode but that are not directly accessible to us. Thus, they provide testable hypotheses on how the brain may represent and encode different processes relevant to cognitive control. For example, performance monitoring requires not only monitoring the outcome of an action, but also a representation of the goal of the action, local trial history, and strategy. This can be formally expressed in models that predict the influence of prior information, *w*, on neural activity, *y*, on a given trial via the unobserved but modeled hidden process. Thus, rather than simply correlating neural activity, *y*, with the presence or absence of a certain stimulus, *w* (figure 23.1a), we aim to estimate the value of the hidden variables mediating this relationship, *z* (figure 23.1b).

The basic procedure for model-based analyses is then as follows (figure 23.1c, see Mars et al.[33] and Daw[11] for an in-depth discussion). First, one has to create a model that can emulate the task in the way hypothesized. This model should describe the transformation of stimuli to the observable behavioral responses and contain the not directly observable variables that affect this transformation (indicated by z in figure 23.1b). One advantage of this approach is that not just one candidate model, but any set of candidate models can be created and compared by fitting the output of these models to the behavioral or neural data from each participant. Often, models have some free parameters—for example, the learning rate in simple reinforcement learning models—which need to be fitted to the individual dataset before one assesses the model fit. These free parameters can, for instance, reflect individual differences between participants. However, one should be cautious not to employ too many free parameters, since this reduces the specificity of the model.

A critical advantage of using formal models is that they permit model comparison; model comparison techniques can account for the number of parameters in a model.[7,51] As formal models encapsulate hypotheses about how different cognitive processes cause the observed activity (or behavior), one can now test whether alternative models (hypotheses) provide more parsimonious explanations of the observed data. A model perfectly emulating the hidden states, z, should perfectly predict the observed data, y, and given these data, the evidence of a model can be used to assess its usefulness. This is quite different from merely assessing the goodness of fit of one model to the data, as in classical statistics. Moreover, it is the formal structure of such models that is appealing: this makes it easy to modify or expand models, but also provides a high level of transparency about the assumptions being made. Because one can, in principle, account for different degrees of model complexity, models of varying structure and complexity can be directly compared. Increasing the complexity of a model can lead to overfitting, and one can assess whether increasing the complexity of a model provides a more parsimonious explanation of the observed data. But perhaps more important, one can in principle compare models that may be very different in their spirit and architecture, and may embellish very different hypotheses on how the data was caused. This may be particularly relevant for studies of cognitive control, where several competing hypotheses (and therefore models) about the processes involved often exist.

An Example: The Use of Information Theory

One essential requirement for quick and successful action selection is having a representation of the previous history and the current state of the environment in order to make predictions about forthcoming events. For example, attention may be allocated to events that are unexpected in the current context, that is, "surprising" events. Fewer resources might therefore be required to process predicted events, which in turn may free resources to respond to unexpected surprising events. Thus, it has been suggested that the cortex may have evolved to predict regularities in the environment, in which surprising events play a central role.[28,39] This might allow for flexible and efficient action selection in the face of an uncertain environment. Indeed, a mechanism of predicting and detecting prediction violations has been suggested as a principle computational mechanism throughout the cortex.[17]

First evidence that observers' responses depend on their estimation of the probability of an event occurring comes from the work of Hick[24] and Hyman.[27] These authors showed a linear mapping from the number of options in a forced-choice task to observed reaction time. This suggests that a statistical model could be used to form hypotheses as to how humans encode uncertainty to make informed decisions and select their actions accordingly. The probabilities of events can be viewed as representing "causes," in that they are used to generate sequences of these events to which an observer has to react. As Hick[24] and Hyman[27] suggest, an observer may track the statistics of these causes over time. These statistics can therefore form the basis of a computational model whose purpose is to explain observed responses of humans to uncertainty. One way to achieve this is to use information theory,[41] which provides explanatory variables that are a function of the observers' estimate of the probability distribution responsible for generating samples.[3,23,32,44]

For example, given samples of an event, the objective is to estimate the probability of the kth event occurring and a measure of uncertainty over it. The number of "counts" of the kth event type, α_k, is updated according to the following formula

$$\alpha_k(N) = \sum_{i=1}^{N} \exp((t_N - t_i)/\tau)\delta(x_i = k)$$

where t_i is the time of the ith observation and $\delta(x_i = k)$ equals 1 if the ith observation was of the kth symbol. The count variables for time point t_N are therefore based on all previous observations, but they are exponentially weighted depending on recency. If we assume that $\tau = \infty$ (in this case the exponential terms reduce to unity), the model never forgets and all past observations are taken into account. The counts are all initialized to 1 at the first time point.

The posterior probability of the kth event occurring is given by the kth parameter of a multinomial distribution[4]

$$\rho_k(N) = \frac{\alpha_k(N) + \alpha_k^0}{\sum_{j=1}^{K} \alpha_j(N) + \sum_{j=1}^{K} \alpha_j^0}$$

The information content or "surprise" of the Nth trial is given by

$$l(N) = -\log \rho_k(N)$$

Thus the occurrence of a low probability event is more surprising. The entropy (average information content) is given by

$$H(N) = -\sum_{k=1}^{K} \rho_k(N) \log \rho_k(N)$$

This procedure generates a series of effective counts which increases by one with each sample and provides a model of what an observer might be encoding when observing a sequence of events to which he has to respond. These can then be used to explain behavioral or neuronal responses, such as reaction time,[3,23,32,44] corticospinal excitability,[3] or fMRI and EEG data[23,32,44] (figure 23.2a). Intuitively, the lower the probability of the kth event occurring, the more surprised an individual is when it occurs. The more equiprobable the events are, the higher the uncertainty about the upcoming event, that is, the higher the entropy. For example, there is greater uncertainty in a fair coin toss than in one that is biased. Consequently, learning to select an appropriate action in response to uncertain and/or more surprising events may require more time. Such a simple computational model can therefore be used to capture the between-trial structure in a sequence of events (stimuli) and corresponding changes in neural or behavioral data.

In the following, we illustrate the model-based approach by presenting recent studies that use an information theoretic approach to investigate whether the brain might use a predictive strategy in action selection in simple choice RT tasks, whether it can be used to explain neural responses related to learning of contextual uncertainty, and whether one can apply this approach to predict electrophysiological response related to contextual surprise.

Action Preparation and Contextual Uncertainty

It is well established that prior information influences action preparation. For example, in monkeys, modulating response probability modulates reaction times and preparatory activity for eye[15] and arm movements.[29] In humans, preparatory activity is modulated by the probability of responding at the end of trial,[47] and by the probability that a particular movement will have to be executed at a given time.[48,50] These results suggest that activity in the motor system can reflect the uncertainty conveyed by visual information required for successful action selection. However, inferring action preparation as the underlying process for this reaction time effect was previously based on the average difference between the a priori known probabilities, thereby ignoring to a large degree the dynamical changes in the context and prior information that need to be learned in order to facilitate action selection. Using quantitative indices of uncertainty enables the analysis of such dynamic between-trial changes, and their influence on preparatory activity. In

a)

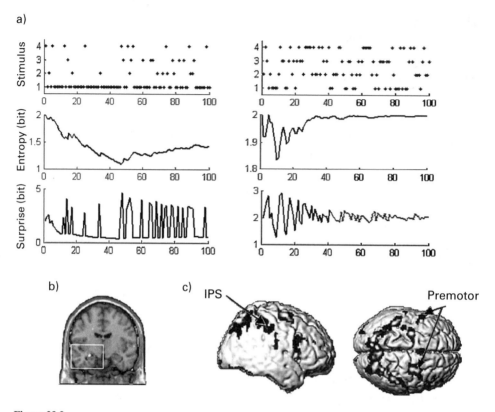

Figure 23.2
(a) Information theoretic measures of uncertainty and surprise. Left-hand panels show situation for highly predictable environment, right-hand panels for a poorly predictable environment. Top row shows occurrence of each of four stimuli during a block of 100 trials. It can be seen that in the highly predictable environment, the first stimulus occurs on most trials, whereas in the poorly predictable environment all stimuli are equiprobable over the course of the block. In the highly predictable environment, entropy diminishes over time, but stimuli occurring with a small probability will be surprising. (b) Activity in the anterior hippocampus correlates with entropy, suggesting that this region encodes the predictability of sequences of events. (c) Surprise correlated with activity in a widespread parietal-premotor network (IPS, intraparietal sulcus). Adapted from Strange et al.[44] with permission.

humans, one can investigate the dynamic changes in preparatory activity, and their correspondence with internal state variables such as uncertainty, using transcranial magnetic stimulation. This technique assesses changes in corticospinal excitability (CSE) during, for example, an instructed delay period. Prior work has established the use of this approach for measuring the physiological signature of action preparation in human motor cortex.[31,49]

In a first study investigating whether the predictive information theoretic models provided a good index of CSE during choice RT tasks, Bestmann and colleagues[3] measured CSE during a probabilistic action preparation task. In this instructed delay task, an instruction cue provided information about the forthcoming move-ment that participants had to make on presentation of a subsequent imperative cue presented about one second later. However, in different blocks of trials, the instruction cue predicted the identity of the imperative cue only with 85%, 70%, or 55% validity, respectively. In other words, in different blocks there were different degrees of uncertainty about the required action, given the instruction cue. These regularities were unknown to the participants and thus had to be learned on each block. As expected, behavioral data showed that participants reacted faster in trials in which the instruction cue was more reliable, yet this observation does not account for the dynamic process through which participants may have learned these underly-ing regularities.

The authors therefore quantified the contextual uncertainty within each block on a trial-by-trial basis using the formulas described previously to ask whether these quantities might predict subject's responses and their preparatory state prior to these (as measured through CSE). RTs and muscle-specific CSE changes were indeed influenced by both entropy and surprise: High uncertainty (high entropy) about the upcoming imperative cue was associated with decreases in CSE during the preparatory period. Moreover, a surprising imperative cue on the preceding trial resulted in a similar decrease in CSE. Thus, delay-period CSE, which provides an index of the preparatory state of a subject was lower when preparatory cues resolved less uncertainty (entropy), and when surprise in the preceding trigger cues was large.[3] Similar results were seen in the reaction time data. Bayesian model comparison furthermore showed that there was more evidence supporting this information theoretic model, given the RT and the CSE data, compared to a small group of alternative models that did not, or not fully, account for the contextual uncertainty inherent in the sequence of trials. Based on these results, the authors concluded that human motor cortex is dynamically biased according to (inferred) contextual probabilities inherent in visual events, which are represented dynami-cally in the brain.

The Encoding of Entropy and Surprise in the Human Brain

The preceding study showed that CSE was influenced by both entropy and surprise. However, the use of single-pulse TMS precludes inferences about brain regions outside primary motor cortex that may be involved in representing the stimulus environment, compute parameters such as surprise and entropy, and update the brain's model of the environment. This issue is better addressed using whole-brain fMRI, which allows the identification of neural activity changes related to contex-tual uncertainty. In a recent study by Strange and colleagues,[44] participants per-formed a simple choice RT task, in which four stimuli were matched to four responses and presented at different frequencies in different blocks (see figure 23.2a). In some blocks, some stimuli were presented more often than others, thus decreasing entropy, while surprise associated with more infrequent stimuli increased. In other blocks, the probability of occurrence was similar for each of the stimuli. In these cases, entropy was high whereas the surprise associated to each stimulus remained relatively low. Inferring these relative probabilities of occurrence may allow for preparing for the appropriate response in advance of a stimulus.

As in the study by Bestmann and colleagues,[3] a significant part of the variance in trial-by-trial fluctuations in reaction time was explained by entropy and surprise.[44] The authors then tested for neural activity explained by either entropy or surprise as a parametric modulation of stimulus occurrence. Activity in the hippocampus, although not showing a significant mean response to stimulus presentation, was modulated by entropy (figure 23.2b). Greater entropy, that is, more random stimulus occurrence, was associated with more hippocampal activity. Thus, although a simple main effect of task (stimulus presentation versus rest) would suggest that the hippocampus is not involved in this task, a model-based approach shows that the hippocampus may encode the expectation of an event before it occurs. In contrast, surprise was associated with activity in a network including bilateral parietal, premotor, inferior frontal, and thalamic regions (figure 23.2c). These results show the allocation of neural resources to surprising events and that less processing is required when events can be predicted.

Neural Signatures of Contextual Updating

It has previously been suggested that a number of salient neural phenomena, such as the P300, the error-related negativity, and the mismatch negativity, represent violations of predictions. Either in visual perception,[45] auditory perception,[20] or reward-based learning,[25] prediction errors or related processes such as surprise indeed seem to account for much of the variance in neural responses.[17,18] The P300 in particular has been described as a component of the event-related brain potential that indexes how surprising a stimulus is according to the brain's internal model of the environment, or the updating of the brain's model in light of novel evidence.[14] A prominent recent theory suggests that the P300 reflects the response of the locus coeruleus-norepinephrine system to the outcome of internal decision-making processes and the consequent effects of noradrenergic potentiation of information processing[35] (see chapter 12, this volume).

One prediction then is that the P300 in a probabilistic choice RT task can be described as a reflection of the trial-by-trial surprise conveyed by visual events. Mars and colleagues[32] tested this hypothesis by asking participants to perform a simple choice RT task similar to the one used by the study of Strange et al.[44] described earlier. During each block of 60 trials, the probability of occurrence of each stimulus varied. Thus, participants had to learn about this underlying structure in order to respond as fast as possible to these events. Again, entropy and surprise were calculated for an ideal Bayesian learner.

The authors first replicated previous work showing that a larger P300 amplitude is associated with less frequent stimuli (figure 23.3). However, the novel question was whether the dynamic changes in surprise would capture how this difference in P300 amplitude to the stimuli with different probabilities evolved. Mars and colleagues showed that the surprise model indeed provided the best explanation of trial-by-trial change in P300 amplitude. One interesting finding was that surprise captured well-known behaviors of the P300, for example, that as an infrequent stimuli is presented twice in succession, the P300 to the second presentation is smaller.[42] This is consistent with the "context-updating" hypothesis, suggesting that

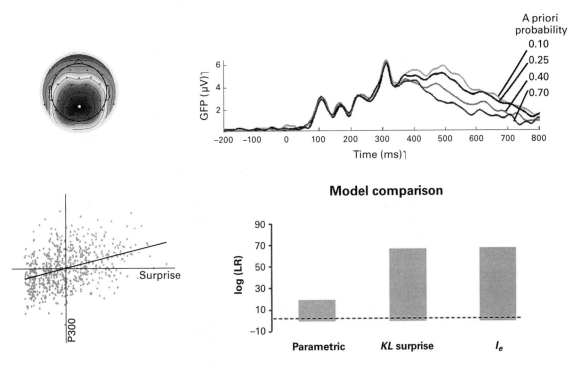

Figure 23.3
P300 and surprise. Top shows scalp distribution and modulation in the P300 by a priori stimulus probability, showing the central-parietal scalp distribution and increasing amplitude for less frequent stimuli commonly reported for P300. Bottom shows modulation of P300 by surprise for data from one participant. Bar graph indicates evidence in favor of a surprise model compared to alternative models that simply model a prior stimulus probability ("Parametric"), an alternative information theoretic measure of surprise ("*KL* surprise"), and surprise with an infinite memory over the whole experiment (i.e., participants assume that the stimulus probabilities remain unchanged between blocks, I_e). Adapted from Mars et al.[32] with permission.

participants update their mental schema following presentation of the first stimulus[13,14] (see chapter 12, this volume, for a discussion).

The Effects of Surprise

An important issue not addressed in the study of Mars and colleagues[32] was what kind of influence the surprise has on subsequent information processing. According to most models of the P300, and indeed most predictive coding models, the surprising stimulus or prediction error will affect the internal model of the environment. This issue was addressed in a recent study by Den Ouden and colleagues, in which the authors asked participants to perform an associative learning task while their brain activity was probed using fMRI.[12] Participants were required to classify a visual stimulus as either a house or a face. Auditory cues predicted the type of visual stimulus with a degree of validity that changed over time. Participants' behavior was modeled by a Bayesian learner that accounts for trial-by-trial updates of probability estimates.[2] Prediction errors were found in response to faces and houses in the fusiform face area (FFA) and the parahippocampal place area (PPA), respectively. Stimulus-independent prediction errors were found in the premotor cortex and the putamen. Importantly, prediction error responses in the putamen modulated the strength of interactions from FFA and PPA to the premotor cortex, illustrating the role of prediction errors in modulating subsequent information processing in relation to the selection of forthcoming actions.

The influence of changes in interaction strength was assessed using dynamic causal modeling (DCM). This technique uses biophysical modeling to generate predictions about the causal effects that generated observed neural data. Its aim is to determine which of several prespecified anatomical models best fits the data, that is, to explain regional BOLD responses in terms of interregional connectivity and its experimentally induced modulation. DCM calculates the statistical likelihood that an evoked response is driven by the flow of information from another, directly or indirectly connected brain region. The basic idea is to estimate the parameters of a reasonably realistic neural model such that the *predicted* regional BOLD signals, which result from converting the modeled neural dynamics into hemodynamic responses, correspond as closely as possible to the *observed* BOLD signals. DCM has been instrumental in providing new insight into the organization of brain systems, including action selection and perceptual inference and associative learning.[19,45] The study by Den Ouden et al. demonstrates the mutual benefits of the model-based approach described above and another form of model-based approach, namely the DCM. In combination, they allow the researcher to ask topical questions about effective connectivity changes and how these are influenced by computational processes that the brain needs to encode, such as prediction error.

Model-Based Approaches to Cognitive Control

The preceding example studies illustrate how a model-based approach, in this case employing information theory, can shed new light on neural data in even simple choice reaction time tasks, by providing trial-by-trial predictions about the causes of observed behavioral and neural data. Research on cognitive control has a strong tradition of employing computational models, as evident from the previous section of this volume. For instance, the error-related negativity (ERN) has been likened to a prediction error in reinforcement learning models. The original papers that put forward this theory focused on a qualitative comparison of the behavior of the ERN during task performance and the changes in the prediction error, as given by an implementation of an actor-critic reinforcement architecture.[1] The average prediction errors given by the model and the average ERPs recorded from healthy human participants showed the same modulation during learning.[25] Furthermore, they showed that changes in dopamine during normal aging could be simulated with the model, by changing the value of a single parameter. This influenced the modulation of the simulated prediction error; analog changes were reported in the ERN recorded from healthy aging participants.[36] Furthermore, it has been shown that individual differences in the value of fitted model parameters relate to differences in participants' choice behavior and neural activity in limbic and prefrontal areas[9] (see also chapter 14, this volume, for illustrations of the use of model-based approaches to individual differences). The original reinforcement learning model of the ERN has been extended substantially. In chapter 18 of the present volume, Holroyd and Yeung propose a hierarchical reinforcement learning model that makes prediction for ACC function, but also relates a number of other model parameters to specific neural areas. A model-based approach to imaging data, in which the trial-by-trial variations in these parameters are evaluated with respect to the fMRI data could now assess whether activity in the ACC is indeed explained by this newly extended model, compared to previously proposed models of ACC function.

The use of model-based approaches to tackle questions about cognitive control is likely to involve a plethora of competing models that formalize the various processes required for cognitive control, as illustrated by the existence of a number of competing models aimed at explaining the function of the anterior cingulate cortex in cognitive control.[5,6,25,26] Answering questions about their neural basis and influence on effective connectivity among brain regions involved in cognitive control, for example, is likely to require the ability to compare a large number of models. In computational fMRI,[19,37] computational models provide predictors that are fitted to behavioral and brain imaging data. The use of model comparison maps in addition to model-based fMRI now allows for differentiating between different computation models.[40] This is now possible through the recently developed Bayesian spatial models and Bayesian Model Selection (BMS) maps. These replace the classical approach to fMRI because competing models can now be compared, at each voxel, by measuring the model evidence for each model, given data (i.e., each voxel).[38] One critical advantage over the use of F-contrasts is that, in principle, any number of models, not restricted to linear, can be compared. Thus, BMS can address questions about different computational models and their functional representation, including non-nested designs that address questions about the best model, given brain responses.[10,33,37] The combination of computational models together with the use of BMS can therefore distinguish the representation of different computational models of, for example, value updating,[34,52] reinforcement learning,[22] or perceptual decision making,[16] and we expect this to be an important direction for future studies on cognitive control.

Acknowledgments

S.B. is supported by the Biotechnology and Biological Sciences Research Council (BBSRC) UK, R.B.M. is supported by the Medical Research Council (MRC) UK.

Outstanding Questions

• Previous model-based studies on cognitive control have largely focused on one specific aspect required for successful interaction with the world. Examples include the information theoretic models presented here to quantify probabilistic relationships among visual events in the context of action selection, or studies that employ models of prediction error in the context of reward processing and reward-based learning. In many cases, many processes (and models) are represented in the brain at the same time, including other important processes such as attention. Future work on cognitive control will require models that incorporate these different cognitive processes that often occur in parallel.

• What are the time courses over which our brain integrates past information to predict future events? The fact that we need to forget distant events appeals to intuition, but little work has been done on how distant information is discarded or weighted to generate predictions about future events.

• Model-based approaches have largely focused on functional data. To what extent is the degree with which these models can predict individual behavior paralleled by structural markers?

Further Reading

Friston KJ, Dolan RJ. 2010. Computational and dynamic models in neuroimaging. *NeuroImage* 52: 752–765. A recent review illustrating the use of computational models in neuroimaging. Contrasts this approach of using computational models of brain function with another recent trend of using computational models of the biophysics of hemodynamics and eletrophysiological time series.

Corrado G, Doya K. 2007. Understanding neural coding through the model-based analysis of decision making. *J Neurosci* 27: 8187–8180. Mini-review providing a nice introduction to the model-based approach to neuroimaging data.

References

1. Barto AG. 1995. Adaptive critics and the basal ganglia. In: Models of Information Processing in the Basal Ganglia (Houck JC, Davis J, Beiser D, eds), pp 215–232. Cambridge, MA: MIT Press.

2. Behrens TE, Woolrich MW, Walton ME, Rushworth MF. 2007. Learning the value of information in an uncertain world. *Nat Neurosci* 10: 1214–1221.

3. Bestmann S, Harrison LM, Blankenburg F, Mars RB, Haggard P, Friston KJ, Rothwell JC. 2008. Influence of uncertainty and surprise on human corticospinal excitability during preparation for action. *Curr Biol* 18: 775–780.

4. Bishop CM. 2006. Pattern Recognition and Machine Learning. New York: Springer.

5. Botvinick MM, Cohen JD, Carter CS. 2004. Conflict monitoring and anterior cingulate cortex: an update. *Trends Cogn Sci* 8: 539–546.

6. Brown JW, Braver TS. 2005. Learned predictions of error likelihood in the anterior cingulate cortex. *Science* 307: 1118–1121.

7. Burnham KP, Anderson DR. 2002. Model Selection and Multimodel Inference: A Practical Information-Theoretic Approach. New York: Springer.

8. Camerer CF. 2003. Behavioral Game Theory: Experiments in Strategic Interaction. Princeton, NJ: Princeton University Press.

9. Cohen MX. 2007. Individual differences and the neural representations of reward expectation and reward prediction error. *Soc Cogn Affect Neurosci* 2: 20–30.

10. Corrado G, Doya K. 2007. Understanding neural coding through the model-based analysis of decision making. *J Neurosci* 27: 8178–8180.

11. Daw N. in press. Trial by trial data analysis using computational models. In: Attention & Performance XIII: Decision Making, Affect, and Learning (Delgado MR, Phelps EA, Robbins TW, eds). Oxford: Oxford University Press.

12. Den Ouden HEM, Daunizeau J, Roiser J, Friston KJ, Stephan KE. 2010. Striatal prediction error modulates cortical coupling. *J Neurosci* 30: 3210–3219.

13. Donchin E. 1981. Surprise! . . . Surprise? *Psychophysiology* 18: 493–513.

14. Donchin E, Coles MGH. 1988. Is the P300 component a manifestation of context updating? *Psychophysiology* 11: 357–374.

15. Dorris MC, Munoz DP. 1998. Saccadic probability influences motor preparation signals and time to saccadic initiation. *J Neurosci* 18: 7015–7026.

16. Forstmann BU, Brown S, Dutilh G, Neumann J, Wagenmakers EJ. 2010. The neural substrate of prior information in perceptual decision making: a model-based analysis. *Front Hum Neurosci* 4: 40.

17. Friston K. 2005. A theory of cortical responses. *Philos Trans R Soc Lond B Biol Sci* 360: 815–836.

18. Friston K. 2009. The free-energy principle: a rough guide to the brain? *Trends Cogn Sci* 13: 293–301.

19. Friston KJ, Dolan RJ. 2010. Computational and dynamic models in neuroimaging. *Neuroimage* 52: 752–765.

20. Furl N, Kumar S, Alter K, Durrant S, Shawe-Taylor JS, Griffiths TD. 2011. Neural prediction of higher-order auditory sequence statistics. *Neuroimage* 54: 2267–2277.

21. Giraldeau LA, Caraco T. 2000. Social Foraging Theory. Princeton, NJ: Princeton University Press.

22. Glascher J, Daw N, Dayan P, O'Doherty JP. 2010. States versus rewards: dissociable neural prediction error signals underlying model-based and model-free reinforcement learning. *Neuron* 66: 585–595.

23. Harrison LM, Duggins A, Friston KJ. 2006. Encoding uncertainty in the hippocampus. *Neural Netw* 19: 535–546.

24. Hick WE. 1952. On the rate of gain of information. *Q J Exp Psychol* 4: 11–26.

25. Holroyd CB, Coles MG. 2002. The neural basis of human error processing: reinforcement learning, dopamine, and the error-related negativity. *Psychol Rev* 109: 679–709.

26. Holroyd CB, Nieuwenhuis S, Mars RB, Coles MGH. 2004. Anterior cingulate cortex, selection for action, and error processing. In: Cognitive Neuroscience of Attention (Posner MI, ed), pp 219–231. New York: Guilford Press.

27. Hyman R. 1953. Stimulus information as a determinant of reaction time. *J Exp Psychol* 45: 175–182.

28. Itti L, Baldi P. 2009. Bayesian surprise attracts human attention. *Vision Res* 49: 1295–1306.

29. Kalaska JF, Crammond DJ. 1995. Deciding not to GO: neuronal correlates of response selection in a GO/NOGO task in primate premotor and parietal cortex. *Cereb Cortex* 5: 410–428.

30. MacKay DJC. 1992. Bayesian interpolation. *Neural Comput* 4: 415–447.

31. Mars RB, Bestmann S, Rothwell JC, Haggard P. 2007. Effects of motor preparation and spatial attention on corticospinal excitability in a delayed-response paradigm. *Exp Brain Res* 182: 125–129.

32. Mars RB, Debener S, Gladwin TE, Harrison LM, Haggard P, Rothwell JC, Bestmann S. 2008. Trial-by-trial fluctuations in the event-related electroencephalogram reflect dynamic changes in the degree of surprise. *J Neurosci* 28: 12539–12545.

33. Mars RB, Shea NJ, Kolling N, Rushworth MFS. in press Model-based analyses: promises, pitfalls, and example applications to the study of cognitive control. *Q J Exp Psychol.*

34. Montague PR, McClure SM, Baldwin PR, Phillips PE, Budygin EA, Stuber GD, Kilpatrick MR, Wightman RM. 2004. Dynamic gain control of dopamine delivery in freely moving animals. *J Neurosci* 24: 1754–1759.

35. Nieuwenhuis S, Aston-Jones G, Cohen JD. 2005. Decision making, the P3, and the locus coeruleus-norepinephrine system. *Psychol Bull* 131: 510–532.

36. Nieuwenhuis S, Ridderinkhof KR, Talsma D, Coles MG, Holroyd CB, Kok A, van der Molen MW. 2002. A computational account of altered error processing in older age: dopamine and the error-related negativity. *Cogn Affect Behav Neurosci* 2: 19–36.

37. O'Doherty JP, Hampton A, Kim H. 2007. Model-based fMRI and its application to reward learning and decision making. *Ann N Y Acad Sci* 1104: 35–53.

38. Penny W, Flandin G, Trujillo-Barreto N. 2007. Bayesian comparison of spatially regularised general linear models. *Hum Brain Mapp* 28: 275–293.

39. Rao RPN, Ballard DH. 1999. Predictive coding in the visual cortex: a functional interpretation of some extra-classical receptive-field effects. *Nat Neurosci* 2: 79–87.

40. Rosa MJ, Bestmann S, Harrison L, Penny W. 2010. Bayesian model selection maps for group studies. *Neuroimage* 49: 217–224.

41. Shannon CE. 1948. A mathematical theory of communication. *Bell Syst Tech J* 27: 379–423.

42. Squires KC, Wickens C, Squires NK, Donchin E. 1976. The effect of stimulus sequence on the waveform of the cortical event-related potential. *Science* 193: 1142–1146.

43. Stephens DW, Krebs JR. 1986. Foraging Theory. Princeton, NJ: Princeton University Press.

44. Strange BA, Duggins A, Penny W, Dolan RJ, Friston KJ. 2005. Information theory, novelty and hippocampal responses: unpredicted or unpredictable? *Neural Netw* 18: 225–230.

45. Summerfield C, Koechlin E. 2008. A neural representation of prior information during perceptual inference. *Neuron* 59: 336–347.

46. Sutton RS, Barto AG. 1998. Reinforcement Learning: An Introduction. Cambridge, MA: MIT Press.

47. Thoenissen D, Zilles K, Toni I. 2002. Differential involvement of parietal and precentral regions in movement preparation and motor intention. *J Neurosci* 22: 9024–9034.

48. Trillenberg P, Verleger R, Wascher E, Wauschkuhn B, Wessel K. 2000. CNV and temporal uncertainty with 'ageing' and 'non-ageing' S1–S2 intervals. *Clin Neurophysiol* 111: 1216–1226.

49. Van den Hurk P, Mars RB, van Elswijk G, Hegeman J, Pasman JW, Bloem BR, Toni I. 2007. Online maintenance of sensory and motor representations: effects on corticospinal excitability. *J Neurophysiol* 97: 1642–1648.

50. Van Elswijk G, Kleine BU, Overeem S, Stegeman DF. 2007. Expectancy induces dynamic modulation of corticospinal excitability. *J Cogn Neurosci* 19: 121–131.

51. Wagenmakers EJ, Waldorp L. 2006. Editor's introduction to the special issue on model selection: theoretical developments and applications. *J Math Psychol* 50: 99–100.

52. Wunderlich K, Rangel A, O'Doherty JP. 2009. Neural computations underlying action-based decision making in the human brain. *Proc Natl Acad Sci USA* 106: 17199–17204.

Contributors

Adam R. Aron Department of Psychology, University of California–San Diego, La Jolla, CA

Timothy E. J. Behrens Centre for Functional MRI of the Brain, University of Oxford, Oxford, United Kingdom

Sven Bestmann Sobell Department of Motor Neuroscience and Movement Disorders, University College London, London, United Kingdom

Erie D. Boorman Computation and Neural Systems, California Institute of Technology, Pasadena, CA

Matthew M. Botvinick Princeton Neuroscience Institute, Princeton University, Princeton, NJ

Gabriele Chierchia Center for Mind/Brain Sciences, University of Trento, Rovereto, Italy

Jeffrey Cockburn Cognitive, Linguistic and Psychological Science, Brown University, Providence, RI

Michael X Cohen Department of Psychology, University of Amsterdam, Amsterdam, The Netherlands

Giorgio Coricelli Department of Economics, University of Southern California, Los Angeles, CA

Eveline A. Crone Department of Psychology, Leiden University, Leiden, The Netherlands

Ellen R. A. de Bruijn Donders Institute for Brain, Cognition and Behaviour, Radboud University Nijmegen, Nijmegen, The Netherlands

Peter F. Dominey Stem Cell and Brain Research Institute, INSERM U846, Bron, France

Birte U. Forstmann Department of Psychology, University of Amsterdam, Amsterdam, The Netherlands

Michael Frank Cognitive, Linguistic and Psychological Science, Brown University, Providence, RI

Jerylin O. Gan Department of Psychiatry & Behavioral Science, University of Washington, Seattle, WA

Ian Greenhouse   Department of Psychology, University of California–San Diego, La Jolla, CA

Suzanne N. Haber   Department of Pharmacology and Physiology, University of Rochester School of Medicine, Rochester, NY

Benjamin Y. Hayden   Department of Neurobiology, Duke University School of Medicine, Durham, NC

Clay B. Holroyd   Department of Psychology, University of Victoria, Victoria, Canada

Laurence T. Hunt   Centre for Functional MRI of the Brain, University of Oxford, Oxford, United Kingdom

Steven W. Kennerley   Institute of Neurology, University College London, London, United Kingdom

Mehdi Khamassi   Stem Cell and Brain Research Institute, INSERM U846, Bron, France

Mark Laubach   Department of Neurobiology, Yale University School of Medicine, New Haven, CT

Mimi Liljeholm   Division of Humanities and Social Sciences, California Institute of Technology, Pasadena, CA

Rogier B. Mars   Department of Experimental Psychology, University of Oxford, Oxford, United Kingdom

Franz-Xaver Neubert   Department of Experimental Psychology, University of Oxford, Oxford, United Kingdom

Sander Nieuwenhuis   Institute of Psychology, Leiden University, Leiden, The Netherlands

Yael Niv   Princeton Neuroscience Institute, Princeton University, Princeton, NJ

MaryAnn P. Noonan   Department of Experimental Psychology, University of Oxford, Oxford, United Kingdom

John P. O'Doherty   Division of Humanities and Social Sciences, California Institute of Technology, Pasadena, CA

John M. Pearson   Department of Neurobiology, Duke University School of Medicine, Durham, NC

Michael Petrides   Montreal Neurological Institute, McGill University, Montreal, Canada

Paul E. M. Phillips   Department of Psychiatry & Behavioral Science, University of Washington, Seattle, WA

Michael L. Platt   Department of Neurobiology, Duke University School of Medicine, Durham, NC

Emmanuel Procyk   Stem Cell and Brain Research Institute, INSERM U846, Bron, France

René Quilodran   Stem Cell and Brain Research Institute, INSERM U846, Bron, France

José J. F. Ribas-Fernandes Princeton Neuroscience Institute, Princeton University, Princeton, NJ

K. Richard Ridderinkhof Department of Psychology, University of Amsterdam, Amsterdam, The Netherlands

Marie Rothé Stem Cell and Brain Research Institute, INSERM U846, Bron, France

Matthew F. S. Rushworth Department of Experimental Psychology, University of Oxford, Oxford, United Kingdom

Jérôme Sallet Department of Experimental Psychology, University of Oxford, Oxford, United Kingdom

Pradeep Shenoy Department of Cognitive Science, University of California–San Diego, La Jolla, CA

Nicole C. Swann Department of Psychology, University of California–San Diego, La Jolla, CA

Philippe N. Tobler Department of Experimental Psychology, University of Oxford, Oxford, United Kingdom

Markus Ullsperger Donders Institute for Brain, Cognition and Behaviour, Radboud University Nijmegen, Nijmegen, The Netherlands

Wouter van den Bos Department of Psychology, Leiden University, Leiden, The Netherlands

Mark E. Walton Department of Experimental Psychology, University of Oxford, Oxford, United Kingdom

Charles R. E. Wilson Stem Cell and Brain Research Institute, INSERM U846, Bron, France

Nick Yeung Department of Experimental Psychology, University of Oxford, Oxford, United Kingdom

Angela J. Yu Department of Cognitive Science, University of California–San Diego, La Jolla, CA

Index